HANDBOOK OF
NEUROLOGICAL SPORTS MEDICINE

Concussion and Other Nervous System Injuries in the Athlete

Anthony L. Petraglia, MD

Julian E. Bailes, MD

Arthur L. Day, MD

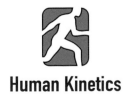

Human Kinetics

Library of Congress Cataloging-in-Publication Data

Petraglia, Anthony L., 1980- author.
 Handbook of neurological sports medicine: concussion and other nervous system injuries in the athlete /
 Anthony L. Petraglia, Julian E. Bailes, Arthur L. Day.
      p. ; cm.
 Includes bibliographical references and index.
 I. Bailes, Julian E., author. II. Day, Arthur L., author. III. Title.
 [DNLM: 1. Athletic Injuries. 2. Brain Injuries. 3. Trauma, Nervous System. QT 261]
 RD97.P4816 2015
 617.1'027--dc23

                            2014009602

ISBN: 978-1-4504-4181-0 (print)

The web addresses cited in this text were current as of May 2014, unless otherwise noted.

Acquisitions Editors: Karalyn Thompson and Joshua J. Stone; **Developmental Editor:** Kevin Matz; **Associate Managing Editor:** Anne E. Mrozek; **Copyeditor:** Joyce Sexton; **Indexer:** Susan Danzi Hernandez; **Permissions Manager:** Dalene Reeder; **Senior Graphic Designer:** Fred Starbird; **Graphic Designer:** Dawn Sills; **Cover Designer:** Sangwon Yeo; **Photographs (interior):** © Human Kinetics, unless otherwise noted; **Photo Asset Manager:** Laura Fitch; **Visual Production Assistant:** Joyce Brumfield; **Photo Production Manager:** Jason Allen; **Art Manager:** Kelly Hendren; **Associate Art Manager:** Alan L. Wilborn; **Illustrations:** © Human Kinetics, unless otherwise noted; **Printer:** Courier Companies, Inc.

Printed in the United States of America   10   9   8   7   6   5   4   3   2   1

The paper in this book was manufactured using responsible forestry methods.

Human Kinetics
Website: www.HumanKinetics.com

United States: Human Kinetics
P.O. Box 5076
Champaign, IL 61825-5076
800-747-4457
e-mail: humank@hkusa.com

Canada: Human Kinetics
475 Devonshire Road Unit 100
Windsor, ON N8Y 2L5
800-465-7301 (in Canada only)
e-mail: info@hkcanada.com

Europe: Human Kinetics
107 Bradford Road
Stanningley
Leeds LS28 6AT, United Kingdom
+44 (0) 113 255 5665
e-mail: hk@hkeurope.com

Australia: Human Kinetics
57A Price Avenue
Lower Mitcham, South Australia 5062
08 8372 0999
e-mail: info@hkaustralia.com

New Zealand: Human Kinetics
P.O. Box 80
Torrens Park, South Australia 5062
0800 222 062
e-mail: info@hknewzealand.com

E5835

Contents

Part III SPORT-RELATED INJURIES OF THE SPINE AND PERIPHERAL NERVOUS SYSTEM

Chapter 16 Cervical, Thoracic, and Lumbar Spine Injuries: Types, Causal Mechanisms, and Clinical Features

Chapter 17 Management of Spine Injuries, Including Rehabilitation, Surgical Considerations, and Return to Play

Chapter 18 Peripheral Nerve Injuries in Athletes

Contributors

Clayton J. Fitzsimmons, Esq.
Fitzsimmons Law Firm
Wheeling, West Virginia

Robert P. Fitzsimmons, Esq.
Fitzsimmons Law Firm
Wheeling, West Virginia

Jennifer Hammers, DO
Department of Forensic Medicine
New York University
New York, New York

Wesley H. Jones, MD
Department of Neurosurgery
University of Texas at Houston
Houston, Texas

Saint-Aaron L. Morris, MD
Department of Neurosurgery
University of Texas at Houston
Houston, Texas

Bennet I. Omalu, MD, MBA, MPH
Department of Medical Pathology
and Laboratory Medicine
University of California Davis Medical
Center
Sacramento, California

Elizabeth M. Pieroth, PsyD, ABPP
Department of Psychiatry
NorthShore University HealthSystem
Evanston, Illinois

Fabio V. C. Sparapani, MD, PhD
Department of Neurological Surgery
Federal University of São Paulo
São Paulo, Brasil

Robert J. Spinner, MD
Department of Neurosurgery
Mayo Clinic
Rochester, Minnesota

Corey T. Walker, MD
Department of Neurosurgery
Barrow Neurological Institute
Phoenix, Arizona

Ethan A. Winkler, MD, PhD
Department of Neurosurgery
University of California, San Francisco
San Francisco, California

Preface

Sports medicine is an exciting specialty concerned with the care of injury and illness in athletes, and it is a specialty that crosses various medical disciplines. Sport-related neurological injuries are among the most complex and dreaded injuries that an athlete can sustain. Without a doubt, recent years have been filled with major cultural and scientific shifts in the way athletes, coaches, parents, and physicians view sport-related neurological injuries, particularly concussion. The enormous public health impact is in part due to the large scope of athletes susceptible to such injuries, from the world-class athlete to the weekend warrior and those participating in youth sports.

There is clearly an increased need for further neurological expertise and training for those practitioners caring for athletes with sport-related neurological injuries. As neurosurgeons, we are typically involved with the treatment of the most serious and catastrophic of athletic injuries. Traditionally, though, we have been trained clinically to deal with the entire spectrum of trauma and illness in both the central and peripheral nervous system. We have now come to realize that injuries once considered mild or minor can have serious acute and long-term effects requiring proper attention. Skyrocketing levels of public awareness have allowed our society to gain a better understanding of these neurological injuries; but we, as a medical community, still have a long way to go. There is still a great need for continued prevention programs and improved systematic and evidence-based approaches to the athlete with neurological injuries.

An explosion in research initiatives has led to significant advances in the field of neurological sports medicine; there is a greater understanding of the causation, diagnosis, and treatment of sports-related neurological injuries than ever before. We have come to appreciate the wide spectrum of spinal injuries in the athlete and their implications for return-to-play decisions. Sophisticated nonoperative and operative techniques are being refined and used in the management of athletic spinal injuries. Often overshadowed by other types of injuries, peripheral nerve injuries affect athletes of all ages and can be equally devastating. A better understanding of these injuries has led to more accurate diagnoses and timely, appropriate interventions.

The on-field management of acute traumatic brain injury in the athlete, specifically concussion, has evolved. Our ability to diagnose concussion has improved with the use of ancillary measures including computerized neuropsychological assessment, balance testing, and advanced neuroimaging techniques. There has been an increased emphasis on developing appropriate return-to-play criteria, and these decisions continue to mature. Although still in its infancy, we also have a better understanding of the long-term sequelae of repetitive head injury and are developing ways to better diagnose and treat these individuals.

For centuries, teams of people with multiple skill sets, experience levels, and technical competencies have consistently outperformed individuals acting alone in trying to solve a problem or complete a task. Similarly, the effective assessment and management of sport-related neurological injuries require a coordinated, interdisciplinary approach, with all team members seeking to collaboratively achieve common objectives. Paramount to efficient and effective care of the athlete is a sound understanding, on the part of all practitioners, of the issues pertinent to neurological injury and illness. This can be challenging in an expansive and constantly evolving field like neurological sports medicine; however, this book aims to facilitate just that.

As a concise and complete guide to the recognition, evaluation, and care of athletes with neurological injuries, this book serves as the definitive handbook of neurological sports medicine and provides the foundation for the clinical decisions that all sports medicine practitioners must make. The text begins by highlighting the scope of neurological injury in sport and provides a thorough overview of some general key concepts in neurological sports medicine, including a unique review of the medicolegal considerations encountered in this area.

The book then guides the practitioner through a complete yet practical review of how far we've come, where we are, and where we are going regarding sport-related head injuries. A review of the biomechanics and pathophysiology underlying concussion sets the stage for a better understanding of the clinical presentation. The acute evaluation of the concussed athlete is covered, including the role of neuroimaging and other adjunct measures of assessment such as neuropsychological evaluation. Emphasis is then placed on bringing the practitioner up to speed on current return-to-play recommendations and the role of education in the management of concussion. A review of participation recommendations for patients with preexisting neurological conditions or structural lesions is also provided. The long-term effects of concussion are also stressed, and the most up-to-date evidence for pharmacotherapy in concussion is reviewed. More catastrophic sport-related head injuries

are considered as well, and attention is given to the emerging concept of subconcussion. Closing out the section on sport-related head injuries is a unique review of cutting-edge, translational research that has investigated the potential acute and chronic neuroprotective benefits of many naturally occurring compounds and herbs as well as other natural treatment approaches.

Attention then turns toward covering the breadth and depth of athletic injuries to the cervical, thoracic, and lumbar spine, as well as the peripheral nervous system. Special consideration is given to other sport-related neurological issues including headache and heatstroke. Several appendixes at the end of the book provide the practitioner with essential resources to aid in the care of any athlete.

Encompassing the full range of neurological sports-related issues, this text provides athletic trainers, physical therapists, emergency medical technicians, students, and physicians of all specialties with an authoritative, comprehensive review of current literature and bridges the gap between principles and practice. We hope that it serves as a practical reference for practitioners caring for athletes and acts as a stimulus for continued advancements in the field of neurological sports medicine.

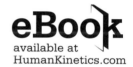

eBook
available at
HumanKinetics.com

Acknowledgments

The authors would like to thank their families; without their endless support this book would not have been written. Deepest gratitude is also due to the other contributors in the book, whose knowledge and assistance have greatly strengthened its content.

This effort was also supported, in part, by a grant from the Houston Texans and the McNair Foundation, organizations committed to research into and protection from lasting effects of athletic-related injuries.

GENERAL CONCEPTS

Sports medicine is a branch of medicine that deals with physical fitness and the treatment and prevention of injuries related to sport and exercise. Neurological injury has always been a potential risk of participation in sport. Care of those with neurological injury has evolved significantly over the years. Neurological injuries can occur in just about any sport, and a sound understanding of the breadth of these injuries allows the sports medicine practitioner to provide comprehensive, efficient care.

In this section we present an overview of the spectrum of neurological injury in sport, covering the pertinent epidemiology and types of injuries observed. We then review some of the general medicolegal concepts that any sports medicine practitioner should be familiar with. Topics such as negligence, duty and breach, standard of care, and proximate cause are discussed, as are cases of interest. Additionally, anyone involved in the care of athletes should be aware of the importance of emergency planning. We review the salient aspects of developing an effective and practical action plan for the coverage of athletic events.

Athletes and Neurological Injuries
A View From 10,000 Feet

Sports and athletics have been around as long as humankind has existed. Their origins can likely be traced to the practice of hunting and the training of combat skills necessary to feed and protect one's family and tribe. As leisure time developed, such activities evolved into athletic contests for their own sake, with games that involved wrestling and the throwing of spears, stakes, and rocks. Early reference to such practice can be found in the book of Genesis: "Jacob was left there alone. Then a man wrestled with him until the break of dawn. When the man saw that he could not prevail over him, he struck Jacob's hip at its socket, so that Jacob's socket was dislocated as he wrestled with him. . . . At sunrise, as he left Penuel, Jacob limped along because of his hip" (New American Bible, Gen. 32:25-26, 32:32). This is some of the earliest documentation of sports-related injury as well.

The recognition of injury and illness with physical activity led to the earliest forms of sports medicine in ancient Greece and Rome. In an effort to improve athletic training and overall supervision, physical education was implemented. Just as physical education became a necessary part of a Greek youth's training, athletic contests became a standard part of Greek life. While these games were originally associated with religious observances, they became increas-ingly popular and ultimately grew into events in themselves, with the first Olympic Games held in 776 BC. Those who excelled at such sporting events quickly gained eminence similar to that of today's elite athletes. In many cases, athletic ability enabled people to improve their social status by becoming a coach or trainer.

At that time, athletic trainers were expected to be experts on massage, diet, physical therapy, and hygiene, as well as proficient in coaching athletes in the techniques of boxing, wrestling, jumping, and the other sports.[305] By the 5th century BC, the trainer-coach had become a significant force in the development of athletics. This influence continued throughout the Roman Empire. Around 444 BC, Iccus of Tarentum, a former pentathlon champion, wrote the first textbook on athletic training and paved the way for others to document their experiences in a similar fashion. [95] One of the most famous trainers was Milo of Croton, who was a heroic athletic figure in his own right. One of his documented training methods for gaining strength was to lift a bull daily, beginning on the day of its birth. He felt that in doing so, one would be able to lift the animal when it was full grown—probably the earliest record of progressive resistance exercise.[305]

Professional conflict between doctors and trainers at the time led to the physician having less involvement in preventive training and care and only being used if an injury occurred. It wasn't until Claudius Galen of Pergamum was appointed physician and surgeon to the gladiators in Pergamum in the 2nd century AD that the physician became increasingly involved in the care of the athlete. Galen used his experiences in the care of athletes to gain considerable skill and knowledge in anatomy and surgery; and once settled in Rome, he became the personal physician to the emperor Marcus Aurelius. Widely considered one of the greatest physicians of ancient Rome, Galen engaged in teaching, publishing, systematic observations, and aggressive pursuit of improved treatment methods that paved the way for practitioners of sports medicine today.

THE PRESENT

Just as sport and athletic competition have evolved over the years in response to economic, social, and political change, so too has the practice of sports medicine. While the basic tenets of athletic care have persisted, sports medicine has evolved from its ancient roots to a more multidisciplinary team effort that includes parents, coaches, athletic trainers, therapists, and physicians. New sports, superior performance, and increased levels of competition have all led to changes in the way athletes are cared for. Never before have the physiological and psychological effects of sport on the human body been as carefully scientifically examined and researched as they are today. Neurological sports medicine has witnessed growth in research initiatives and public awareness unlike that of any other aspect of sports medicine.

Sport-related neurological injuries are among the most complex and dreaded injuries that an athlete can sustain. While the rates and types of neurological injury vary and are dependent on the sporting activity, age of the participants, and level of competition,[335, 336] the risk of neurological injury derives primarily from the nature of the sport (contact vs. collision vs. noncontact) and the specific activities associated with participation. For most sports, there seems to be a higher risk of injury during competition than during practice sessions; however, greater reporting of injury within sport in recent years has highlighted the need for increased attention at all times.

SPECTRUM OF NEUROLOGICAL INJURY IN SPORT

Increased awareness and medical advances have certainly led to a greater understanding of the causation, diagnosis, and treatment of sports-related neurological injuries, although it is clear that there is still much to learn. To grasp the enormous public health impact these injuries have, it is paramount to appreciate that neurological injury can occur in just about any type of sport. It is important to keep in mind that a wealth of data on neurological injuries exist for some sports whereas there is a paucity of literature for others. Additionally, the epidemiological data for some injuries, such as concussion, are widely variable, in part due to the significant change in awareness and diagnosis of athletic neurological injuries over the past few decades. The following sections provide a broad overview of neurological injuries across a spectrum of sports ranging from recreational activities to organized athletic competition.

American Football

The history of American football can be traced to early versions of rugby football and soccer. The first game of intercollegiate football was played on November 6, 1869, between Rutgers University and Princeton University. The popularity of collegiate football grew as it became the dominant version of the sport for the first half of the 20th century. The origin of professional football, though, can be traced back to 1892 when William "Pudge" Heffelfinger accepted $500 to play in a game for the Allegheny Athletic Association against the Pittsburgh Athletic Club, marking the first known time a player was paid for participating in the sport.

The sport has undergone much growth and change over the past century, becoming one of the most popular in the United States. Prior reports cited 1,800,000 participants in all levels of football.[72] However, new participation numbers gathered by the National Operating Committee for Standards in Athletic Equipment (NOCSAE), the National Federation of State High School Associations (NFHS), and USA Football are higher. The NFHS has estimated that there are approximately 1.1 million high school players (grades 9 through 12).[227] Reports also indicate that there are approximately 100,000 post–high school players in organizations including the National Football League (NFL), National Collegiate Athletic Association (NCAA), National Association of Intercollegiate Athletics (NAIA), National Junior College Athletic Association (NJCAA), Arena Football, and semiprofessional football.[227] Additionally, USA Football estimates that there are 3 million youth football players in the United States.[227] Thus, according to these figures, the 2011 football season saw an estimated 4.2 million participants in the United States.

Catastrophic injuries constitute an uncommon but nonetheless devastating occurrence in football.[10] There were four fatalities directly related to football during the 2011 football season, with two in high school football, one in college football, and one in sandlot football.[227] Both of the high school fatalities resulted from injuries to the brain; the youth injury was a cervical vertebra fracture, and the collegiate death was due to brain trauma. Thus, for the approximately 4.2 million participants in 2011, the rate of direct fatalities was 0.10 per 100,000 participants.

Work in the mid-1960s focusing on football-related head and neck injuries resulted in a significant reduction in the incidence of these accidents owing to improvements in equipment, education in proper techniques, offseason conditioning, and rule changes. The rate of injuries with incomplete neurological recovery in high school and junior high school football was 0.33 per 100,000 players, and the rate at the college level was 2.66 per 100,000 players.[226] Cervical cord neurapraxia and the various types of fractures seen in football are covered in greater detail later in the book.

Concussions are a frequent injury in football. The rate of concussion in football participants reported in the literature is widely variable, in large part due to the changes in concussion awareness and diagnosis in the past few decades. One study evaluated concussions in high school football players that were reported to medical professionals over a three-season time span.[254] In this study the concussion rate in high school football players was found to be 3.66 concussions per 100 player-seasons, meaning that there were 3.66 concussions every season for every 100 players. That being said, another study surveyed 233 high school football players after one season and

found that 110 players (47.2%) had experienced at least one concussion and 81 players (34.9%) reported having experienced multiple concussions during the season, a much higher rate than in the former study.[178] A more recent report found the concussion rate in high school football players to be 0.21 per 1,000 athletic exposures in practice and 1.55 per 1,000 athletic exposures in games.[114] Collectively, the concussion rate was 0.47 per 1,000 athletic exposures. An athletic exposure is defined as participation in a single practice, competition, or event.

The concussion rate in collegiate football players studied over a 16-year study period was found to be 0.37 per 1,000 athletic exposures.[135] As with high school football players, though, other studies have suggested a higher rate of concussions in collegiate football players. Another study found a concussion injury rate of 0.39 per 1,000 athletic exposures in practice and 3.02 per 1,000 athletic exposures in games (an overall rate of 0.61 concussions per 1,000 athletic exposures).[114] It is important to note that although it may seem that the rate of concussion is significantly greater in college compared to high school football, this may be due to the greater access to medical care, reporting, and oversight provided at the college level and not necessarily a reflection of a difference in the actual number of concussions. Thus a continued emphasis on concussion awareness at the youth and high school levels is paramount, considering that younger athletes may experience more symptoms and recover more slowly than collegiate and professional athletes.[72, 201] There is now a greater awareness of the potential for chronic brain injury with repetitive head injuries, in part due to the increased numbers of football players diagnosed with chronic traumatic encephalopathy.[206, 241, 313] Chronic neurodegenerative diseases, including dementia pugilistica, chronic traumatic encephalopathy, and mild cognitive impairment, are covered further in later chapters.

Brachial plexus injury is one of the most common peripheral nerve injuries in football. Initially called "pinched nerve syndrome," this phenomenon is colloquially referred to as a "burner" or "stinger."[52, 91, 310, 335] It has been reported to account for approximately 36% of all neurological upper extremity injuries in football.[171] The incidence of transient brachial plexus injury is significant over the course of a high school, college, or professional football player's career.[157] Peripheral nerve injuries in football may also occur as a result of blocking or tackling techniques. One study reported that football was the sport that most commonly caused injury necessitating referral for electrodiagnostic testing.[172] Mononeuropathies in football have been reported to involve the axillary, suprascapular, ulnar, median, long thoracic, and radial nerves.[172] Peroneal neuropathy has been reported to occur in 24% of football players in whom complete knee dislocation and ligamentous injury have taken place.[172] Even in the absence of serious musculoskeletal injury, the superficial course of the peroneal nerve lends itself to injury or even neurapraxia with transient deficits in situations of contact to the lower extremity.

Archery and Bow Hunting

Archaeological evidence dates archery back over 25,000 years, with the sport first appearing as an organized event in the Olympic Games in Paris in 1900. Similarly, hunting with bow and arrow has always been a popular recreational sport for outdoor enthusiasts. Undoubtedly the most common cause of neurological injury associated with the sport is accidental falls from hunting tree stands. Hunting tree stands are typically small platforms elevated approximately 15 to 30 feet (4.6-9 m) above the ground, providing hunters with a greater field of view and decreasing the odds of their scent being detected by game at the ground level. Falls from this height can result in speeds in excess of 30 miles per hour (48 km/h) and a broad spectrum of neurological injury. Despite several studies[64, 65, 88, 111, 211, 255, 262, 346] demonstrating that falls represent a significant proportion of hunting-related injuries, tree stands are still not widely appreciated as one of the most dangerous pieces of equipment a hunter owns.

Crites and colleagues[64] retrospectively reviewed the types of spinal injuries that resulted from falls from hunting tree stands. Of the 27 patients included in the study, 44% sustained significant neurological deficits. In total there were 17 burst fractures, eight wedge compression fractures, four fractures involving the posterior elements, and one coronal fracture of the sacral body. A significant percentage of patients had associated injuries. Thirty-three percent of

patients required surgical intervention for their spinal injuries. In 1994, Price and Mallonee studied the Oklahoma State Department of Health spinal cord injury (SCI) surveillance data in an attempt to describe the incidence and circumstances surrounding hunting-related spinal cord injuries.[255] They found that all of the hunting-related injuries in the SCI database resulted from falls from trees or tree stands. The incidence rate of injury in the study was less than 1 per 100,000 licensed hunters. Urquhart and colleagues also analyzed patients with injuries related to falls from hunting tree stands.[346] Of the 19 patients in the cohort, there was one death, and eight of the 18 survivors were either paralyzed or permanently disabled.

More recent studies[65, 88, 211] have reminded us that hunting tree stands are a persistent cause of neurological sport injury, despite many years of awareness. Additionally, Metz and colleagues highlighted in their study of 51 patients that brain injuries can also occur in falls from tree stands.[211] The most common injuries were spinal fractures (51% of patients in the study); however, closed head injuries were identified in 24% of patients and included concussions and intracranial hemorrhages, in addition to skull and facial fractures. All three of the patients in the study who died had intracranial hemorrhages. It is clear that tree stand falls are associated with high morbidity and mortality, and their treatment is associated with a significant utilization of patient care resources. Increased attention to hunter education regarding the safe and proper use of tree stands is critical to decreasing the incidence of hunting-related injuries.

Falls aside, the other type of neurological injury for which the archer is at risk is peripheral nerve injury in the upper extremity.[259] It is possible for the archer to lacerate a digital nerve and artery with the razor-sharp broad head used for bow hunting. Rayan also has described patients with compression neuropathies of the digital nerves from the bowstring and median nerve compression at the elbow as well as the wrist.[259] A case of isolated long thoracic nerve palsy has been described.[296] The patient presented with classic winging of the scapula and atrophy of the serratus anterior muscle, presumably due to recurrent compression and overstretching of the long thoracic nerve with repetitive practice.

Another archer presented with atrophy of the infraspinatus muscle secondary to suprascapular nerve palsy.[130]

Another interesting risk for injury in archery is bow hunter's stroke. The condition results from vertebrobasilar insufficiency caused by vertebral artery spasm or mechanical injury secondary to the repeated cervical rotations associated with the sport.[308] Although it is an unusual condition usually caused by structural abnormalities at the craniocervical junction, cases have been reported secondary to lateral intervertebral disc herniations as well.[348]

Australian Rules Football and Rugby

Rugby originated in England in 1823 and became a professional sport in 1895. It is an international sport in which protective gear is at a minimum and aggressive tackling is an integral part of the game.[336] Likewise, Australian rules football is an aggressive sport, with similarities to both rugby and American football, that began in Melbourne, Australia, in 1858. Competitions seem to result in more injuries per exposure, while practice accounts for a greater percentage of the total number of injuries. The majority of injuries occur during the scrum and tackles. Forwards, who are more physically involved during the game, seem to be at the greatest risk.[205]

A significant number of injuries are to the head and neck. Overall, the rate of head, neck, and orofacial injuries in Australian rules football is 2.6 injuries per 1,000 participation-hours.[36] McIntosh and colleagues studied the incidence of injury in youth rugby over two seasons and found the rate to be 19.2 injuries per 1,000 hours of player–game exposure.[205] Thirty percent of the injuries were to the head, face, and neck; and of the 234 head injuries, 85% were concussions. A recent systematic review found that the highest incidence of concussion for adolescent rugby was 3.3 per 1,000 playing hours.[27] Adams reviewed 1,000 injuries due to rugby and found a 14.0% incidence of head injuries.[3] Another study retrospectively examined Australian rules football–related fatalities over 9 years.[202] The authors identified 25 mortalities associated with the sport; and of these, nine were secondary to brain injury. They identified intracranial hemorrhage in eight of those nine athletes, as well as traumatic subarachnoid hemorrhage secondary to vertebral artery injury in three players.

Injuries to the spine are not infrequent in rugby and Australian rules football.[18, 61, 82, 106, 257, 278] The average annual incidence of acute spinal cord injuries in these sports has been reported to be between 1.5 and 3.2 per 100,000 players.[18] The incidence of spinal injuries in professional rugby players is 10.9 per 1,000 player match-hours; it seems to be lower during practice, with an incidence of 0.37 per 1,000 player training hours.[106] The most common mechanism of injury seems to be cervical spine hyperflexion, producing fracture dislocations.[257] Transient quadriparesis has also been reported in rugby.[278]

Automobile Racing

Automobile racing boasts some of the largest attendance figures in all of sport. The types of auto racing can be classified in a variety of ways (e.g., open- vs. closed-wheel) and can range from go-kart to stock car racing. The course style and speeds can vary as well. In Formula 1 racing, cars often reach speeds in excess of 240 miles per hour (386 km/h) on tortuous circuits, whereas in drag racing the vehicles can exceed speeds of 300 miles per hour (483 km/h) on a straight racing strip. Evolution of the sport and the use of helmets, safety restraints, and safety cells and cages have resulted in a significant reduction in the severity of injury. More than 90% of the neurological injuries that occur in the sport are to the head.

The full spectrum of brain injury has been observed, from concussion to diffuse axonal injury and intracranial hemorrhage. One study retrospectively reviewed open-wheel racing accidents at Indianapolis Raceway Park during six seasons.[312] During 61 open-wheel racing events, 57 drivers were evaluated at Indianapolis Raceway Park after crashes, and only two required an ICU admission due to head injury. In Indy car events from 1985 to 1989, 367 crashes occurred, involving 413 drivers, with 38 of these drivers sustaining 48 injuries.[338] According to this report, 29.2% of the injuries were closed head injuries despite the use of helmets and other safety equipment. Trammell and colleagues also reported that open head injuries occurred in only 5% of these cases.[338] Weaver and coauthors analyzed data regarding Indy Racing League car crashes from 1996 to 2003, comparing the likelihood of head injury in drivers in a vehicle that sustained an impact greater than or equal to 50 g versus those sustaining a lesser impact. [359] They found that drivers in a crash with an impact greater than or equal to 50 g developed a head injury 16% of the time versus 1.6% for those involved in crashes with a lesser impact.

Peripheral nerve injuries can occasionally occur in racing. Some drivers have reported symptoms consistent with brachial plexus injury. They describe transient upper extremity paresthesias secondary to the safety straps looped tightly around their arms. These straps are also connected to their helmets to combat the high forces the racers experience. Ulnar, peroneal, and sciatic nerve injuries can result from the constant pressure against the seat or other objects in the car during long races. Heatstroke has even been reported to occur, although rarely. [147]

Spinal cord injury, spinal fractures, and cervical sprains and strains have also been described in automobile racing. [335] One study investigated racing injuries in either single-seat or formula cars or saloon cars between 1996 and 2000 at Fuji Speedway in Japan. [222] While extremity bruising accounted for the majority of injuries in single-seat car racing, 53.2% of the injuries in saloon car racing were neck sprains. Another report found that spinal injuries composed 20% of injuries experienced by professional automobile drivers. [338] In this review, injuries most commonly occurred during a vehicular rollover and usually led to cervical spine or spinal cord injury. In general, thoracolumbar injuries are uncommon, mainly due to the driver's being so well restrained. The HANS (head and neck support) device is a safety item in many car racing sports (figure 1.1). It reduces the likelihood of head and neck injuries, such as a basilar skull fracture, in the event of a crash. The device is primarily made of carbon-fiber and is U-shaped. The back of the U sits behind the nape of the neck, and the two arms lie flat along the top of the chest over the pectoral muscles. The device is attached only to the helmet, by two anchors on either side, and not to the belts, driver's body, or seat. Therefore it is secured with the body of the driver only. The purpose is to stop the head from whipping forward in a crash without otherwise restricting movement of the neck. In a crash, the device maintains the relative position of the head to the

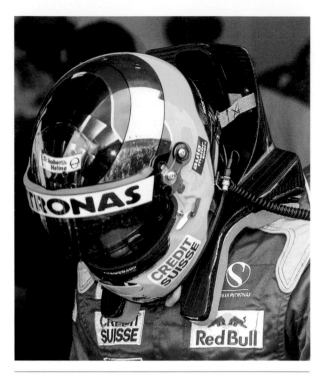

Figure 1.1 The head and neck support (HANS) device reduces the likelihood of head and neck injuries in the event of a crash.
Picture Alliance/Photoshot

body, transferring energy to the much stronger chest, torso, shoulder, seat belts, and seat as the head is decelerated.

Ballet and Dance

Dance has been an important part of life since ancient civilization. An extraordinary range of styles exists, from classical ballet and ballroom to modern dance and breakdancing. Although typically thought of as an art form, many forms of dance are physically taxing and can be considered sport. Additionally, dance is incorporated into a variety of sports including gymnastics, figure skating, synchronized swimming, and even martial arts kata. Regardless of style, all types of dance have something in common—they involve not only flexibility, athleticism, and body movement, but also physics. If the proper physics are not taken into consideration, injuries can occur. Many dance movements require extreme positions that can place the body at risk for acute, subacute, or chronic injury. In general, though, neurological injuries seen in many forms of dance, such as ballet, result from chronic microtrauma or overuse, as opposed to the acute injury seen in other sports. It is important to remember that as with other athletes, dancers are often highly motivated to suppress pain and ignore injury until it affects their performance; this creates a need for increased awareness.

Dancers are vulnerable to various stress-related injuries, and muscle strains represent more than a third of all injuries. Injuries particularly affect the lumbar spine and the peripheral nerves and, to a lesser extent, the cervical spine. In one study, the National Organization of Dance and Mime surveyed 141 dancers from seven professional ballet and modern dance companies regarding their injuries.[35] Forty-eight percent had experienced a chronic injury, and 42% reported a more recent injury within the previous 6 months that had affected their performance. Garrick and Requa[109] reported 2.97 injuries per injured dancer in a large professional ballet company, with the lumbar spine the second most frequently involved region. Back problems are fairly prevalent in dance, with 10% to 17% of injuries occurring in the vertebral column.[218] Spondylolysis is a form of overuse injury secondary to chronic hyperextension and hyperlordosis of the lumbar spine. Microfractures of the vertebral bodies can occur, especially with repetitive flexion. This can result in wedging and Schmorl's nodes at the thoracolumbar junction, a condition known as atypical Scheuermann's disease. This condition can also result from lumbar extension contracture with excessive flexion demands transferred to the thoracic spine and resultant anterior end plate fractures and secondary bony formation.[30, 182] Fractures of the pars interarticularis and pedicles, arthritic degeneration, premature arthrosis, scoliosis, and discogenic as well as mechanical back pain are also common in dancers. Peripheral nerve injuries including nerve entrapment, neuropathy, and nerve dysfunction in the legs, ankles, and feet frequently occur in dancers.[219, 270-273]

It should also be noted that neurologic injuries can occur in more recreational forms of dance. Breakdancing, for instance, involves athletic moves and spinning on various parts of the body, including the head and hands. One study described a breakdancer who presented with headaches and papilledema and was found to have multiple subdural hematomas.[208] Head banging, a popular dance form accompanying heavy metal music, involves extreme flexion, extension, and rotation of the head and cervical spine. The motions can be performed so violently as to cause mild traumatic brain injury, whiplash injury to the cervical spine, or even subdural hematomas.[75, 158, 246] In 2008, Patton and McIntosh performed an observational study and biomechanical analysis of head banging.[246] They determined that an average head banging song has a tempo of about 146 beats per minute, which is predicted to cause mild head injury when the range of motion is greater than 75 degrees. Similarly, at higher tempos and greater ranges of motion, they found a greater risk of neck injury. Another study reported on a group of thirty-seven 8th graders participating in a dance marathon in which head banging occurred; 82% of the girls and 17% of the boys had resultant cervical spine pain that lasted 1 to 3 days.[158]

Baseball and Softball

Baseball and softball are extremely popular sports. Between the fall of 1982 and the spring of 2008, approximately 10.9 million high school men and 23,517 high school women competed in baseball.[47, 72, 225] Over that time frame, an additional 616,947 men played baseball at the collegiate level.[225] Approximately 419,000 males and 900 females participate in baseball at the high school level annually.[72, 225] In the United States it is estimated that 23 million organized softball games are played each year. In 2008, Mueller and Cantu reported that between the fall of 1982 and the spring of 2008, approximately 30,000 men and 8.1 million women played high school softball.[225] An additional 323,000 collegiate women played softball over that time frame. Around 1,100 men and 313,000 women compete in softball at the high school level each year.[225]

Injuries resulting from playing recreational baseball and softball are among the most frequent causes of sport-related emergency room visits, accounting for an estimated 286,708 injuries in 2009.[345] Minor injuries are fairly common in both sports, but catastrophic injuries can occur as well. Acute neurologic injuries are typically more common than chronic ones. Pasternack and colleagues studied patterns of injury in 2,861 Little League baseball players aged 7 to 18 years and reported 81 total injuries.[245] Eighty-one percent were found to be acute, and 19% were reported to be secondary to overuse. The authors found that 62% of the acute injuries were due to being struck by the ball. Interestingly, in softball, base sliding was found to be responsible for 71% of the injuries in one study.[146]

These studies are consistent with other studies that have found the main mechanisms of injury to be related to being struck by a ball, repetitive motions or overuse such as throwing or swinging, collisions, sliding, and, much more rarely, being struck by a bat. As mentioned previously, severe neurologic injuries such as epidural hematomas or intracranial hemorrhages and catastrophic fatalities can occur but are rarer than mild brain injury. One study reported catastrophic injury rates in baseball of 0.37 per 100,000 high school player-games and 1.7 per 100,000 college player-games.[32] This study also found the fatality rates in baseball to be 0.067 per 100,000 high school baseball players and 0.86 per 100,000 college baseball players.

Powell and Barber-Foss studied 10 different high school sports over the course of 3 years, identifying mild traumatic brain injuries, and found that softball and baseball accounted for only 2.1% and 1.2% of these injuries, respectively.[254] Two hundred forty-six certified athletic trainers reported a rate of 0.23 concussions per 100 player-seasons in high school baseball players, meaning that 0.23 concussions occurred every season for every 100 athletes. The same study found that the rate of concussion in high school softball was 0.46 per 100 player-seasons. Covassin and colleagues[63] studied NCAA athletic injuries over a 3-year time span and reported that concussions accounted for 2.9% of all injuries that occurred in practice and 4.2% of all injuries that occurred in games. In softball, concussions that occurred in practice accounted for 4.1% of all softball injuries, whereas in games, concussions accounted for 6.4% of all injuries. A more recent study investigated injuries in NCAA athletes over 16 years and found the rate of concussion in baseball to be 0.07 per 1,000 athletic exposures.[135] This survey also revealed a concussion rate in softball of 0.14 per 1,000 athletic exposures. These rates of concussion in collegiate softball are higher than those reported in a recent 1-year study of high school softball athletes, in which the overall concussion rate was 0.07 per 1,000 athletic exposures.[114]

Injuries to the spine are rare but can occur, usually secondary to collisions or headfirst sliding. While the use of breakaway bases and rules against headfirst sliding (at the youth level) have helped to substantially reduce the occurrence of sliding-related injuries, the risk for catastrophic spinal cord injury still exists. With headfirst slides, the top of the runner's head can collide with the body or leg of the defensive player, creating a significant amount of axial load to the vertebral column. Baseball and softball players also are at risk for injury to their peripheral nervous system in addition to injuries of the brain and spine.

A pitcher's arms in baseball and softball withstand tremendous repetitive stress throughout a season. Long and colleagues[189] reported that every major league baseball pitcher, most minor league pitchers, and a few amateur pitchers they had studied had had reduced sensory nerve action potentials in the throwing arm. This is probably due to overuse and is a manifestation of brachial plexus injury. Although they throw underhand, fast-pitch softball pitchers withstand maximum compressive forces at the elbow and shoulder equivalent to 70% to 98% of their total body weight.[15] The more common peripheral nerve injuries in baseball and softball include suprascapular, axillary, and ulnar nerve injuries, although more infrequent injuries to the radial, musculocutaneous, and median nerves have been described.[140, 174, 301, 337]

Basketball

Originally developed in 1891 by Dr. James Naismith at the International YMCA Training School in Springfield, Massachusetts, basketball has grown into a tremendously popular sport enjoyed worldwide and equally by men and women. Approximately 13.8 million high school men, 11 million high school women, 375,000 college men, and 328,000 college women participated in basketball between 1982 and 2008.[225] Most basketball injuries are musculoskeletal, affecting primarily the lower extremity; however, neurologic injuries can occur to the head, spine, and peripheral nerves.

Head injuries in basketball can be caused by the sudden deceleration of the head when the player strikes an immobile object, such as the floor, another player, or a basketball pole or rim. These forces can cause direct contusions to the brain or even result in tears of arteries and bridging veins, subsequently causing epidural and subdural hematomas. Several reports of acute subdural and epidural hematoma related to playing basketball are in the literature.[73, 160, 341] In their 16-year study, Hootman and colleagues found in college basketball that men experienced a rate of 0.16 concussions per 1,000 athletic exposures compared to a rate of 0.22 concussions per 1,000 athletic exposures in women.[135] Powell and Barber-Foss demonstrated that in high school basketball, the rate of concussion was 0.75 and 1.04 concussions per 100 player-seasons in men and women, respectively.[254] Additionally, in men's high school basketball, concussions accounted for 4.1% and 5.0% of all the injuries sustained during practices and games, respectively.[114] While this was not significantly different for men, they did note that in women's high school basketball, concussions accounted for 4.7% and 8.5% of the injuries sustained during practice and games, respectively; and this was significantly different. This subtle significant difference was also confirmed in a separate study.[261]

Injuries to the spine are more common in basketball than other forms of neurologic injury. Basketball involves rapid, repetitive changes in direction and explosive movements that put significant stresses on the spine, resulting in a spectrum of spinal disease including lumbar sprains, contusions, facet hypertrophy, pars interarticularis fractures, spinal stenosis, spondylolisthesis, and disc herniations or degenerative disc disease.[4, 66, 141, 209, 213, 234, 311, 321] Cases of cervical cord neurapraxia have been reported in basketball players as well.[332]

Although typically thought of as a football injury, burners or stingers have been reported in basketball secondary to acute head, neck, or shoulder trauma.[91, 92] Suprascapular, musculocutaneous, ulnar, median, peroneal, and sciatic nerves are all susceptible to entrapment neuropathies.[56, 68, 92, 152, 326, 340] Compression neuropathies of the arms are common injuries in a unique subgroup of basketball players—those who participate in wheelchair basketball.[43]

Bowling

Bowling can be traced back more than 5,000 years ago to Egypt. In the 1930s, a British anthropologist named Sir Flinders Petrie discovered a collection of objects in a child's tomb in Egypt that appeared to have been used for a primitive form of bowling. A crude version of a bowling ball and primitive pins were all sized for a child. A similar game evolved during the Roman Empire that entailed tossing stone objects as close as possible to other stone objects. This game became popular with soldiers and eventually evolved into Italian bocce (considered a form of outdoor bowling). The game has continued to evolve and today is a sport enjoyed by more than 100 million people in more than 90 countries each year and is considered a timeless sport.[97]

Although not typically thought of as a sport with a high risk of injury, bowling can be both physically and psychologically demanding. Tremendous force is applied to the body throughout a bowler's stance, approach, pivot step, arm swing, release, and follow-through. Repetitive stress is applied to the entire upper extremity including the fingers, wrist, and elbow. Injuries may vary by age as well. A recent study examined bowling-related injuries presenting to U.S. emergency departments between 1990 and 2008. [162] The authors analyzed data from the U.S. Consumer Product Safety Commission's National Electronic Injury Surveillance System and found that children younger than 7 years had a higher proportion of finger injuries and injuries from dropping the ball than individuals older than 7 years. On the other hand, bowlers more than 65 years old sustained a greater proportion of injuries related to falling, slipping, or tripping.

While the annual incidence of injury is extremely low, the sport can cause a spectrum of neurologic hand and upper extremity injuries, either acute or due to overuse. Injuries to the fingers and digital nerves can occur. One report described a bowler with a rare traumatic dislocation of the four long fingers.[197] More commonly, though, the repetitive nature of bowling can lead to injuries to the digital nerve of the thumb, which most bowlers place inside the ball holes; this is referred to as "cherry pitter's thumb"[337] (figure 1.2). Perineural fibrosis of the digital nerve of the thumb[297, 351] and even cases of thumb neuromas have been described. [164, 165] Dobyns and colleagues reported on one of the largest series of these patients.[78] Patients may present with a positive Tinel's sign and skin atrophy or callusing over the neuroma. The nerve may ultimately become atrophied with fibrous

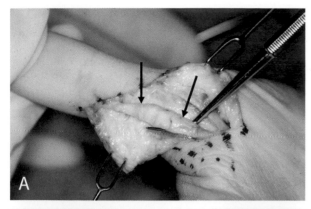

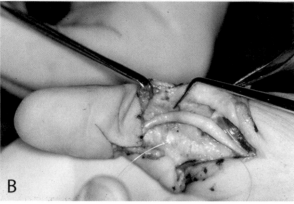

Figure 1.2 Bowler's thumb. This patient was taken to surgery because he did not respond to conservative therapy after a clinical diagnosis of bowler's thumb. At surgery, the digital nerve was markedly enlarged secondary to perineural fibrosis. (a) The enlarged ulnar digital nerve (arrows) is surrounded by perineural fibrosis producing an irregular rather than a normal smooth contour. Definitive surgical therapy consisted of neurolysis with careful removal of perineural fibrotic tissue. (b) The nerve is smaller and has a smoother contour following neurolysis. The patient had an uneventful postoperative course and was able to eventually return to bowling.

Reprinted from M.F. Showalter, D.H. Flemming, and S.A. Bernard, 2010, "MRI manifestations of bowler's thumb," *Radiology Case Reports* 6: 458. By permission of D.H. Flemming.

tissue proliferation at the site of injury. Not to be forgotten, neck and back pain can also occur in bowling and is often the result of discogenic injury.[228]

Boxing

Unorganized hand-to-hand combat can be traced back to prehistoric man, and sparring activity of one sort or another, in general, can be observed in most animals. The earliest form of boxing can be traced back to 1500 BC in what is known today as Ethiopia; it then spread to ancient Egypt and throughout the Mediterranean. Grecian boxers would fight to the death, and Onomastos of Smyrna has been credited with first defining the rules of the sport:

Onomastos' Rules of Boxing

- No time limits or pauses unless agreed upon by both fighters
- No ring
- Matches open to all comers
- Fighters not matched by weight
- Won by disabling the opponent

Eventually the sport was introduced to the Olympics in 688 BC. Great Britain is given credit, though, for turning boxing into the sport we know today, with its first formal set of boxing rules introduced in 1743 by Jack Broughton, who has since been referred to as the father of English boxing. Today it is a popular sport enjoyed by spectators and athletes of all levels.

One must take a couple of important considerations into account to understand the types of neurological injuries that occur in boxing. For starters is the level of competition, which can be broken down into two simple subgroups: amateur and professional boxing. Amateur boxing differs from professional boxing in many regards. To begin with, amateur boxing contests feature a shorter length and fewer rounds. In amateur boxing the primary objective is to score points. The force of a blow or its effect on the opponent does not count as it receives the same credit as any regular blow. Hence, the knockout is a byproduct in amateur boxing. In contrast, in professional boxing, added weight is given to a blow based on its impact or effect on one's opponent, and thus the knockdown and knockout are objectives in the pros. In amateur boxing, in contrast to professional, headgear is worn, and boxers use 10-ounce (0.28 kg) gloves for all weight classes. Professional boxers use 8-ounce gloves (0.22 kg) and less padding. These differences have a large effect on the spectrum of injury seen in boxing as a sport. Another consideration is that injuries in boxing can be classified as acute or chronic. While acute injuries can typically be recognized and appreciated at the time the sport is played, the chronic manifestation of nervous system injury secondary to repetitive trauma may not be realized until years after one has stopped boxing.

The most commonly injured sites in boxing are the head, neck, face, and hands. Because the head is one of two primary targets, neurological injury, both acute and chronic, is the greatest potential risk that a participant accepts. Head injuries generally occur secondary to contact between the fist and head, head and head, or head and some part of the boxing ring. Concussions are by far the most common acute neurological injury in boxing. However, well-designed studies to assess the incidence of concussion in boxing have not been published. Some studies have estimated the rate of concussion to be 0.58 and 1.5 to 3 per 100 athletic exposures in amateur and professional boxing, respectively.[29, 151] Zazryn and colleagues retrospectively sought to investigate the risk of injury to professional boxers in a 16-year study in the state of Victoria, Australia.[375] A total of 107 injuries were recorded from 427 fight participations; concussions were common and accounted for approximately 15.9% of the injuries. To further explore the epidemiology of injury to both amateur and professional boxers in Victoria, the same group performed a prospective cohort study with 1-year follow-up from 2004 to 2005.[374] Thirty-three amateur and 14 active professional boxers sustained 21 injuries during the study period; most were to the head region, with concussion being the most common (33%). A recent study investigated the epidemiology of boxing injuries presenting to U.S. emergency departments between 1990 and 2008.[253] The study demonstrated that an estimated 165,602 individuals sustained boxing injuries resulting in a visit to a U.S. hospital emergency department during this time period, which amounted to an average of 8,716 injuries occurring annually. When a subgroup analysis was done according to age, the percentage of injuries that were concussions or closed head injuries in the group aged 12 to 17 years (8.9%) was similar to that in the group aged 18 to 24 years (8.1%) and the group aged 25 to 34 years (8.5%).

While a knockout in boxing is synonymous with concussion, the majority of concussions in boxing are not associated with a loss of consciousness and are more commonly associated with transient cognitive impairment, loss of motor tone, or both; future studies are certainly needed

to better define the true rate of concussion in this population of athletes. The true incidence of acute intracranial hemorrhage is also largely unknown. The full spectrum of acute neurological injury can be seen: brain contusion or intraparenchymal hemorrhage, traumatic subarachnoid hemorrhage, acute subdural hematoma (the most common form of serious and lethal boxing brain injuries), epidural hematoma, diffuse axonal injury, carotid or vertebral artery dissection, and second impact syndrome.[148, 150, 216, 217] As noted earlier, chronic neurological injuries from boxing tend to have an insidious onset and often present and progress once a boxer's career is over. Chronic neurodegenerative disease including mild cognitive impairment (MCI), chronic traumatic encephalopathy (CTE), and dementia pugilistica (DP) have all been described in boxers, although it is still unknown why certain boxers go on to develop these conditions and others do not.[200, 201, 206, 241, 313] These individual acute and chronic injuries are more thoroughly discussed in later chapters.

There is a paucity of validated epidemiological data on which to accurately base boxing fatality rates. Instead, many of the reported fatality data have been obtained from a combination of media sources, industry reports, and individual case reports. A recent review of fatalities in boxing showed that based on the data analyzed between the control and fatal-bout groups, a computerized method of counting landed blows at ringside could provide sufficient data to stop matches that might result in fatalities.[215] However, such a process would become less effective as matches become more competitive, and implementing such a change would significantly decrease the competitive nature of the sport. From what can be ascertained based on the available reviews of boxing deaths, it appears that the rate of boxing fatalities has declined over the last few decades and that this can in part be attributed to rule changes as well as medical advances improving both the diagnosis and treatment of the acutely injured fighter.[11]

A couple of final general concepts regarding the risk for sustaining acute neurological injury in boxing are worth noting. The literature contains studies reporting conflicting results regarding age, sex, experience, and various measures of exposures as risk factors for acute neurological injuries in combat sports. Several groups of boxers, though, have a theoretically higher risk of sustaining neurological injuries—including those who are fatigued or dehydrated. A large number of brain injuries in boxing occur as a result of fatigue. As participants fatigue, they tend to rely more on instinct and become increasingly oblivious to the amount of trauma they are receiving. Also as they fatigue, they have a decreased ability to maintain good balance and block or avoid punches. They are also less able to move with a punch when struck. This loss of defensive ability makes the fatigued boxer more vulnerable to acute neurological injuries.

Dehydration in boxers can occur as a result of perspiration as a match progresses or intentional weight loss before a fight in order to meet a weight requirement, and it can increase a boxer's vulnerability to injury. Dehydration can contribute to and accentuate fatigue, affecting a boxer in the ways already mentioned. Additionally, dehydration can decrease the amount of cerebrospinal fluid (CSF) surrounding the brain, which normally provides the brain with a buffer from trauma. Also, this decrease in CSF enlarges the potential space around the brain, increasing the likelihood of developing hemorrhages such as subdural hematomas.

Bungee Jumping

Bungee jumping has quite an old origin. This way of jumping comes from the ancient ritual known as Gkol, performed on the Pentecost Island in the Pacific archipelago of Vanuatu, where young men would jump from tall wooden platforms with vines tied to their ankles as a test of their courage and passage into manhood. The first modern bungee jumps were made on April 1, 1979, from the 250-foot (76 m) Clifton Suspension Bridge in Bristol, England, by members of the Oxford University Dangerous Sports Club. The jumpers were arrested shortly afterward, but they continued with jumps in the United States, and the concept spread worldwide soon thereafter. Over 1 million jumps have been made since that time.

Bungee jumping injuries can be grouped into those that occur secondary to equipment failure or technical misjudgment and those that occur regardless of safety measures. In the first instance, catastrophic injury can occur if the safety harness fails, the cord elasticity is miscalculated, or the cord is not properly connected to the jump plat-

form. There are several reports of quadriplegia and death secondary to these errors.[127, 129, 134, 191] In one case report of a bungee cord attachment apparatus malfunctioning, a jumper experienced a free fall of approximately 240 feet (73 m) and avoided a catastrophic outcome, sustaining only minor injury, because of the presence of an air cushion on the ground below.[288] Catastrophic injury can also occur if the jump height is miscalculated or if it changes. In 1997, a member of a 16-person professional bungee jumping team died of significant traumatic brain injury when she jumped from the top level of the Louisiana Superdome and collided headfirst into the concrete-based playing field while practicing for a performance that was to take place during the halftime show of Super Bowl XXXI. Hot air balloon–based launching sites are vulnerable to undetected changes in altitude, which can cause the cord length to be greater than the distance to the ground. However, jumps from fixed sites, such as bridges, have resulted in catastrophic injury as well, secondary to striking the platform on rebound. There have also been reports of jumpers whose cord becomes tangled around their neck after a jump.

Even when appropriate safety measures are taken, there can be risk for neurological injury. A case of peroneal nerve palsy was diagnosed in a bungee jumper presenting with foot drop and paresthesias, presumably secondary to repetitive compression from the safety harness around the ankles.[334] More recently, a bungee jumper suffered a traumatic carotid artery dissection due to the force created by the free fall and rebound motion associated with the jump.[377] Fortunately for thrill seekers, despite all of the risks involved, bungee jumping is still considered one of the safest of the "extreme sports."

Canoeing and Kayaking

Canoeing originated to meet the simple needs of transportation across and along waterways and was the primary mode of long-distance transportation at one time. As a method of water transportation, canoes have generally been replaced by motorized boats and sailboats, although they remain popular as recreational or sporting watercraft. Canoeing as recreation and sport is often attributed to Scottish explorer John MacGregor, who was introduced to canoes on a camping trip in Canada and the United States in 1858. Upon returning to the United Kingdom, he constructed his own canoes and used them on waterways in various parts of Britain, Europe, and the Middle East; he subsequently founded the Royal Canoe Club, the world's oldest canoe club, in 1866.[260] The first canoeing competition was held by the club in 1874, and by 1936 canoeing had become an Olympic sport. The International Canoe Federation (ICF) is the umbrella organization for all canoe organizations worldwide and oversees the various disciplines, including canoe marathon, canoe slalom, canoe sprint, whitewater racing, canoe polo, canoe sailing, freestyle kayaking, surfski, and dragon boat racing.

Lower back pain and injury are the most common complaints of athletes who are injured during canoeing or kayaking.[355] Those who train harder are obviously at a greater risk in these sports. Kameyama and colleagues surveyed 821 active canoeists and performed a medical check of 63 top competitive canoeists, including physical and laboratory tests and radiographic examinations of the chest, spine, shoulder, elbow, and wrist joints.[153] Completed questionnaires were returned by 417 canoeists, whose reported racing styles were kayak, 324; Canadian canoe, 71; slalom, 13; and not specified, 9. Of the 417 respondents, 94 canoeists (22. 5%) reported that they experienced low back pain. On medical examinations, the lower back pain was found to be mainly of myofascial origin or due to spondylolysis.[153] Catastrophic cervical spine injury or head injury is also possible and can occur particularly in kayakers who flip their vessel in shallow water.[289] Participants are also prone to median nerve entrapment secondary to the significant torque that wrists are subjected to with paddling.[355]

Cheerleading

Cheerleading originated as squads aimed at getting the crowd at a sporting event to cheer louder. Today, however, it has evolved into an athletic activity that incorporates elements of dance and gymnastics along with stunts and pyramid formations. An estimated 3.5 million people participate as cheerleaders each year, from 6-year-olds to adults who cheerlead for professional athletic teams. While cheerleading is meant to support an athletic team, its intense competitions at the high school and collegiate levels have created a new dynamic, including increased risk for injury.

The increase in cheerleading-related injuries in recent years can be attributed to the increase in the number of athletes engaged in the sport. The rise in catastrophic injuries, though, appears to be related to the increasing difficulty of the acrobatic routines that cheerleaders perform and the daring skills of prospective cheerleaders trying to make a cheering squad. Modern cheerleading involves high team throws and daring aerial drills that frequently lead to accidents, particularly during pyramid building (figure 1.3).[31, 291-293] Mortalities in cheerleading have been reported. [31] Severe neurological injuries have included skull fractures, intracranial hemorrhages, and diffuse cerebral edema. Additionally, major spine injuries have ranged from cervical fractures to spinal cord contusion and paralysis.[31, 336]

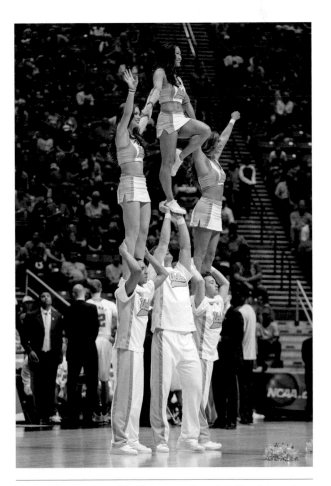

Figure 1.3 Pyramid building in cheerleading is particularly dangerous.
© Ric Tapia/Icon SMI

A recent study described the epidemiology of cheerleading-related strain and sprain injuries. [294] Athletic exposure and injury data were collected from 412 U.S. cheerleading teams via the Cheerleading Reporting Information Online surveillance tool; spotting or basing other cheerleaders was the most common mechanism of injury and was more likely to result in a lower back strain or sprain than other mechanisms. Another study investigated a cohort of 9,022 cheerleaders on U.S. cheerleading teams.[292] Of the 567 cheerleading injuries reported during the 1-year study, 83% occurred during practice as opposed to competition; specifically, 52% occurred while the cheerleader was attempting a stunt, and 24% occurred while the cheerleader was basing or spotting one or more team members. The authors also noted that collegiate cheerleaders were more likely to sustain a concussion or closed head injury than were cheerleaders at other levels. One prospective cohort study of high school cheerleaders found that 6.3% of all injuries were concussions.[283] Cheerleading can be associated with median palmar digital neuropathy as a result of chronic trauma to the palm during cheerleading activities, although this is rare.[295]

Cricket

Although cricket has been long heralded as a "gentleman's game," the game's evolution has resulted in shorter and more competitive matches involving greater aggression, more stressful training programs, and a workload on par with that of other professional athletes.[13] Thus it is no surprise that an increase in the number of cricketing injuries has been observed recently, with players exposed to risk of impact (ball or bat), collision (other players, fences), slips and falls, and repetitive and overuse injuries. While well-designed studies critically investigating the incidence of neurological injury are lacking, neurological injuries can and do occur.

Epidemiological studies undertaken in Australia, South Africa, England, and the West Indies have repeatedly demonstrated that fast bowlers have the highest risk of injury in cricket, with the lower back being most susceptible to both traumatic and overuse injuries.[116, 181, 195, 242, 315] A 1-year study prospectively surveyed all injuries occurring in all major matches of the West Indies Cricket Board and found that injuries to the head,

cervical spine, and lumbar spine accounted for 8%, 4%, and 20% of the total, respectively.[195] Another recent study reviewed injuries in cricket players of all levels over a 6-year period and indentified 498 cases.[354] Head injuries accounted for 20% of injuries in this study, and of those, 77% were the result of being struck by a ball or bat. The head injuries involved fractures (35%), contusions (18%), and concussion (10%).

As with other sports, injury mechanisms seem to vary with age. In one study, players less than 10 years of age were most commonly injured by being struck by the bat; for those aged 10 to 50 years, being struck by the ball or the bat was most common; and for those >50 years of age, the most common mechanisms were overexertion, strenuous or repetitive movements, or falls.[354] The injury pattern also changed with age. Fifty percent of all injuries to those younger than 10 years occurred to the head; players aged 10 to 19 years sustained mostly injuries to the head, as well as upper and lower extremities; and those older than 20 years mainly sustained extremity injury. These figures are important when one considers how to tailor protective equipment and injury prevention education to these athletes.

Cycling and BMX

Participation in the sport of cycling has grown significantly in the past several years. The first competitive bicycle race was held in France in 1869. Since that time the sport has expanded to include recreational riding, road and off-road cycling, track racing, BMX, and cyclocross competition. The sport is associated with a wide range of neurological injuries affecting both the central and peripheral nervous systems.

While at first glance one might expect the incidence of injury to be greater in BMX biking versus other forms of cycling, the reported incidences appear to be similar.[370] A comparison of various groups of cyclists showed that a large number of head injuries needed admission to a hospital, but interestingly, BMX riders had fewer head injuries than the other groups. Concussions account for about 7% of the injuries in BMX racing.[145] Off-road racing carries a high risk for musculoskeletal injury; however, in several reports the incidence of concussion was quite small, less than 1%.[173, 265] Regardless of the type of cycling, injuries to the head are common in accidents. Each year, more than 500,000 people in the United States are treated in emergency departments, and more than 700 people die as a result of bicycle-related injuries.[51] The rate of fatalities in children from bicycle accidents exceeds that from causes such as falls, poisoning, suffocation, and firearms—problems that typically receive much more attention.[360] The majority of fatal accidents are due to intracranial hemorrhages and subdural hematomas. Helmet use has significantly helped to reduce the incidence of catastrophic injury.

Neck and back pain are extremely common complaints in cyclists, occurring in up to 60% of participants.[361] In one recent descriptive epidemiological study, 109 elite cyclists in the training camps of seven professional teams were interviewed regarding overuse injuries they had experienced in the previous 12 months.[58] Injuries that required attention from medical personnel or involved time loss from cycling were registered. Of the 94 injuries registered, 45% were in the lower back. Additionally, 58% of all cyclists had experienced lower back pain at some point in the prior 12 months, and interestingly, only 41% had sought medical attention for it. Another study of overuse injuries in cyclists found that the most common anatomical site was the neck (49%) and that the lower back accounted for 30% of complaints.[362] It is thought that one mechanistic etiology might be the hyperextension of the neck and forward-bent riding position. Also, if the bicycle is not fitted appropriately for the participant, the cyclist may need to reach farther forward for the handlebars, exacerbating the hyperextension of the neck and extreme flexion of the back needed to ride. Spinal cord injuries and disc herniations have also been associated with cycling accidents.[79, 169, 350]

Injuries to the peripheral nerves can occur with cycling as well. The most common peripheral nerve deficits associated with the sport include injuries to the pudendal, genitofemoral, and ulnar nerves. Neuropathies with symptoms in the distribution of the pudendal and genitofemoral nerves are common and can occur in as many as 50% of male cyclists competing in long-distance rides.[33] Goldberg, Peylan, and Amit described a cyclist with injury to the pudendal nerves who presented with numbness of the buttocks and genitalia, associated with difficulty in achieving an erection.[118]

Cessation of cycling for a few weeks resulted in a spontaneous resolution of the patient's symptoms, fortunately without residual deficit. The injury is thought to occur from overuse or improper or poor positioning of the seat. Less frequently, the shape of the seat is the root of the problem. Ulnar nerve injury secondary to chronic compression at the handlebar interface has been recognized for over 100 years.[105] One study reported 117 cases over a 4-year period.[139] This condition, often referred to as cyclist's or handlebar palsy, can result in both motor and sensory symptoms and most commonly occurs during a long ride, often over rough terrain. Although much less common than ulnar neuropathy, median nerve involvement has been described in cyclists as well.[37]

Darts and Lawn Darts

The sharp point on the dart used in recreational indoor dart competition as well as outdoor lawn darts can be a cause for neurological injury. Lawn darts are typically 12 inches (30 cm) long with a weighted metal or plastic tip on one end and three plastic fins on a rod at the other end, basically an oversized version of the traditional indoor dart. The darts are tossed underhand toward a horizontal ground target, where the weighted end hits first and sticks into the ground, similarly to a horseshoe. While injuries are typically rare with the use of indoor darts, several reports have documented the neurological injury risk with lawn darts. One of the largest series reported 76 patients who presented to the hospital with lawn dart injuries.[309] The patients ranged from 1 to 18 years of age and were predominantly male. The most common sites of injury were the head (54%), eye (17%), and face (11%), and hospitalization was required for nearly 54% of these patients. Two other reports corroborated the risk for penetrating brain injury with these darts.[128, 325] The U.S. Consumer Product Safety Commission banned the sale of lawn darts in December 1988,[344] and Canada followed in similar suit shortly thereafter.[132] Despite the ban on the sale of lawn darts, there remain millions of sets in circulation. These dangerous products may still be in garages, basements, or secondhand stores, and the U.S. Consumer Product Safety Commission has urged consumers to discard or destroy all lawn darts immediately.[344]

Diving and Swimming

In the 1800s, diving evolved from a sport called plunging. It became a part of the Olympic Games in St. Louis, Missouri, in 1904. As a sport, it has always carried a risk of catastrophic cervical spine injury. It was recognized as early as 1948 that unsafe diving is the leading cause of spinal cord injuries associated with aquatic activities.[20, 71] Diving is the fourth leading cause of spinal cord injury in the United States[239] and is also responsible for significant proportions of spinal cord injury worldwide.[20, 26, 71, 221] These devastating injuries can occur when divers strike the springboard or platform with their head during a dive or when the head contacts the bottom surface of the pool. Most injuries do not happen in elite divers but rather occur in recreational athletes who dive into shallow water (in swimming pools, ponds, or lakes), often with disastrous results.[76] Spinal cord injuries are most commonly associated with either fracture dislocations or compression fractures of the spinal column forced into hyperflexion.

One study investigated 220 patients with spinal cord injury secondary to diving accidents who were admitted to the Midwest Regional Spinal Injury Center in Chicago.[8] Of the total patients, 70% had neurological injury; and among these, 47% had complete spinal injuries with loss of all motor and sensory function below the level of injury. The rest of the patients sustained incomplete injuries: 62% anterior cord syndrome, 17% central cord syndrome, and 20% Brown-Sequard syndrome.[8] The most common levels of injury were at the C-5 and C-6 levels. In another large retrospective study, all spinal cord injuries associated with diving were at the cervical level.[280]

The incidence of spinal cord injury in diving is heavily dependent on patient factors, agent factors (i.e., that which imparts force on the diver), physical environmental factors (e.g., warning signs, depth indicators, lighting), and social factors (e.g., absence of lifeguards or presence of alcohol).[71] Given the burden and rates of these injuries, as well as the fact that they appear to be (for the most part) preventable, efforts at multifaceted prevention programs are urgently needed.[71]

The sport of swimming per se is generally felt to be one of the safest with regard to nervous system injury, with a low incidence of head, spine, and peripheral nerve injuries. Most catastrophic injuries in swimming are related to diving into the water. That being said, in swimmers, neurogenic thoracic outlet syndrome may develop in association with hypertrophied pectoralis minor muscles.[155, 316]

Dodgeball

Dodgeball is a well-known form of team sport that is best known as a game played in physical education classes. While the game is typically played among children in elementary school, the sport has emerged internationally as a popular middle school, high school, and college sport. It is also popular in informal settings and can be played on a playground, in a gym, or in organized recreational leagues. There are no standards for the measurements or materials of the balls used; however, most dodgeballs are roughly the size of a volleyball and are composed of foam with a thin plastic or rubber shell. Although dodgeball is typically thought of as a benign activity, the risk for concussion or other severe head injury exists. A recent report described a 9-year-old child who was found to have a chronic subdural hematoma due to repeated minor dodgeball head impacts.[356] No altered mental status or focal neurological deficits were observed; however, the child presented with intermittent severe headache associated with nausea and vomiting.

Equestrian Sports

Horses were first domesticated in 4500 BC by tribesmen in Central Asia. The horse has played an important role throughout human history, all over the world, both in warfare and in peaceful pursuits such as transportation, trade, and agriculture. While horses were initially trained and ridden for practical working purposes, equestrianism has since evolved to include a wide range of sports including, but not limited to, endurance riding, show jumping, harness racing, vaulting, polo, thoroughbred horse racing, steeplechase racing, rodeo, and recreational riding.

Equestrian-related injuries are a serious occurrence, and horseback riding is recognized as more dangerous than skiing and motorcycle or automobile racing.[14] In the United States, an estimated 30 million people ride horses each year, resulting in 50,000 emergency room visits (1 visit per 600 riders per year).[49, 170] Children participating in equestrian activities are at risk for substantial injury, and pediatric care providers must maintain a high index of suspicion when evaluating these children.[25, 70, 235] Females tend to have a higher rate of injury than males, but this is partly due to the female predominance in the sport.[22, 23, 235] Riding carries with it an implicit risk of injury associated with the unpredictability of the animals, the weight of the horse, the positioning of the rider's head as high as 10 feet (3 m) off the ground, and travel at speeds up to 40 miles per hour (64 km/h).[131] The most common mechanism of injury is falling or being thrown from the horse, followed by being kicked, trampled, and bitten.[83, 131, 170, 186] One study reviewed a national database of equestrian injuries over a 2-year period to identify predictors of significant injury.[186] The authors found that the injuries occurred at home (36%), in a recreation or sporting facility (30%), on a farm (19%), and on other public property (12%). The injuries were due to a fall (59%) or to being thrown from or bucked off the horse (22%), or they occurred while on the horse (9%).

Neurological injury in particular is a common consequence of these activities; it ranges in severity from concussions and degenerative spine disease to spinal cord injury and debilitating closed head injuries, and can even result in death.[14, 24, 131, 185, 266, 339] Chronic neurodegenerative disease, in the form of dementia pugilistica, has been reported in steeplechase jockeys. For professional jockeys, head trauma is one of the most common types of career-ending injuries.[12] Helmets have helped to decrease the incidence of catastrophic injury; however, helmet use (particularly during recreational riding) remains low.[34] One possible obstacle to helmet use in equestrian sports may be the cost. However, while helmets traditionally have been quite expensive, many approved helmets can now be found for less than $50.

Golf

Although golf may trace its origins to ancient Rome, it has been fairly well established that the modern game was actually devised in Scotland in the late 14th or 15th century. Today, more than 26 million people in the United States alone play golf. Golf is considered a safe sport, and although they are uncommon, injuries incurred during golfing are an increasing problem. A number of studies have examined the occurrence of injuries in amateur as well as elite or professional golfers. In professional male golfers, the most common site of injury is the lower back.[204] For professional female golfers, the lower back is the second most common site of injury.[198] The most common mechanism of injury for professional golfers is the highly repetitive practice, followed by hitting an object other than the ball with the club.[198, 204] The amount of practice places this group of golfers at risk for overuse injuries; and often they continue to play, making them more likely to aggravate the injury compared to amateur golfers. In amateur golfers, the lower back is an extremely common site of injury. The literature is conflicting regarding the most common site of injury, as some studies report that the wrist is more commonly injured than the lower back.[16, 199] In amateur golfers, the most common mechanisms of injury are overuse, poor biomechanics of the swing, and hitting the ground or an object other than the ball during the swing.[199, 204]

One study reviewed golf-related injuries that occurred in 300 patients attending emergency departments over a 6.5-year period.[363] Most of these injuries involved the head. The main mechanisms of injury were being hit by a club (37%), being hit by a ball (28%), sprains or strains (9.67%), and slips or falls (7%). When the data were broken down by age, the main source of injury in adults was being hit by a ball, whereas for children and adolescents, being struck by a golf club accounted for 77% of hospital presentations. Catastrophic injury can occur as a result of being struck by either a club or a ball, although each of these occurs rarely.[204] Standing behind someone who unexpectedly takes a practice swing or standing too close to another player who is swinging is the most common source of this injury. Freak accidents have also been described—for example, the golf club shaft breaks, resulting in a penetrating head injury. Some golf-related neurological injuries are due to golf cart accidents or falls out of a cart, often involving inebriated passengers and drivers.[193, 204, 335, 342]

Gymnastics and Trampoline

Although gymnastics began more than 2,000 years ago, it was seen originally as an activity, not a sport. It has evolved into a widely popular sport today with significant increases in participation in the last two decades. Approximately 3,800 men and 24,500 women participate in gymnastics annually.[225] The increase in numbers has exposed a larger number of athletes to acute and chronic injuries. Many studies place the overall injury rate as high as in football, wrestling, and softball.[335]

One study sought to describe the epidemiology of gymnastics-related injuries among children ages 6 to 17 years in the United States over a 15-year period.[300] This retrospective review revealed an estimated 425,900 children treated in U.S. hospital emergency departments for gymnastics-related injuries during the 16-year period, with the number of injuries averaging 26,600 annually. The places where injuries occurred included schools (40.0%), places of recreation or sport (39.7%), homes (14.5%), and other public property (5.8%).

The required maneuvers and postures are difficult and place the body at risk for neurological injury, particularly spine injury (figure 1.4). Degenerative disc disease and spondylolysis are common injuries in gymnasts. Most spinal cord injuries occur at the midcervical levels.[7, 9, 237] With most gymnastics activities, the incidence of catastrophic brain injury is relatively low; most of these injuries occur during a dismount in which an athlete lands on the head. Milder head injuries such as concussion occur more frequently. In their 15-year study of children ages 6 to 17 years, Singh and colleagues found that head and neck injuries accounted for 12.9% of all injuries.[300] Strain and sprain injuries were most common (44.5%), and concussion or closed head injury occurred in only 1.7% of the cases.[300] The concussions in that study were more likely to occur while participants were performing headstands versus other skills. In a 16-year survey of collegiate gymnasts, the concussion rate was found to be 0.16 per 1,000 athletic exposures.[135] Although extremely rare, peripheral nerve injuries involving the femoral, lateral femoral cutaneous, and distal posterior interosseus nerves have all been reported.[5, 41, 115, 119]

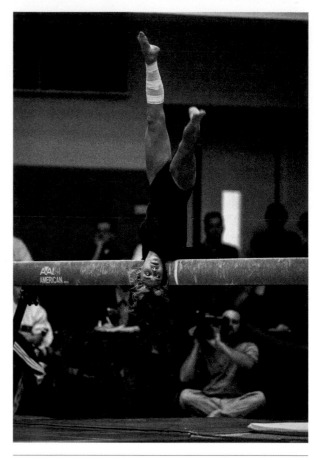

Figure 1.4 The maneuvers and postures involved in gymnastics can place the body at risk for neurological injury.

Trampolines have evolved only over the last 50 years, with an unprecedented surge in popularity recently. They are used both as a part of gymnastics events and for recreational activity. Trampolines have been identified as a common cause of injury—spinal cord injury in particular—with many studies documenting the risk.[144, 240, 274, 317, 369] Participants can be projected many feet in the air and fall back to the trampoline or the ground, landing on their head or neck, putting them at risk for catastrophic injury. One study demonstrated that in the United States, trampolines accounted for greater than 6,500 pediatric cervical spine injuries in 1998.[40, 107] This was a fivefold increase in trampoline-related injuries compared with the previous 10 years. While fractures are the most common injury, spinal injuries reportedly account for 12% of trampoline-related injuries.[107] These occur frequently in children;

however, teenagers and young adults have sustained spinal cord injuries as well.[183, 298]

Hang Gliding

Thousands in the United States participate in hang gliding despite the risks inherent to the sport. Hang gliders are kite-like crafts to which the flier is attached via a harness and supported on a swing-like frame. By shifting their body weight, fliers can steer the craft in various directions. The sport has continued to grow, with competitions held at both the national and international levels. The potential for neurological injury, particularly catastrophic injury, is fairly obvious and has been noted in the literature.[17, 367] Usual causes of injury include misjudgment of landing speed and altitude, resulting in injurious landing forces. An earlier study noted that most of the hang gliding injuries examined occurred as a result of in-flight errors in judgment versus equipment failure.[331] Another study showed that the majority of all injuries (60%) occurred during landing.[180] In that same study, spinal injuries were the most common type, accounting for 36% of the total.[180] The majority of hang gliding injuries reportedly occur in young adults age 20 to 40 years.[100] Another study noted that of nonfatal injuries, 16% were head injuries and 17% involved the spine.[331]

Hockey (Field and Ice)

Native North Americans played variations of stickball such as tabé or shinny, which are similar in some ways to modern field hockey. For well over 1,000 years, though, the Daur people of Inner Mongolia have been playing a game called beikou, which entails whacking around a ball-like knob of apricot root with long wooden branches.[203] For night games, they use an ignitable ball covered in felt.[203] The modern game of field hockey grew from English public schools in the early 19th century, and the game was codified for use in the Olympics shortly thereafter. One study showed that between 1982 and 2008, approximately 3,000 men and 1.43 million women competed in high school field hockey, with an additional 145,000 women competing at the college level.[225] Most believe that ice hockey evolved from outdoor stick-and-ball games as

well. It is thought that these games were adapted to the icy conditions of Canada in the 19th century and later evolved into a game played on ice skates, often with a puck. Ice hockey is a sport that is widely popular today, and an average of approximately 27,800 men and 2,800 women play it each year.[72, 225]

Both sports use a hard object (ball or puck) and sticks and are played in an aggressive manner. Neurological injuries in both forms of hockey most commonly consist of concussions and spinal cord injuries, with peripheral nerve injuries much less common. Possible mechanisms include falls during ball or puck handling, collisions with other players or inanimate objects (bench, goal, boards), and checking.[72, 335] Although there are many similarities between ice and field hockey, the proportions of concussions differ between the sports. Considering the lower number of participants compared to other sports, both forms of hockey are associated with relatively higher rates of concussion. In a 13-year study comparing injuries in male and female pediatric (ages 2 through 18 years) ice and field hockey participants, the proportion of concussion was higher in ice hockey players (3.9%) than in field hockey players (1.4%).[373]

Concussions in high school field hockey have been reported at a rate of 0.46 per 100 player-seasons.[254] Collegiate field hockey athletes had a rate of 0.18 concussions per 1,000 athletic exposures in one large 16-year study.[135] In that same study, the rate of concussions in male and female collegiate ice hockey participants was 0.41 and 0.91 per 1,000 athletic exposures, respectively.[135] The relationship between age and concussion in ice hockey in uncertain; however, studies in youth hockey players seem to suggest that Bantam and Pee-Wee ice hockey players (ages 11-14 years) have a greater rate of concussion than Atom players (age 9-10 years).[84, 85] Nonetheless, with increased awareness and reporting in recent years, concussion appears much more common than we once thought across all levels of ice hockey competition.

Hockey-related spinal injuries have seen an increased occurrence, although this may be in part due to the larger number of players, better diagnostic skills, or increased reporting.[323, 335] An earlier study looked at the SportSmart Registry for the years 1966 to 1996.[324] The authors examined the nature and incidence of major spinal injuries in ice hockey players and identified 300 players worldwide who had sustained spinal injuries, of which approximately 250 occurred in Canada, 35 in the United States, and 15 in Europe. Complete motor injuries were suffered in approximately 25% of players, and 75% of the injuries occurred during organized games as opposed to practice.[324] Burst fractures and fracture dislocations are the most common vertebral injuries and carry with them an increased risk for spinal cord injury. The most frequently reported mechanism of injury is a push or a check from behind, sending the unsuspecting player hurling into the boards headfirst. Spinal injury can also occur when a player is hit while looking down at the puck, delivering an axial loading force to the head and spine. Rule changes, education, neck strengthening exercises, and conditioning have all been important aspects of injury prevention in these athletes.

As mentioned previously, peripheral nerve injury in both forms of hockey is rare but can occur.[337] Although more commonly reported in football players, burners or stingers have been described in hockey players.[91] Direct trauma or orthopedic injuries always carry a risk for peripheral neuropathy. Axillary nerve injury secondary to direct trauma associated with shoulder dislocation has been reported in two hockey players.[247, 248] Similarly, peroneal neuropathy has occurred in hockey players, though rarely, secondary to laceration of the nerve with a skate blade or as a result of direct blunt nerve trauma.[192, 290]

Hurling

Hurling is one of the three national games of Ireland and has prehistoric origins, having been played for at least 3,000 years. It is a fast-paced game that combines elements of baseball, field hockey, and lacrosse. A similar game for women is called camogie. Players hurl a small, hard, 100- to 130-gram leather ball (sliotar) with a long tapered stick (hurley). They score points by propelling the ball over or under the crossbar of the goal. This is a contact sport that differs from other "stick" games in that the majority of play is above the participants' heads in the air. As a result, injuries to the head are common and are usually due to contact with the ball, the stick, or another player.[229] Two studies found that hurling

injuries occurred to the head or face 36% to 40% of the time.[67, 69, 229] As of 2010, all players must wear helmets with face guards, and a resultant decrease in injuries is apparent. Before this time, helmet use during game play was optional, and resistance to helmet use certainly contributed to the high injury rates.

An earlier prospective study investigated hurling injuries in 74 players over the 8 months of one season.[358] The most common types of injuries were muscle strains. Back and head injuries accounted for 11% and 9% of the total, respectively. Concussions accounted for 3% of the total. Interestingly, 41% of the injuries were attributed to foul play, making a case for the need for better rule enforcement. Even though it is one of the all-around fastest field sports, catastrophic injury in hurling is quite rare.

In-Line Skating, Roller Skating, and Skateboarding

The first recorded use of roller skates was in 1743 during a London stage performance, although the inventor of this skate is largely unknown. John Joseph Merlin is credited as the inventor of the skate in 1760, which was actually a primitive in-line skate with metal wheels. Roller skating saw rapid growth throughout the early 1900s and immediately became a popular pastime for both men and women. In-line skating evolved from roller skating; some believe it was developed to occupy ice hockey players during the months when there was no ice. The first in-line skate, featuring three in-line wheels attached to a wooden plate, was patented in Paris in 1819. Several renditions appeared over the next century. In-line skating has since become one of the fastest-growing recreational sports for children and teenagers in the United States. The low cost and various health benefits have allowed the sport to thrive beyond the limits of a fad, as evidenced by the existence of professional leagues and international competitions (roller hockey, roller derby, aggressive in-line). Millions of participants have gravitated toward skating as a means of recreation, competition, fitness, training, or transportation. Skateboarding is also a popular recreational activity and part of a lifestyle among many young people.[103, 263] The most common injuries among all of these skate sports are musculoskeletal, with ankle strains and sprains and extremity fractures.[1, 90, 101, 103, 159, 175, 263, 277, 279] The incidence of injury with roller skating and in-line skating is less than that in ice skating. For skateboarding, the incidence of injuries is estimated to be 10 injuries per year, per skateboarder.[263]

A total of 65% of injured adolescent skate-boarders sustain injuries on public roads, on foot-paths, and in parking lots.[103, 159] Furthermore, injuries seem to occur more frequently while people are performing a trick.[263] Helmet use has helped to reduce the incidence of severe head injury, but head injuries still do occur.[117, 138, 167, 187] "Truck surfing" or "skitching" refers to skating behind or alongside a vehicle while holding on to the vehicle. This results in a skater's travel-ing at the same speed as the vehicle. Such risky behavior can be very dangerous, particularly if the skater cannot slow down fast enough to prevent colliding with the vehicle or if the skater is thrown into oncoming traffic or the roadbed should the vehicle suddenly slow down, stop, or turn. The enhanced momentum results in a greater force of impact and consequently a more severe injury. Death is not uncommon with these severe injuries.

Lacrosse

The native North Americans used to play a game called baggataway in order to train for battle.[299] Many tribes played games with carefully shaped sticks made of hickory and other spiritu-ally important woods that had nets on the end, generally made of elm bark, leather, or deer hide. The National Lacrosse Association came into being in 1867, and the game evolved over time into the modern sport we know today. It is a fast-paced contact sport, played in close quarters, using sticks to propel a hard ball at high speeds. Neurological injuries can occur when a player falls or is struck by another player, the ball, or a stick, or when colliding with fixed objects such as the goal or a bench. Men's lacrosse is considered a contact sport and women's lacrosse is consid-ered noncontact, which may be a reason why protective gear, including helmets, is used only occasionally or not at all in women's lacrosse. High school lacrosse has approximately 33,000 male and 22,000 female participants each year.[72, 225] An additional 5,800 collegiate men and 4,000 collegiate women play lacrosse annually, as well.[72, 225]

In one study of scholastic women's lacrosse, the reported rate of head and face injury was 1.1 per 1,000 athletic exposures.[121] Head injuries are frequent in lacrosse players. In one 10-year study, closed head injuries composed 6% of all lacrosse-related injuries.[77] An earlier study of college athletes found that of all major women's collegiate sports, lacrosse appeared to have the highest percentage of concussive injuries (14%) and that this was higher than the proportion of concussion seen in male lacrosse players (10%).[63] Hootman and colleagues, in their 16-year study, reported the rate of concussion in col-legiate athletes to be 0.26 and 0.25 per 1,000 athletic exposures for men and women lacrosse players, respectively. Injuries are more common in games than in practice, likely due to the more aggressive play during competition.[121] In one study, concussions accounted for 8.6% of all inju-ries in lacrosse competitions, with athletes nine times more likely to experience a concussion in a game compared with practice.[135] Catastrophic injury can occur, as well. There is one report of an epidural hematoma resulting from a strike to the head from a lacrosse stick.[264] At the institu-tion of one of the authors, a teen lacrosse player presented to the trauma bay after being struck in the back of the neck with a lacrosse ball. The com-puted tomography (CT) scan of his head demon-strated diffuse subarachnoid and intraventricular hemorrhage secondary to a significant vertebral artery dissection. The patient died shortly after admission to the hospital.

Martial Arts and Mixed Martial Arts

Martial arts are ancient forms of combat modified for modern sport and exercise. Participation in martial arts is increasing, with millions of people practicing each year. In general, martial arts pro-vide health-promoting and meaningful exercise and have been shown to improve participants' overall cardiovascular endurance, strength, bal-ance, flexibility, body fat composition, stress and relaxation, confidence, and socialization.[258] Mixed martial arts (MMA) competition, also referred to as no-holds-barred (NHB) fighting, ultimate fighting, and cage fighting, has its roots in ancient Greece. In 648 BC, it was referred to as pankration and was featured at the 33rd ancient Olympics.[44, 252, 258] Pankration, which is Greek for "all powerful," was the hybridization of boxing and wrestling and was spawned from unarmed combat on the battlefield.[252] It became an extremely popular freestyle fighting sport and served as the climactic event of the Olympics for centuries. Despite the attempts by legislators and the medical community to ban it, MMA grew in the early 1990s from an underground spectacle into an internationally sanctioned sport with many of the same health benefits as traditional martial arts. In addition to these health benefits, however, all forms of martial arts activities carry an obvious risk of injury.

The incidence of injuries among the various individual disciplines seems to be roughly similar, at least between karate, taekwondo, and Muay Thai kickboxing.[110, 335] Martial arts styles that involve striking, such as kickboxing, karate, and taekwondo, have been shown to have a higher incidence of injury than styles that involve grappling alone, such as judo, sumo, and Brazilian jiu-jitsu. One large study sought to determine the rate and types of injuries occurring to registered professional kickboxers in Victoria, Australia, over a 16-year period.[376] Of the 382 injuries recorded from 3,481 fight participations, the body region most commonly injured was the head-neck-face (52.5%), with intracranial injury specifically occurring 17.2% of the time. Another study assessed the conditions under which concussions occurred in full-contact taekwondo competition.[250] The incidence of concussion in this study was high and was greater in men (7.04 per 1,000 athletic exposures) than in women (2.42 per 1,000 athletic exposures).

Initially promoted as a violent and brutal sport, MMA has dramatically changed, with revised rules and improved regulations to minimize the risk of injury. With regard to safety, MMA has been compared to other combat sports, such as boxing; however, MMA may actually have a safer track record with respect to serious injury and death. This difference may be due largely to the competitive structure of MMA events. Mixed martial arts competitions consist of three 5-minute rounds (for nonchampionship bouts) or five 5-minute rounds (for championship bouts), followed by 1-minute rest periods between rounds.[258] Competitors are matched according to designated weight classes and experience levels and wear protective equipment consisting of a mouth guard, groin protector, and 4- to 6-ounce (0.11-0.17 kg) MMA gloves.

Limited studies have investigated injury incidence in MMA.[28, 236, 258, 285, 286] Based on the data available, closed head injuries, lacerations, and orthopedic injuries are commonly experienced by competitors.[286] Knockout rates are lower in MMA competitions than in boxing, suggesting a reduced risk of brain injury in MMA competitions compared to other events involving striking. Since the inception of MMA in the modern era, only four deaths have been documented, with three of the four occurring outside of the United States in unsanctioned fights.[258] As a comparison, one study documented 71 deaths in boxing from 1993 to 2007, with a total of 1,355 deaths from 1890 to 2007, averaging 11.6 deaths per year during the modern history of the sport.[320] The incidence of concussion in MMA matches has ranged from 1% to 3%, with almost 25% of the matches stopped secondary to impact to the head; however, the incidence of concussion may be underreported. Injuries to the peripheral nerves are possible, with both acute and chronic symptoms reported.[161] Neuropathic symptoms can occur in individuals as a result of strikes on pressure points or exposed peripheral nerves. Although the majority of symptoms resolve within 1 year, individuals with repetitive exposure strikes may be more likely to have chronic symptoms.[161] Injuries to the spine can occur, although they are rare.[21, 251, 343] Studies using mathematical models of the biomechanics of maneuvers in MMA have shown that the forces involved are of the same order as those involved in whiplash injuries and of the same magnitude as compression injuries of the cervical spine.[168]

Motorcycle Racing

The International Motorcycling Federation (FIM) is the governing body of motorcycle racing. It represents 103 national motorcycle federations, divided into six regional continental unions, and oversees the various motorcycle racing disciplines including road racing, motocross, endure and cross-country rallies, and track racing. Other forms of motorcycle racing include drag racing, hill climb, and land speed racing. Although extremity injuries are the most common type of injury, motorcycle racers frequently sustain significant spine and head trauma, as well.[53, 123, 124,

[136, 330, 347] Studies have reported that head injuries account for 10% to 30% of injuries and that 25% of these are severe, with associated intracranial hemorrhage or mortality.[136, 347] In one study, the mortality rate in motorcycle racing was estimated at 9% of all injuries.[347] Spinal injuries are uncommon but can occur.[136, 179]

Mountain and Rock Climbing and Hiking

High-altitude travel for mountain climbing, trekking, or sightseeing has become very popular. Mountaineering is a sport that requires experience, athletic ability, and technical knowledge to maintain safety. In general, injury rates among mountain climbers and hikers are low, estimated at two cases per 1,000 climbers.[335] Falls during climbing represent one of the more common causes of serious injury, although acute and chronic musculoskeletal injuries of the hands and extremities are also frequent.[303] While catastrophic neurological injury can occur as with most sports, a unique form of sport-related neurological injury is associated with the condition referred to as acute mountain sickness (AMS). Acute mountain sickness is an illness that can affect mountain climbers, hikers, travelers, or even skiers at high altitudes (typically above 8,000 feet or 2,400 m). It is thought to be due to a combination of reduced air pressure and lower oxygen levels at high altitudes. The faster one climbs to a high altitude, the more likely acute mountain sickness becomes. The symptoms depend on the speed of the climb and the level of exertion. Headache is one of the cardinal symptoms of AMS and is presumed to be due to the development of cerebral edema.[42, 99, 102, 142] It may also be related to vascular dilation secondary to hypercapnea before the development of hypoxia-induced hyperventilation.[102] Dyspnea, weakness, asthenia, and nausea are also commonly associated with AMS. Acute mountain sickness can progress to high-altitude pulmonary edema (HAPE) or high-altitude cerebral edema (HACE), which is potentially fatal. Acute mountain sickness has been reported without headache, making it important for mountaineers to maintain awareness that the rapid onset of HAPE with subsequent severe desaturation may lead to the development of HACE even in the absence of headache.[328]

While traveling too high too fast is one factor relating to the development of AMS, individual susceptibility to high altitude–related illness is a further risk factor that can be recognized only in persons who have traveled to high altitudes in the past. One study found that in an unselected group of mountain climbers, 50% had AMS at 4,500 meters, while 0.5% to 1% had HACE and 6% had HAPE at the same altitude.[282] Magnetic resonance imaging (MRI) changes have been noted in several studies.[87, 126] One study recruited 35 climbers (12 were professional and 23 were amateur) in four expeditions without supplementary oxygen.[87] Twelve professionals and one amateur went to Mount Everest (8,848 meters), eight amateurs to Mount Aconcagua (6,959 meters), seven amateurs to Mont Blanc (4,810 meters), and seven amateurs to Mount Kilimanjaro (5,895 meters). Interestingly, only one of the 13 Everest climbers had a normal MRI; the amateur showed frontal subcortical lesions, and the remainder had cortical atrophy and enlargement of Virchow-Robin spaces but no lesions.[87] Among the remaining amateurs, 13 showed symptoms of high-altitude illness, five had irreversible subcortical lesions, and 10 had innumerable widened Virchow-Robin spaces.[87] No changes were noted on the MRI of a control group.

Mountain climbers and hikers can be subject to certain sport-specific peripheral nerve injuries. Tarsal tunnel syndrome can occur in mountaineers and is attributable to repetitive dorsiflexion of the ankle, causing injury to the tibial nerve.[190] Rucksack paralysis refers to a syndrome of brachial plexus injury at the upper and middle trunk that occurs with the use of a hiking backpack.[19, 62, 122, 149, 166] Injury of the suprascapular, axillary, and long thoracic nerves can also occur with rucksack use.[62, 220] Brachial plexus traction is thought to be the underlying mechanism, and the use of a backpack without waist support may exacerbate such traction.

Racket Sports

Racket sports are those sports in which players use rackets to hit a ball or other object; tennis, badminton, paddleball, and squash are a few examples. These sports are played by millions of people annually. Neurological injuries sustained in racket sports primarily involve the peripheral nervous system. All racket sports involve repetitive arm swinging, which can lead to several musculoskeletal overuse injuries, although the symptoms may mimic a nerve entrapment syndrome.[337] Specific nerve entrapments are possible, however. Posterior interosseous nerve entrapment is relatively common in tennis players secondary to compression at the arcade of Frohse.[190] Suprascapular injury can also occur in tennis players, likely secondary to the repetitive overhead swinging during serving, with compression at the suprascapular or supraglenoid notches.[74, 267] Long thoracic nerve injury can occur via the same repetitive serving mechanism.[337] Radial nerve palsy has been reported in tennis players, most usually as a result of compression from the fibrous bands at the lateral head of the triceps.[256, 314] Compression of the lateral cutaneous nerve of the forearm has also been described in a tennis player thought to have used the forehand swing excessively.[93]

Rodeo

Rodeo originated in the mid-19th century as informal events in the western United States and northern Mexico, with cowboys and cattle ranchers testing their work skills against one another.[125] Although Deer Trail, Colorado, lays claim to the first rodeo in 1869, the first true formal rodeo was held in Cheyenne, Wyoming, in 1872.[125] Many rodeo events are based on the tasks required in cattle ranching. Today, events include saddle bronco riding, steer wrestling, team roping, bareback bronco riding, calf roping, and bull riding. The rates of injury vary by rodeo event but are highest in bull riding and bareback and saddle bronco riding.[45] The sport involves contact, collision, and repetitive forces, not to mention the risk secondary to the size, strength, and unpredictability of the animals. Bull riders appear to be most at risk. In bull riding, the incidence of injury is reported at 32.2 injuries per 1,000 athletic exposures.[80] While a number of different injuries can occur during bull riding, concussions are often the most alarming. Concussions have been reported to account for 9% to 14% of all reported rodeo-related injuries.[45, 212] More serious head injuries can occur, and cervical as well as lumbar injuries and sprains have been reported. Injuries can occur secondary to violent dismounts, contact

with the animal, or equipment failure.[45] That being said, experience may also account for the incidence of injury at various levels of competition, although further studies are needed to delineate this.[46]

Rowing

Competitive rowing is a taxing sport that dates back to ancient Rome and Egypt. Even since the earliest recorded references to rowing, the sporting element has been present. The first known "modern" rowing races began from competition among the professional watermen who provided ferry and taxi service on the River Thames in London. Today the sport has evolved to include races on rivers, on lakes, or on the ocean, depending on the type of race and the discipline. The sport requires both strength and aerobic conditioning. There is a significant injury rate among competitive participants. The extensive training and repetitive technique place the rower at risk for overuse injury.[207, 249]

The most frequently injured region is the low back, mainly due to excessive hyperflexion and twisting, and can include specific injuries such as spondylolysis, sacroiliac joint dysfunction, and disc herniation.[268] One study found a 17% incidence of spondylolysis in high-level rowers.[307] Smoljanovic and colleagues investigated injuries in 398 international elite-level junior rowers.[304] Overall, 290 (73.8%) injuries involved overuse, and 103 (26.2%) were related to a single traumatic event. Female rowers were injured more frequently than male rowers; and in both sexes, the most common injury site was the low back, followed by the knee and the forearm-wrist. Interestingly, the rowers with traumatic injuries had less rowing experience than the uninjured rowers, and the incidence of traumatic injuries was significantly lower in rowers who regularly performed more than 10 minutes of posttraining stretching. Another recent study prospectively followed 20 international rowers who were competing as part of the Irish Amateur Rowing Union squad system over the course of 12 months.[366] The mean number of injuries sustained per athlete was 2.2 over the 12-month period. The most frequent injury involved the lumbar spine (31.82% of total injuries), and cervical spine injuries accounted for 11.36% of the total number of injuries.[366]

Injuries to the peripheral nerves can occur and are usually the result of improper technique or poorly fitting equipment. The repetitive rowing technique predisposes rowers to carpal tunnel syndrome secondary to entrapment of the median nerve. Additionally, pressure from an improperly fitted seat can cause sciatic nerve injury.[156]

Shooting Sports

The sport of shooting was introduced to the Olympics in 1896. The sport is competitive and involves tests of accuracy and speed using various types of guns including rifle, handgun, shotgun, action gun, 3-gun, submachine gun, and crossbow gun. Musculoskeletal complaints are common in competitive shooters, with lower back pain the most frequent complaint. An older screening study found that nearly 80% of shooters experience back pain during a competition and 63% suffer back pain after a competition.[352] It is thought that lower back pain in shooters may be secondary to the prolonged hyperextension and rotation of the spine during aiming. Peripheral nerves are also at risk for injury in shooting sports. Injury to the long thoracic nerve with subsequent weakness of the serratus anterior muscle has been reported in shooters.[368] Hearing loss is a common complaint among shooters and can be addressed with the use of protective earpieces. The right ear tends to be more affected than the left simply because of the positioning of guns in right-handed individuals. The longer an athlete is exposed to shooting, particularly without protective earpieces, the greater the risk of developing hearing deficits.[54] Finally, lead absorption and intoxication with resultant symptomatic neuropathy may be of concern for shooters, particularly in users of indoor small-bore rifle or pistol ranges.[98, 113, 177, 238, 319] This can occur at outdoor ranges as well.[120]

Skiing and Snowboarding

Some of the earliest people to ski may have been prehistoric Nordic people. The Norwegians transformed skiing from a mode of transportation to a competitive sport that is enjoyed today by millions. The various types of skiing including freestyle, alpine (slalom, giant slalom, super-G, and downhill), and Nordic or cross-country skiing. Skiing attracts more than 200 million participants worldwide each year,[143] with an estimated 11.5 million participating in the United States alone.[163] In the United States, another 8.2 million people annually participate in snowboarding, a winter sport that was pioneered in the 1960s and 1970s as an alternative to alpine skiing.[163] Snowboarding is one of the fastest-growing winter sports in the world and in 1998 became an official part of the Winter Olympic Games in Nagano, Japan. Although most skiing- and snowboarding-related injuries are orthopedic, both are high-speed sports with an associated high risk of injury to the nervous system. In general, older skiers tend to have the highest skiing-related injury rates.[371] In contrast, snowboarding-related injuries are more associated with younger participants, which is likely a reflection of the greater number of young snowboarders.[371] Intermediate or expert snowboarders tend to be more likely to sustain injury than beginners, usually because of the jumps attempted at this level of experience.[333, 353, 372] In one study, intentional jumping was the cause of injury in 77% of snowboarders compared with 20% of skiers.[322] Numerous studies have examined differences in injuries between snowboarding and alpine skiing.[2, 133, 163, 184, 371] While injury rates have fluctuated over time, in general, snowboarding is associated with higher injury rates than skiing.[163]

Most spinal injuries in skiing and snowboarding result from a simple fall or from striking a tree.[230, 372] In contrast to the situation with other sports, most skiing-related spinal injury occurs in the thoracolumbar region, followed by the cervical region.[89] Snowboarding-related spinal injuries occur most commonly in the cervical spine.[112, 372] While they may not receive as much publicity as spinal cord injuries, traumatic brain injuries are also common in skiing and snowboarding.[231, 335] It has been estimated that 15% to 20% of the annually reported skiing and snowboarding injuries are head injuries.[224] Most of these occur early in the season; and in one study, mild injuries were more common than severe brain injuries.[184] Concussions have been reported to represent 9.6% of all injuries in skiers and 14.7% of all injuries in snowboarders.[39, 72] One study examined 5 years of trauma registry data to compare skiers and snowboarders and showed that the rate of head injury for the two sports was similar.[133] A concussion was present in 60% of the skiers and 21% of the snowboarders.[133] Additionally, snowboarders suffered an intracranial hemorrhage in 71% of the cases compared to 28% of the skiers.[133] In summary, this study seemed to show that skiers sustain a greater proportion of concussions whereas snowboarders may experience a greater number of severe brain injuries.

Snowmobiling and All-Terrain Vehicles

All-terrain vehicles (ATVs) are popular recreational and utility vehicles. Snowmobiles are a type of all-terrain vehicle intended as a winter utility vehicle to be used where other vehicles cannot go. The evolution of the snowmobile is not the work of any one inventor but more a process of advances in engines for the propulsion of vehicles and supporting devices over snow. Snowmobiles appealed to hunters and workers transporting personnel and materials across snow-covered land, frozen lakes, and rivers. In the later part of the 20th century, though, they were put to use for recreational purposes as well. Contemporary types of recreational riding include snowcross and racing, trail riding, freestyle, and mountain climbing. Summertime activities for snowmobile enthusiasts include drag racing on grass, on asphalt strips, or even across water. Operating both ATVs and snowmobiles requires skill and physical strength, given their inherent maneuverability, acceleration, and top speed capabilities. These same characteristics increase the risk of injury with operation of these vehicles.

Many studies have documented the inherent risks of operating these fun recreational vehicles. [48, 96, 188, 196, 275, 276, 302, 327, 349] One study reviewed experience at a children's hospital over 10 years. [194] The authors retrospectively analyzed 185 pediatric cases involving ATV-related accidents. Sixty-two patients (33.5%) suffered neurological injuries, and the most common injuries included skull fracture (37 cases) and closed head injury (30 cases). There were 39 cases of intracranial hemorrhage and 11 patients with spinal fractures. A recent study identified different radiologically diagnosed injuries in 512 consecutive children suffering from ATV-related injuries who were treated at a tertiary care pediatric hospital.[287] Head injuries occurred in 244 children (48%) and accounted for five of six deaths. Calvarial skull fractures occurred in 104 children and were associated with intraparenchymal, subdural, and epidural hematomas. [287] Extremity injuries were common as well. In another study, four statewide trauma and hospital databases were queried to obtain data on hospital visits by patients with ATV-related neurological injuries in Utah from 2001 to 2005. [96] Seven hundred forty-one patients with ATV-related head and spinal injuries were identified. Five hundred fifty-nine patients experienced head trauma, and 328 patients sustained spinal trauma. Vehicle rollover was the most common mechanism of injury (28.6%), followed by loss of control and separation of rider and vehicle (20.1%) and collisions with stationary objects (6.1%) or other vehicles (4.1%).[96] Other common mechanisms of injury include being thrown to the ground, striking a tree, and flipping backward.[269]

In most studies, helmet use is inconsistently documented or just not known; however, as would be expected, patients without helmets are more likely to have a head injury.[96, 269, 349] While people of all ages use snowmobiles and ATVs, adolescent riders tend to have more severe injuries and more head injuries than other age groups.[302] Another study profiled ATV crash victims with neurological injuries who were treated at a level I trauma center over 10 years; only 22% of all patients had been wearing helmets. [48] Interestingly, alcohol or drugs or both were involved in almost one-half of all incidents in that same study. Fifty-five of 238 patients sustained spinal axis injuries.[48]

Other studies have focused on describing some of the spinal injuries that can occur. In one report, spinal injury occurred in 7.4% of patients. [276] The most common level of fracture was thoracic (39%), followed by lumbar (29%) and cervical (16%).[276] Snowmobile- and ATV-related trauma is associated with a higher incidence of axial compression and burst-type fracture morphologies than in the general spinal cord injury population.[275]

Peripheral nerve injuries attributable to snowmobiling and ATV use are common. Brachial plexus injuries occur in 4.8% of snowmobile accident victims.[214] Severe injury with complete brachial plexopathy occurs in 67% of patients with brachial plexus injuries who have had snowmobile accidents.[38]

Soccer

Soccer originated more than 2,000 years ago in China, where the sport started with kicking a basic ball around. Modern football, otherwise called soccer, started in 1863 when the English Football Association was founded, and today the sport remains one of the most popular worldwide with over 200 million participants. While most soccer-related injuries are musculoskeletal, neurological injuries can occur, particularly concussion.

A 2-year study found the concussion rates in soccer to be 0.92 and 1.14 injuries per 100 player-seasons in high school men and women, respectively.[254] A separate study found that high school men and women playing soccer experienced a rate of 0.04 and 0.09 concussions per 1,000 athletic exposures, respectively, in practice, and 0.59 and 0.97 concussions per 1,000 athletic exposures, respectively, in games.[114] The rate of concussion in collegiate male and female soccer players has been reported as 0.28 and 0.41 per 1,000 athletic exposures.[135] In another study, college male soccer players experienced 0.24 and 1.38 concussions per 1,000 athletic exposures in practice and games, respectively.[114] In that same study, collegiate female soccer players experienced 0.25 and 2.8 concussions per 1,000 athletic exposures in practices and games, respectively.[114] Both men and women appear to be at a greater risk of suffering a concussion in games as opposed to practice.[261]

Concussions in both male and female soccer players typically occur as a result of head-to-head collisions sustained in the act of heading the ball (figure 1.5). In male soccer players, another common cause of concussions is contact with another person. Male goalies seem to be significantly more likely to experience a concussion than other players.[114] Women experience fewer concussions as a result of contact with another player; however, they sustain more concussions than men as a result of contact with the ground and contact with the ball.[114]

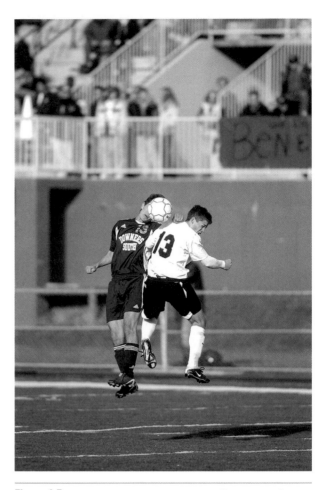

Figure 1.5 Concussion in soccer usually occurs during the act of heading the ball.

Surfing and Skimboarding

Compared with other sports, surfing is relatively safe. Contact with the surfboard, rocks, coral, or sand causes most injuries. Environmental factors such as sun exposure and marine animal bites and stings are other causes of injury.[232, 318] Various types of surfing injuries have been described in the medical literature, with lacerations and contusions occurring most commonly. Head injuries that can result from striking the surfboard represent the full spectrum of injury, from skull fractures and concussions to catastrophic brain injury and fatality. Spinal fractures and spinal cord injury are also possible. One study examined the relative frequency, pattern, and mechanisms of surfing injuries.[233] Fifty-five percent of injuries resulted from contact with one's own board, 12% with another surfer's board, and 17%

with the sea floor. Thirty-seven percent of acute injuries were to the head and neck. The authors identified seven cases of cervical spine fractures due to the surfer's head striking the ocean floor, three of which resulted in permanent neurological deficits and four of which resulted in thoracic spine fractures.

Surfer's myelopathy is a unique form of spinal cord injury associated with surfing.[6, 57, 154, 329] This relatively new condition is a nontraumatic myelopathy that was first described in 2004.[329] Fewer than 20 cases have been discussed in the literature since that time. The proposed mechanism of injury is an ischemic event to the watershed zones of the spinal cord and is thought to occur in surfers who, while paddling their board in a hyperextended position, perform a Valsalva maneuver while attempting to stand up on the boards. This is postulated to increase intraspinal pressure and bring about an ischemic myelopathy. Peripheral nerve injuries can occur as well. Prolonged surfing can result in repetitive microtrauma that can cause common peroneal or saphenous neuropathy in young surfers.[86, 357] Long-duration riding can lead to compression on the inner leg and stretching of the peroneal nerve due to prolonged leg abduction.

Skimboarding is another sport that has grown in popularity. As the maneuvers have become more "extreme" and technically difficult, the injury rates have been growing. There are two distinct styles of skimboarding. Both begin with the skimboarder's running and jumping on the moving board as it hydroplanes in the surf.[60] The skimboarder can either ride along the beach in the receding water or ride away from the beach into the oncoming waves. With the latter style, they can make a 180-degree turn and ride the wave back to shore or choose to incorporate aerial tricks such as jumps, flips, and twists once they hit the wave.[60] Injuries can occur with the sudden deceleration of the board as it transitions from water to land or with falls into shallow water. Studies have demonstrated that upper and lower extremity fractures are most common.[210, 284, 365] Certainly, though, the combination of high speed and height (especially with tricky maneuvers or jumps) increases the risk of significant injury from landing headfirst in shallow water with subsequent head or spinal cord injury.[60]

Volleyball

Volleyball originated in 1895 in Holyoke, Massachusetts, as a game termed Mintonette. It was developed by William G. Morgan, a YMCA physical education director, and later came to be known as volleyball. Overall, the sport is one of the safest competitive and recreational activities played by high school and collegiate athletes.[335] The rate of concussion in high school volleyball players has been reported as 0.14 per 100 player-seasons.[254] A 16-year study of collegiate volleyball players found a concussion rate of 0.09 per 1,000 athletic exposures.[135] An additional study reported that concussions accounted for 1.3% of all volleyball injuries reported during practices and 4.1% of injuries reported during games.[63]

Peripheral nerve injuries tend to occur frequently in volleyball players.[337] The most common form of peripheral nerve entrapment is an isolated entrapment of the suprascapular nerve related to the overhand motion of serving[81, 94, 176, 223, 243] (figure 1.6). This neuropathy typically occurs in the serving, or dominant, arm of the volleyball player. Isolated mononeuropathies of the axillary nerve have been reported in younger volleyball players as well.[244]

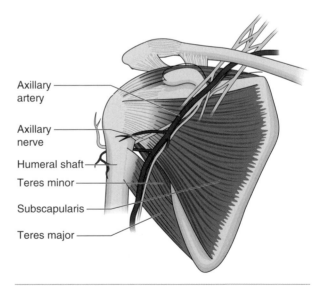

Figure 1.6 Peripheral nerve injuries are common in volleyball. Suprascapular nerve entrapment may be due to repetitive trauma from the repeated overhand loading with serving.

Wakeboarding and Water Skiing

Wakeboarding is a popular water sport but one that has significant potential for trauma due to the high velocities, rotational maneuvers, acceleratory forces, water obstacles, and general lack of protective equipment used. This surface water sport, involving riding a wakeboard over the surface of a body of water, was developed from a combination of water skiing, snowboarding, and surfing techniques. Riders are usually towed behind a motorboat, typically at speeds of 17 to 24 miles per hour (27-38 km/h); however, they can also be towed by other means, including closed-course cable systems, which have increased significantly in popularity worldwide as of late.[281]

The most common injuries reported are anterior cruciate ligament (ACL) tears, shoulder dislocations, contusions, fractures, and ankle sprains. [50] Head or neck trauma is a concern and may be even more common in wakeboarding than in other water sports, but the true trauma incidence is unknown and probably underreported. One study analyzed data on water skiing– and wakeboarding-related injuries presenting to 98 hospital emergency departments in the United States between 2001 and 2003.[137] Head injuries represented the largest percentage of injuries for wakeboarders (28.8% of all injuries) and the smallest percentage for water skiers (4.3%). Traumatic brain injury with intracranial hemorrhage has been reported to occur during wakeboarding as well.[55] Additionally, an unusual case of central nervous system injury occurred in a wakeboarder who developed a carotid artery dissection and stroke shortly following a wakeboarding accident. [104] Similarly, a carotid dissection was recently reported in an athlete who sustained a whiplash-type injury while water skiing.[364]

Wrestling

Wrestling is one of the oldest forms of recreational combat. The wide range of styles includes both traditional and more modern styles, with varying rules. Annually, there are approximately 239,000 male and 1,700 female high school wrestlers, as well as 6,700 male collegiate wrestlers.[225] This is an aggressive sport with a fairly high injury rate

considering the lower number of participants, particularly at the high school level. As seen in most other sports, the injury rate is higher during competition than during practice.

Concussions occur frequently in wrestling. The concussion rate in high school wrestling has been reported as 1.58 per 100 player-seasons. [254] A more recent survey of athletic trainers from the 2005 to 2006 season found that concussions occurred at a rate of 0.13 per 1,000 athletic exposures and 0.32 per 1,000 athletic exposures in practices and games, respectively. [114] That same study found that takedowns were the most common cause of concussion and were more likely than other wrestling maneuvers to lead to a concussion. Approximately 60% of the concussions occurred as a result of contact with another wrestler; the remainder occurred as a result of contact with the mat.[114] The rate of concussion in collegiate wrestlers has been reported at around 0.25 to 0.35 concussions per 1,000 athletic exposures.[114, 135] Another study found that concussions accounted for 6.6% of all injuries occurring during matches and 4.5% of those occurring during practice.[63]

An older survey of wrestling injuries showed that severe injuries can include cervical spinal fractures, spinal cord injury, cervical cord neurapraxia, severe closed head injury, and acute disc herniation with quadriplegia and that they rarely lead to death.[306] Severe injuries can result from head-to-head collisions during takedown attempts or slams to the mat. In a study of 63 patients who sustained cervical spinal injuries while participating in organized sporting events, wrestling accounted for the second highest number of injuries, preceded only by football.[7] Additionally, cases of chronic traumatic encephalopathy have been described in professional wrestlers, raising awareness about the potential for chronic neurodegenerative disease with repetitive head trauma in this sport.[108]

Brachial plexus injury occurs relatively commonly in wrestling compared with other sports; such injuries occur typically as a result of the grappling holds. Some reports have shown that burners or stingers account for 37% of all head and neck injuries in competitive wrestlers.[91, 337] Other forms of peripheral nerve injuries have been reported, albeit less frequently, including axillary neuropathy; ulnar neuropathy; and long thoracic, median, suprascapular, and spinal accessory nerve injuries.[59, 172]

CONCLUDING THOUGHTS

Injuries are obviously a common occurrence in sport and can result from acute trauma or from overuse of a particular body part. It is easy to appreciate that neurological injury can occur in just about any type of sport. Injuries to the brain, spine, and peripheral nerves can be devastating.

Sports medicine practitioners should familiarize themselves with the potential neurological injuries characteristic of each individual sport. While we have a good sense of the epidemiology underlying neurological injury in some sports, we are lacking data in others. Such data would highlight areas requiring increased focus. An understanding of the risks inherent in any sport would also allow for the development of injury prevention strategies and serve as a starting point for effective educational programs.

REFERENCES

1. AAP. Committee on injury and poison prevention: skateboard and scooter injuries. Pediatrics 2002;109(3):542-543.

2. Ackery A, Hagel BE, Provvidenza C, Tator CH. An international review of head and spinal cord injuries in alpine skiing and snowboarding. Inj Prev 2007;13(6):368-375.

3. Adams ID. Rugby football injuries. Br J Sports Med 1977;11(1):4-6.

4. Anakwenze OA, Namdari S, Auerbach JD, Baldwin K, Weidner ZD, Lonner BS, et al. Athletic performance outcomes following lumbar discectomy in professional basketball players. Spine (Phila Pa 1976) 2010;35(7):825-828.

5. Aulicino PL. Neurovascular injuries in the hands of athletes. Hand Clin 1990;6(3):455-466.

6. Aviles-Hernandez I, Garcia-Zozaya I, DeVillasante JM. Nontraumatic myelopathy associated with surfing. J Spinal Cord Med 2007;30(3):288-293.

7. Bailes JE, Hadley MN, Quigley MR, Sonntag VK, Cerullo LJ. Management of athletic injuries of the cervical spine and spinal cord. Neurosurgery 1991;29(4):491-497.

8. Bailes JE, Herman JM, Quigley MR, Cerullo LJ, Meyer PR Jr. Diving injuries of the cervical spine. Surg Neurol 1990;34(3):155-158.

9. Bailes JE, Maroon JC. Spinal cord injuries in athletes. N Y State J Med 1991;91(2):44-45.

10. Bailes JE, Petschauer M, Guskiewicz KM, Marano G. Management of cervical spine injuries in athletes. J Athl Train 2007;42(1):126-134.

11. Baird LC, Newman CB, Volk H, Svinth JR, Conklin J, Levy ML. Mortality resulting from head injury in professional boxing. Neurosurgery 2010;67(5):1444-1450; discussion 1450.

12. Balendra G, Turner M, McCrory P. Career-ending injuries to professional jockeys in British horse racing (1991-2005). Br J Sports Med 2008;42(1):22-24.

13. Bali K, Kumar V, Krishnan V, Meena D, Rawall S. Multiple lumbar transverse process stress fractures as a cause of chronic low back ache in a young fast bowler - a case report. Sports Med Arthrosc Rehabil Ther Technol 2011;3(1):8.

14. Ball CG, Ball JE, Kirkpatrick AW, Mulloy RH. Equestrian injuries: incidence, injury patterns, and risk factors for 10 years of major traumatic injuries. Am J Surg 2007;193(5):636-640.

15. Barrentine SW, Fleisig GS, Whiteside JA, Escamilla RF, Andrews JR. Biomechanics of windmill softball pitching with implications about injury mechanisms at the shoulder and elbow. J Orthop Sports Phys Ther 1998;28(6):405-415.

16. Batt ME. A survey of golf injuries in amateur golfers. Br J Sports Med 1992;26(1):63-65.

17. Bentley TA, Page SJ, Macky KA. Adventure tourism and adventure sports injury: the New Zealand experience. Appl Ergon 2007;38(6):791-796.

18. Berry JG, Harrison JE, Yeo JD, Cripps RA, Stephenson SC. Cervical spinal cord injury in rugby union and rugby league: are incidence rates declining in NSW? Aust N Z J Public Health 2006;30(3):268-274.

19. Bessen RJ, Belcher VW, Franklin RJ. Rucksack paralysis with and without rucksack frames. Mil Med 1987;152(7):372-375.

20. Bhide VM, Edmonds VE, Tator CH. Prevention of spinal cord injuries caused by diving: evaluation of the distribution and usage of a diving safety video in high schools. Inj Prev 2000;6(2):154-156.

21. Birrer RB. Trauma epidemiology in the martial arts. The results of an eighteen-year international survey. Am J Sports Med 1996;24(6 Suppl):S72-79.

22. Bixby-Hammett D, Brooks WH. Common injuries in horseback riding. A review. Sports Med 1990;9(1):36-47.

23. Bixby-Hammett DM. Accidents in equestrian sports. Am Fam Physician 1987;36(3):209-214.

24. Bixby-Hammett DM. Horse-related injuries and deaths in North Carolina, 1995-1999. N C Med J 2006;67(2):161-162.

25. Bixby-Hammett DM. Pediatric equestrian injuries. Pediatrics 1992;89(6 Pt 2):1173-1176.

26. Blanksby BA, Wearne FK, Elliott BC, Blitvich JD. Aetiology and occurrence of diving inju-

ries. A review of diving safety. Sports Med 1997;23(4):228-246.

27. Bleakley C, Tully M, O'Connor S. Epidemiology of adolescent rugby injuries: a systematic review. J Athl Train 2011;46(5):555-565.

28. Bledsoe GH, Hsu EB, Grabowski JG, Brill JD, Li G. Incidence of injury in professional mixed martial arts competitions. J Sports Sci Med 2006;5:136-142.

29. Blonstein JL, Clarke E. Further observations on the medical aspects of amateur boxing. Br Med J 1957;1(5015):362-364.

30. Blumenthal SL, Roach J, Herring JA. Lumbar Scheuermann's. A clinical series and classification. Spine (Phila Pa 1976) 1987;12(9):929-932.

31. Boden BP, Tacchetti R, Mueller FO. Catastrophic cheerleading injuries. Am J Sports Med 2003;31(6):881-888.

32. Boden BP, Tacchetti R, Mueller FO. Catastrophic injuries in high school and college baseball players. Am J Sports Med 2004;32(5):1189-1196.

33. Bohlmann T. Injuries in competitive cycling. Phys Sportmed 1981;9:118.

34. Bond GR, Christoph RA, Rodgers BM. Pediatric equestrian injuries: assessing the impact of helmet use. Pediatrics 1995;95(4):487-489.

35. Bowling A. Injuries to dancers: prevalence, treatment, and perceptions of causes. BMJ 1989;298(6675):731-734.

36. Braham R, Finch CF, McCrory P. The incidence of head/neck/orofacial injuries in non-elite Australian football. J Sci Med Sport 2004;7(4):451-453.

37. Braithwaite IJ. Bilateral median nerve palsy in a cyclist. Br J Sports Med 1992;26(1):27-28.

38. Braun BL, Meyers B, Dulebohn SC, Eyer SD. Severe brachial plexus injury as a result of snowmobiling: a case series. J Trauma 1998;44(4):726-730.

39. Bridges EJ, Rouah F, Johnston KM. Snowblading injuries in Eastern Canada. Br J Sports Med 2003;37(6):511-515.

40. Brown PG, Lee M. Trampoline injuries of the cervical spine. Pediatr Neurosurg 2000;32(4):170-175.

41. Brozin IH, Martfel J, Goldberg I, Kuritzky A. Traumatic closed femoral nerve neuropathy. J Trauma 1982;22(2):158-160.

42. Brundrett G. Sickness at high altitude: a literature review. J R Soc Promot Health 2002;122(1):14-20.

43. Burnham RS, Steadward RD. Upper extremity peripheral nerve entrapments among wheelchair athletes: prevalence, location, and risk factors. Arch Phys Med Rehabil 1994;75(5):519-524.

44. Buse GJ. No holds barred sport fighting: a 10 year review of mixed martial arts competition. Br J Sports Med 2006;40(2):169-172.

45. Butterwick DJ, Hagel B, Nelson DS, LeFave MR, Meeuwisse WH. Epidemiologic analysis of injury

in five years of Canadian professional rodeo. Am J Sports Med 2002;30(2):193-198.

46. Butterwick DJ, Meeuwisse WH. Effect of experience on rodeo injury. Clin J Sport Med 2002;12(1):30-35.

47. Cantu RC, Mueller FO. The prevention of catastrophic head and spine injuries in high school and college sports. Br J Sports Med 2009;43(13):981-986.

48. Carr AM, Bailes JE, Helmkamp JC, Rosen CL, Miele VJ. Neurological injury and death in all-terrain vehicle crashes in West Virginia: a 10-year retrospective review. Neurosurgery 2004;54(4):861-866; discussion 866-867.

49. Carrillo EH, Varnagy D, Bragg SM, Levy J, Riordan K. Traumatic injuries associated with horseback riding. Scand J Surg 2007;96(1):79-82.

50. Carson WG Jr. Wakeboarding injuries. Am J Sports Med 2004;32(1):164-173.

51. CDC. Centers for Disease Control and Prevention: Bicycle Related Injuries. 2009. Available from: http://www.cdc.gov/HomeandRecreationalSafety/Bicycle/index.html.

52. Chao S, Pacella MJ, Torg JS. The pathomechanics, pathophysiology and prevention of cervical spinal cord and brachial plexus injuries in athletics. Sports Med 2010;40(1):59-75.

53. Chapman MA, Oni J. Motor racing accidents at Brands Hatch, 1988/9. Br J Sports Med 1991;25(3):121-123.

54. Charakorn C, Amatyakul P. Hearing impairment in Thais due to sport shooting: a preliminary report. J Med Assoc Thai 1998;81(5):344-351.

55. Chia JK, Goh KY, Chan C. An unusual case of traumatic intracranial hemorrhage caused by wakeboarding. Pediatr Neurosurg 2000;32(6):291-294.

56. Cho D, Saetia K, Lee S, Kline DG, Kim DH. Peroneal nerve injury associated with sports-related knee injury. Neurosurg Focus 2011;31(5):E11.

57. Chung HY, Sun SF, Wang JL, Lai PH, Hwang CW. Non-traumatic anterior spinal cord infarction in a novice surfer: a case report. J Neurol Sci 2011;302(1-2):118-120.

58. Clarsen B, Krosshaug T, Bahr R. Overuse injuries in professional road cyclists. Am J Sports Med 2010;38(12):2494-2501.

59. Cohn BT, Brahms MA, Cohn M. Injury to the eleventh cranial nerve in a high school wrestler. Orthop Rev 1986;15(9):590-595.

60. Collier TR, Jones ML, Murray HH. Skimboarding: a new cause of water sport spinal cord injury. Spinal Cord 2010;48(4):349-351.

61. Collins CL, Micheli LJ, Yard EE, Comstock RD. Injuries sustained by high school rugby players in the United States, 2005-2006. Arch Pediatr Adolesc Med 2008;162(1):49-54.

62. Corkill G, Lieberman JS, Taylor RG. Pack palsy in backpackers. West J Med 1980;132(6):569-572.

63. Covassin T, Swanik CB, Sachs ML. Epidemiological considerations of concussions among intercollegiate athletes. Appl Neuropsychol 2003;10(1):12-22.

64. Crites BM, Moorman CT III, Hardaker WT Jr. Spine injuries associated with falls from hunting tree stands. J South Orthop Assoc 1998;7(4):241-245.

65. Crockett A, Stawicki SP, Thomas YM, Jarvis AM, Wang CF, Beery PR, et al. Tree stands, not guns, are the midwestern hunter's most dangerous weapon. Am Surg 2010;76(9):1006-1010.

66. Crockett HC, Wright JM, Madsen MW, Bates JE, Potter HG, Warren RF. Sacral stress fracture in an elite college basketball player after the use of a jumping machine. Am J Sports Med 1999;27(4):526-528.

67. Crowley PJ, Condon KC. Analysis of hurling and camogie injuries. Br J Sports Med 1989;23(3):183-185.

68. Cruz Martinez A, Arpa J. Carpal tunnel syndrome in childhood: study of 6 cases. Electroencephalogr Clin Neurophysiol 1998;109(4):304-308.

69. Cuddihy B, Hurley M. Contact sports and injury. Ir Med J 1990;83(3):98-100.

70. Cuenca AG, Wiggins A, Chen MK, Kays DW, Islam S, Beierle EA. Equestrian injuries in children. J Pediatr Surg 2009;44(1):148-150.

71. Cusimano MD, Mascarenhas AM, Manoranjan B. Spinal cord injuries due to diving: a framework and call for prevention. J Trauma 2008;65(5):1180-1185.

72. Daneshvar DH, Nowinski CJ, McKee AC, Cantu RC. The epidemiology of sport-related concussion. Clin Sports Med 2011;30(1):1-17, vii.

73. Datti R, Gentile SL, Pisani R. Acute intracranial epidural haematoma in a basketball player: a case report. Br J Sports Med 1995;29(2):95-96.

74. Daubinet G, Rodineau J. Paralysis of the suprascapular nerve and tennis. Apropos of 3 groups of professional players. Schweiz Z Sportmed 1991;39(3):113-118.

75. De Cauwer H, Van Giel R, Mortelmans L, van den Hauwe L. An uncommon cause of headache after headbanging at a party. Eur J Emerg Med 2009;16(4):212-213.

76. DeVivo MJ, Sekar P. Prevention of spinal cord injuries that occur in swimming pools. Spinal Cord 1997;35(8):509-515.

77. Diamond PT, Gale SD. Head injuries in men's and women's lacrosse: a 10 year analysis of the NEISS database. National Electronic Injury Surveillance System. Brain Inj 2001;15(6):537-544.

78. Dobyns JH, O'Brien ET, Linscheid RL, Farrow GM. Bowler's thumb: diagnosis and treatment. A review of seventeen cases. J Bone Joint Surg Am 1972;54(4):751-755.

79. Dodwell ER, Kwon BK, Hughes B, Koo D, Townson A, Aludino A, et al. Spinal column and spinal cord injuries in mountain bikers: a 13-year review. Am J Sports Med 2010;38(8):1647-1652.

80. Downey DJ. Rodeo injuries and prevention. Curr Sports Med Rep 2007;6(5):328-332.

81. Dramis A, Pimpalnerkar A. Suprascapular neuropathy in volleyball players. Acta Orthop Belg 2005;71(3):269-272.

82. Dunn RN, van der Spuy D. Rugby and cervical spine injuries - has anything changed? A 5-year review in the Western Cape. S Afr Med J 2010;100(4):235-238.

83. Eckert V, Lockemann U, Puschel K, Meenen NM, Hessler C. Equestrian injuries caused by horse kicks: first results of a prospective multicenter study. Clin J Sport Med 2011;21(4):353-355.

84. Emery CA, Hagel B, Decloe M, Carly M. Risk factors for injury and severe injury in youth ice hockey: a systematic review of the literature. Inj Prev 2010;16(2):113-118.

85. Emery CA, Meeuwisse WH. Injury rates, risk factors, and mechanisms of injury in minor hockey. Am J Sports Med 2006;34(12):1960-1969.

86. Fabian RH, Norcross KA, Hancock MB. Surfer's neuropathy. N Engl J Med 1987;316(9):555.

87. Fayed N, Modrego PJ, Morales H. Evidence of brain damage after high-altitude climbing by means of magnetic resonance imaging. Am J Med 2006;119(2):168 e161-166.

88. Fayssoux RS, Tally W, Sanfilippo JA, Stock G, Ratliff JK, Anderson G, et al. Spinal injuries after falls from hunting tree stands. Spine J 2008;8(3):522-528.

89. Federiuk CS, Schlueter JL, Adams AL. Skiing, snowboarding, and sledding injuries in a northwestern state. Wilderness Environ Med 2002;13(4):245-249.

90. Feiler S, Frank M. Pattern of injuries and risk of injury in skateboarding. Sportverletz Sportschaden 2000;14(2):59-64.

91. Feinberg JH. Burners and stingers. Phys Med Rehabil Clin N Am 2000;11(4):771-784.

92. Feinberg JH, Nadler SF, Krivickas LS. Peripheral nerve injuries in the athlete. Sports Med 1997;24(6):385-408.

93. Felsenthal G, Mondell DL, Reischer MA, Mack RH. Forearm pain secondary to compression syndrome of the lateral cutaneous nerve of the forearm. Arch Phys Med Rehabil 1984;65(3):139-141.

94. Ferretti A, Cerullo G, Russo G. Suprascapular neuropathy in volleyball players. J Bone Joint Surg Am 1987;69(2):260-263.

95. Finley MI, Pleket HW. The Olympic Games: The First Thousand Years. London: Chatto and Windus; 1976.

96. Finn MA, MacDonald JD. A population-based study of all-terrain vehicle-related head and spinal injuries. Neurosurgery 2010;67(4):993-997; discussion 997.

97. FIQ. Fédération Internationale des Quilleurs. Available from: www.fiq.org/index.php.

98. Fischbein A, Rice C, Sarkozi L, Kon SH, Petrocci M, Selikoff IJ. Exposure to lead in firing ranges. JAMA 1979;241(11):1141-1144.

99. Fischer R. Hazards of mountain climbing and hiking. MMW Fortschr Med 2005;147(38):28-30, 32.

100. Foray J, Abrassart S, Femmy T, Aldilli M. Hang-gliding accidents in high mountains. Apropos of 200 cases. Chirurgie 1991;117(8):613-617.

101. Forsmann L, Eriksson A. Skateboard injuries of today. Br J Sports Med 2001;35:325-328.

102. Foulke GE. Altitude-related illness. Am J Emerg Med 1985;3(3):217-226.

103. Fountain JL, Meyers MC. Skateboarding injuries. Sports Med 1996;22(6):360-366.

104. Fridley J, Mackey J, Hampton C, Duckworth E, Bershad E. Internal carotid artery dissection and stroke associated with wakeboarding. J Clin Neurosci 2011;18(9):1258-1260.

105. Frontera WR. Cyclist's palsy: clinical and electrodiagnostic findings. Br J Sports Med 1983;17(2):91-93.

106. Fuller CW, Brooks JH, Kemp SP. Spinal injuries in professional rugby union: a prospective cohort study. Clin J Sport Med 2007;17(1):10-16.

107. Furnival RA, Street KA, Schunk JE. Too many pediatric trampoline injuries. Pediatrics 1999;103(5):e57.

108. Garber G. Doctors: Wrestler had brain damage. ESPN. 2009. Available from: http://sports.espn.go.com/espn/otl/news/story?id=4724912.

109. Garrick JG, Requa RK. Ballet injuries. An analysis of epidemiology and financial outcome. Am J Sports Med 1993;21(4):586-590.

110. Gartland S, Malik MH, Lovell ME. Injury and injury rates in Muay Thai kick boxing. Br J Sports Med 2001;35(5):308-313.

111. Gates RL, Helmkamp JC, Wilson SL, Denning DA, Beaver BL. Deer stand-related trauma in West Virginia: 1994 through 1999. J Trauma 2002;53(4):705-708.

112. Genelin A, Kathrein A, Daniaux A, Lang T, Seykora P. Current status of spinal injuries in winter sports. Schweiz Z Med Traumatol 1994(1):17-20.

113. George PM, Walmsley TA, Currie D, Wells JE. Lead exposure during recreational use of small bore rifle ranges. N Z Med J 1993;106(965):422-424.

114. Gessel LM, Fields SK, Collins CL, Dick RW, Comstock RD. Concussions among United States high school and collegiate athletes. J Athl Train 2007;42(4):495-503.

115. Giuliani G, Poppi M, Acciarri N, Forti A. CT scan and surgical treatment of traumatic iliacus hematoma with femoral neuropathy: case report. J Trauma 1990;30(2):229-231.

116. Glazier PS. Is the "crunch factor" an important consideration in the aetiology of lumbar spine pathology in cricket fast bowlers? Sports Med 2010;40(10):809-815.

117. Goh SH, Tan HK, Yong WS, Low BY. Spectrum of roller-blading injuries. Ann Acad Med Singapore 1996;25(4):547-549.

118. Goldberg I, Peylan J, Amit S. Nerve injuries in bicycle riders. Harefuah 1991;121(5-6):159-161.

119. Goldberg MJ. Gymnastic injuries. Orthop Clin North Am 1980;11(4):717-726.

120. Goldberg RL, Hicks AM, O'Leary LM, London S. Lead exposure at uncovered outdoor firing ranges. J Occup Med 1991;33(6):718-719.

121. Goldenberg MS, Hossler PH. Head and facial injuries in interscholastic women's lacrosse. J Athl Train 1995;30(1):37-41.

122. Goodson JD. Brachial plexus injury from light tight backpack straps. N Engl J Med 1981;305(9):524-525.

123. Grange JT, Bodnar JA, Corbett SW. Motocross medicine. Curr Sports Med Rep 2009;8(3):125-130.

124. Grant T, Whipp JA. Injuries resulting from motorcycle desert racing. Am J Sports Med 1976;4(4):170-172.

125. Groves M. Ropes, Reins, and Rawhide: All About Rodeo. Albuquerque, NM. University of New Mexico Press; 2006:3-4.

126. Hackett PH, Yarnell PR, Hill R, Reynard K, Heit J, McCormick J. High-altitude cerebral edema evaluated with magnetic resonance imaging: clinical correlation and pathophysiology. JAMA 1998;280(22):1920-1925.

127. Hanbury PH. Bungy jumping. Aust N Z J Ophthalmol 1990;18(2):229.

128. Hanigan WC, Olivero WC, Duffy JJ, Peterson R. Lawn dart injury in children: report of two cases. Pediatr Emerg Care 1986;2(4):247-249.

129. Harries M. The ups and down of bungee jumping. BMJ 1992;305(6868):1520.

130. Hashimoto K, Oda K, Kuroda Y, Shibasaki H. Case of suprascapular nerve palsy manifesting as selective atrophy of the infraspinatus muscle in an archery player. Rinsho Shinkeigaku 1983;23(11):970-973.

131. Havlik HS. Equestrian sport-related injuries: a review of current literature. Curr Sports Med Rep 2010;9(5):299-302.

132. Health-Canada. Requirements of the Hazardous Products Act and Controlled Products Regulations: SOR/2001-270. Canada. 2001. Available from: www.hc-sc.gc.ca/ewh-semt/alt_formats/hecs-sesc/pdf/pubs/occup-travail/ref_man/hpa_schedule-annexes_lpd-eng.pdf.

133. Hentschel S, Hader W, Boyd M. Head injuries in skiers and snowboarders in British Columbia. Can J Neurol Sci 2001;28(1):42-46.

134. Hite PR, Greene KA, Levy DI, Jackimczyk K. Injuries resulting from bungee-cord jumping. Ann Emerg Med 1993;22(6):1060-1063.

135. Hootman JM, Dick R, Agel J. Epidemiology of collegiate injuries for 15 sports: summary and recommendations for injury prevention initiatives. J Athl Train 2007;42(2):311-319.

136. Horner CH, O'Brien AA. Motorcycle racing injuries on track and road circuits in Ireland. Br J Sports Med 1986;20(4):157-158.

137. Hostetler SG, Hostetler TL, Smith GA, Xiang H. Characteristics of water skiing-related and wakeboarding-related injuries treated in emergency departments in the United States, 2001-2003. Am J Sports Med 2005;33(7):1065-1070.

138. Houshian S, Herold N, Rock ND. Roller skating injuries. Ugeskr Laeger 1997;159(23):3580-3582.

139. Hoyt CS. Letter: Ulnar neuropathy in bicycle riders. Arch Neurol 1976;33(5):372.

140. Hsu JC, Paletta GA Jr, Gambardella RA, Jobe FW. Musculocutaneous nerve injury in major league baseball pitchers: a report of 2 cases. Am J Sports Med 2007;35(6):1003-1006.

141. Hsu WK, McCarthy KJ, Savage JW, Roberts DW, Roc GC, Micev AJ, et al. The Professional Athlete Spine Initiative: outcomes after lumbar disc herniation in 342 elite professional athletes. Spine J 2011;11(3):180-186.

142. Hultgren HN. High altitude medical problems. West J Med 1979;131(1):8-23.

143. Hunter RE. Skiing injuries. Am J Sports Med 1999;27(3):381-389.

144. Hurson C, Browne K, Callender O, O'Donnell T, O'Neill A, Moore DP, et al. Pediatric trampoline injuries. J Pediatr Orthop 2007;27(7):729-732.

145. Illingworth CM. BMX compared with ordinary bicycle accidents. Arch Dis Child 1985;60(5):461-464.

146. Janda DH, Hankin FM, Wojtys EM. Softball injuries: cost, cause and prevention. Am Fam Physician 1986;33(6):143-144.

147. Jareno A, de la Serna JL, Cercas A, Lobato A, Uya A. Heat stroke in motor car racing drivers. Br J Sports Med 1987;21(1):48.

148. Jayarao M, Chin LS, Cantu RC. Boxing-related head injuries. Phys Sportsmed 2010;38(3):18-26.

149. Johnson RJ. Anatomy of backpack-strap injury. N Engl J Med 1981;305(26):1594.

150. Jordan BD. Brain injury in boxing. Clin Sports Med 2009;28(4):561-578, vi.

151. Jordan BD, Campbell EH. Acute boxing injuries among professional boxers in New York State: a two year survey. Phys Sportmed 1988;12:53-67.

152. Juel VC, Kiely JM, Leone KV, Morgan RF, Smith T, Phillips LH II. Isolated musculocutaneous neuropathy caused by a proximal humeral exostosis. Neurology 2000;54(2):494-496.

153. Kameyama O, Shibano K, Kawakita H, Ogawa R, Kumamoto M. Medical check of competitive canoeists. J Orthop Sci 1999;4(4):243-249.

154. Karabegovic A, Strachan-Jackman S, Carr D. Surfer's myelopathy: case report and review. CJEM 2011;13(5):357-360.

155. Karas SE. Thoracic outlet syndrome. Clin Sports Med 1990;9(2):297-310.

156. Karlson K. Rowing injuries. Phys Sportmed 2000;28:40-50.

157. Kasow DB, Curl WW. "Stingers" in adolescent athletes. Instr Course Lect 2006;55:711-716.

158. Kassirer MR, Manon N. Head banger's whiplash. Clin J Pain 1993;9(2):138-141.

159. Keilani M, Krall C, Lipowec L, Posch M, Komanadj TS, Crevenna R. Skateboarding injuries in Vienna: location, frequency, and severity. PM R 2010;2(7):619-624.

160. Keller TM, Holland MC. Chronic subdural haematoma, an unusual injury from playing basketball. Br J Sports Med 1998;32(4):338-339.

161. Kelly MD. Traumatic neuralgia from pressure-point strikes in the martial arts: results from a retrospective online survey. J Am Osteopath Assoc 2008;108(6):284-287.

162. Kerr ZY, Collins CL, Comstock RD. Epidemiology of bowling-related injuries presenting to US emergency departments, 1990-2008. Clin Pediatr (Phila) 2011;50(8):738-746.

163. Kim S, Endres NK, Johnson RJ, Ettlinger CF, Shealy JE. Snowboarding injuries: trends over time and comparisons with alpine skiing injuries. Am J Sports Med 2012.

164. Kisner WH. Thumb neuroma: a hazard of ten pin bowling. Br J Plast Surg 1976;29(3):225-226.

165. Kitagawa T, Kimura S, Ogata H. Fatigue fracture. Seikei Geka 1966;17(7):564-566.

166. Knapik JJ, Reynolds KL, Harman E. Soldier load carriage: historical, physiological, biomechanical, and medical aspects. Mil Med 2004;169(1):45-56.

167. Knox CL, Comstock RD, McGeehan J, Smith GA. Differences in the risk associated with head injury for pediatric ice skaters, roller skaters, and in-line skaters. Pediatrics 2006;118(2):549-554.

168. Kochhar T, Back DL, Mann B, Skinner J. Risk of cervical injuries in mixed martial arts. Br J Sports Med 2005;39(7):444-447.

169. Konkin DE, Garraway N, Hameed SM, Brown DR, Granger R, Wheeler S, et al. Population-based analysis of severe injuries from nonmotorized wheeled vehicles. Am J Surg 2006;191(5):615-618.

170. Kriss TC, Kriss VM. Equine-related neurosurgical trauma: a prospective series of 30 patients. J Trauma 1997;43(1):97-99.

171. Krivickas LS, Wilbourn AJ. Peripheral nerve injuries in athletes: a case series of over 200 injuries. Semin Neurol 2000;20(2):225-232.

172. Krivickas LS, Wilbourn AJ. Sports and peripheral nerve injuries: report of 190 injuries evaluated in a single electromyography laboratory. Muscle Nerve 1998;21(8):1092-1094.

173. Kronisch RL, Chow TK, Simon LM, Wong PF. Acute injuries in off-road bicycle racing. Am J Sports Med 1996;24(1):88-93.

174. Kuschner SH, Lane CS. Recurrent fracture of the humerus in a softball player. Am J Orthop (Belle Mead NJ) 1999;28(11):654-656.

175. Kyle SB, Nance ML, Rutherford GW Jr, Winston FK. Skateboard-associated injuries: participation-based estimates and injury characteristics. J Trauma 2002;53(4):686-690.

176. Lajtai G, Pfirrmann CW, Aitzetmuller G, Pirkl C, Gerber C, Jost B. The shoulders of professional beach volleyball players: high prevalence of infraspinatus muscle atrophy. Am J Sports Med 2009;37(7):1375-1383.

177. Landrigan PJ, McKinney AS, Hopkins LC, Rhodes WW Jr, Price WA, Cox DH. Chronic lead absorption. Result of poor ventilation in an indoor pistol range. JAMA 1975;234(4):394-397.

178. Langburt W, Cohen B, Akhthar N, O'Neill K, Lee JC. Incidence of concussion in high school football players of Ohio and Pennsylvania. J Child Neurol 2001;16(2):83-85.

179. Larson AN, Stans AA, Shaughnessy WJ, Dekutoski MB, Quinn MJ, McIntosh AL. Motocross morbidity: economic cost and injury distribution in children. J Pediatr Orthop 2009;29(8):847-850.

180. Lautenschlager S, Karli U, Matter P. Paragliding accidents—a prospective analysis in Swiss mountain regions. Z Unfallchir Versicherungsmed 1993;Suppl 1:55-65.

181. Leary T, White JA. Acute injury incidence in professional county club cricket players (1985-1995). Br J Sports Med 2000;34(2):145-147.

182. Lemire JJ, Mierau DR, Crawford CM, Dzus AK. Scheuermann's juvenile kyphosis. J Manipulative Physiol Ther 1996;19(3):195-201.

183. Leonard H, Joffe AR. Children presenting to a Canadian hospital with trampoline-related cervical spine injuries. Paediatr Child Health 2009;14(2):84-88.

184. Levy AS, Hawkes AP, Hemminger LM, Knight S. An analysis of head injuries among skiers and snowboarders. J Trauma 2002;53(4):695-704.

185. Lin CY, Wright J, Bushnik T, Shem K. Traumatic spinal cord injuries in horseback riding: a 35-year review. Am J Sports Med 2011;39(11):2441-2446.

186. Loder RT. The demographics of equestrian-related injuries in the United States: injury patterns, orthopedic specific injuries, and avenues for injury prevention. J Trauma 2008;65(2):447-460.

187. Lohmann M, Petersen AO, Pedersen OD. Skateboard and rollerskate accidents. Ugeskr Laeger 1990;152(22):1591-1593.

188. Long G, Thompson TM, Storm B, Graham J. Cranial impalement in a child driving an all-terrain vehicle. Pediatr Emerg Care 2011;27(5):409-410.

189. Long RR, Sargent JC, Pappas AM, Hammer K. Pitcher's arm: an electrodiagnostic enigma. Muscle Nerve 1996;19(10):1276-1281.

190. Lorei MP, Hershman EB. Peripheral nerve injuries in athletes. Treatment and prevention. Sports Med 1993;16(2):130-147.

191. Louw D, Reddy KK, Lauryssen C, Louw G. Pitfalls of bungee jumping. Case report and review of the literature. J Neurosurg 1998;89(6):1040-1042.

192. MacDonald PB, Strange G, Hodgkinson R, Dyck M. Injuries to the peroneal nerve in professional hockey. Clin J Sport Med 2002;12(1):39-40.

193. Macgregor DM. Golf related head injuries in children. Emerg Med J 2002;19(6):576-577.

194. Mangano FT, Menendez JA, Smyth MD, Leonard JR, Narayan P, Park TS. Pediatric neurosurgical injuries associated with all-terrain vehicle accidents: a 10-year experience at St. Louis Children's Hospital. J Neurosurg 2006;105(1 Suppl):2-5.

195. Mansingh A, Harper L, Headley S, King-Mowatt J, Mansingh G. Injuries in West Indies cricket 2003-2004. Br J Sports Med 2006;40(2):119-123; discussion 119-123.

196. Matejka J, Zeman J, Belatka J, Nepras P, Houcek P, Linhart M. Seat-belt and chance fractures of the thoracolumbar spine. Zentralbl Chir 2010;135(2):149-153.

197. Mauch F, Bauer G. Traumatic dislocation of long fingers at the metacarpophalangeal joint while bowling—case report of an extremely rare injury. Sportverletz Sportschaden 1999;13(3):76-78.

198. McCarroll JR, Gioe TJ. Professional golfers and the price they pay. Phys Sportsmed 1982;10(7):64-70.

199. McCarroll JR, Retting AC, Shelbourne KD. Injuries in the amateur golfer. Phys Sportsmed 1990;18(3):122-126.

200. McCrory P. Sports concussion and the risk of chronic neurological impairment. Clin J Sport Med 2011;21(1):6-12.

201. McCrory P, Meeuwisse W, Johnston K, Dvorak J, Aubry M, Molloy M, et al. Consensus statement on concussion in sport: the 3rd International Conference on Concussion in Sport held in Zurich, November 2008. J Athl Train 2009;44(4):434-448.

202. McCrory PR, Berkovic SF, Cordner SM. Deaths due to brain injury among footballers in Victoria, 1968-1999. Med J Aust 2000;172(5):217-219.

203. Mcgrath C. A Chinese hinterland, fertile with field hockey. New York Times. August 23, 2008;Sect. D1.

204. McHardy A, Pollard H, Luo K. Golf injuries: a review of the literature. Sports Med 2006;36(2):171-187.

205. McIntosh AS, McCrory P, Finch CF, Wolfe R. Head, face and neck injury in youth rugby: incidence and risk factors. Br J Sports Med 2010;44(3):188-193.

206. McKee AC, Cantu RC, Nowinski CJ, Hedley-Whyte ET, Gavett BE, Budson AE, et al. Chronic traumatic encephalopathy in athletes: progressive tauopathy after repetitive head injury. J Neuropathol Exp Neurol 2009;68(7):709-735.

207. McNally E, Wilson D, Seiler S. Rowing injuries. Semin Musculoskelet Radiol 2005;9(4):379-396.

208. McNeil SL, Spruill WA, Langley RL, Shuping JR, Leonard JR III. Multiple subdural hematomas associated with breakdancing. Ann Emerg Med 1987;16(1):114-116.

209. Meeuwisse WH, Sellmer R, Hagel BE. Rates and risks of injury during intercollegiate basketball. Am J Sports Med 2003;31(3):379-385.

210. Merriman D, Carmichael K, Battle SC. Skimboard injuries. J Trauma 2008;65(2):487-490.

211. Metz M, Kross M, Abt P, Bankey P, Koniaris LG. Tree stand falls: a persistent cause of sports injury. South Med J 2004;97(8):715-719.

212. Meyers MC, Elledge JR, Sterling JC, Tolson H. Injuries in intercollegiate rodeo athletes. Am J Sports Med 1990;18(1):87-91.

213. Micheli LJ, Hall JE, Miller ME. Use of modified Boston brace for back injuries in athletes. Am J Sports Med 1980;8(5):351-356.

214. Midha R. Epidemiology of brachial plexus injuries in a multitrauma population. Neurosurgery 1997;40(6):1182-1188; discussion 1188-1189.

215. Miele VJ, Bailes JE. Objectifying when to halt a boxing match: a video analysis of fatalities. Neurosurgery 2007;60(2):307-315; discussion 315-306.

216. Miele VJ, Bailes JE, Cantu RC, Rabb CH. Subdural hematomas in boxing: the spectrum of consequences. Neurosurg Focus 2006;21(4):E10.

217. Miele VJ, Bailes JE, Voelker JL. Boxing and the neurosurgeon. Clin Neurosurg 2002;49:396-406.

218. Milan KR. Injury in ballet: a review of relevant topics for the physical therapist. J Orthop Sports Phys Ther 1994;19(2):121-129.

219. Miller EH, Benedict FE. Stretch of the femoral nerve in a dancer. A case report. J Bone Joint Surg Am 1985;67(2):315-317.

220. Millesi-Eberhard D, Konig B, Millesi H. Compression syndromes of the axillary nerve and the suprascapular nerve. Handchir Mikrochir Plast Chir 1999;31(5):311-316.

221. Minaire P, Demolin P, Bourret J, Girard R, Berard E, Deidier C, et al. Life expectancy following spinal cord injury: a ten-years survey in the Rhone-Alpes region, France, 1969-1980. Paraplegia 1983;21(1):11-15.

222. Minoyama O, Tsuchida H. Injuries in professional motor car racing drivers at a racing circuit between 1996 and 2000. Br J Sports Med 2004;38(5):613-616.

223. Montagna P, Colonna S. Suprascapular neuropathy restricted to the infraspinatus muscle in volleyball players. Acta Neurol Scand 1993;87(3):248-250.

224. Mueller BA, Cummings P, Rivara FP, Brooks MA, Terasaki RD. Injuries of the head, face, and neck in relation to ski helmet use. Epidemiology 2008;19(2):270-276.

225. Mueller FO, Cantu RC. Catastrophic Sport Injury Research Annual Report (2008). Chapel Hill, NC: National Center for Catastrophic Injury Research; 2008. Available from: www.unc.edu/depts/nccsi/AllSport.pdf.

226. Mueller FO, Cantu RC. Catastrophic Sport Injury Research Annual Report (2010). Chapel Hill, NC: National Center for Catastrophic Injury Research; 2010.

227. Mueller FO, Colgate B. Annual Survey of Football Injury Research (2011 Report). Chapel Hill, NC: National Center for Catastrophic Injury Research; 2012. Available from: www.unc.edu/depts/nccsi/2011FBAnnual.pdf.

228. Mundt DJ, Kelsey JL, Golden AL, Panjabi MM, Pastides H, Berg AT, et al. An epidemiologic study of sports and weight lifting as possible risk factors for herniated lumbar and cervical discs. The Northeast Collaborative Group on Low Back Pain. Am J Sports Med 1993;21(6):854-860.

229. Murphy JC, Gissane C, Blake C. Injury in elite county-level hurling: a prospective study. Br J Sports Med 2012;46(2):138-142.

230. Myles ST, Mohtadi NG, Schnittker J. Injuries to the nervous system and spine in downhill skiing. Can J Surg 1992;35(6):643-648.

231. Nakaguchi H, Fujimaki T, Ueki K, Takahashi M, Yoshida H, Kirino T. Snowboard head injury: prospective study in Chino, Nagano, for two seasons from 1995 to 1997. J Trauma 1999;46(6):1066-1069.

232. Nathanson A, Bird S, Dao L, Tam-Sing K. Competitive surfing injuries: a prospective study of surfing-related injuries among contest surfers. Am J Sports Med 2007;35(1):113-117.

233. Nathanson A, Haynes P, Galanis D. Surfing injuries. Am J Emerg Med 2002;20(3):155-160.

234. NBTA. National Basketball Trainers' Association: Injury Reporting System. New York: National Basketball Association; 1991.

235. Nelson DE, Bixby-Hammett D. Equestrian injuries in children and young adults. Am J Dis Child 1992;146(5):611-614.

236. Ngai KM, Levy F, Hsu EB. Injury trends in sanctioned mixed martial arts competition: a 5-year review from 2002 to 2007. Br J Sports Med 2008;42(8):686-689.

237. Noguchi T. A survey of spinal cord injuries resulting from sport. Paraplegia 1994;32(3):170-173.

238. Novotny T, Cook M, Hughes J, Lee SA. Lead exposure in a firing range. Am J Public Health 1987;77(9):1225-1226.

239. NSCISC. 2010 NSCISC Annual Statistical Report. Birmingham, AL: NSCISC; 2010.

240. Nysted M, Drogset JO. Trampoline injuries. Br J Sports Med 2006;40(12):984-987.

241. Omalu B, Bailes J, Hamilton RL, Kamboh MI, Hammers J, Case M, et al. Emerging histomorphologic phenotypes of chronic traumatic encephalopathy in American athletes. Neurosurgery 2011;69(1):173-183; discussion 183.

242. Orchard JW, James T, Portus MR. Injuries to elite male cricketers in Australia over a 10-year period. J Sci Med Sport 2006;9(6):459-467.

243. Ozer D, Baltaci G, Leblebicioglu G. Rehabilitation and shoulder function after suprascapular nerve entrapment operation in a volleyball player. Arch Orthop Trauma Surg 2007;127(9):759-761.

244. Paladini D, Dellantonio R, Cinti A, Angeleri F. Axillary neuropathy in volleyball players: report of two cases and literature review. J Neurol Neurosurg Psychiatry 1996;60(3):345-347.

245. Pasternack JS, Veenema KR, Callahan CM. Baseball injuries: a Little League survey. Pediatrics 1996;98(3 Pt 1):445-448.

246. Patton D, McIntosh A. Head and neck injury risks in heavy metal: head bangers stuck between rock and a hard bass. BMJ 2008;337:a2825.

247. Perlmutter GS, Apruzzese W. Axillary nerve injuries in contact sports: recommendations for treatment and rehabilitation. Sports Med 1998;26(5):351-361.

248. Perlmutter GS, Leffert RD, Zarins B. Direct injury to the axillary nerve in athletes playing contact sports. Am J Sports Med 1997;25(1):65-68.

249. Perrin AE. Rowing injuries. Conn Med 2010;74(8):481-484.

250. Pieter W, Zemper ED. Incidence of reported cerebral concussion in adult taekwondo athletes. J R Soc Promot Health 1998;118(5):272-279.

251. Pieter W, Zemper ED. Injury rates in children participating in taekwondo competition. J Trauma 1997;43(1):89-95; discussion 95-86.

252. Poliakoff M. Combat Sports in the Ancient World: Competition, Violence, and Culture. New Haven, CT: Yale University Press; 1995.

253. Potter MR, Snyder AJ, Smith GA. Boxing injuries presenting to U.S. emergency departments, 1990-2008. Am J Prev Med 2011;40(4):462-467.

254. Powell JW, Barber-Foss KD. Traumatic brain injury in high school athletes. JAMA 1999;282(10):958-963.

255. Price C, Mallonee S. Hunting-related spinal cord injuries among Oklahoma residents. J Okla State Med Assoc 1994;87(6):270-273.

256. Prochaska V, Crosby LA, Murphy RP. High radial nerve palsy in a tennis player. Orthop Rev 1993;22(1):90-92.

257. Quarrie KL, Cantu RC, Chalmers DJ. Rugby union injuries to the cervical spine and spinal cord. Sports Med 2002;32(10):633-653.

258. Rainey CE. Determining the prevalence and assessing the severity of injuries in mixed martial arts athletes. N Am J Sports Phys Ther 2009;4(4):190-199.

259. Rayan GM. Archery-related injuries of the hand, forearm, and elbow. South Med J 1992;85(10):961-964.

260. RCC. Royal Canoe Club. Available from: www.royalcanoeclub.com/.

261. Rechel JA, Yard EE, Comstock RD. An epidemiologic comparison of high school sports injuries sustained in practice and competition. J Athl Train 2008;43(2):197-204.

262. Reishus AD. Injuries and illnesses of big game hunters in western Colorado: a 9-year analysis. Wilderness Environ Med 2007;18(1):20-25.

263. Rethnam U, Yesupalan RS, Sinha A. Skateboards: are they really perilous? a retrospective study from a district hospital. BMC Res Notes 2008;1:59.

264. Rimel R, Nelson W, Persing J. Epidural hematoma in lacrosse. Phys Sportmed 1983;11:140-144.

265. Rivara FP, Thompson DC, Thompson RS, Rebolledo V. Injuries involving off-road cycling. J Fam Pract 1997;44(5):481-485.

266. Roe JP, Taylor TK, Edmunds IA, Cumming RG, Ruff SJ, Plunkett-Cole MD, et al. Spinal and spinal cord injuries in horse riding: the New South Wales experience 1976-1996. ANZ J Surg 2003;73(5):331-334.

267. Romeo AA, Rotenberg DD, Bach BR Jr. Suprascapular neuropathy. J Am Acad Orthop Surg 1999;7(6):358-367.

268. Rumball JS, Lebrun CM, Di Ciacca SR, Orlando K. Rowing injuries. Sports Med 2005;35(6):537-555.

269. Russell A, Boop FA, Cherny WB, Ligon BL. Neurologic injuries associated with all-terrain vehicles and recommendations for protective measures for the pediatric population. Pediatr Emerg Care 1998;14(1):31-35.

270. Sammarco GJ. Dance medicine. Foot Ankle 1982;3(2):63-64.

271. Sammarco GJ, Miller EH. Forefoot conditions in dancers: part I. Foot Ankle 1982;3(2):85-92.

272. Sammarco GJ, Miller EH. Forefoot conditions in dancers: part II. Foot Ankle 1982;3(2):93-98.

273. Sammarco GJ, Stephens MM. Neurapraxia of the femoral nerve in a modern dancer. Am J Sports Med 1991;19(4):413-414.

274. Sandler G, Nguyen L, Lam L, Manglick MP, Soundappan SS, Holland AJ. Trampoline trauma in children: is it preventable? Pediatr Emerg Care 2011;27(11):1052-1056.

275. Sanfilippo JA, Winegar CD, Harrop JS, Albert TJ, Vaccaro AR. All-terrain vehicles and associated spinal injuries. Spine (Phila Pa 1976) 2008;33(18):1982-1985.

276. Sawyer JR, Bernard MS, Schroeder RJ, Kelly DM, Warner WC Jr. Trends in all-terrain vehicle-related

spinal injuries in children and adolescents. J Pediatr Orthop 2011;31(6):623-627.

277. Schalamon J, Sarkola T, Nietosvaara Y. Injuries in children associated with the use of nonmotorized scooters. J Pediatr Surg 2003;38(11):1612-1615.

278. Scher AT. Rugby injuries to the cervical spine and spinal cord: a 10-year review. Clin Sports Med 1998;17(1):195-206.

279. Schieber RA, Branche-Dorsey CM, Ryan GW, Rutherford GW Jr, Stevens JA, O'Neil J. Risk factors for injuries from in-line skating and the effectiveness of safety gear. N Engl J Med 1996;335(22):1630-1635.

280. Schmitt H, Gerner HJ. Paralysis from sport and diving accidents. Clin J Sport Med 2001;11(1):17-22.

281. Schofer MD, Hrabal SA, Timmesfeld N, Fuchs-Winkelmann S, Patzer T. Cable wakeboarding, a new trendy sport: analysis of injuries with regard to injury prevention. Scand J Med Sci Sports 2010.

282. Schommer K, Bartsch P. Basic medical advice for travelers to high altitudes. Dtsch Arztebl Int 2011;108(49):839-848.

283. Schulz MR, Marshall SW, Yang J, Mueller FO, Weaver NL, Bowling JM. A prospective cohort study of injury incidence and risk factors in North Carolina high school competitive cheerleaders. Am J Sports Med 2004;32(2):396-405.

284. Sciarretta KH, McKenna MJ, Riccio AI. Orthopaedic injuries associated with skimboarding. Am J Sports Med 2009;37(7):1425-1428.

285. Scoggin JF III, Brusovanik G, Pi M, Izuka B, Pang P, Tokumura S, et al. Assessment of injuries sustained in mixed martial arts competition. Am J Orthop (Belle Mead NJ) 2010;39(5):247-251.

286. Seidenberg PH. Mixed martial arts: injury patterns and issues for the ringside physician. Curr Sports Med Rep 2011;10(3):147-150.

287. Shah CC, Ramakrishnaiah RH, Bhutta ST, Parnell-Beasley DN, Greenberg BS. Imaging findings in 512 children following all-terrain vehicle injuries. Pediatr Radiol 2009;39(7):677-684.

288. Shapiro MJ, Marts B, Berni A, Keegan MJ. The perils of bungee jumping. J Emerg Med 1995;13(5):629-631.

289. Shephard RJ. Science and medicine of canoeing and kayaking. Sports Med 1987;4(1):19-33.

290. Shevell MI, Stewart JD. Laceration of the common peroneal nerve by a skate blade. CMAJ 1988;139(4):311-312.

291. Shields BJ, Fernandez SA, Smith GA. Epidemiology of cheerleading stunt-related injuries in the United States. J Athl Train 2009;44(6):586-594.

292. Shields BJ, Smith GA. Cheerleading-related injuries in the United States: a prospective surveillance study. J Athl Train 2009;44(6):567-577.

293. Shields BJ, Smith GA. Epidemiology of cheerleading fall-related injuries in the United States. J Athl Train 2009;44(6):578-585.

294. Shields BJ, Smith GA. Epidemiology of strain/sprain injuries among cheerleaders in the United States. Am J Emerg Med 2011;29(9):1003-1012.

295. Shields RW Jr, Jacobs IB. Median palmar digital neuropathy in a cheerleader. Arch Phys Med Rehabil 1986;67(11):824-826.

296. Shimizu J, Nishiyama K, Takeda K, Ichiba T, Sakuta M. A case of long thoracic nerve palsy, with winged scapula, as a result of prolonged exertion on practicing archery. Rinsho Shinkeigaku 1990;30(8):873-876.

297. Showalter MF, Flemming DH, Bernard SA. MRI manifestations of bowler's thumb. Radiol Case Rep 2011;6(1).

298. Silver JR, Silver DD, Godfrey JJ. Trampolining injuries of the spine. Injury 1986;17(2):117-124.

299. SimplyLacrosse. Who Invented Lacrosse. 2011. Available from: www.simplylacrosse.com/who-invented-lacrosse.html.

300. Singh S, Smith GA, Fields SK, McKenzie LB. Gymnastics-related injuries to children treated in emergency departments in the United States, 1990-2005. Pediatrics 2008;121(4):e954-960.

301. Sinson G, Zager EL, Kline DG. Windmill pitcher's radial neuropathy. Neurosurgery 1994;34(6):1087-1089; discussion 1089-1090.

302. Smith LM, Pittman MA, Marr AB, Swan K, Singh S, Akin SJ, et al. Unsafe at any age: a retrospective review of all-terrain vehicle injuries in two level I trauma centers from 1995 to 2003. J Trauma 2005;58(4):783-788.

303. Smith LO. Alpine climbing: injuries and illness. Phys Med Rehabil Clin N Am 2006;17(3):633-644.

304. Smoljanovic T, Bojanic I, Hannafin JA, Hren D, Delimar D, Pecina M. Traumatic and overuse injuries among international elite junior rowers. Am J Sports Med 2009;37(6):1193-1199.

305. Snook GA. The history of sports medicine. Part I. Am J Sports Med 1984;12(4):252-254.

306. Snook GA. A survey of wrestling injuries. Am J Sports Med 1980;8(6):450-453.

307. Soler T, Calderon C. The prevalence of spondylolysis in the Spanish elite athlete. Am J Sports Med 2000;28(1):57-62.

308. Sorensen BF. Bow hunter's stroke. Neurosurgery 1978;2(3):259-261.

309. Sotiropoulos SV, Jackson MA, Tremblay GF, Burry VF, Olson LC. Childhood lawn dart injuries. Summary of 75 patients and patient report. Am J Dis Child 1990;144(9):980-982.

310. Standaert CJ, Schofferman JA, Herring SA. Expert opinion and controversies in musculoskeletal and sports medicine: conflict of interest. Arch Phys Med Rehabil 2009;90(10):1647-1651.

311. Starkey C. Injuries and illnesses in the national basketball association: a 10-year perspective. J Athl Train 2000;35(2):161-167.

312. Steele AG. Emergency medical care for open wheel racing events at Indianapolis Raceway Park. Ann Emerg Med 1994;24(2):264-268.

313. Stern RA, Riley DO, Daneshvar DH, Nowinski CJ, Cantu RC, McKee AC. Long-term consequences of repetitive brain trauma: chronic traumatic encephalopathy. PM R 2011;3(10 Suppl 2):S460-467.

314. Streib E. Upper arm radial nerve palsy after muscular effort: report of three cases. Neurology 1992;42(8):1632-1634.

315. Stretch RA. Cricket injuries: a longitudinal study of the nature of injuries to South African cricketers. Br J Sports Med 2003;37(3):250-253; discussion 253.

316. Strukel RJ, Garrick JG. Thoracic outlet compression in athletes: a report of four cases. Am J Sports Med 1978;6(2):35-39.

317. Sukeik M, Haddad FS. Trampolining injuries. Br J Hosp Med (Lond) 2011;72(1):23-25.

318. Sunshine S. Surfing injuries. Curr Sports Med Rep 2003;2(3):136-141.

319. Svensson BG, Schutz A, Nilsson A, Skerfving S. Lead exposure in indoor firing ranges. Int Arch Occup Environ Health 1992;64(4):219-221.

320. Svinth JR. Death under the stoplight: The Manuel Velazquez boxing fatality collection. Journal of Combative Sport [serial on the Internet]. 2007. Available from: http://ejmas.com/jcs/jcsart_svinth_a_0700.htm.

321. Sward L. The thoracolumbar spine in young elite athletes. Current concepts on the effects of physical training. Sports Med 1992;13(5):357-364.

322. Tarazi F, Dvorak MF, Wing PC. Spinal injuries in skiers and snowboarders. Am J Sports Med 1999;27(2):177-180.

323. Tator CH, Carson JD, Cushman R. Hockey injuries of the spine in Canada, 1966-1996. CMAJ 2000;162(6):787-788.

324. Tator CH, Carson JD, Edmonds VE. New spinal injuries in hockey. Clin J Sport Med 1997;7(1):17-21.

325. Tay JS, Garland JS. Serious head injuries from lawn darts. Pediatrics 1987;79(2):261-263.

326. Tennent TD, Chambler AF, Rossouw DJ. Posterior dislocation of the hip while playing basketball. Br J Sports Med 1998;32(4):342-343.

327. Thepyasuwan N, Wan XT, Davis VJ. All-terrain vehicle injuries at Arrowhead Regional Medical Center (Level II): epidemiology, risks, and outcome. Am Surg 2009;75(10):1004-1008.

328. Thomassen O, Skaiaa SC. High-altitude cerebral edema with absence of headache. Wilderness Environ Med 2007;18(1):45-47.

329. Thompson TP, Pearce J, Chang G, Madamba J. Surfer's myelopathy. Spine (Phila Pa 1976) 2004;29(16):E353-356.

330. Tomida Y, Hirata H, Fukuda A, Tsujii M, Kato K, Fujisawa K, et al. Injuries in elite motorcycle racing in Japan. Br J Sports Med 2005;39(8):508-511.

331. Tongue JR. Hang gliding injuries in California. J Trauma 1977;17(12):898-902.

332. Torg JS, Corcoran TA, Thibault LE, Pavlov H, Sennett BJ, Naranja RJ Jr, et al. Cervical cord neurapraxia: classification, pathomechanics, morbidity, and management guidelines. J Neurosurg 1997;87(6):843-850.

333. Torjussen J, Bahr R. Injuries among competitive snowboarders at the national elite level. Am J Sports Med 2005;33(3):370-377.

334. Torre PR, Williams GG, Blackwell T, Davis CP. Bungee jumper's foot drop peroneal nerve palsy caused by bungee cord jumping. Ann Emerg Med 1993;22(11):1766-1767.

335. Toth C. The epidemiology of injuries to the nervous system resulting from sport and recreation. Neurol Clin 2008;26(1):1-31, vii.

336. Toth C, McNeil S, Feasby T. Central nervous system injuries in sport and recreation: a systematic review. Sports Med 2005;35(8):685-715.

337. Toth C, McNeil S, Feasby T. Peripheral nervous system injuries in sport and recreation: a systematic review. Sports Med 2005;35(8):717-738.

338. Trammell TR, Olvey SE, Reed DB. Championship car racing accidents and injuries. Phys Sportsmed 1986;14:114-120.

339. Tsirikos A, Papagelopoulos PJ, Giannakopoulos PN, Boscainos PJ, Zoubos AB, Kasseta M, et al. Degenerative spondyloarthropathy of the cervical and lumbar spine in jockeys. Orthopedics 2001;24(6):561-564.

340. Tsur A, Shahin R. Suprascapular nerve entrapment in a basketball player. Harefuah 1997;133(5-6):190-192, 247.

341. Tudor RB. Acute subdural hematoma following a blow from a basketball. Am J Sports Med 1979;7(2):136.

342. Tung MY, Hong A, Chan C. Golf buggy related head injuries. Singapore Med J 2000;41(10):504-505.

343. Tuominen R. Injuries in national karate competitions in Finland. Scand J Med Sci Sports 1995;5(1):44-48.

344. U.S. CPSC. Following Recent Injury CPSC Reissues Warning: Lawn Darts Are Banned and Should Be Destroyed. Washington, DC: U.S. Consumer Product Safety Commission; 1997. Available from: www.cpsc.gov/CPSCPUB/PREREL/PRHTML97/97122.html.

345. U.S. CPSC. National Electronic Injury Surveillance System (NEISS) 2009 Data Highlights. 2009. Available from: www.cpsc.gov/neiss/2009highlights.pdf.

346. Urquhart CK, Hawkins ML, Howdieshell TR, Mansberger AR Jr. Deer stands: a significant

cause of injury and mortality. South Med J 1991;84(6):686-688.

347. Varley GW, Spencer-Jones R, Thomas P, Andrews D, Green AD, Stevens DB. Injury patterns in motorcycle road racers: experience on the Isle of Man 1989-1991. Injury 1993;24(7):443-446.

348. Vates GE, Wang KC, Bonovich D, Dowd CF, Lawton MT. Bow hunter stroke caused by cervical disc herniation. Case report. J Neurosurg 2002;96(1 Suppl):90-93.

349. Vegeler RC, Young WF. All-terrain vehicle accidents at a level II trauma center in Indiana: an 8-year retrospective review. Int Surg 2009;94(1):84-87.

350. Veisten K, Saelensminde K, Alvaer K, Bjornskau T, Elvik R, Schistad T, et al. Total costs of bicycle injuries in Norway: correcting injury figures and indicating data needs. Accid Anal Prev 2007;39(6):1162-1169.

351. Viegas SF, Torres FG. Cherry pitter's thumb. Case report and review of the literature. Orthop Rev 1989;18(3):336-338.

352. Volski R, Bourguignon G, Rodriguez H. Lower spine screening in the shooting sports. Phys Sportmed 1986;14:101-106.

353. Wakahara K, Matsumoto K, Sumi H, Sumi Y, Shimizu K. Traumatic spinal cord injuries from snowboarding. Am J Sports Med 2006;34(10):1670-1674.

354. Walker HL, Carr DJ, Chalmers DJ, Wilson CA. Injury to recreational and professional cricket players: circumstances, type and potential for intervention. Accid Anal Prev 2010;42(6):2094-2098.

355. Walsh M. Preventing injury in competitive canoeists. Phys Sportmed 1985;13:120-128.

356. Wang HK, Chen HJ, Lu K, Liliang PC, Liang CL, Tsai YD, et al. A pediatric chronic subdural hematoma after dodgeball head injury. Pediatr Emerg Care 2010;26(9):667-668.

357. Watemberg N, Amsel S, Sadeh M, Lerman-Sagie T. Common peroneal neuropathy due to surfing. J Child Neurol 2000;15(6):420-421.

358. Watson AW. Sports injuries in the game of hurling. A one-year prospective study. Am J Sports Med 1996;24(3):323-328.

359. Weaver CS, Sloan BK, Brizendine EJ, Bock H. An analysis of maximum vehicle G forces and brain injury in motorsports crashes. Med Sci Sports Exerc 2006;38(2):246-249.

360. Weiss BD. Bicycle-related head injuries. Clin Sports Med 1994;13(1):99-112.

361. Weiss BD. Nontraumatic injuries in amateur long distance bicyclists. Am J Sports Med 1985;13(3):187-192.

362. Wilber CA, Holland GJ, Madison RE, Loy SF. An epidemiological analysis of overuse injuries among recreational cyclists. Int J Sports Med 1995;16(3):201-206.

363. Wilks J, Jones D. Golf-related injuries seen at hospital emergency departments. Aust J Sci Med Sport 1996;28(2):43-45.

364. Willett GM, Wachholtz NA. A patient with internal carotid artery dissection. Phys Ther 2011;91(8):1266-1274.

365. Williams MR, Poulter RJ, Fern ED. Skimboarding: a new danger in the surf? Emerg Med J 2006;23(2):137.

366. Wilson F, Gissane C, Gormley J, Simms C. A 12-month prospective cohort study of injury in international rowers. Br J Sports Med 2010;44(3):207-214.

367. Windsor JS, Firth PG, Grocott MP, Rodway GW, Montgomery HE. Mountain mortality: a review of deaths that occur during recreational activities in the mountains. Postgrad Med J 2009;85(1004):316-321.

368. Woodhead AB III. Paralysis of the serratus anterior in a world class marksman. A case study. Am J Sports Med 1985;13(5):359-362.

369. Wootton M, Harris D. Trampolining injuries presenting to a children's emergency department. Emerg Med J 2009;26(10):728-731.

370. Worrell J. BMX bicycles: accident comparison with other models. Arch Emerg Med 1985;2(4):209-213.

371. Xiang H, Kelleher K, Shields BJ, Brown KJ, Smith GA. Skiing- and snowboarding-related injuries treated in U.S. emergency departments, 2002. J Trauma 2005;58(1):112-118.

372. Yamakawa H, Murase S, Sakai H, Iwama T, Katada M, Niikawa S, et al. Spinal injuries in snowboarders: risk of jumping as an integral part of snowboarding. J Trauma 2001;50(6):1101-1105.

373. Yard EE, Comstock RD. Injuries sustained by pediatric ice hockey, lacrosse, and field hockey athletes presenting to United States emergency departments, 1990-2003. J Athl Train 2006;41(4):441-449.

374. Zazryn T, Cameron P, McCrory P. A prospective cohort study of injury in amateur and professional boxing. Br J Sports Med 2006;40(8):670-674.

375. Zazryn TR, Finch CF, McCrory P. A 16 year study of injuries to professional boxers in the state of Victoria, Australia. Br J Sports Med 2003;37(4):321-324.

376. Zazryn TR, Finch CF, McCrory P. A 16 year study of injuries to professional kickboxers in the state of Victoria, Australia. Br J Sports Med 2003;37(5):448-451.

377. Zhou W, Huynh TT, Kougias P, El Sayed HF, Lin PH. Traumatic carotid artery dissection caused by bungee jumping. J Vasc Surg 2007;46(5):1044-1046.

Medicolegal Considerations in Neurological Sports Medicine

In collaboration with
Robert P. Fitzsimmons, Esq. • Clayton J. Fitzsimmons, Esq.

In 1999, Pittsburgh Steelers Hall of Famer Mike Webster filed a disability claim with the National Football League (NFL) alleging that he was totally and permanently disabled as a result of repetitive brain trauma, concussions, and subconcussive blows he received over the course of his 17-year NFL playing career. A PhD psychologist and four doctors, including a hand-picked neurologist retained by the NFL, unanimously found that Mike Webster was totally and permanently disabled from football-related head trauma. The NFL's pension board granted total and permanent disability for football-related head trauma but denied that it had existed at the time of Webster's retirement. Webster appealed the pension board's decision to the U.S. District Court of Maryland (Baltimore), which reversed the NFL's ruling. That ruling was subsequently affirmed on appeal in 2006 by the U.S. Court of Appeals for the 4th Circuit.[1] Sadly, "Iron" Mike Webster died in 2002 and was never able to fully enjoy his victory over the NFL.

Mike Webster's battle with the NFL and his life story after football garnered significant publicity and propelled the issue of concussions and closed head injuries to the forefront of the sporting and medical worlds. After Webster's death, a brilliant forensic pathologist and neuropathologist, Bennet Omalu, MD, examined and autopsied Mike Webster's brain and discovered the condi-tion of chronic traumatic encephalopathy (CTE). Chronic traumatic encephalopathy is a progressive degenerative disease, diagnosed postmortem,[2] in individuals with a history of concussive and subconcussive impacts. Subsequent deaths (many of which were suicides) of star athletes, such as Chris Henry and Chris Benoit, together with numerous other NFL players, National Hockey League players, boxers, and high school and college athletes, further heightened the attention surrounding concussions in contact sports. Because of this increased awareness, the public is more informed today about the dangers of concussions, which for many years were significantly underappreciated and undertreated.

WITH INCREASED AWARENESS COMES INCREASED SCRUTINY

The risk of traumatic brain injury and concussions is inherent in all contact sports. This is especially true for children and adolescents, who have an increased risk of neurological injury with greater morbidity and mortality. According to the National Center for Sports Safety, 62% of sport injuries occur during practice, and 3.5 million children under the age of 14 receive medical treatment each year as a result of injuries sustained during sporting or recreational activities.[3]

Additionally, the Centers for Disease Control and Prevention estimates that as many as 3,900,000 sport-related and recreation-related concussions occur in the United States every year.[4] Undoubtedly, football is the most visible and publicized contact sport with the highest rate of concussions, but concussions also frequently occur in basketball, soccer, hockey, lacrosse, rugby, wrestling, and bull riding. In fact, any sport or activity in which an individual can contact an opposing player or a hard surface, such as a floor, goalpost, or backboard, is considered a contact sport.

Concussions and head injuries have always existed in contact sports, but society has not given proper deference to their serious consequences until recently. As a result of this increased attention, individuals and entities overseeing and supervising contact sports will be subjected to closer scrutiny and will be expected to use and implement standards of care that are more expansive and stringent. Team doctors, trainers, and subsequent treatment personnel need to be fully acquainted with preparticipation testing, eligibility, on-field evaluations, treatment, and return-to-play standards.

From a neurological standpoint, this chapter attempts to provide a legal overview of the laws and principles that govern the conduct of individuals who are responsible for athletes exposed to potential neurological injuries from sporting activities. Because of recent and emerging research on concussions and their dire consequences, concussions are used as the basic injury in this chapter for purposes of illustration and explanation. The principles in this chapter are equally applicable to all neurological injuries, including all forms of trauma to the brain or spinal cord.

THE KING OF CONCUSSIONS

Mike Webster's lawsuit and Dr. Omalu's discovery of CTE are credited with energizing the present movement to strengthen the diagnosis of concussions, require proper treatment for those affected by head injuries, and fully inform participants about the risks of permanent brain damage associated with concussions and closed head injuries. Although Mike Webster was the first person actually diagnosed with CTE (also referred to as Mike Webster's disease), he was by no means the first person to suffer from the effects of multiple concussions or head trauma.

King Henry VIII is one of the most well-known figures in world history. In addition to being considered an intellectual, Henry VIII was an accomplished musician, author, and poet who also enjoyed one of the most extreme contact sports of all time—jousting. For those unfamiliar with it, two riders charge horses directly at each other; the horsemen are armed with long wooden lances (9-14 feet long [2.7-4.3 meters]) and equipped with metal chest armor and a helmet called a helm. Contact is so severe that even the horses wear head shields. The object of the match is to drive the lance into the torso or head of the opponent to unhorse him. Such contact often results in serious injuries, including concussions, and death.

During the course of his jousting career, King Henry VIII sustained at least two suspected severe concussions.[5] In 1524, Henry was struck with an opponent's lance above his right eye, after which he constantly and regularly complained of serious headaches. On January 24, 1536, while engaged in a jousting tournament at Greenwich Palace, King Henry VIII was knocked off his horse, which then fell on him, thereby rendering him unconscious for a reported 2 hours.

According to some accounts, King Henry VIII suffered from personality changes, obesity (to the extent that he had to be moved by mechanical means), and anger problems. He also reportedly experienced psychological difficulties. The king had six wives, most of whom he had executed and one of whom he declared was the product of witchcraft. King Henry's abnormal behavior is perhaps best captured by John Denham's poem "Cooper's Hill," which asks, "Tell me (my muse) what monstrous dire offence, what crime could any Christian King [Henry] incense, to such a rage?" There is a strong probability that these psychological issues were caused, at least in part, by the multiple head traumas sustained in the jousting arenas.[6]

NEGLIGENCE

The essence of negligence is conduct that creates unreasonable danger to others.[7] Negligence claims arise from one's conduct, that is, an act or a failure to act. In order to prove liability for negligence, the law requires a claimant to prove all four of the following elements by a preponderance of evidence, that is, "more probably than not"[8] or 51% vs. 49%:

1. A duty, or obligation, recognized by the law, requiring the person to conform to a certain standard of conduct, for the protection of others against unreasonable risk
2. A breach of the duty by failing to conform to the standard of care
3. Proximate cause, that is, the breach of duty must have caused or contributed to the damage or injury
4. Actual loss or damage[9]

The entire concept of negligence is based on a uniform standard of behavior. It is impossible to affix a specific standard that fits all scenarios because of the multitude of situations encountered in life. The law, therefore, uses an objective standard to judge all conduct that is equally applicable to all persons. This standard is called the reasonable person standard and is the standard under which all negligence claims are evaluated.[10] According to the reasonable person standard, each person has a duty to behave as a reasonable person would under the same or similar circumstances.[11] Thus, this standard is flexible enough to cover any individual or class of individuals. This fictional "reasonable person" is aptly described by the following quote: "This excellent but odious character stands like a monument in our courts of justice, vainly appealing to his fellow citizens to order their lives after his own example."[12]

DUTY AND BREACH

The initial inquiry in all negligence cases is whether the defendant owed a legal duty of care to protect the plaintiff.[13] A legal duty is "an obligation, to which the law will give recognition and effect, to conform to a particular standard of conduct toward another."[14] The duty is defined by the nature of the relationship itself (e.g., doctor–patient; coach–player; trainer–player; team doctor–player–patients) together with the conduct of the individual(s).

Generally, a legal duty is created in one of two ways. First, as a basic principle of tort law,

every person has a legal duty to exercise reasonable care to avoid physical harm to others.[15] The scope of this duty is limited by the foreseeability of the resulting harm. "The ultimate test of the existence of a duty to use care is found in the foreseeability that harm may result if it is not exercised. The test is, would the ordinary man in the defendant's position, knowing what he knew or should have known, anticipate that the harm of the general nature of that suffered was likely to result."[16] No person is expected to protect against harm from events that one cannot reasonably anticipate or foresee or that are so unlikely to occur that the risk, although recognizable, would commonly be disregarded.[17]

Additionally, a legal duty may be created by a statute or case law, which may exist separate and apart from, or in place of, the duty to exercise reasonable care.

Once it is determined that a duty of care exists, a defendant may be liable only if she breached this duty by an act or omission that exposed others to an unreasonable risk of harm.[18] This requires a claimant to demonstrate that the defendant acted unreasonably under the circumstances.[19] What is unreasonable is a very fact-specific inquiry and requires a balancing of the risks and benefits of the conduct.[20] Typically an analysis is undertaken to compare the "magnitude of the risk" versus the "utility of the conduct."[21]

Hypothetically, you are the team doctor of King Henry's jousting team, the Canterbury Knights. You are asked to determine the king's medical eligibility for an upcoming match against the Tudor Dragons, in which Henry will be pitted against Richard the Lionheart. Whether paid or not, you would clearly owe a duty of care to the members of the team, which would include, at a minimum, conducting a full physical, together with a detailed medical history with specific questions relating to concussions. That would be the duty owed by you to Henry. If you failed to perform this duty, you would likely be executed or, in today's legal system, be found to have breached your duty and therefore be found negligent.

VIOLATION OF STATUTORY DUTY

Anyone associated with sporting activities should be familiar with all state laws that regulate the activity, if any, as well as all laws regulating the profession, job, or skill being performed. These laws may establish, in whole or in part, a standard of care applicable to your conduct.[22] If it can be shown that the state law was meant to protect the safety of individuals, like athletes in contact sports, and that the law was intended to regulate the specific conduct under scrutiny, a violation of this law will result in a finding that you were "per se" negligent (presumptively negligent or negligent as a matter of law).[23]

Approximately 49 states have now passed concussion legislation following the lead of the State of Washington.[24] Generally these laws require athletes to be removed from play if they are **suspected** of having suffered a concussion; require athletes to obtain written medical authorization before returning to physical activity; and require some form of concussion education, typically for coaches, parents, and athletes.

Assume that the City of Canterbury has enacted a concussion law similar to the ones discussed here. The coach of the Canterbury Knights is told that King Henry got his "bell rung" during the last joust. Upon inquiry, Henry admits to being dazed but claims that he is fine now and wants to ride again in order to win the last jousting match for the team. The coach has no discretion and must follow Canterbury's concussion law. If he does not, he will be found "per se" negligent.

STANDARD OF CARE DEFINED BY EXPERTS

The reasonable person standard is the minimum standard by which a person will be judged. However, if the potential defendant has knowledge or skill superior to that of the ordinary person, the law adjusts the standard and requires that the reasonable person be one within the same profession or with the same skill set as the defendant.[25]

In litigation, an expert of the same or a similar profession or skill set will often be permitted to render an opinion as to what the applicable standard of care is in the same or similar circumstances and whether the person on trial breached that standard. An expert does not testify as to what he would have done, but rather as to what a reasonable and competent person (coach, trainer, team doctor, and so on) would have done under the same or similar circumstances. Thus,

experienced or trained team doctors, subsequent caretakers, athletic directors, coaches, or trainers will be judged by the reasonable person standard of a person in the same or a similar profession or skill set that is revealed through the testimony of an expert witness.[26]

Before being allowed to render any such opinions, however, the expert must first be determined to be truly qualified, which will be based on her knowledge, education, training, and experience. In order for an expert's testimony to be admissible at trial, it must further satisfy certain rules of evidence, case authority, or both, which generally require the following:

- The expert is qualified by knowledge, skill, experience, training, or education.
- The expert's scientific, technical, or other specialized knowledge will help the jury or finder of fact to understand the evidence.
- The testimony is based on sufficient facts or data.
- The testimony is the product of reliable principles and methods.
- The expert has reliably applied principles and methods to the facts.[27]

The requirement that an expert's principles and methods be reliable was designed to disqualify opinions based on junk science. This standard is commonly referred to as the Daubert rule (named after the case that established the law).[28] If an expert's testimony is based on an assertion or inference derived from scientific methodology, there must first be an assessment as to (a) whether the scientific theory or conclusion has been tested, (b) whether it has been subjected to peer review and publication, (c) whether its rate of error is known, and (d) whether it is generally accepted within the scientific community.[28]

For example, the Daubert rule may be used to disqualify a proposed expert who claims he conducted personal noncontrolled impact studies in a courtyard where he had lanced the heads of 10 knights riding horses and none sustained a concussion. Standing alone, such a study would probably fail every criteria of Daubert and therefore be inadmissible at trial.

The strength or weakness of an expert generally hinges on the effectiveness or ineffectiveness of cross-examination by opposing counsel and the established expertise of the expert. This is critical because the success or failure of a professional or medical negligence claim is largely affected by the testimony of each side's expert witness.

STANDARD OF CARE ESTABLISHED THROUGH LITERATURE, RULES, PROTOCOLS, AND TEXTBOOKS

As previously discussed, experts are frequently called upon to render opinions on duty (standard of care), breach, causation, and past and future damages in cases involving serious injuries from a sport-related accident. During the course of an expert's direct examination or on cross-examination, the questioner (or interrogator as this person is referred to by some experts) may reference a statement, passage, or chart contained in a treatise, periodical, journal, or pamphlet. If permitted by the court, the statement may be used to impeach an opposing expert (or defendant). Before this occurs, however, the treatise, journal, or pamphlet must first be shown to be reliably authoritative. This can be established by the witness's acknowledgement of reliability or by another expert's testimony that the document is reliably authoritative. If the statement or passage is admitted into evidence, it can be used as substantive proof of the standard of care.[29] The benefit of this type of evidence is that the opinions expressed by the author in the treatise, journal, or pamphlet are allowed into evidence without being subjected to cross-examination, and the party using the written statement gains the benefit of an additional expert opinion.

You are the team physician for the Canterbury Knights, accused of negligently allowing King Henry to return to jousting following a concussion. The facts reveal that 7 days ago, Henry sustained a concussion, which caused severe headaches for 5 days. On the seventh day post-concussion, Henry tells you that he feels much better and that the headaches have been only mild over the last 2 days. He wants to joust today and, despite no testing, you give Henry the green light. At the match, Henry is struck in the head and receives a second major concussion within 7 days.

At trial, your expert, Dr. Butts, a graduate of King's College of Medicine, comes to save the day and testifies that your decision to let Henry joust was within the applicable standard of care because the headaches had improved and there was no need for neuropsych testing. Henry's attorney, Cromwell, confronts your expert with a 5-year study of jousting concussions published in the peer-reviewed *Journal of Oxford Brain Surgeries* (JOBS). The authors of the article studied 300 jousting concussions and concluded that "following a concussion, a knight should never be permitted to return to jousting if any symptoms remain, including mild headaches, and until proper neuropsych testing has been performed." This type of impeachment can be devastating to your expert's credibility, and it aligns the entire study and its authors against you and your expert. What do you do besides pray? Instruct your attorney to settle the case.

In addition to learned treatises and articles, numerous organizations publish policies, procedures, and protocols that can also come into play in negligence claims. For example, the American Academy of Family Physicians collaborated with multiple organizations and put together several team physician consensus statements. These statements are an obvious source of quality information and guidance and provide information on such topics as concussion and the team physician,[30] sideline preparedness,[31] and return-to-play issues.[32]

Each consensus statement advises the reader on the first page that "[it] is not intended as a standard of care and should not be interpreted as such." However, few lawyers or juries will buy in to such a disclaimer. Not to pick on the AAFP, but aren't these statements ones that the AAFP feels are representative of what a qualified, competent team physician should do in these circumstances? Of course they are. Furthermore, the existence of the multiple disclaimers probably has the exact opposite effect of their intended purpose by bringing attention to the standards and highlighting them as the applicable standards of care. Juries are smart and would see such disclaimers as a blatant attempt to avoid obvious responsibility. After all, the word "consensus" means "the judgment arrived at by most of those concerned," that is, reasonable team physicians! A good cross-examiner would feast upon such statements.

Other publications by professional or trade organizations that are relevant to the subject matter may help establish the standard of care governing your conduct and the way you practice your profession. A must-read for any team physician is the article "Heads Up: Concussions in High School Sports."[33] Athletic trainers should also familiarize themselves with the position statement of the National Athletic Trainers' Association, "Preventing Sudden Death in Sports."[34]

GOOD SAMARITAN LAWS

When there is no duty to go to the assistance of a person in peril or danger, there is at least a duty to avoid any affirmative act that would make the person's situation worse.[35] This general principle of law discourages persons from voluntarily rendering aid in times of need. Over the years, medical groups have lobbied to change this harsh rule and have been successful. In most states, there are now laws that absolve a doctor who gratuitously renders aid in an emergency from all liability for negligence. These types of laws are commonly referred to as the "Good Samaritan Law." However, these laws do not immunize a health care provider if her conduct was beyond negligent and was willful, wanton, or reckless.[36] Many state laws have extended the immunity provided under the Good Samaritan Law to other professions rendering emergency aid. All providers of care should check the law in their individual state to determine whether rendering emergency aid could potentially subject them to liability.

PROXIMATE CAUSE

In addition to proving that the defendant breached a duty of care owed to the plaintiff, the claimant must also demonstrate that his injuries and damages were a proximate cause of the negligent act. "Proximate cause" is a legal term that means there must be some reasonable connection between the act of negligence and the damages that the plaintiff claims.[37] Many courts today define proximate cause in terms of whether the negligent conduct "caused or contributed to" the injury and damages. There may be more than one proximate cause for an injury, which means that two or more negligent acts may each

be a proximate cause of an injury. A limitation to proximate cause is that the injury resulting from the negligent conduct must be foreseeable.[38]

With regard to King Henry, it was certainly foreseeable that he could sustain a second major concussion within a few days that would cause him to suffer permanent neurological damage. Thus, if you were the team doctor for the Canterbury Knights who permitted Henry to joust on the seventh day postconcussion and he sustained permanent neurological damage, your negligent act would be a proximate cause of Henry's injuries and damages.

ASSUMPTION OF THE RISK

Because contact sports involve some risk of injury, a discussion about the defense of assumption of the risk is appropriate. "Assumption of the risk" generally means that a potential claimant has given her express or implied consent to the risk of injuries inherent in a particular activity before engaging in said activity.[39] In such circumstances, the plaintiff is held to have assumed the risk and is therefore prohibited from any recovery for negligence. For example, in **Higgins v. Pfeiffer**, the plaintiff was an amateur baseball player who was struck in the eye by a baseball thrown by a teammate during warm-ups.[40] The Higgins court held that the injury sustained by the player was within the scope of his consent implicit in the game and attendant circumstances and therefore that the teammate, catcher, and coach were not liable.[41] In reaching its decision, the Higgins court stated, "Participants in sporting activity are assumed to be aware of hazards inherent in the playing of the game and have consented to the risk of injury inherent in the contest, other than breaches of contest rules designed to protect safety of the players as opposed to integrity of the contest."[42]

Importantly, the doctrine or defense is limited to known, inherent risks and would typically not serve as a bar to a claim for injuries from unsportsmanlike conduct, which is not within the scope of the game's rules with the possible exception of hockey.[43] Additionally, it must be shown that the injured individual recognized and understood the particular risk or danger involved and voluntarily chose to encounter it.[44] In the context of concussions, the dangers and risks associated with multiple concussions were not fully appreciated until recently, which makes it an issue whether a player could knowingly and voluntarily assume the risk of concussions. This defense will likely play an instrumental part in any future NFL or National Collegiate Athletic Association (NCAA) player's lawsuits, as discussed later in this chapter.

THEORIES OF NEGLIGENCE

Many different theories of negligence have arisen over the years in litigation concerning injuries sustained during contact sports. These theories are limited only by the innovative thought processes of skilled attorneys. Nonetheless, final judgment is always decided by our judiciary, which is charged with ensuring compliance with the law. Although the system is not perfect (none are), our civil justice system allows theories regulated by rules of procedure and evidence to be subjected to a judgment by our peers with constant judicial oversight. An additional safeguard is provided through appellate review.

The following negligence claims frequently appear in sports-related injury cases:

- Failure to properly train
- Failure to be properly credentialed
- Inadequate supervision[45]
- Failure to properly observe, refer, or stabilize the injured player
- Unequal matching of opponents (boxing)
- Improper return to play[46, 47]
- Improper equipment or fitting
- Improper screening or physicals
- Failure to warn of risks
- Failure to enact proper rules for concussions or return to play
- Failure to stop or curtail risky or violent conduct
- Medical malpractice[48]
- Negligent hiring or retention of personnel
- Improper design or maintenance of playing field or premises
- Failure to have an emergency medical plan[49]
- Improper medical clearance[50]

This list of claims is not meant to be all-inclusive, but rather sets forth various examples of claims that have been made in recent years. Irrespective of the type of claim, there must always be evidence sufficient to support a finding of each of the four elements of negligence, that is, duty, breach, causation, and damages.

Product liability cases stand alone in a separate category. These claims are typically filed against the manufacturer or distributor of the equipment, alleging that the product was defective in design or manufacture or that the manufacturer failed to warn of known dangers with the use of the product. Some product cases may also include an allegation that the product was unsafe for its intended purpose.[51] An example of a products liability claim is **Daniels v. Rawlings Sporting Goods Company, Inc.,**[52] wherein a high school football player sustained permanent brain damage when his helmet "caved in" during a collision with another player. The injured player brought a products liability and negligence claim against the helmet manufacturer. The jury found that the helmet was defectively manufactured and that the manufacturer had a duty to warn that the helmet would not protect a player against head and brain injuries. A judgment was rendered against the manufacturer for $750,000 in compensatory damages and $750,000 in punitive damages.

CASES OF INTEREST

It is impossible to predict all of the factual scenarios people will encounter that could subject them to potential liability arising from a sport-related contact or neurological injury. Examining prior legal cases and their results, however, can provide guidance as to what is and is not acceptable conduct when one is confronted with a sport-related injury. The doctrine of **stare decisis** requires courts of law "to follow earlier judicial decisions when the same points arise again in litigation."[53, 54] Courts of law adhere to **stare decisis** because it provides continuity and predictability in our legal system and further provides notice to society as to what one's rights, duties, and obligations are.[55, 56]

As noted previously, the public has only recently begun to learn about the serious consequences of concussions and head trauma in contact sports. Because of this, there are limited published legal opinions addressing these issues as compared to other traditional areas of tort law. It can be expected that the law on this subject will continue to develop rapidly to keep pace with advancing research and science. The following cases are a sample of judicial opinions from across the country that demonstrate how courts have addressed various issues relating to neurological sports injuries. These cases are not intended to cover the full litany of factual patterns that may lead to allegations of liability, and they do not cover all the legal issues implicated in sport injuries. Rather, these cases have been selected to allow the reader to gain insight into how the law is applied to varying factual scenarios.

Harvey v. Ouchita Parish School Board

During his sophomore and junior years, Michael Harvey had established himself as a star player on the West Monroe High School football team in Ouachita Parish, Louisiana. Before the start of his senior year, he sustained two minor neck injuries during football.[57] Harvey's father, a chiropractor, treated his son for these injuries and told Michael's coach that Michael had to wear a neck roll in all practices and games for an indefinite period of time to protect his neck from further injury.[58]

During the second game of his senior season, Michael's neck roll was torn off his shoulder pads and was damaged to the extent it could not be reattached. During halftime of the game, Michael inquired about an extra neck roll with the student trainer, who indicated that there were none. Michael did not ask any of the coaches for a neck roll and returned to play in the third quarter without a neck roll. After making an interception, Michael was tackled by the face mask during the return and sustained a ruptured disc at C4-5. Michael was treated with a discectomy and fusion.

Michael filed suit against his high school football coach and the school board as a result of the injuries he sustained. At trial, the court found the coach and staff negligent for failing to require a "player to wear available protective equipment to minimize the risk of a player being injured when tackled, even by actions that violate game rules, such as the 'face mask' and 'late hit' infractions for which penalty flags are thrown."[59] The judgment totaled $215,000 including $35,000 for "loss of opportunity to play college football." The total judgment was reduced by 20% for Michael's portion of his comparative fault.[60]

Maldonado v. Gateway Hotel Holdings, L.L.C.

A 23-year-old professional boxer, Fernando Maldonado, was knocked out in a fight at the Gateway Hotel in St. Louis in 1999. After being revived, Maldonado walked to his dressing room, where he lost consciousness. There was no ambulance on-site or on standby, nor was medical monitoring provided. Maldonado alleged that the hotel, as the landowner, failed to have an ambulance and medical monitoring on-site, which delayed his treatment, thereby causing significant brain injury and numerous motor and cognitive deficits. The jury found the hotel negligent and awarded $13.7 million in compensatory damages. Although a request for punitive damages was not made, the jury, on its own, assessed punitive damages in the amount of $27.4 million to the verdict, which was later struck by the judge.[61]

Cerny v. Cedar Bluffs Junior/Senior Public School

In September 1995, Brent Cerny struck his head against the ground while attempting to make a tackle in a football game. Reports indicated that Cerny was dizzy and disoriented but remained in the game for a couple of plays before taking himself out. Cerny returned to the game in the third quarter and played to its conclusion. He participated in practice the following week and was injured again when his helmet struck another player during practice drills. Cerny's doctor testified that he suffered a closed head injury with second concussion syndrome.

In his lawsuit, Cerny advanced several theories of negligence against his coach, including failing to adequately examine, failing to obtain qualified medical attention, and improperly allowing him to return to play. Critical testimony during the trial was conflicting. The judge found that the coach's conduct in evaluating Cerny and permitting him to reenter the game and participate in subsequent practices was consistent with what a reasonable coach would do under like or similar circumstances. The judge's verdict found that the coach was not negligent.[62]

Pinson v. State of Tennessee

In 1984, Michael Pinson received a blow to his head in a football practice. Shortly afterward, he collapsed and remained unconscious for 10 minutes. The school's athletic trainer examined Pinson and found facial palsy; no control on the left side of the body; unequal pupils; and no response to pain, sound, or movement. Pinson was thereafter immediately rushed to the hospital. The team trainer did not accompany Pinson to the hospital and instead sent a student trainer. Hospital records revealed that the student trainer informed hospital personnel that Pinson had been unconscious for 2 minutes. The school's trainer later appeared at the hospital but never conveyed to hospital personnel the significant neurological findings he had made on the field. Pinson's subsequent symptoms of headache, known by the trainer, together with the trainer's original findings, were never relayed to Pinson's treating doctor, who ultimately allowed Pinson to return to play.

Three weeks after the concussion, Pinson was "kicked in the head" and collapsed unconscious at practice. Surgery revealed a chronic subdural hematoma that had been present likely for 3 to 4 weeks. Pinson remained in a coma for several weeks following his brain surgery and became hemiparetic.

At a commissioner's trial, the school's trainer was found negligent for failing to communicate Pinson's neurological signs and symptoms to the emergency room and treating physician. Damages of $300,000 were assessed against the school trainer and the school.[63]

Rosada v. State of New York

John Rosado, a state detainee, filed suit against the state as a result of a fractured skull he sustained when he fell while playing basketball at the detention center. Rosado alleged that the state was negligent for using concrete floors instead of hardwood. The court found that no duty existed to use wooden basketball floors, and judgment was entered against Rosado.[64]

Regan v. State of New York

In Regan v. State of New York, a young college rugby player suffered a broken neck while practicing as a member of the rugby club and was rendered quadriplegic. The player filed a lawsuit against the state university alleging inter alia, negligent supervision of the practice. The court dismissed the claim, finding that the player had assumed the risk of "those injury-causing events which are known, apparent, or reasonably foreseeable consequences of their own participation."[65]

Fox v. Board of Supervisors of Louisiana State University and Agricultural and Mechanical College

In another rugby club lawsuit, a visiting club member sued the host school as a result of injuries he sustained during a match which rendered him quadriplegic. Interestingly, the player alleged that his injuries resulted from fatigue caused by the host school's actions. The claimant asserted that the host team had provided a cocktail party the evening before (in which he had participated); scheduled two matches on the next day; and had failed to ascertain whether the invitees were properly trained, coached, and supervised. In denying the claim against the host university, the court found that the "fact that a Rugby Club at a State University invited the [visiting team's] player who was injured during a game at the University did not make the University guardian of all participants' safety."[66]

Pahulu v. University of Kansas

Alani Pahulu, a University of Kansas scholarship football player, suffered a hit to his head during a tackle, which briefly dazed him and caused numbness and tingling in his arms and legs. Team doctors described this episode as transient quadriplegia, and Pahulu was not allowed to return to play. A team physician subsequently diagnosed Pahulu with a congenitally narrow cervical canal. In consultation with a neurosurgeon, the team physician concluded that based on the "one previous episode of transient quadriplegia and markedly stenotic cervical canal, [Pahulu was] at extremely high risk for subsequent and potentially permanent severe neurological injury including permanent quadriplegia." The team physician then disqualified Pahulu from participation in intercollegiate football.

Pahulu objected to the school's decision and consulted three specialists who concluded that he could participate in intercollegiate football with no more risk of permanent paralysis than any other player.[67] Pahulu, who was entering his last year of eligibility to play intercollegiate football, sought an injunction under Section 504 of the Rehabilitation Act of 1973[68] and asserted that he was an "individual with a disability" (previously referred to as a handicap). Under this act, a person must show that he has a physical or mental impairment that substantially limits one or more major life activities.[69]

Pahulu's case demonstrates the extreme difficulty in determining return-to-play eligibility. Here, the player had a perceived disability but still sought eligibility under a federal act that was designed to give equal protection to persons with disabilities.[70] Despite a brilliant argument by Pahulu's attorneys, the court ultimately affirmed the university's decision of disqualification.

Kyriazis v. University of West Virginia

West Virginia University, a rugby coach, and a faculty advisor of a rugby club were all sued when a rugby player claimed to have been injured during a match.[71] The player had been required to sign a release before being allowed to participate as a club member. The release indicated that the player accepted "any and all risks of . . . personal injury or death" and released the university and others "from any present and future claims including negligence, for . . . personal injury, or wrongful death, arising from my participation in rugby club activities."[72] The court held that this release was void because the university possessed a decisive bargaining advantage over the student and the release was not freely and fairly made between the parties.

Lessons to Be Learned

As demonstrated by the previously discussed cases, the application of the law is not a mechanical approach. The outcome of each case is dependent on its own unique facts. As such, there is no bright-line rule or specific course of conduct that the law prescribes to avoid liability completely. As in all negligence claims, in a claim against a medical provider or responsible person involving a sport-related injury, the defendant will be evaluated under the "reasonable person" standard. Thus, in order to avoid liability, she must act as a reasonable medical provider, trainer, coach, or other professional would under the same or similar circumstances.

NFL AND NCAA CONCUSSION LITIGATION

The highly publicized class action lawsuit filed by former players against the NFL was settled in September 2013. The lawsuit sought damages for football-related brain injuries as a result of concussions and subconcussive traumas. The class action complaint generally alleged two types of wrongful conduct by the NFL, namely, negligence and fraud. The theories underlying the negligence claims were failing to disclose the harmful effects of concussions, failing to properly treat concussions, and failing to establish rules governing tackling techniques and return to play. The more serious allegations against the NFL, however, were that it fraudulently concealed knowledge of the harmful effects of concussions and misrepresented material facts relating to the dangers of concussions. Specifically, the lawsuit alleged that the NFL knew as early as the 1920s of the harmful effects of concussions but concealed this knowledge from coaches, trainers, players, and the public until October 2009.

The NFL filed a motion to dismiss the lawsuit, arguing that the plaintiffs' claims were preempted under Section 301 of the Labor Management Relations Act because resolution of the plaintiffs' claims was substantially dependent on or inextricably intertwined with the terms of the collective bargaining agreement (CBA), or arose under the CBA, or both.[73] As such, the NFL argued that the parties must resolve their disputes by the dispute resolution process prescribed by the CBA—which in this case prohibited civil claims and required arbitration. Additionally, the NFL argued that under the terms of the CBA it was not responsible for player safety and that this responsibility fell to each team, the union, the individual players, or some combination of these.[74] While this motion was pending, the parties reached a settlement fully resolving all claims against the NFL.

Under the terms of the settlement, it has been reported that the NFL will pay $765 million, of which approximately $65 million will go toward testing and $10 million will be used to fund education and research. Former players are eligible for compensation only if they have been diagnosed with one of five categories of diseases: (1) ALS or amyotropic lateral sclerosis (Lou Gehrig's disease), (2) Alzheimer disease, (3) Parkinson disease, (4) dementia, or (5) severe cognitive impairment. Additionally, a sixth category of eligibility for compensation is "death from 2006 to the present (September 2013) with a medically diagnosed condition of 1 through 5 while alive, or suicide after 2006 with a diagnosis of CTE by autopsy." Pursuant to these terms of the settlement, some of the most deserving players and their families, such as the families of Mike Webster, Terry Long, and Justin Strzelczyk, will not be compensated.

At first blush, the amount of the settlement may seem to be a large sum. However, considering the damages incurred, that is, brain damage, this amount is potentially inadequate. This is especially true considering the number of claimants (approximately 4,500 players) and the payment conditions, which allow the NFL to pay the money over a 20-year period (reducing the settlement to an actual "present value" of approximately $600 million). Furthermore, the settlement amount is paltry compared to the NFL's anticipated revenue of approximately $180 billion (currently $9 billion per year) during the 20-year payout period.

In addition to the monetary components, two other aspects of the settlement warrant particular attention. First, one of the principal terms of the settlement is that the settlement cannot be considered an admission by the NFL of liability or an admission by the NFL that the plaintiffs' injuries were caused by football. Second, the lawsuit was settled before the plaintiffs were able to conduct discovery. Discovery is the pretrial phase of a lawsuit during which the parties gather information primarily through depositions, interrogatories, requests for documents, and requests for admissions. Because no discovery was undertaken, the plaintiffs never gained access to the NFL's internal documents and never were allowed to cross-examine NFL personnel, executives, or members of the NFL Brain Injury Committee under oath. Thus, the fundamental question underlying this lawsuit remains unanswered: What did the NFL know about concussions and when?[75]

Although the NFL concussion lawsuit appears to have been settled,[76] this is by no means the end of concussion litigation. Because the NFL concussion lawsuit was filed as a class action, members of the class have the opportunity to object to the terms and conditions of the settlement and further may opt out of the class and pursue individual claims. It is impossible to determine whether a significant number of players will opt out. Several factors will certainly influence this decision: (1) the reasonableness of the amount of money actually received, (2) the requirement that the NFL be allowed to maintain that it did nothing wrong, and (3) the fact that no answers have been provided as to what the NFL knew about concussions and when.

Additionally, concussion-related lawsuits have been filed against the NCAA. The NCAA lawsuits assert claims for negligence and fraudulent concealment, as well as claims seeking to establish a trust fund to provide for medical monitoring for all past, present, and future student-athletes who have suffered or will suffer concussion-related symptoms. The complaints against the NCAA specifically allege that the NCAA failed to correct the coaching and teaching of tackling techniques that cause head injuries, failed to educate personnel and players as to what a concussion is, had improper or no return-to-play rules, failed to screen and test for head injuries, and failed to determine that players with multiple concussions were ineligible.

Individual players who opt out of the National Football League Players' Concussion Injury Litigation class action settlement and pursue individual claims and plaintiffs in all future concussion-related litigation, including the NCAA concussion litigation, will need to overcome several barriers in order to prevail on their claims. Besides encountering a general denial of the allegations, one can expect that the NFL and NCAA defendants will assert the Statute of Limitations as a defense. A Statute of Limitations is a law that limits the amount of time a person has to file a claim. There are numerous exceptions to the Statute of Limitations, including time periods when a person was incompetent. The allegation of fraudulent concealment, if proven, would also potentially extend the time periods for filing these claims.

As indicated earlier in the chapter, one of the claimants' biggest hurdles will be to overcome the defense of assumption of the risk, that is, the concept that a "person who participates in sports assumes the risks inherent in that sport."[38] Stated another way, "when parties voluntarily enter a relationship where the plaintiff will assume certain well-known risks, the defendant has no duty to protect the plaintiff from those risks."[38] The defendants are also likely to use a defense borrowed from a skiing accident case, which provides that there is "[i]nherent risk which a [football player] is deemed to have knowledge of and assume is one that cannot be removed through the exercise of due care if the sport is to be enjoyed."[77]

Additionally, it is anticipated that the defendants will claim that many, if not all, of the players intentionally disregarded the known risks of concussions. Troy Polamalu, a four-time All-Pro safety for the Pittsburgh Steelers, is on record as stating that he has "chosen to continue playing injured in games when the team's medical staff would tell him not to."[78] According to ESPN, Polamalu and Chicago Bears Pro-Bowl linebacker Brian Urlacher have admitted that they would hide a head injury to stay on the field.[78]

Another potential defense the NFL and NCAA may raise can be found in the responses and warranties made by the individual players during their yearly qualifying medical examination. These exams typically include a section on past medical history that each player is required to complete. One question regularly asked in this section is whether the player has ever experienced dizziness, headaches, visual disturbances, and so on. These types of questions may be construed as questions relating to the symptoms of concussions and head trauma. Any failure on the part of the player to fully and accurately report

any prior symptoms could potentially hamper his ability to successfully pursue a claim.

As part of these yearly medical exams, the player may have also been required to make certain warranties about his health. For example, the questionnaires may have included language like the following: "I hereby warrant that the information provided herein is true and accurate and I recognize and understand that the team/school/league is relying on the information provided herein as stated." If the information provided by the player was not true, inaccuracies or false answers like these will be aggressively pursued by the defendants as a total bar to the claims.

Another issue and defense that may be raised in the NFL lawsuits is whether the individual players' claims are barred by states' workers' compensation laws. Each state generally has laws that grant employers immunity from civil lawsuits by their employees for work-related injuries. Some states provide an exception to this immunity if it can be shown that the employer acted knowingly, willfully, or both.[79] This issue will also be affected by the status of the player, that is, whether the player qualified as an employee or was an independent contractor.

It is too early to tell what impact these cases will have on the sport we all know and love—football—as well as other contact sports. But one thing is for certain: These lawsuits, together with other claims in the future, will help to provide necessary compensation to persons who have been severely injured. These lawsuits have also had beneficial secondary effects. They have raised awareness about the dangers of concussions, which has enabled others, especially our youth and their parents, to make informed decisions about whether to play contact sports; they have encouraged research aimed at providing a better understanding of the disease and creating improved diagnostics, treatment protocols, and a cure for CTE; and they have been the catalyst behind rules enacted to lessen the incidence and severity of the disease.

CONCLUDING THOUGHTS

Mike Webster's successful claims against the NFL, combined with the brain research done over the last decade and Dr. Omalu's discovery of CTE, has heightened awareness of the disabling effects of concussions. Our understanding of CTE is changing daily. This has resulted in a nationwide response to educate and enact standards and duties to lessen the incidence of concussions and provide proper treatment. As such, the duties, responsibilities, and obligations of those in charge of supervising contact sports and treating injuries sustained in such activities are correspondingly evolving. Future lawsuits, legislatively enacted laws, and our growing experiences with sport-related injuries will define the standards of care that will regulate the conduct and standards for medical providers, trainers, coaches, and others involved in caring for participants in contact sports. As a team doctor, trainer, or subsequent caretaker, for example, it is imperative that you become fully acquainted and stay up to date with all preparticipation testing protocols, eligibility criteria, on-field evaluations, return-to-play standards, and all other standards involved with contact sports.

REFERENCES

1. Jani (Estate of Mike Webster) v. Bell, 209 F. App'x 305 (4th Cir. 2006).
2. Studies are presently under way that show promise in diagnosing CTE through PET scans in living individuals. The study is known as a TauMark scan.
3. National Center for Sports Safety and Safe Kids, U.S.A., 2011.
4. Langlois JA, Rutland-Brown W, Wald M. The epidemiology and impact of traumatic brain injury: a brief overview. Journal of Head Trauma Rehabilitation 2006; 21(5): 375-378.
5. The jousting accident that turned Henry VIII into a tyrant. The Independent, 18 April, 2009.
6. Ibid.
7. Prosser W. Handbook of the Law of Torts §31 (5th ed. 1984).
8. Jackson v. State Farm Mut. Auto. Ins. Co., 600 S.E.2d 346 (2004).
9. Prosser W. Handbook of the Law of Torts, §30 (5th ed. 1984).
10. The "reasonable person" standard traces its roots back to 1837 in the English case of Vaughn v. Menlove, 132 Eng. Rep. 490 (C.P. 1837), which is the leading case articulating support for the reasonable person standard. Vaughn v. Menlove addressed the issue of whether the conduct of someone who built a haystack that caused a fire should be judged against that person's best possible farm work or the farm work that a reasonable person would have done.
11. Brown v. Kendall, 60 Mass. 292 (1850); Restatement (Second) of Torts §283.
12. Herbert AP. Misleading Cases in the Common Law; 1930, 12-16.
13. Epps v. United States, 862 F. Supp. 1460, 1463 (D.S.C. 1994).
14. Prosser W. Handbook of the Law of Torts, p. 356 (5th ed. 1984).
15. Restatement (Second) of Torts §302, comment a (1965).
16. Syl. pt. 3, Sewell v. Gregory, 371 S.E.2d 82 (W.Va. 1988).
17. Prosser W. Handbook of the Law of Torts §31, p. 170 (5th ed. 1984).
18. Osborne v. Montgomery, 234 N.W. 372, 379 (Wis. 1931).
19. Ibid.
20. Restatement (Second) of Torts §291 (1965).
21. United States v. Carroll Towing, 159 F.2d 169 (2nd Cir. 1947).
22. Restatement (Second) of Torts, §285-286 (1965).
23. Martin v. Herzog, 126 N.E. 814 (N.Y. 1920). The court found that the defendant was negligent per se as a result of driving his wagon without lights at night, which was in violation of a traffic statute.
24. See Wash. Rev. Code Ann. §28A.600.194 (also known as the Zackery Lystedt Law), which states: "(1)(a) Concussions are one of the most commonly reported injuries in children and adolescents who participate in sports and recreational activities. The centers for disease control and prevention estimates that as many as three million nine hundred thousand sports-related and recreation-related concussions occur in the United States each year. A concussion is caused by a blow or motion to the head or body that causes the brain to move rapidly inside the skull. The risk of catastrophic injuries or death are significant when a concussion or head injury is not properly evaluated and managed. (b) Concussions are a type of brain injury that can range from mild to severe and can disrupt the way the brain normally works. Concussions can occur in any organized or unorganized sport or recreational activity and can result from a fall or from players colliding with each other, the ground, or with obstacles. Concussions occur with or without loss of consciousness, but the vast majority occurs without loss of consciousness. (c) Continuing to play with a concussion or symptoms of head injury leaves the young athlete especially vulnerable to greater injury and even death. The legislature recognizes that, despite having generally recognized return to play standards for concussion and head injury, some affected youth athletes are prematurely returned to play resulting in actual or potential physical injury or death

to youth athletes in the state of Washington. (2) Each school district's board of directors shall work in concert with the Washington interscholastic activities association to develop the guidelines and other pertinent information and forms to inform and educate coaches, youth athletes, and their parents and/or guardians of the nature and risk of concussion and head injury including continuing to play after concussion or head injury. On a yearly basis, a concussion and head injury information sheet shall be signed and returned by the youth athlete and the athlete's parent and/or guardian prior to the youth athlete's initiating practice or competition. (3) A youth athlete who is suspected of sustaining a concussion or head injury in a practice or game shall be removed from competition at that time. (4) A youth athlete who has been removed from play may not return to play until the athlete is evaluated by a licensed health care provider trained in the evaluation and management of concussion and receives written clearance to return to play from that health care provider. The health care provider may be a volunteer. A volunteer who authorizes a youth athlete to return to play is not liable for civil damages resulting from any act or omission in the rendering of such care, other than acts or omissions constituting gross negligence or willful or wanton misconduct. (5) This section may be known and cited as the Zackery Lystedt law."

25. Everett v. Bucky Warren Inc., 380 N.E.2d 653, 659 (Mass. 1978) (stating that the hockey coach, "as a person with substantial experience in the game of hockey, may be held to a higher standard of care and knowledge than would an average person"); McCoid AH, The Care Requirement of Medical Practitioners, 12 Vand. L. Rev. 549 (1959).

26. Prosser W. Handbook of the Law of Torts, p. 185-189 (5th ed. 1984).

27. Fed. R. Evid. 702; Hardin v. Ski Venture, Inc., 50 F.3d 1291 (4th Cir. 1995).

28. Daubert v. Merrell Dow Pharmaceuticals, Inc., 509 U.S. 579 (1993).

29. Fed. R. Evid. 803(18), which provides that the following is not excluded by the rule against hearsay: "To the extent called to the attention of an expert witness upon cross-examination or relied upon by the expert witness in direct examination, statements contained in published treatises, periodicals or pamphlets on a subject of history, medicine, or other science or art, established as a reliable authority by the testimony or admission of the witness or by other expert testimony or by judicial notice. If admitted, the statements may be read into evidence but may not be received as exhibits."

30. American Academy of Family Practitioners. Concussion (mild traumatic brain injury) and the team physician: a consensus statement, 2005.

31. American Academy of Family Practitioners. Sideline preparedness for the team physician: a consensus statement, 2001.

32. American Academy of Family Practitioners. The team physician and return-to-play issues: a consensus statement, 2002.

33. Heads up: concussions in high school sports. In: Guide for Coaches, U.S. Department of Health and Human Services Centers for Disease Control and Prevention. June 2010.

34. Casa D, Guskiewicz K, Anderson S, et al. National Athletic Trainers' Association position statement: preventing sudden death in sports. Journal of Athletic Training, 2012: 47(1): 96-118.

35. Prosser W. Handbook of the Law of Torts, §56, pp. 343-344 (4th ed. 1978).

36. See Minn. Stat. §604A.01 subd.2(a); West's F.S.A. §768.13.

37. Prosser W. Handbook of the Law of Torts, p. 378 (5th ed. 1984)

38. Prosser W. Handbook of the Law of Torts, p. 480, 481 (5th ed. 1984).

39. Prosser W. Handbook of the Law of Torts §68 (5th ed. 1984); see also Weistart J, Lowell C, The Law of Sports, 1979, ch. 8; Annots., 1977, 77 A.L.R. 3d 1300 for overview of the doctrine of assumption of risk in sports and, in particular, contact sports.

40. Higgins v. Pfeiffer, 546 N.W.2d 645 (Mich. Ct. App. 1996).

41. Ibid.

42. Ibid.

43. See Nabozny v. Barnhill, 334 N.E.2d 258 (Ill. App. Ct. 1975) (holding "that when athletes are engaged in an athletic competition; all teams involved are trained and coached by knowledgeable personnel; a recognized set of rules governs the conduct of the competition; and a safety rule is contained therein which is primarily designed to protect players from serious injury, a player is then charged with a legal duty to every other player on the field to refrain from conduct proscribed by a safety rule"); Hackbart v. Cincinnati Bengals, Inc., 435 F. Supp. 352 (Dist. Colo. 1977), reversed, 601 F.2d 516 (10th Cir., 1979) (a football player struck another player on the head and neck in anger and frustration following an interception); Karas v. Strevell, 884 N.E.2d 122 (Ill. 2008).

44. Ventura v. Winegardner, 357 S.E.2d 764 (W.Va. 1987).

45. Wahrer v. San Bernadino City Unified School District, E036671, 2006 WL 350461 (Cal. Ct. App. Feb. 16, 2006) (unpublished).

46. Serrell v. Connetquot Central School District of Islip, 798 N.Y.S.2d 493 (N.Y. App. Div. 2005).

47. Cerney v. Cedar Bluffs Public School, 679 N.W.2d 198 (Neb. 2004).

48. Coonradt v. Averill Park Central School Dist., 414 N.Y.S. 2d 242 (N.Y. App. Div. 1979).

49. Mogabgab v. Orleans Parish School Board, 239 So.2d 456 (La. Ct. App. 1970).

50. Knapp v. Northwestern University, 101 F.3d 473 (7th Cir. 1996); see also Paterick TE, Paterick TJ, Fletcher GF, Maron BJ, Medical and legal issues in the cardiovascular evaluation of competitive athletes, JAMA 2005; 294: 3011-3018.

51. Austria v. Bike Athletic Co., 810 P.2d 1312 (Or. Ct. App. 1991) (parents of football player severely injured by blow to the head during football practice brought suit against designer and manufacturer of football helmet alleging defective design).

52. Rawlings Sporting Goods Company, Inc. v. Daniels, 619 S.W.2d 435 (Tex. Civ. App. 1981).

53. Black's Law Dictionary (8th ed. 2004) 1443.

54. Stare decisis is an abridged version of the Latin phrase stare decisis et non quieta movera, which means "[t]o stand by things decided, and not to disturb settled points." City of Rocky River v. State Employment Relations Bd., 539 N.E.2d 103 (Ohio 1989) (citing Black's Law Dictionary [5th ed. rev. 1979] 1261).

55. Westfield Ins. Co. v. Galatis, 797 N.E.2d 1256, 1268 (Ohio 2003).

56. Stare decisis is a judicial policy and is not an absolute rule of law. Courts of law will part ways with precedent that is not legally sound and when the decisions were based on reasoning that has become outdated or fallen into disfavor. Cherrington v. Erie Ins. Property and Cas. Co., 745 S.E.2d 508, 519 (W.Va. 2013).

57. Harvey v. Ouachita Parish Sch. Bd., 674 So. 2d 372, 375(La. Ct. App. 1996), writ denied, 681 So. 2d 1260 (1996).

58. Ibid.

59. Harvey, 674 So.2d at 376.

60. Harvey, 674 So.2d at 375, 376.

61. Maldonado v. Gateway Hotel Holdings, L.L.C., 154 S.W.3d 303 (Mo. Ct. App. 2003).

62. Cerny v. Cedar Bluffs Junior/Senior Public School, 628 N.W.2d 697 (Neb. 2001).

63. Pinson v. State of Tennessee, C.A. No. 02A01-9409-BC-00210, 1995 WL 739820 (Tenn. Ct. App. 1995).

64. Rosado v. State of New York, 527 N.Y.S.2d 314 (N.Y. App. Div. 1988).

65. Regan v. State of New York, 654 N.Y.S.2d 488, (N.Y. App. Div. 1997).

66. Fox v. Board of Sup'rs of Louisiana State University and Agr. and Mechanical College, 576 So.2d 978 (La. 1991).

67. Pahulu v. University of Kansas, 897 F. Supp. 1387 (D.C. Kan. 1995).

68. 29 U.S.C. §706 et seq.

69. Welsh v. City of Tulsa, Okla., 977 F.2d 1415 (10th Cir. 1992).

70. Mitten MJ. Amateur athletes with handicaps or physical abnormalities: who makes the participation decision, 71 Neb. L. Rev. 987 (1992).

71. The plaintiff became dizzy, lost his balance, and was later diagnosed with a basilar-artery thrombosis. The case does not describe how, if at all, this condition was caused by any act of negligence.

72. Kyriazis v. University of West Virginia, 450 S.E.2d 649 (W.Va. 1994).

73. Mem. of Law of Def. Mot. to Dismiss, In re: National Football League Players' Concussion Injury Litigation, No. 2:12-md-02323, MDL No. 2323 (Aug. 30, 2012).

74. Ibid.

75. For additional information on this subject, see Fainaru-Wade M, Fainaru S, League of Denial: The NFL, Concussions, and the Battle for Truth, Crown: 2013.

76. Another component of the NFL class action lawsuit is product liability claims asserted against helmet manufacturer Riddell Inc./All American Sports Corporation. These claims include negligent design, manufacturing defects, failure to warn, and negligence. Whether these claims will be pursued post-NFL settlement is yet to be seen, but they still exist within the NFL concussion litigation.

77. Brett v. Great American Recreation, Inc., 677 A.2d 705 (N.J. 1996).

78. Polamalu T. I've hid concussions, ESPN.com News Services, July 18, 2012.

79. For example, in West Virginia an employer is stripped of its immunity if it is proven that the employer acted with "deliberate intention." W.Va. Code §23-4-2(d)(2). There are two ways to prove that an employer acted with "deliberate intention": (1) by proving a "consciously formed" deliberate intent to bring about the specific result of injury or (2) by proving the existence of the five statutory elements set forth in W.Va. Code §23-4-2(d)(2)(ii), which establish a prima facie case of "deliberate intent" essentially requiring an employee to demonstrate that the employer intentionally disregarded a known safety violation.

Having a Game Plan

Organizations or institutions that sponsor athletic activities or events must establish emergency response plans. Written emergency plans should be coordinated in consultation with local emergency medical services. Everyone should know his respective responsibilities. Emphasis should be on education and training of school athletic trainers, coaches, and school staff. In addition, the maintenance of emergency equipment and supplies at schools for prevention and treatment of sports-related emergencies is of ultimate importance. This chapter reviews the formation and implementation of a comprehensive, practical, and flexible game plan.

DEVELOPING AN EMERGENCY ACTION PLAN

While most injuries sustained during athletics or other physical activity are relatively mild, it is evident that emergencies can and do occur. The relatively low incidence rate of catastrophic injury may create a false sense of security among athletic program personnel, and the consequences of a lack of preparedness can be disastrous.[3, 14, 23] Injuries of this nature are often unpredictable and occur without warning. One of the more demanding medical decisions in athletics today occurs immediately following a neurological injury in the athlete, particularly to the head or spine. Proper care of an athlete with a neurological injury (or any injury for that matter)

requires preparation for response to emergencies, including education and training, appropriate use of personnel, and the formation and implementation of an emergency action plan. The "Sideline Preparedness Statement" was developed by a collaboration of six major professional associations concerned about clinical sports medicine issues (American Academy of Family Physicians, American Academy of Orthopaedic Surgeons, American College of Sports Medicine, American Medical Society for Sports Medicine, American Orthopaedic Society for Sports Medicine, and the American Osteopathic Academy of Sports Medicine). The goal was to provide physicians who are responsible for making decisions regarding the medical care of athletes with guidelines for identifying and planning for medical care and services at the site of practice or competition.[1] The document was not intended as a standard of care but rather only a guide, and it can serve as a very valuable resource. The National Athletic Trainers' Association (NATA) issued an excellent position statement regarding emergency planning in athletics that should be read by anyone involved in the care of an athlete.[3]

Need for a Plan

The concept may seem rather intuitive, but it is important to consider the need for emergency planning in athletics. As with other accidents or natural disasters, emergencies in sport are usually not expected; however, when they do occur, a controlled response makes all the difference.

This is not unique to athletic events, as such plans provide the foundation for law enforcement, fire and rescue, pilots, and other military and government agencies to effectively respond to emergencies. Emergency planning should be a dynamic rather than a static process, because many lessons that are gleaned from major events can be used to help improve or refine an existing emergency plan. Several points of consideration are unique to emergency management in athletics, though. Typically, at any one time, only a single athletic participant is requiring response for a possible internal injury, bleeding, cardiac event, or traumatic head or spine injury. That being said, multiple injuries can happen all at once, requiring simultaneous triage and management. Additionally, the possibility for injury to a game official, a fan, or other sideline participant should be accounted for. In addition to providing responders with an organized approach to reacting to an untoward event, the need for emergency plans in athletics can be thought of from two major vantage points—professional and legal.[3]

Professional Need

Any practitioners caring and providing oversight for athletes have an organizational and professional responsibility to provide an emergency plan. Governing bodies associated with all levels of athletic competition have stated that access to emergency medical care should be provided in the event of an emergency. The National Collegiate Athletic Association (NCAA) and the National Federation of State High School Associations (NFHS) both recommend that all member institutions develop an emergency plan for their athletic programs.[24, 25] Both organizations reinforce that coverage should be provided for any aspect of athletic activity, including practices and contests during both in-season and off-season activities. Similar plans have been recommended at the youth sport level as well.[28]

Interestingly, despite the aforementioned oversight, several studies have demonstrated less than 100% adherence to these recommendations. One survey of NCAA member institutions revealed that at least 10% of the institutions do not maintain any form of emergency plan.[5] A more recent study surveyed 1,000 randomly selected members of NATA and included questions on the clinical background of the athletic trainer, the demographic features of the school,

the preparedness of the school to manage life-threatening athletic emergencies, the presence of preventive measures to avoid potential sport-related emergencies, and the immediate availability of emergency equipment.[26] Ultimately 521 of the returned questionnaires were eligible for analysis. The results showed that 70% of schools have a written emergency plan (WEP), although 36% of schools with a WEP did not practice the plan. Only 34% of schools had an athletic trainer present during all athletic events. Interestingly, the sports typically with higher rates of fatalities or injuries based on published literature, such as ice hockey and gymnastics, had less coverage by athletic trainers compared with other sports with lower rates of fatalities or injuries.[26] So, again, emergency plans are not used 100% of the time across the board. Additionally, even though some schools are in compliance with many of the recommendations for school-based athletic emergency preparedness, there are still many specific areas for improvement, including practicing the emergency plan, linking all areas of the school directly with emergency medical services, and increasing the presence of athletic trainers at athletic events.

Several national organizations, such as NATA and the American College of Sports Medicine, recognize the professional need for emergency preparedness and have incorporated such competencies into their educational curriculum. Such competencies justify the need for any health care practitioner involved in the care of athletes to be involved with the development and application of emergency plans as a fulfillment of her professional obligations. Ultimately, the burden of planning for such untoward events rests on those most intimately involved with the athletes, as it should.

Legal Need

The other major point of consideration is the legal need for the development and application of an emergency plan. All organizational medical personnel, from trainers to physicians, have a legal duty as reasonable and prudent professionals to ensure high-quality care of the participating athlete. From a legal standpoint, even more important is the precedence for the standard of care by which health professionals are measured.[27, 29] It is this standard of care that sets the umbrella of accountability for both the practitioners and the governing bodies that oversee these practitioners. The emergency plan has been categorized as a written document that defines the standard of care required during an emergency situation.[19] In addition to the essentially legal requirement that sports medicine programs have a well-formulated, adequately written, and periodically rehearsed emergency action plan, it has been stated that the lack of an emergency plan is frequently the basis for claims and suits based on negligence.[19]

One factor that comes into play from the legal standpoint is the concept of foreseeability. Administrators, organizations, and members of the sports medicine team must question whether a particular emergency situation has a reasonable possibility of occurring during the sport in question; if the answer is yes, then a previously prepared emergency plan must be in place.[3] Several legal claims and suits have set precedence as to the need for emergency plans, alluding to a lack thereof as resulting in a delayed response and subsequent catastrophic consequences.[32]

Therefore, there clearly exists both a professional and legal obligation to provide an emergency action plan in order to protect the interests of all parties involved. A failure to provide an emergency plan results at a minimum in inefficient care for the athlete and at worst allows for potential negligence and subsequent catastrophic ramifications for the injured athlete and all personnel involved.

Team Approach to Neurological Sports Medicine

The overarching goal of the sports medicine team is the delivery of the highest possible quality health care to the athlete; paramount to achieving this goal is solid teamwork. Just as with an athletic team, athletic trainers, students, emergency medical personnel, coaches, and physicians need to work together as an efficient unit in emergency situations, because time is crucial.[22] Sometimes a few seconds or a single move here or there can mean the difference between life and death or permanent disability. Whether in a stadium with 60,000 fans or at a local high school game with stands of concerned parents watching your every move, it is important to remember that the environment can often become chaotic

very quickly and that emotions can run high when an athletic emergency occurs. Herein lies the importance of having an emergency plan to provide an organized structure to the sports medicine team response.

In an athletic environment, the first person to respond in an emergency situation may vary widely.[22] In most settings, athletic trainers represent the workforce in the trenches, able to provide immediate care for most injuries sustained; and they are often the first responders to most injuries during a game. This may even be the case in settings where team physicians are available on the sidelines. In the case of certain neurological injuries, such as concussion, this may prove to be extremely valuable, as athletic trainers have the advantage of knowing the personalities and habits of their athletes because of the amount of time spent with them on a regular basis.[17] Such intimate knowledge of the athletes allows for the sensitive detection of subtle signs that someone may have experienced a concussion. However, once a concussion is identified, a physician needs to be involved in the overall management and return-to-play decisions; and the same goes for more severe neurological injuries to the head, spine, or peripheral nervous system.

It is important to remember, though, that the first responder may also be a coach, a game official, or an emergency medical technician. It is this variation that makes it imperative for an emergency plan to be in place and well rehearsed.[3] With a plan in place, people with different training levels and skills sets will be able to work effectively together when responding to an emergency situation. All personnel involved with athletes should also have basic cardiopulmonary response and first aid training, as well as familiarity with the use of automatic external defibrillators.[3] With regard to neurological injuries specifically, it would be ideal for every sports medicine team member, as well as the athletes, parents, school officials, and coaches, to be educated about concussion and spine injury.

The emergency plan should outline and clarify an understanding regarding team member responsibilities. For example, who will be responsible for on-field responses? Who will handle the emergency assessment and handle communication if more advanced help is needed? Who will observe and care for the athlete on the sideline following an injury should the player not need to be transferred? Who will communicate with the parents and coaches? In an ideal situation, all members of the team would be involved in some aspect of the care, although a team leader should be identified, particularly for emergency situations.

Implementation

Implementing an emergency plan involves writing, education, and rehearsal. First, committing a protocol to writing provides a clear response mechanism and allows for continuity among all team members.[19] Flow sheets or algorithmic charts can be helpful in projecting a clear protocol for emergency events. It is important to have separate plans or modified versions for different athletic venues and for practices versus games. Additionally, the different versions and protocols should be flexible and should account for the personnel available at different times. For instance, the team physician may be present for games but not necessarily for practices, so plans may vary dependent on these changes. Also the location and type of equipment as well as communication devices may differ among sports, venues, and level of athletic participation.[3] The take-home point is that one size does not fit all; and to be thorough, all possible versions should be put into writing.

Once the protocol is set in writing, the next step to implementing an emergency plan is educating all members of the team. Any and all personnel should be very familiar with the current system in place for responding to an athletic catastrophe. The coordinated response is only as good as the weakest link, so each team member should have a written copy of the entire emergency plan, as well as documentation with that individual's specific roles and responsibilities in emergency situations. The same rule of thumb applies for institutional and organizational administrators. It is also helpful if a venue-specific plan is posted in clear sight at each venue, as well.[3]

Finally, once all members of the sports medicine team are educated, the plan needs to be rehearsed. Championship teams at any level do not just "wing" things—they practice. By rehearsing the emergency plan, team members are able to maintain their skills at a high level of competency and gain comfort within a specific system. Before a game, the preparation should

include mock episodes of catastrophic neurological injuries such as spinal injuries. All team members should have an understanding of all responsibilities of each member of the staff. Cross-training staff members allows for proper care in the event of an absent staff member. Dry runs also allow for working through potential pitfalls and challenges that could be encountered in a real emergency situation, in the comfort of a practice session. Rehearsals can also be accomplished through annual or biannual in-service meetings and through preseasonal debriefings, with reviews performed as needed throughout any given sport season, to compensate for potential personnel turnover.

Equipment

All specialized equipment for emergency care should be checked on a regular basis for wear, safety, and loss and should be in good operating condition.[16] The necessary equipment should be at the site and quickly accessible.[31, 38] All staff should be well versed in the application of all equipment associated with emergency injury management and should be trained in advance to use it properly. The equipment should be comprehensive but also appropriate for the level of training of the emergency medical providers available and the venue being considered. For spine injury, typical equipment includes a spine board, scoop stretcher, rigid collar, and support padding for immobilization. Improvements in technology and emergency training, however, require personnel to also become familiar with the use of automatic external defibrillators, oxygen, and advanced airways, especially for use in the setting of catastrophic head or spine injury.

Communication

An important part of ensuring a thorough emergency plan is securing access to a working telephone or other telecommunications device, whether fixed or mobile.[3, 16, 22, 32] The designated communications system should be checked before each practice or competition to ensure that everything is in working condition, and a backup plan should be in place should a failure occur with the primary communication device.[16] A list of emergency contact numbers, in addition to a copy of the overall emergency plan, should be posted near the communication system. Clear details regarding the venue location, directions, and any other pertinent information can help facilitate the effective communication of coordinated and accurate information in the event of an emergency and should also be readily available.

Transportation

A clear plan for transportation of the injured athlete is essential to the overall emergency protocol. In an ideal situation, an ambulance should be available on-site for athletic events; however, this is not always realistic given multiple events at the same time and overall logistics. Thus, at a minimum, emphasis should definitely be placed on ensuring ambulance availability on-site for high-risk events. The type of transportation service, equipment available, and training level of the personnel staffing the ambulance or other transportation means should be identified and taken into consideration when the emergency plan is put together. If an ambulance will be available on-site, a location should be designated with rapid access to the site and a cleared route for exiting and entering the venue.[3] A plan should also be put into place to account for and allow athletic medical coverage at the venue, should the emergency care provider and ambulance need to leave the site to transport an injured athlete.

Venue Location

As mentioned previously, the emergency plan should be not only activity specific but venue specific as well. The plan for the venue should take into account and encompass all aspects of the emergency plan, including accessibility to emergency medical transportation, equipment, communication, and proximity to medical care facilities. The host and visiting medical staff should communicate about the venue, in particular regarding the location of equipment and the communications system in place at the site.

Medical Care Facilities

An emergency medical facility should be identified for all athletic events. In selecting an appropriate facility, consideration should be given to the location of the facility with respect to the athletic venue and the level of service available to deliver appropriate care to an injured athlete. [3, 16] There should be clear communication with the designated medical care facility in advance of athletic events. Additionally, it is recommended that the emergency plan be reviewed with the medical staff present at the designated facility and that any issues pertinent to athletic medical care discussed, such as the proper removal of athletic equipment.[3, 22]

Documentation and Establishing Policy

The protocol is different from the policy in that it specifically outlines the clinical tests and steps that will be used for assessments and overall management. The policy outlines the steps to be put in place, including roles and responsibilities of the team, athlete, and organization. It is important to involve institutional and organizational administration and coaching staff in the planning and documentation process, as this creates a sense of individual ownership and "buy-in" of the policy, in addition to fostering a sense of teamwork across the board. The policy should, at the very least, consider four components:

1. Preseason planning
2. On-field and sideline evaluation
3. Removal from play
4. Graduated return-to-play progression[17]

Sample concussion policies can be found readily online, and most policies include information regarding the implementation of educational programs for all players, parents, and team staff.

Other important documentation should include the following:[3, 19]

- Delineation of the person or group (or both) responsible for documenting the emergency situation
- Follow-up documentation on evaluation of response to the emergency situation
- Documentation of regular rehearsal of the emergency plan
- Documentation and records of personnel training
- Documentation of maintenance of emergency equipment

CARING FOR ATHLETIC INJURIES

To ensure adequate and timely care of athletic injuries, proper triage is important. While on the sideline, when able, the team physician and athletic trainers can watch the activity intently and have a unique opportunity to see the injury occur. In contrast to receiving a patient in the hospital setting, having the chance to see the mechanics of the injury as it occurs provides the opportunity to respond to the athlete immediately without need for extensive subjective assessment. The proper steps in evaluating an injured athlete include the primary survey, resuscitation, the secondary survey, and then sideline assessment to include any other necessary first aid.

Primary Survey

Immediately following an injury, a primary survey is taken, beginning with an assessment of the athlete's level of consciousness. A team approach is used; however, there should always be one person in charge while performing any on-field maneuvers, particularly those involving a potential spine-injured athlete. The person in charge varies from situation to situation but is often the team physician. That being said, in most situations, especially at the youth and high school levels, the athletic trainers not only are the first responders to an injury but also assume the role of team leader. The conscious athlete is obviously much easier to assess, as the unconscious athlete poses a variety of additional challenges for the health care provider. In the event that an athlete is rendered unconscious, the clinician should also suspect a concomitant cervical spine injury when approaching him on the field. In the conscious patient, a spinal fracture or cord injury may be accompanied by severe muscle spasm and pain, which may indicate the nature of the injury. However, if the mechanism of injury is not known or if a cervical spine injury cannot be ruled out, one still needs to assume initially that the neck is injured. Guidelines stress that any athlete suspected of having a spinal injury should not be moved,[34] and in a short period of time the primary survey can be conducted.

Responders should immediately attempt to expose the airway. One can rapidly assess the airway by just talking to the patient. If the athlete is able to communicate, then the airway is patent; however, care must be taken to ensure that the airway is kept open and patent. Foreign debris should be removed, and a jaw thrust (preferred over a chin lift due to the potential for neck movement) can be performed as needed. This assessment should be performed with as little motion as possible. Should the athlete be unconscious, one should obtain access to the airway by removing any existing barriers, such as a protective face mask if one is present (figure 3.1). Otherwise, in a conscious athlete with a stable airway, face mask removal can be initiated once the decision to immobilize and transport has been made. Responders should be aware of and well trained in established face mask removal techniques. Many tools are available for this purpose, and the goal should be to perform this quickly and with as minimal movement and difficulty as possible (figure 3.2). A powered (cordless) screwdriver is generally faster, produces less head movement, and is easier to use than cutting tools; it should be the first tool used in an attempt to remove a face mask attached with loop straps that are secured with screws.[10, 33, 34, 36] A backup cutting tool, specifically matched to the sport equipment used, should be available in case screw removal fails. Examples of such cutting tools include the Trainers Angel (Riverside, CA) and the FM Extractor (Sports Medicine Concepts, Inc., Livonia, NY). This is referred to as a combined-tool approach.[6, 15] Having helmets undergo regular maintenance, reconditioning, and recertification throughout a season can increase the likelihood that face mask screws can be removed successfully.[6, 35]

Once the airway has been quickly inspected, the athlete's breathing is assessed with a "look, listen, and feel" method and circulation assessed by palpating for peripheral pulses. If rescue breathing becomes necessary, the individual with the most training and experience should establish an airway and commence rescue breathing using the safest technique. All aspects of assessment and management should be performed in accordance with the American Heart Association guidelines for cardiopulmonary resuscitation (CPR) and basic life support (BLS),[2, 37] which all team members should be familiar with and certified in. Often the athlete with a head or spine injury is found lying prone or on the side. It cannot be stressed enough that the initial assessment of airway, breathing, and circulation should be performed with the athlete in the position she

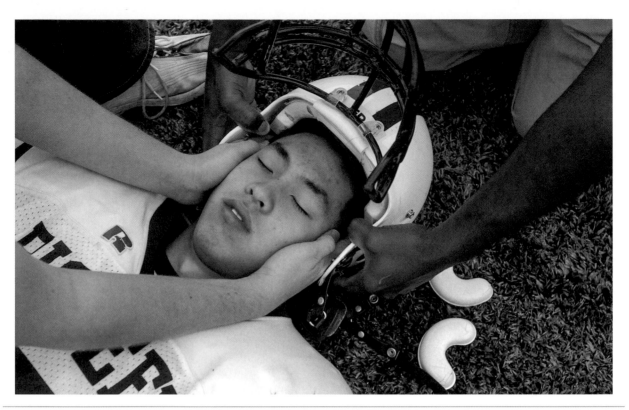

Figure 3.1 If the athlete is unconscious, the face mask should be removed while maintaining in-line immobilization. In a conscious athlete with a stable airway, face mask removal can be initiated once the decision to immobilize and transport has been made.

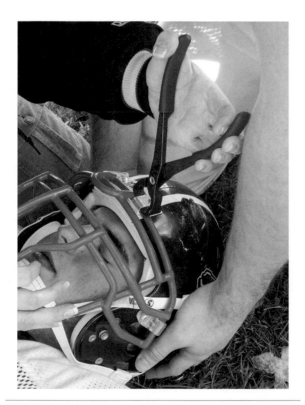

Figure 3.2 A variety of face mask removal tools are available.

was found in. In the conscious prone athlete, if vital signs are present and stable, there is no significant rush to move the athlete to the supine position. Following the primary survey, any other necessary resuscitative measures must be implemented or continued, including CPR, fluid replacement for dehydration (with intravenous line if needed), immediate cooling of the athlete (in the case of heatstroke or exhaustion), splinting of fractures, or stopping any bleeding with direct pressure.

Spine Boarding and Stabilization

If the athlete must be moved from a prone to supine position, or if the patient is requiring transfer and spine boarding, care has to be taken to keep the spine immobilized during this process. The head, neck, and trunk are moved as one unit, with avoidance of any movement of the cervical spine or any rotation, flexion, extension, or lateral flexion of the rest of the spine. The sports medicine team should be prepared to immobilize athletes with suspected spine injuries on a long spine board or other full-body immobilization device[18, 21, 34] (figure 3.3). The traditional spine board represents the most common device used for full-body immobilization; however, devices such as the full-body vacuum splint are more comfortable for athletes, reduce superficial irritation and sores over bony prominences, and may be used in appropriate situations.[18, 21] One study comparing these two types of spine board immobilization concluded that although the vacuum splint was applied more easily and quickly, the efficacy of cervical immobilization required additional padding to support the spine.[21] So these points should be taken into consideration when the type of spine board is chosen. There are also improved models that include a winged-type apparatus to compensate for larger athletes or athletes with bulky equipment.

Selection of the appropriate transfer technique is also critical. The log roll technique requires four or five rescuers: one to control the head and cervical spine, two or three to roll the patient on command, and one to position the spine board. [34, 39] The lift-and-slide technique is a lift requiring six or more people that involves lifting the athlete to allow for spine board placement.[34] This

technique is effective in minimizing structural interference that could result in unwanted spinal column movements. The straddle lift-and-slide technique requires only four responders to lift the body and shift the athlete onto a spine board.[34] For the prone athlete, the log roll technique is the only option. For the supine athlete, any of these techniques may be used; however, the lift-and-slide technique has been reported to produce less motion at the head and in the cervical spine than the log roll technique and thus should be used when possible.[4, 11-13] Interestingly, the same has been reported in studies looking at the removal of patients off of a spine board, despite the fact that most patients in hospitals are still log-rolled.[20]

Manual stabilization of the head and cervical spine should be converted to immobilization using external devices such as rigid cervical collars before transfer to a spine board. In equipment-laden sports, this may be difficult or impossible, although a cervical vacuum immobilization device has been shown to limit cervical spine range of motion in the fully equipped football player.[30, 34] Tape, foam blocks, and towels can complement the basic items and improve

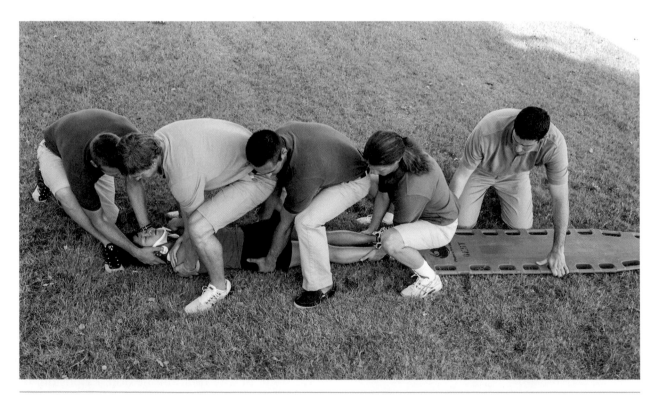

Figure 3.3   Athletes with a suspected spine injury should be immobilized on a long spine board or other full-body immobilization device.

stability.[7] Stabilization of the cervical spine should be continued, until a destabilizing injury has been ruled out, using appropriate diagnostic testing or exam or both; and whenever possible, manual stabilization should be resumed after the application of external devices.[9] Studies have also compared the effectiveness of different manual cervical spine stabilization techniques. One study compared head motions that occurred when trained professionals performed the head squeeze (HS) and trap squeeze (TS) cervical spine stabilization techniques.[4] The authors compared peak head and neck motion with both HS and TS during lift-and-slide and log roll placement of a simulated cooperative patient on a spinal board and did the same in a simulated agitated patient trying to sit up or rotate his head. They concluded that there was little overall difference between HS and TS techniques in a cooperative patient; however, when a patient was confused and agitated, the HS was much worse than the TS at minimizing cervical spine motion.[4]

Regarding positioning of the cervical spine, a nice neutral alignment should be sought. Studies have demonstrated that in healthy individuals, a slight degree of flexion equivalent to 2 cm of occiput elevation produces a favorable increase in the spinal canal/spinal cord ratio, opening the angle within the spinal canal.[8, 9] In unhelmeted athletes, some posterior padding may be required to maintain neutral spinal positioning; however, this alignment is usually achieved by the typical football, hockey, or lacrosse helmet and thus is another reason to not remove an athlete's helmet right away. Because of the unwanted movement that could occur in the cervical spine with the removal of athletic equipment such as a helmet and shoulder pads, removal should be deferred until the athlete has been transported to an emergency medical facility except under extenuating circumstances such as the following[34]:

- If a helmet is not securely fitted and is affecting immobilization of the head and neck
- If the face mask cannot be removed safely in a reasonable amount of time to gain access to an athlete's airway
- If the helmet impedes the ability to provide ventilation, if required, even after removal of the face mask

- If the equipment prevents neutral alignment of the cervical spine or forces the head and neck to rotate, extend, or flex unsafely

It is also important to remember and educate those caring for athletes that shoulder pads and helmets are best removed simultaneously in order to preserve anatomical alignment of the neck. Again, teamwork is essential!

Secondary Survey

Once the primary survey is completed and the athlete is stabilized, the secondary survey begins. The secondary survey involves assessing the whole body from head to toe to check for injuries and simultaneously measuring vital signs including blood pressure and heart rate. Testing should sequentially evaluate the head and neck, pupil size and reactivity, chest, abdomen, pelvis, and extremities. Specific to neurological injuries, a thorough pertinent neurological exam in the secondary survey involves examining the cranial nerves (table 3.1) and performing a formal motor strength assessment (table 3.2) and sensory testing (figures 3.4-3.6) to detect any signs of a head injury, as well as to address and rule out any motor or sensory dysfunction. The secondary survey may not always be feasible at the site of the event and may need to be done once the patient is at the designated emergency medical facility or even in the ambulance while on the way to the hospital. For most athletes, though, the secondary exam can continue on the sideline, or the patient can be taken to the locker room (if available) for further assessment.

Sideline Assessment

Athletes who have not lost consciousness and have been deemed stable via a thorough on-field evaluation may frequently be moved to the sidelines where management can continue and should focus on the injuries sustained. Many personnel have adopted the routine of taking the athlete to the locker room (rather than the sidelines) to perform the postconcussion assessment in order to get away from the crowd, teammates, and commotion of the game. This is preferable, when possible, in order to perform a thorough assessment free of distraction. Once

Table 3.1   Cranial Nerves and Examination

Cranial nerve (CN)	Name	Function	Method of testing
CN I	Olfactory	Special sensory: smell	• Test sense of smell (oranges, coffee)
CN II	Optic	Special sensory: sight	• Visual acuity (Snellen chart) • Visual fields (covering an eye, bring finger toward midline from above, below, sides)
CN III	Oculomotor	Somatic motor: superior and medial inferior rectus, inferior oblique Visceral motor: sphincter pupillae	• Pupillary response to light and accommodation • Ask patient to look medially
CN IV	Trochlear	Somatic motor: superior oblique	• Ask patient to look medially and then downward
CN V	Trigeminal	Somatic sensory: face and anterior 2/3 of tongue Somatic motor: muscles of mastication, tensor tympani, tensor palatini	• Test patient's sensation to touch over all areas of face • Afferent arm of corneal reflex • Ask patient to clench teeth, feel muscles bilaterally • Jaw jerk reflex
CN VI	Abducens	Somatic motor: lateral rectus	• Ask patient to look laterally
CN VII	Facial	Somatic sensory: posterior external ear canal Special sensory: taste, anterior 2/3 of tongue Somatic motor: muscles of facial expression Visceral motor: salivary glands, lacrimal glands	• Ask patient to identify tastes • Ask patient to smile, raise eyebrows, and squeeze eyes tight while observing facial symmetry
CN VIII	Vestibulo-cochlear	Special sensory: auditory, balance	• Weber's test, Rinne's test • Balance examination
CN IX	Glossopha-ryngeal	Somatic sensory: posterior 1/3 of tongue, middle ear Special sensory: taste, posterior 1/3 of tongue Visceral sensory: carotid body, sinus Somatic motor: stylopharyngeus Visceral motor: parotid gland	• CN IX and X usually tested together by asking patient to say "Ah" and observing uvula and soft palate • Uvula and soft palate should demonstrate symmetric elevation • *Note:* Uvula will deviate away from the side of a lesion or injury (toward intact side)
CN X	Vagus	Somatic sensory: external ear Special sensory: taste over epiglottis Visceral sensory: aortic arch, body Somatic motor: soft palate, pharynx, larynx Visceral motor: bronchoconstriction, peristalsis, bradycardia, vomiting	
CN XI	Spinal accessory	Somatic motor: trapezius, sternocleidomastoid	• Ask patient to shrug shoulders against resistance • Ask patient to turn head from side to side against resistance

Cranial nerve (CN)	Name	Function	Method of testing
CN XII	Hypo-glossal	Somatic motor: tongue	• Inspect tongue for size and any abnormal movements (i.e., fasciculations) • Ask patient to protrude tongue in midline • *Note:* Tongue will deviate toward the side of a lesion or injury

Table 3.2   Spinal Nerve Motor Root Distribution and Examination

Segment	Muscle	Action to test	Reflex
C1-C4	Neck muscles	–	–
C3, C4, C5	Diaphragm	Inspiration, forced expiratory volume (FEV$_1$)	–
C5, C6	Deltoid Biceps	Abduct arm >90 degrees Elbow flexion	Biceps reflex
C6, C7	Extensor carpi radialis	Wrist extension	Supinator reflex
C7, C8	Triceps Extensor digitorum	Elbow extension Finger extension	Triceps reflex
C8, T1	Flexor digitorum profundus Hand intrinsics	Grasp Abduct little finger	–
T2-T9	Intercostals	–	–
T9, T10	Upper abdominal muscles	Beevor's sign	Abdominal cutaneous reflex
T11, T12	Lower abdominal muscles	Beevor's sign	Abdominal cutaneous reflex
L2, L3	Iliopsoas	Hip flexion	Cremasteric reflex
L3, L4	Quadriceps	Knee extension	Quadriceps reflex (knee jerk)
L4, L5	Medial hamstrings Tibialis anterior	 Ankle dorsiflexion	–
L5, S1	Lateral hamstrings Posterior tibialis Extensor hallucis longus	Knee flexion Foot inversion Great toe extension	–
S1, S2	Gastrocnemius	Ankle plantar flexion	Achilles reflex (ankle jerk)
S2, S3	Flexor digitorum	–	–
S2-S4	Bladder, lower bowel, anal sphincter	Clamp down during rectal exam	Anal cutaneous reflex (anal wink), bulbocaver-nosus reflex

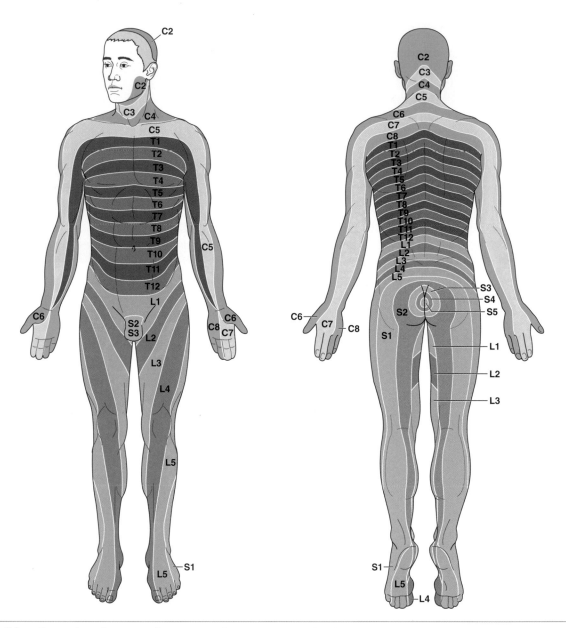

Figure 3.4 Illustration of sensory dermatomes for sensory examination.

the athlete is on the sidelines or in the locker room, if a spinal injury is no longer a concern, the helmet should be taken off and given to the equipment personnel. In this way, one can prevent the athlete from being inadvertently returned to the game without any clearance from the medical team. Symptoms in head-injured athletes may not be obvious during the first few minutes postinjury. Thus, any form of head trauma should be monitored continuously on the sidelines with serial exams. The highly variable nature of concussion requires an individualized approach to injury management, and this is described in further detail in a subsequent chapter. The same close attention should be paid to patients who experience burners or stingers or other peripheral nerve injuries. If the athlete is found to have a normal neurological assessment and is cleared to return to play, the medical staff should still maintain direct contact with the athlete during the remainder of the contest and reassess afterward, as well.

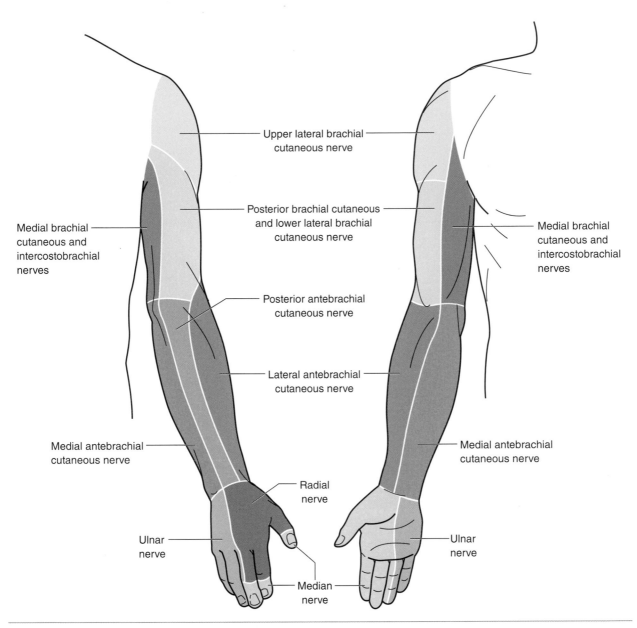

Upper lateral brachial
cutaneous nerve

Posterior brachial cutaneous
and lower lateral brachial
cutaneous nerve

Medial brachial
cutaneous and
intercostobrachial
nerves

Medial brachial
cutaneous and
intercostobrachial
nerves

Posterior antebrachial
cutaneous nerve

Lateral antebrachial
cutaneous nerve

Medial antebrachial
cutaneous nerve

Medial antebrachial
cutaneous nerve

Radial
nerve

Ulnar
nerve

Ulnar
nerve

Median
nerve

Figure 3.5 Cutaneous nerve distribution of the upper limb.

RESPONSIBILITIES OF HOST AND VISITING MEDICAL STAFF

The responsibilities of the host medical and athletic training staff are usually completed before the athletic season. Many of these responsibilities are folded into the formation of the emergency action plan. In general, effective medical coverage for athletic events requires creating a sound working relationship with the medical community in one's area. As mentioned previously, the designated emergency medical facility should be provided with a list of dates, times, and locations of annual athletic events. This direct communication should occur before the start of each season. Often the team physician facilitates this process because of familiarity with hospital personnel and policy.

The host medical staff is responsible for arranging the transportation of an injured athlete to an emergency medical facility, usually securing an

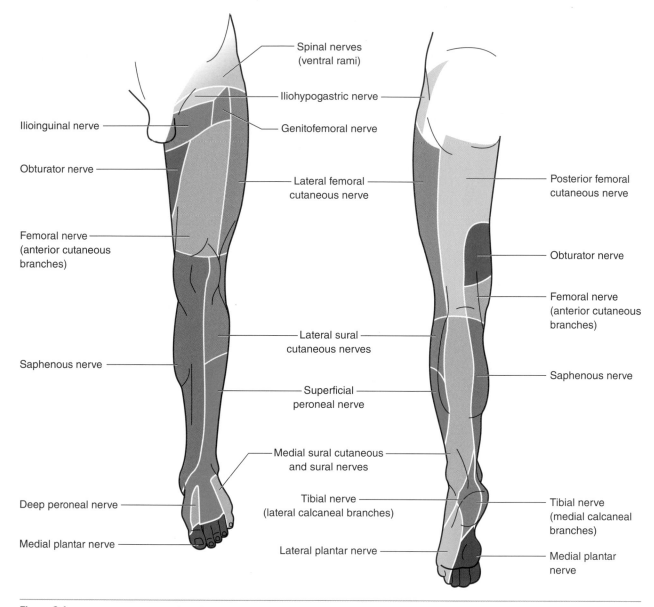

Figure 3.6 Cutaneous nerve distribution of the lower limb.

ambulance on-site or at least having one readily available. Therefore relationships and contractual arrangements need to be made with emergency medical services specialists and ambulance companies before the season starts, as well. Finally, the host medical staff should contact the visiting staff to address any needs that they may have before or during the contest. This may allow the visiting team to make adjustments to the type and amount of equipment and staff needed during travel. In many cases there is a limit to the equipment the traveling medical staff can bring, so communication in advance is helpful. This is

usually less of a concern at the collegiate and professional levels than it is at the high school and youth levels. International venues can add additional complexity in that there may be technology gaps that need to be accounted for.

The visiting medical staff is responsible for communicating with the host upon arrival at the venue. Athletic trainers, physicians, and other medical personnel should meet to discuss the emergency plan and any other pertinent details. The visiting medical staff should also take the time to familiarize themselves with the facility and the venue in its entirety. At the end of an athletic event, the medical staff and trainers from the host and visiting teams typically shake hands and "close the loop" on any outstanding issues or injuries that occurred during the game.

CONCLUDING THOUGHTS

An emergency action plan needs to be developed for any athletic event. All involved with the care and oversight of athletes should be familiarized with the plan so that it can be implemented immediately when necessary and in order to provide appropriate standards of emergency care to all sport participants. The plan should coordinate communication, proper coverage of events, maintenance of appropriate emergency equipment and supplies, use of appropriate emergency medical personnel, and continuing education in the area of emergency medicine and planning. Similarly, once an injury does occur, the approach to the athlete should be a focused, coordinated effort that runs through the primary and secondary surveys in a standard fashion. Hopefully, through careful preparticipation planning, adequate medical coverage, safe practice and training techniques, and other safety measures, potential emergencies will be handled appropriately or even averted.

REFERENCES

1. Sideline preparedness for the team physician: consensus statement. Med Sci Sports Exerc 2001;33(5):846-849.
2. AHA. American Heart Association: Basic Life Support. 2010. Available from: www.heart.org/HEARTORG/CPRAndECC/HealthcareTraining/BasicLifeSupportBLS/Basic-Life-Support-BLS_UCM_001281_SubHomePage.jsp.
3. Andersen J, Courson RW, Kleiner DM, McLoda TA. National Athletic Trainers' Association position statement: emergency planning in athletics. J Athl Train 2002;37(1):99-104.
4. Boissy P, Shrier I, Briere S, Mellete J, Fecteau L, Matheson GO, et al. Effectiveness of cervical spine stabilization techniques. Clin J Sport Med 2011;21(2):80-88.
5. Brown GT. NCAA group raising awareness on medical coverage. NCAA News 1999;15:6-7.
6. Copeland AJ, Decoster LC, Swartz EE, Gattie ER, Gale SD. Combined tool approach is 100% successful for emergency football face mask removal. Clin J Sport Med 2007;17(6):452-457.
7. De Lorenzo RA. A review of spinal immobilization techniques. J Emerg Med 1996;14(5):603-613.
8. De Lorenzo RA, Augustine JJ. Patient positioning. Laying out the options. JEMS 1996;21(2):72-74, 77-82; quiz 88-79.
9. De Lorenzo RA, Olson JE, Boska M, Johnston R, Hamilton GC, Augustine J, et al. Optimal positioning for cervical immobilization. Ann Emerg Med 1996;28(3):301-308.
10. Decoster LC, Shirley CP, Swartz EE. Football face-mask removal with a cordless screwdriver on helmets used for at least one season of play. J Athl Train 2005;40(3):169-173.
11. Del Rossi G, Horodyski M, Conrad BP, Dipaola CP, Dipaola MJ, Rechtine GR. Transferring patients with thoracolumbar spinal instability: are there alternatives to the log roll maneuver? Spine (Phila Pa 1976) 2008;33(14):1611-1615.
12. Del Rossi G, Horodyski M, Heffernan TP, Powers ME, Siders R, Brunt D, et al. Spine-board transfer techniques and the unstable cervical spine. Spine (Phila Pa 1976) 2004;29(7):E134-138.
13. Del Rossi G, Horodyski MH, Conrad BP, Di Paola CP, Di Paola MJ, Rechtine GR. The 6-plus-person lift transfer technique compared with other methods of spine boarding. J Athl Train 2008;43(1):6-13.
14. Dolan MG. Emergency care: planning for the worst. Athl Ther Today 1998;3(1):12-13.
15. Gale SD, Decoster LC, Swartz EE. The combined tool approach for face mask removal during on-field conditions. J Athl Train 2008;43(1):14-20.
16. Griffin LY. Emergency preparedness: things to consider before the game starts. Instr Course Lect 2006;55:677-686.
17. Guskiewicz KM, Broglio SP. Sport-related concussion: on-field and sideline assessment. Phys Med Rehabil Clin N Am 2011;22(4):603-617, vii.
18. Hamilton RS, Pons PT. The efficacy and comfort of full-body vacuum splints for cervical-spine immobilization. J Emerg Med 1996;14(5):553-559.
19. Herbert DL. Legal Aspects of Sports Medicine. Canton, OH: Professional Reports; 1990.
20. Horodyski M, Conrad BP, Del Rossi G, DiPaola CP, Rechtine GR II. Removing a patient from the spine board: is the lift and slide safer than the log roll? J Trauma 2011;70(5):1282-1285; discussion 1285.
21. Johnson DR, Hauswald M, Stockhoff C. Comparison of a vacuum splint device to a rigid backboard for spinal immobilization. Am J Emerg Med 1996;14(4):369-372.
22. Kleiner DM. Emergency management of athletic trauma: roles and responsibilities. Emerg Med Serv 1998;27(10):33-36.
23. Kleiner DM, Glickman SE. Medical considerations and planning for short distance road races. J Athl Train 1994;29(2):145-151.

24. NCAA. 2011-2012 NCAA Sports Medicine Handbook. 22nd ed. Indianapolis: National Collegiate Athletic Association; 2011.

25. NFHS. NFHS Sports Medicine Handbook. 4th ed. Indianapolis: National Federation of State High School Associations; 2011.

26. Olympia RP, Dixon T, Brady J, Avner JR. Emergency planning in school-based athletics: a national survey of athletic trainers. Pediatr Emerg Care 2007;23(10):703-708.

27. Osborne B. Principles of liability for athletic trainers: managing sport-related concussion. J Athl Train 2001;36(3):316-321.

28. Pop Warner. 2012 Coaches Risk Management Handbook. Pop Warner Little Scholars (updated March 19, 2012). Available from: www.popwarner.com/forms.htm.

29. Quandt EF, Mitten MJ, Black JS. Legal liability in covering athletic events. Sports Health 2009;1(1):84-90.

30. Ransone J, Kersey R, Walsh K. The efficacy of the rapid form cervical vacuum immobilizer in cervical spine immobilization of the equipped football player. J Athl Train 2000;35(1):65-69.

31. Rubin A. Emergency equipment: what to keep on the sidelines. Phys Sportsmed 1993;21(9):47-54.

32. Shea JF. Duties of care owed to university athletes in light of Kleinecht. J Coll Univ Law 1995;21:591-614.

33. Swartz EE, Armstrong CW, Rankin JM, Rogers B. A 3-dimensional analysis of face-mask removal tools in inducing helmet movement. J Athl Train 2002;37(2):178-184.

34. Swartz EE, Boden BP, Courson RW, Decoster LC, Horodyski M, Norkus SA, et al. National Athletic Trainers' Association position statement: acute management of the cervical spine-injured athlete. J Athl Train 2009;44(3):306-331.

35. Swartz EE, Decoster LC, Norkus SA, Cappaert TA. The influence of various factors on high school football helmet face mask removal: a retrospective, cross-sectional analysis. J Athl Train 2007;42(1):11-19; discussion 20.

36. Swartz EE, Norkus SA, Cappaert T, Decoster LC. Football equipment design affects face mask removal efficiency. Am J Sports Med 2005;33(8):1210-1219.

37. Travers AH, Rea TD, Bobrow BJ, Edelson DP, Berg RA, Sayre MR, et al. Part 4: CPR overview: 2010 American Heart Association guidelines for cardiopulmonary resuscitation and emergency cardiovascular care. Circulation 2010;122(18 Suppl 3):S676-684.

38. Waeckerle JF. Planning for emergencies. Phys Sportsmed 1991;19(2):35-38.

39. Watkins RG. Neck injuries in football players. Clin Sports Med 1986;5(2):215-246.

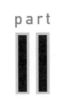
SPORTS-RELATED HEAD INJURIES

In recent years, societal attention to the occurrence of head injuries in athletes has been increasing. Catastrophic brain injuries at all levels of play, as well as concern about the association of chronic neurodegenerative disease with repetitive mild traumatic brain injury, have highlighted some of the well-publicized coverage of this issue. Head injuries can be considered in two broad categories. The first comprises severe traumatic brain injuries, which occur rarely but nevertheless constitute a reproducible number of cases of severe neurologic impairment and death on an annual basis. The second broad category includes mild traumatic brain injury or concussion. These injuries have made the most profound impact on neurologic sports medicine lately. Such injuries are a significant public health issue, in part due to the sheer number of players who potentially sustain a concussion each year, as well as the cumulative effects and potential for long-term sequelae.

Our understanding of the pathophysiology underlying traumatic brain injury, particularly concussion, has improved. We start this section of the book by reviewing the most up-to-date literature regarding the biomechanics and pathophysiology of concussion. Similarly, the evaluation and management of sport-related head injuries have matured and improved at an unprecedented rate. We first discuss the acute assessment of the head-injured athlete. The on-field evaluation, "in the trenches," is the most critical moment for the athlete, as efficient care begins with appropriate identification that a head injury has even occurred. We then provide an overview of the various neuroimaging sequences used to assess the head-injured patient. Additionally, we review the role of neuropsychological testing, balance testing, and other adjunct measures of assessment.

In addition to talking about subconcussion and severe brain injury, we discuss the subacute and chronic sequelae of sport-related brain injury. Finally, we review the literature regarding the management of these injuries, including the pharmacologic management of concussion, natural treatment approaches, the role of rehabilitation, and return-to-play guidelines.

Biomechanics, Pathophysiology, and Classification of Concussion

In collaboration with
Corey T. Walker, MD

For centuries, neurological injuries have occurred in sport. Often, impacts to the head are considered merely part of the game, and in many instances, a player's ability to withstand or "shake off" such blows has been a mark of toughness. It was not until the past few decades that minor hits were recognized as potentially damaging to the brain. A large proportion of head injuries that would be diagnosed as concussions today would have been dismissed 10 years ago as inappreciable impacts of no consequence. Hence, we are still in an upswing of mindfulness and attentiveness among athletes, coaches, trainers, and caregivers regarding concussion in sport. We are also amid an explosion in research and a scientific understanding of how concussions occur, as well as the neurologic alterations that result from them.

In this chapter, we first describe the biomechanics of concussion. That is, how does something colliding with the head change the head's physical properties in space? After this macroscopic study of forces and accelerations, we will be in a position to see how such forces affect single neurons and other cells of the central nervous system on a microscopic level. In turn, this will allow for an exploration of current pathophysiological concepts and studies to date. Lastly, we will take a step back and examine classification systems that have been in place to

grade concussion. This will not only demonstrate some of the clinical aspects of concussion but also provide a historical reference for how diagnostic changes have occurred in the past couple of decades.

BIOMECHANICS AND BASIC CONCEPTS

One of the most complex aspects of concussion as a disease is the uniqueness of each incident. Every concussive insult is slightly different from the last; no two head impacts occur at exactly the same speed or with the same direction, or contain the same mass or occur at exactly the same anatomical location. It is no wonder, then, that the field of concussion research has focused much of its attention on the biomechanical parameters that contribute to head injury. Augmenting the body of knowledge in this area may allow for improved clinical injury identification, as well as advanced prevention and more accurate animal models for research.

Newton's Second Law of Motion

In order to understand the biomechanics of concussion, it is vital that one have sufficient comprehension of the fundamental physics underlying collisions. Specifically, laws of energy transfer, force, acceleration, and momentum play governing roles in injury mechanisms. At the most basic level, Newton's Second Law of Motion enables the visualization of how the forces of head impacts result in head and consequently brain acceleration.

$$\text{Force} = \text{Mass} \times \text{Acceleration}$$

Given this rudimentary equation, and assuming a purely linear impact (no rotation), it can be seen that as the impacting force (e.g., striking player, ball, punch) increases, so will the acceleration of the head, since its mass is constant. Similarly, in instances of rotational force (figure 4.1), or torque, we have

$$\text{Torque} = \text{Moment of Inertia} \times \text{Angular Acceleration.}$$

Therefore, just as with linear forces, increased rotational forces result in a greater amount of rotational head acceleration, as the moment of inertia is also constant. Armed only with these two simple physics concepts, we can appreciate a great deal about concussion biomechanics, as many experts believe linear and angular brain accelerations to be the most predictive variables of head injury.[27]

It can be assumed in most cases of head injury that there are components of both linear and angular forces at work. In order to understand how these two variables come together, the laws relating to conservation of energy need to be examined. That is, the total energy entering a closed system (like that of an insulting blow to the head) is equal to that leaving the system. Therefore, the sum of the kinetic energies of the striking object and of the struck player is equal to the total linear and angular energy imparted to the head plus that energy dissipated to the head. This also includes small amounts of energy emitted as heat and vibration. Determining the degree to which the output energy is linear relative to angular relies on the directionality of the vector forces and the point of impact in relation to the fulcrum point around which the head is rotating (neck). Hence, the speed of the object hitting the head, the velocity of the struck player, and the point of impact on the head are critical values that one must consider when investigating hits to the head.

Law of Momentum Conservation

Likewise, we can institute the Law of Momentum Conservation to witness how muscle contraction and body alignment affect brain velocities. Here we define this law using the following equation, where i refers to initial conditions, or those before impact, and f refers to final conditions, or those after impact:

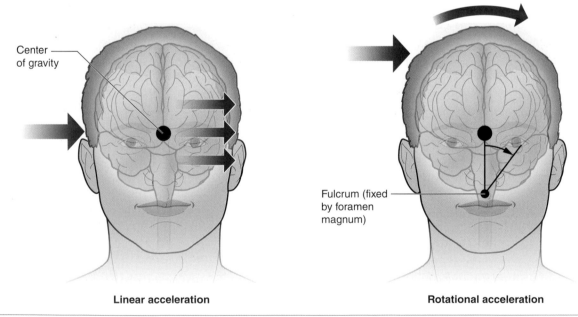

Center of gravity

Linear acceleration

Fulcrum (fixed by foramen magnum)

Rotational acceleration

Figure 4.1 The difference between linear and rotational acceleration with respect to the human brain.

$$v_{object,i} \, m_{object} + v_{player,i} \, (m_{body} + m_{head})$$
$$= v_{object,f} \, m_{object} + v_{body,f} \, m_{body} + v_{head,f} \, m_{head}$$

From this equation, it can be seen that the larger the mass (m) of the striking object (or person) and the faster the velocity (v) it strikes with, the more momentum that will be transferred to the player's head and body. One instance of this that is practically demonstrable in contact sports relates to the relative **effective** mass of a striking player. When a player strikes with his head, neck, and body in alignment, the mass behind the strike is 1.67 times larger than if the hit was made from an upright position. As one can imagine, this imparts much more momentum to the struck player's head and greatly augments the risk for injury.[153]

Conversely, if one looks at increasing the mass of the struck player by coupling his body weight to that of the head ($m_{body} + m_{head}$) during collisions, the effective weight through which the striking momentum can be dispersed is increased. Therefore, by precontracting the neck muscles (to make the head and neck one unit) before a head impact, one can dramatically reduce final head velocities. This implies that if an athlete is struck on the head before he has had a chance to do this, the value of m_{body} in the equation approaches zero, and consequently, all of the momentum of the inciting force is transferred directly to the head. Such theoretical suggestions have been reproduced in the laboratory setting using test dummies: Viano and colleagues showed that increased neck stiffness reduced peak head accelerations and a composite concussion risk identification score, which they termed Head Injury Criterion (HIC).[151] Similarly, data from hockey biomechanical studies demonstrate the heightened head impact severity in unanticipated hits, with players clearly unable to contract their neck muscles before contact.[93] This analysis lends support to the notion that neck strengthening and elevated impact awareness in sports with high incidences of head injury could provide preventive protection against brain injury, an example of biomechanical research having direct neurological sports medicine application.

Although much insight can be derived from this simplified version of the law of momentum conservation, one must also consider the anatomical location of impact in order to visualize how it applies spatially. For example, it can be realized that impacts delivered to a player's torso do not impart the same amount of momentum as those of the same magnitude imparted directly to the head. This is why significant focus has been placed on protecting players in the National Football League (NFL) against helmet-to-helmet contact, as this type of tackling technique grossly increases the risk of concussion in football players.[157] In fact, one study analyzed 174 severe impacts from 1996 to 2001 in the NFL and showed that 107 (62%) of them were the result of helmet-to-helmet impacts.[112]

Acceleration–Deceleration Injury

Concussions result largely from the acceleration–deceleration forces placed on the brain during head impacts. As discussed later in this chapter, this places shearing forces on neurons and other cells in the brain, ultimately leading to most of the pathophysiological changes seen in concussion. In models of head injury in which head acceleration is not allowed and the head is fixed (not allowed to move in either a linear or rotational fashion), considerably more force is required to cause a concussion.[29, 107] In experimental animal models, Ommaya and Gennerelli demonstrated the particular importance of rotational acceleration specifically, as animals were placed under high accelerations with their heads either free to rotate or to translate only in a linear plane.[108] The former group experienced concussions across a range of accelerations, while the latter did not. Likewise, the authors showed that wearing a neck collar protected the brain against concussion, presumably by preventing head rotation. More recent studies have corroborated these findings and have demonstrated the importance of both linear and rotational accelerations in the incidence of concussion.[110, 113]

Brain Slosh

Given the importance of acceleration–deceleration injury, certain theories have been proposed to explain how the kinematic dynamics of the **head** result in harm to the **brain**. In clinical pathologic studies of brain contusions, the phenomenon of coup–contrecoup brain injury (figure 4.2) has been shown in which there is an initial injury to the brain below the site of blunt force (coup) and a resulting injury on the opposite side of the

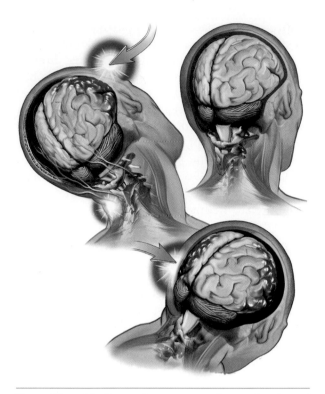

Figure 4.2 This figure demonstrates the mechanism of a coup–contrecoup injury of the brain during impact. As shown, the injury results from the damage produced at the location of direct injury (coup), as well as the damage produced when the momentum of the brain causes it to slam into the opposite side of the bony cranium (contrecoup).

brain (contrecoup) due to what is believed to be the brain's slamming into the other side of the cranial cavity.[48, 98] This contusion pathogenesis helps to depict an important concept, which is that the brain is essentially an object floating in a fluid within a rigid container and has a considerable amount of freedom to move within this compartment. In essence, there is a reserve volume within the cranium filled with cerebrospinal fluid (CSF) through which the brain can accelerate and collide with the skull. This movement has been referred to as brain "slosh" because of the semisolid properties of neural tissue and its surrounding stromal cytoarchitecture.

This notion provides context that enables understanding of the limitations of helmets in preventing concussion. Despite preventing fracture of the skull and limiting the incidence of brain contusion and catastrophic head injury, helmets are unable to mitigate sloshing of the brain. As a result, recent research efforts have focused on reducing this effect by decreasing the volume compliance of the brain. In a study using animal models, Smith and colleagues attempted to do this by increasing intracranial blood volume (blood is much more amenable to changes in volume and pressure) through means of slight compression of the internal jugular vein, thereby reducing this residual volume and increasing intracranial pressure.[137] The results of this methodology showed a significantly reduced extent of axonal injury. The authors posited that decreasing sloshing allows elastic collisions between molecules in the brain rather than imparting frictional, acoustic, and kinetic energies on the cells as a result of the relative motion (shear and collision) between compartments. Though more studies are required to further elucidate the exact mechanisms, such biomechanical interactions likely play a noteworthy role in the mechanism of concussion injury.

LESSONS LEARNED FROM FOOTBALL

As described in the opening chapter of this book, sport-related neurological injuries occur in many sports. However, American football has one of the higher incidences of concussion, largely due to the high rate of impacts and the expanse of participation in this sport.[57] Therefore, the breadth of concussive injuries in football has provided an arena for immense amounts of research. Moreover, due to the mandatory use of helmets, football has an advantage for studying injury biomechanics in that it has a medium by which real-time measurements of impacts can be measured.[27] Hence, it is from this field that we have gained an extensive amount of our knowledge about the forces, velocities, accelerations, and frequencies at which head injuries take place.

Methods of Analysis

In 1994, the NFL formed the Committee on Mild Traumatic Brain Injury. One of the committee's goals was to examine and improve safety equipment. Despite widespread innovation in the helmet industry since the early 1970s, few scientific data existed to predict the amount of protection provided by helmet use. At that point, the committee pursued its own independent research on the biomechanics and causes of mild traumatic brain injury (mTBI) and shared its results with the National Operating Committee on Standards for Athletic Equipment (NOCSAE), helmet manufacturers, researchers, and clinicians in this field.[111]

The first report from this group examined 182 concussive and subconcussive (but severe) hits that occurred in the NFL between 1996 and 2001.[113] Only incidents that were caught on two or more game-time cameras were included. Using this video footage, the group was able to very accurately reconstruct each of the impacts on Hybrid III anthropometric test dummies (Humanetics Innovative Solutions, Plymouth, MI), the same models used previously for safety investigations in the automotive industry. Fitted with football helmets, the anthropometric test devices (ATDs) enabled measurements of translational (linear) acceleration through installation of a standard accelerometer in the center of the head and rotational acceleration with nine linear accelerometers strategically placed in a 3–2–2–2 configuration around the head. Kinematic analysis of these reconstructions was then performed by calculations based on two high-speed cameras to ensure accuracy of the models. Based on their

scrutiny of the methodology used, the group calculated a maximum theoretical error of 15% of peak value, with most measurements falling much below this level.[103]

Despite the relative accuracy of this approach simulating real impacts, certain limitations exist. Certainly, the use of ATDs rather than real players in studies limits some of the conclusions that can be drawn. Furthermore, this dataset dealt with only one specific inciting hit and did not take into account the hits that the players took before getting a concussion. Not only would the latter allow researchers to get quantification of **all** the hits given and received, it would also allow for analysis of cumulative effects and whether previous impact "dosages" cause a predilection for concussive injury. Subsequent studies built off of some of these limitations and furthered the field. Duma and coauthors first reported the use of novel acceleration-measuring helmets that could be used by players during practice and games.[30] This technology, termed the Head Impact Telemetry System (HITS; Simbex LLC, Lebanon, OH), uses the Sideline Response System (Ridell Corp., Elyria, OH) in order to relay measurements of six spring-loaded single-axis accelerometers loaded in the helmets to a computer on the sidelines (figure 4.3). In addition to

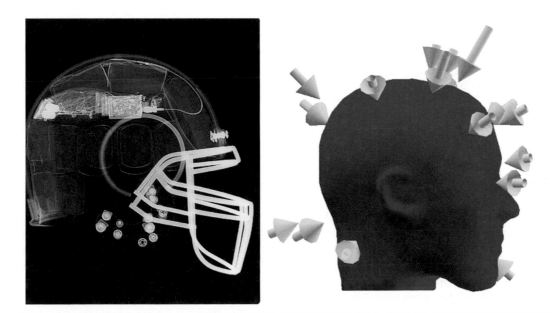

Figure 4.3 X-ray view of the Head Impact Telemetry System fitted into an American football helmet (figure courtesy of Simbex, LLC). The head figure, generated by the HIT System software, indicates impact location and magnitude by arrow placement and length.

reports of accelerations, the HIT System localizes the point of contact on the head. Such data allow researchers to fully compile all the impacts that players incur during a season and to describe variables that may contribute to increased risk for neurological injury. To date, this has been the most widely implemented system to study human impact biomechanics in vivo within sport.

Recent research has looked at modifications of this system in order to allow for direct measurements of angular kinematics given the important role that angular rotation plays in concussion pathogenesis.[126, 127] Though rotational accelerations can be calculated using the HIT System, rotational velocities cannot, making it difficult to measure the temporal component of the impact pulses. Such information has been shown to be important, as rotational head accelerations of great magnitudes can be tolerated over very short durations, but this tolerance decreases as the duration goes up. Therefore, a newly adapted six degrees of freedom (6DOF) system, which uses 12 custom-oriented accelerometers (distinct from the arrangement of the six in the HIT System), has been devised to directly measure both of these factors. Initial studies using these devices have corroborated values seen with the HIT System, thereby demonstrating the overall reliability of these methods.[126]

Impact Frequency

One of the most interesting epidemiological components of impact biomechanics in American football is the sheer number of hits (concussive and subconcussive) a player takes to the head in a given season. This is revisited in chapter 11 on subconcussion. There have been various reports on the number of collisions that the average collegiate player sustains, and there is some amount of variation in the results between studies. This may be due to relative differences in the number of games and contact practices that various teams participate in or opt to study for a given season. Additionally, the threshold point that each study used in order for the minimum force to be considered a hit may be different, thereby creating a slight incongruity in methodologies. In any case, even in the more conservative estimates, college players are experiencing on average 900 to 1,000 hits per season.[23, 30, 92, 130] Two major studies of high school football players found

similar individual player hit frequencies of 520 and 652 per season.[16, 130] This is quite alarming given that in high school players the brain is not fully developed. Emerging evidence is indicating that the minimal amount of damage that occurs with even subconcussive hits could feasibly carry a cumulative injurious effect.

Impact Magnitude

While impact frequency constitutes an important portion of the picture of head injury in football, it is vital to also consider the magnitude of impacts. It is evident that a player can receive a thousand hits in a season and never sustain a concussion, just as easily as a player can get struck only one time in a season and have this be concussive. Therefore, many recent studies have aimed to use the HIT System technology to scrutinize acceleration vectors and compare them for concussive and subconcussive hits.

Interestingly, current results have shown only few differences in average accelerations (linear and angular) over the course of a season between high school and collegiate athletes despite the physical differences in strength and speed between these two levels of play.[16] It is not until one examines the distribution of the magnitudes, and specifically the subset of hardest impacts, that differences in intensity and number emerge, with collegiate athletes experiencing high-acceleration impacts more often.[32, 130] This may create suspicion that collegiate players are at higher risk for concussion than high school athletes. However, that does not appear to be the case based on epidemiological studies, as discussed previously.[51, 116]

As expected, though, a recent study examining impact exposure in even younger players (7- to 8-year-olds) demonstrated that overall accelerations were lower in this population.[25] That being said, linear accelerations ranged from 10 g (threshold to be counted by HIT System) to 100 g and angular accelerations from 52 rad/s^2 to 7,694 rad/s^2, indicating that these players are still at risk of concussive injury. Of note, the authors reported that of the 38 impacts measured in the 95% of linear accelerations (>40 g), 76% of them occurred during practices. Also worth noting is that of those impacts greater than 80 g, all eight took place in practices, as well. Hence, impact exposure in young football players with developing brains can be greatly reduced through evaluation and restructuring of practices so that drills entailing full contact are minimized and emphasis is placed instead on correct tackling techniques and learning fundamentals.

Another key finding from these seasonal impact exposure studies pertains to positional differences in hit frequency and magnitude. One might expect that players on the line consistently experience different impact biomechanics from players in the open field. In a study of 72 collegiate players, Mihalik and colleagues showed that offensive and defensive linemen experienced the brunt of all impacts recorded over two seasons (35.52% and 21.99%, respectively), with offensive backs, defensive backs, linebackers, and wide receivers sustaining many fewer (12.39%, 15.37%, 10.33%, and 4.39%, respectively). [92] Furthermore, a strong association between high-magnitude impacts and position was seen. In particular, offensive backs had a 1.52, 1.41, 1.24, 1.17, and 1.03 times greater probability of receiving an impact of 80 g acceleration than defensive linemen, defensive backs, offensive linemen, linebackers, and wide receivers, respectively. Therefore, it can be seen that while line players have a greater frequency of contact, running backs and receivers are more likely to encounter harder blows to the head. In 20 concussions reported by Eckner and colleagues, only 5 occurred in offensive or defensive linemen compared to 7 among offensive backs and wide receivers or tight ends, a clearly disproportionate amount considering the total number of hits sustained in a given season and the relative number of players at these two positions at any one time.[32]

Additionally, when examining impact locations, one sees variations in frequencies at which different portions of the helmet get hit. As would be expected, hits to the face mask are the most common, followed by those to the back and the top of the head, with the sides being struck the least. More importantly, the average magnitude of impacts differs based on impact location, with the top of the head resulting in the highest linear accelerations (29.22 g). This is compared to the hits to all other portions of the helmet having average accelerations less than 21.71 g.[92] These data correspond to reports of impact locations in concussion. Guskiewicz and coauthors reported on 13 demonstrated concussions in collegiate

players; nearly half (6/13) occurred due to hits to the top of the helmet.[50] Of the other injuries, four were to the face mask, two were to the right side, and only one was to the back of the helmet.

While this research is mostly descriptive, it provides important details that may someday help protect American football players from undue injury. For example, coaches can use such data to aid in teaching their players to lead blocks with their arms rather than their heads in order to minimize the frequency of impacts. All players in general should attempt to avoid leading with their heads down to prevent hits to the top of their helmets. Perhaps this information also will guide safety equipment manufacturers in their design of the next generation of helmets.

Concussion Threshold

As mentioned earlier, many attempts have been made to compare the biomechanics of concussive and subconcussive hits. Ultimately, the goal of such pursuits is to find a threshold of one or more parameters above which a concussion will occur and below which one will not. Given the subtlety or lack of clinical symptoms exhibited by many concussed athletes, this would be tremendously helpful in the screening of injured players on the sidelines, especially if an experienced caregiver is not on-site. However, despite repeated attempts to find this threshold, such cutoffs have proven of little diagnostic value due to their limited sensitivity, specificity, or both. Again, the emerging evidence is indicating that such a distinction may not necessarily be as important as identifying the role that the total impact burden may play in both concussion occurrence and more long-term sequelae.

In animal studies, researchers have tried to recreate head accelerations in order to find a value at which they could consistently generate a mTBI. Hodgson and colleagues used a short-duration impact model in monkeys and found that concussions were caused by linear accelerations of 2,000 to 5,000 g.[55] Along the same lines, Unterharnscheidt reported that he could produce a concussion with rotational accelerations of 200 rad/s^2 in most of his subjects.[146] However, in humans, the range over which concussions and subconcussive injuries occurs varies greatly. In 1964, in an effort to better understand acceleration tolerance in automobile crashes, Gurdjian and coauthors proposed the Wayne State University Concussion Tolerance Curve, which was a functional probability equation based on impact duration and magnitude.[49] It suggested that an impact below 80 g would be "noninjurious," but that impacts greater than 90 g could likely cause a mTBI. Likewise, after performing the previously described studies, Pellman and colleagues claimed that a threshold of 70 to 75 g would likely cause a mTBI based on their recreation of NFL impacts.[113] However, in the study described by Guskiewicz and colleagues,[50] concussions were reported at accelerations as low as 60.5 g and 163.4 rad/s² (range: 60.5-168.7 g, 163.4-8,994.4 rad/s²; mean: 102.8 g, 5,311.6 rad/s²), and only seven of 1,858 (<0.38%) impacts over 80 g produced mTBI.[92] There is an obvious problem, then, with use of these values as a cutoff, as they are highly nonspecific with regard to detection. Still, if one increases the threshold value any further, the sensitivity of the screen decreases, as an 80 g cutoff already misses a fair number of injuries.

Zhang and coauthors also created a brain injury model, one that mimicked the anatomical structures of an average adult male head and was validated against cadaveric data.[164] Using this model, the group was able to apply finite element analysis to predict that linear accelerations of 66, 82, and 106 g or angular accelerations of 4,600 rad/s², 5,900 rad/s², and 7,900 rad/s² were associated with 25%, 50%, and 80% probability of concussion, respectively. Still, the data from actual American football participation suggest that these values overestimate probabilities for injury.[50, 92] Another interesting study by McCaffrey and colleagues casts doubt on the ability to predict clinical outcomes based on an acceleration threshold.[85] Again using collegiate athletes, they took 22 players who sustained a greater than 90 g impact without developing concussion and compared their cognitive and balance scores (against their preinjury baseline) to those of a control group of players who received no impact measuring greater than 60 g acceleration. They found that the high-magnitude impact group did not experience any decline in scores relative to controls, thereby indicating that one should not expect a 90 g impact to automatically indicate functional decreases or concussion even though it is well above purported cutoffs.

Other groups have therefore attempted to incorporate different parameters into predicting injury risks. Greenwald and coauthors applied a principal component analysis to create a predictive variable, called HITsp, based on the weighting of several parameters including linear acceleration, rotational acceleration, Head Injury Criterion, Gadd Severity Index (GSI; another injury severity criterion developed by the automotive industry), and impact location.[47] They found that this equation was a stronger predictor of concussion risk and that a HITsp score greater than 63 was an indication of a 75% injury risk. Still, it is clear from the results of these studies that a single variable threshold remains an elusive goal. It is important for such methods to be highly specific and highly sensitive so that players are not underdiagnosed. More research will be needed before HIT technology can be used for accurate sideline concussion diagnosis or for predicting occurrence. Hence, having a high degree of suspicion and appropriately trained personnel continues to be the most efficacious method of detecting concussion in sports.

LESSONS LEARNED FROM OTHER SPORTS

While American football has drawn a lot of attention, we have learned much regarding the biomechanics of sport-related head injuries from sports such as boxing, hockey, and soccer. Here we review the literature published in these fields.

Boxing

Despite the vast history of boxing and organized fighting, close medical attention to the longstanding changes that exist in the brains of boxers did not arise until the 1980s.[2, 70] It was at that time that growing concern about pathologic changes seen in postmortem brains of boxers led researchers to focus on the pathogenesis of chronic mTBI-mediated brain damage. However, since then, a paucity of studies have focused on the biomechanics of punches. This is somewhat surprising given the readily apparent proclivity for head injury in the sport. One study estimated that of all the punches thrown in boxing, 70% are to the head.[163]

In comparison to American football, one can also readily appreciate that boxing causes a significantly larger number of subdural hematomas and acute brain injury deaths.[146] Indeed, this must be accounted for by differences in protective equipment and impact biomechanics. As in football, initial biomechanical studies in boxing were performed using surrogate dummy models. One of the first studies employing such techniques was reported by Atha and colleagues, who used a ballistic pendulum to estimate forces and accelerations produced by punches of a world-ranked heavyweight boxer.[7] They estimated an impact force of 6,320 N and roughly 53 g of linear acceleration.

More recently, Walilko and colleagues [154] and Viano and colleagues[152] used the same Hybrid III dummies from football reenactments to simulate different boxing punches to the head. Olympic boxers were allowed to warm up and then were instructed to deliver two impacts with four different punch types: straight punches to the jaw and forehead, an uppercut with the dominant hand, and a hook to the temple with the nondominant hand. Impact acceleration, location, and force were determined using force accelerometers in the dummies and high-speed video. Additionally, the authors calculated effective punch mass by measuring the anthropometric data of each boxer's hand. The studies showed that the hook generated the most impact force compared to the other three punch types, a finding not entirely surprising to individuals familiar with the sport. These hits generated on average 71.2 g of linear acceleration and 9,306 rad/s² of rotational acceleration, values well within the concussive range seen in American football injuries. Secondly, the studies demonstrated that by lining up the wrist behind the hand, boxers are able to increase the effective mass of their punches, thereby generating more force. This is analogous to how tackling players in football increase their effective mass by lining up their body behind their point of contact. Still, it is of note that the effective striking mass of a boxer's punch is small compared to that of a football player's body.

Lastly, and perhaps most importantly, these studies demonstrated that boxing tends to generate significantly more rotational acceleration than linear acceleration, especially when compared to impacts in American football.[152] The authors

suggested that this may be the consequence of an increased effective radius from the head's center of gravity and point of origin in rotation. [152] They also suggested that the coefficient of friction between gloved hands and bare skin was greater than that between helmets or between helmets and jersey or skin. This may result in decreased rotational impact forces in football and consequent subconscious adjustments by football players to strike more squarely through the head center of gravity, causing relatively increased linear forces. Such increases in rotational involvement in boxing are significant clinically, as they may explain the increased incidence of subdural hematomas. Enhanced rotational forces may impart shearing strains on the bridging veins of the brain, increasing the likelihood for them to rupture and bleed into the subdural space (figure 4.4).

Despite the intriguing data, these studies were limited, much as those in American football

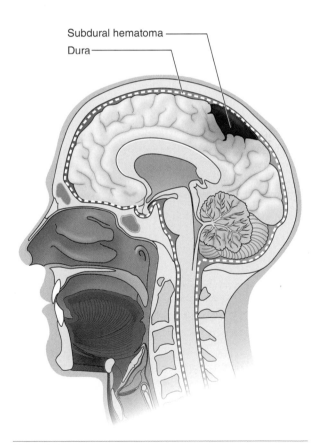

Figure 4.4 Tears in the veins that bridge from the surface of the brain to the dura can result in bleeding and accumulation of blood in the subdural space.

studies were, by their imperfect biofidelity. As a result, Stojsih and colleagues decided to employ HIT technology in boxing headgear (a system called Impact Boxing Headgear [IBH]) to evaluate punch mechanics during sparring sessions in male and female amateur boxers.[141] Overall, they measured somewhat lower average accelerations; 30 g (max: 191 g) and 2,571 rad/s² (max: 17,156 rad/s²) for men and 28 g (max: 184 g) and 2,533 rad/s² (max: 13,113 rad/s²) for women. Therefore, based on their findings, while most punches produced subconcussive blows, peak accelerations were definitely above proposed thresholds for both sexes. Moreover, these authors showed that between-sex differences were seen only with peak accelerations and impact frequency, not with mean accelerations, GSI, or HIC. However, these measurements were taken during sparring bouts and may not be entirely reflective of values seen in actual fights or those bouts in which no headgear is worn.

Further, the study revealed that impacts to the side and back of the head exhibited on average higher accelerations and HIC scores compared to those to the front of the head.[141] It is projected that this may be a result of a lack of neck muscle preactivation as described for American football. Since more than half of the impacts occurred to the front of the head, boxers may be more in anticipation of hits to this location, leaving them vulnerable to punches on opposing parts of the head. Hence, an order of injury prevention in boxing may come from educating participants about protecting themselves from punches to the back and side of the head, as well.

Hockey

Though hockey is not as popular as football in the United States, it is the dominant sport of many geographic regions, including Canada, parts of Europe, Russia, and countries of the former Soviet Union. As in football, despite the required usage of protective equipment and helmets, concussions are common.[156] Fast game play, hard ice, perimeter boards, flying pucks (sometimes moving in excess of 80 miles per hour [128 km/h]), collisions, checking, and illegal on-ice activity all contribute to the risk of playing this physical sport. Additionally, hockey is the only organized sport other than boxing

and mixed martial arts that accepts fighting as part of the game. Consequently, biomechanically analyzing concussion in this sport is difficult due to the heterogeneity of potential insults. In fact, the biomechanics of concussions resulting from fighting may be better understood by examination of the previously discussed data from boxing than from the literature published on hockey. Nevertheless, several studies have examined true game-time impacts. Furthermore, many of these studies have involved children as the subjects, as there is significant contention in many countries over the minimum age at which youth players should be allowed to begin checking, with some allowing it as early as 9 years old. Undoubtedly, significant research must be performed regarding impact biomechanics in these young players in order to determine the potential risks associated with play.

One of the first studies in hockey players fitted a high school defenseman with a helmet containing a triaxial accelerometer and compared game-time impacts to those in age-matched football offensive and defensive linemen.[102] Given the equipment used to measure the impacts, only linear acceleration could be calculated. Likewise, values of acceleration may have been slightly overestimated. Still, the consistency of devices allowed for comparison between the two sports. Interestingly, the authors observed that fewer hits occur per hour in hockey games than in football games. Moreover, they demonstrated that while maximum-impact accelerations were in the same range, the average linear accelerations for the hockey players were larger (35.0 g) than for the football players (29.2 g). The authors also noted that the collisions resulting in the highest accelerations were those between players and the boards. However, the small sample size greatly limited the power of this study.

A more recent study by Gwin and coauthors used HIT technology in the helmets of a small sample of men's National Collegiate Athletic Association (NCAA) hockey players over the course of two seasons.[52] They found that approximately 80% of all impacts sustained were between 10 g and 30 g and that the top 1%, 2%, and 5% of all linear accelerations were 104.9, 90.0, and 62.4 g, respectively. Additionally, they reported that 33.2% of hits were to the back of the head, 32.6% were to the side, 26.5% were to the front, and 7.8% were to the top. Most commonly, the highest-acceleration impacts were to the back of the head; this was consistent with epidemiological data dating back to the 1960s, which showed that this was the most critical area for protection of the head. In contrast, it was found that collisions to the facemask and forehead were consistently of lower magnitude.

Another study of NCAA players, by Brainard and coauthors, sought to compare biomechanics between men and women.[15] In contrast to the situation with men's hockey, NCAA regulations do not allow body and board checking in women's competitions, though significant body contact does still occur. Interestingly, reports from the NCAA on incidences of concussion in both leagues showed higher rates of concussion in women.[3] Yet the study by Brainard and colleagues, using a larger cohort, demonstrated a much higher hit frequency among men than women, thought to be secondary to checking regulations.[15] Furthermore, the highest percentage of linear and angular accelerations experienced in men was higher than that in women. That is, women were 1.1 times as likely to experience an impact of less than 50 g, while men were 1.3 and 1.9 times more likely to experience an impact over 100 g and 5,000 rad/s², respectively. Therefore, despite having a lower impact frequency and intensity, women, for unknown reasons, have higher concussion risks. This suggests that there might be additional extrinsic and intrinsic factors specific to sex that modulate the relationship between mTBI and impact biomechanics. It is speculated that this could be due to physiologic differences between the sexes such as neck strength and hormones, or possibly due to differences in reporting patterns.

A series of other studies focused on youth hockey (Bantam [13-14 years old] and Midget [15-16 years old]) and provided widely applicable information about impact biomechanics.[93-96] Specifically, one of the studies compared impact characteristics for different playing positions, event types, and impact locations.[95, 96] Compared to findings in American football, mean accelerations (18.4 g, 1,464.5 rad/s²) and frequency (223 per season) were slightly lower overall (see above discussion of biomechanics in American football). Likewise, the most severe hits recorded (95% of all hits) were on average still well below puta-

tive concussion thresholds (45.6 g, 4,150.1 rad/s²). Examination of positions, forwards versus defensemen, demonstrated no differences in linear or angular accelerations. However, comparison of event types showed that rotational accelerations and HITsp scores were significantly higher in games than during practices. More striking is the relative frequency of hits in games (61 per game) compared to practices (22 per practice). These data should prompt coaches to emphasize safe contact drills during practices in order to better prepare players for the hard hits that occur in games. Another important finding relating to player safety was that hits to the top of the head resulted in significantly higher linear accelerations than those to other locations on the head. Furthermore, another study showed trends toward greater accelerations in those instances in which an imminent hit was unanticipated.[93] This highlights the need for instruction of younger players to keep their heads up so that they can become aware of their surroundings and skate through impending collisions. Additionally, it highlights the risk that younger players with less skill have for head injuries when checking is permitted.

Another of these studies quantified the additional risk of illegal hits in the setting of Bantam players with allowable checking.[94] Of all 665 hits examined, 17.3% were deemed illegal. Of these, 17.4% were boarding or charging infractions; 16.5% were checks from behind; and 66.1% were due to elbowing, intentional head contact, or high sticking to the head. This is significant, as infractions, especially those in the latter group, resulted in higher HITsp scores than legal collisions did. A similar study by Brust and colleagues showed that 15% of all injuries were deemed intentional and 34% of all injuries happened in games characterized as hostile.[17] Based on these data and a growing body of evidence regarding the recklessness and violence-tolerating nature of youth hockey,[41] significant efforts are required to guide young players away from this mentality. A recent prospective study underlined the importance of doing so and showed that players, if taught, retain such information about injury risks throughout the season.[31] Again, this points to the importance of coaches, trainers, and officials understanding how biomechanics affects concussion risks in order to promote player safety at all levels.

Soccer

Soccer continues to be the world's most popular sport. Just as with the sports previously discussed, head impacts are considered a necessary part of the sport; in this case, heading is used to stop, deflect, or redirect high-speed kicks. However, in soccer, head-to-ball contact is only part of the picture, with player–player, player–ground, and player–goal collisions likely, as well. In fact, only 12.6% of soccer concussions occur from head–ball contact, with head–player (head, arm, and leg of opposing player) composing 40% and head–ground and head–goal making up the remaining 10.3% (roughly one-third of injuries were not specified).[14] Furthermore, the same prospective study of U.S. collegiate players found that none of the head–ball concussions were the result of intentional heading; rather, all were associated with being accidentally struck by a high-speed ball. Therefore, in describing the biomechanics of head injury in soccer, one must inspect the physical characteristics associated with intentional heading of the ball, which is subconcussive, as well the unintentional impacts that ultimately cause concussions.

Heading is a complex maneuver that includes three stages: preimpact, ball contact, and follow-through. It involves an active engagement of multiple muscle groups throughout the body and can involve any portion of the head, though common teaching advocates that impacts be absorbed on an individual's front hairline.[139] In order to prevent the head from recoiling backward, neck flexor and extensor muscles must be contracted at the same time.[73] Therefore, great disparity in heading kinematics exists between players of different size, age, skill, and strength. Moreover, when applying the laws of conservation of momentum and energy to this specific scenario, it is important to look at the relative masses of the head and the object (ball). The human head weighs approximately 5 kg while the regulation soccer ball weighs 0.45 kg. Players who are younger and thus have a smaller head experience higher resulting head velocities and accelerations. Neck contraction has been shown in models of heading to reduce linear head accelerations, thereby highlighting the vulnerability of younger players with reduced neck strength.[133] Therefore, it is especially important that young players use age-appropriate reduced ball sizes.

Naunheim and coauthors sought to characterize some of these accelerations of heading in adults.[101] They found that the heads of players during this movement experience had approximately 15 to 20 g of linear acceleration and 1,000 to 2,000 rad/s^2 of rotational acceleration when the ball approaches at 9 to 12 m/s. These values are roughly similar to those mentioned earlier for hockey and football, especially if one considers that soccer balls can fly two or three times that fast in real game situations. Therefore, these authors also reported impact energies and momentums imparted as 18 to 51 J and 4 to 7 J, which when compared to those seen in professional football (312-916 J, 99-179 N)[152] and hockey checking (121-238 J, 49-68 N)[125] are significantly less powerful, perhaps reflecting the differences in incidences of concussions.

In a study of nonheading head impacts in Fédération Internationale de Football Association (FIFA) matches, Withnall and colleagues reconstructed 62 cases of subconcussive hits.[157] Of these, 38% were contacts with other players' upper extremities and 30% were contacts with other players' heads, percentages similar to those reported by other groups.[4] Within these subsets of impacts, the authors demonstrated that head-to-hand or head-to-forearm impacts produced on average linear accelerations of 20.4 g and rotational accelerations of 1,445 rad/s^2. However, with head-to-head impacts at higher speeds of 3.0 m/s, the linear accelerations generated ranged from 79.0 to 86.7 g and rotational accelerations from 3,100 rad/s^2 to 7,033 rad/s^2, which could certainly put players at risk for concussion. Again, this indicates the need for heightened awareness of the dangers associated with such collisions.

Another interesting finding relates to sex differences in concussion rates among soccer players. As in hockey, women experience significantly higher concussion rates than men; and interestingly, a large proportion of them are due to headers.[40, 42] However, in contrast to findings for hockey, females, according to a study of collegiate soccer players, experienced 10% to 44% larger accelerations during impacts than their male counterparts. It is speculated that this was predominantly due to the measured decreases in their head mass and neck strength, although other unknown variables could contribute as well. The same study showed that the female athletes in the sample did not benefit from protective head equipment. Therefore, surveillance among coaches and trainers working with female soccer players should be augmented as long as concussion rates remain high.

PATHOPHYSIOLOGY OF CONCUSSION

As seen from this discussion of head injury biomechanics, there is a vast array of scenarios in which concussion can occur in sports. However, understanding the kinematics, mechanics, and forces that contribute to mTBI allows for only a gross comprehension of how damage is occurring to the brain. To fully grasp how this happens requires additionally delving into the molecular changes that occur as a result of these accelerations and strains. As discussed in the following sections, the pathophysiology of concussion involves a complex interplay between the cells of the brain, thereby leading to certain clinical manifestations. It should be noted that while sizable gains have been made in our comprehension of what occurs microscopically after head injury, pathological analysis has been difficult to research in humans, and large gaps in our knowledge about this disease remain. Nevertheless, this section presents current theories and study results in order to provide insight into what we know of the pathogenesis of concussion. A recent review by Dashnaw and colleagues covers many of the pathophysiological aspects of concussion.[27]

Neurometabolic Cascade

In 1941, Denny-Brown and Russell first described the lack of neuropathologic changes in a primate model of concussion.[28] Since then, contention has existed over whether the changes that occur in mTBI are short-lived or involve long-term histologic changes.[87] Today, the overwhelming consensus agrees with these authors' original findings and suggests that there are also no macroscopic pathologic findings associated with these injuries, such as the cerebral edema, subarachnoid hemorrhage, contusions, or hematomas that often accompany more severe TBI.[88] Therefore, it is believed that the symptoms of concussion must result largely from a transient functional disturbance of neuronal and parenchymal cells rather than overt neuronal destruction.

As discussed previously, linear and rotational accelerations are pivotal components in our biomechanical understanding of how concussion occurs. It is thought that such changes in velocity result in shear stresses to neurons, thereby resulting in a neurometabolic cascade of events and axonal disruption[91] (figure 4.5). One of the first of such events is a dysregulation of channels within the neuronal plasmalemma (cell membrane) that allows for uncontrolled ion flux.[36] Biochemically, this causes a sudden liberation of potassium, certain neurotransmitters, and excitatory amino acids (EAAs), particularly glutamate.[35, 64] Glutamate then acts on several receptors, including N-methyl-D-aspartate (NMDA) receptors, causing further depolarization and calcium influx into the neuron. As a result, adenosine triphosphate (ATP)-dependent pumps are forced to work in overdrive in order to restore ionic homeostasis. Such compensatory energy expenditure drives glucose hypermetabolism starting approximately 30 minutes after injury.[65, 162] However, after 5 to 6 hours, a transition to a hypometabolic state predominates, lasting up to 5 days or longer with more severe TBIs.[10] Consequently, more glycolysis and anaerobic respiration occur and local extracellular acidosis follows, possibly contributing to further membrane permeability.[62]

In addition to the alterations in cellular metabolism, a neurophysiologic phenomenon occurs due to the sudden depolarization of neurons. In 1944, Leao described the propagation of a wave of electrical activity depression across the cerebral cortex of rabbits, which is termed cortical spreading depression.[72] It is believed that this same spreading depression occurs in the setting of mTBI.[68] Essentially the surge of depolarizations acts as short-circuit waves that rapidly activate neurons and astrocytes en masse and interrupt local cortical function. It has been suggested that such neuronal suppression may be a basis for the migraine and seizure symptoms sometimes associated with concussion.[8, 34, 142] Additionally, a recent report suggests that this neurophysiologic abnormality may be closely tied to cerebral perfusion and may play a role in the secondary neural injury seen after severe TBI.[53]

Another major problem is that the glutamate-mediated accumulation of intracellular calcium ions contributes to mitochondrial oxidative dysfunction.[74, 122, 149, 159] Hovda and coauthors

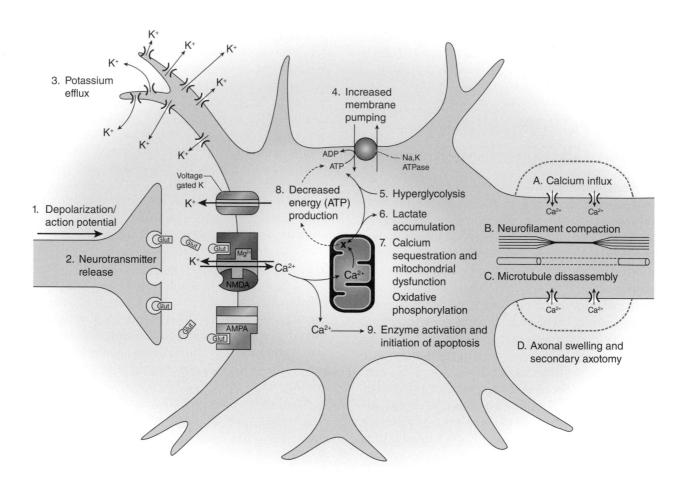

Figure 4.5   Neurometabolic cascade following traumatic injury. (1) Nonspecific depolarization and initiation of action potentials. (2) Release of excitatory neurotransmitters (EAAs). (3) Massive efflux of potassium. (4) Increased activity of membrane ionic pumps to restore homeostasis. (5) Hyperglycolysis to generate more adenosine triphosphate (ATP). (6) Lactate accumulation. (7) Calcium influx and sequestration in mitochondria leading to impaired oxidative metabolism. (8) Decreased energy (ATP) production. (9) Calpain activation and initiation of apoptosis. (A) Axolemmal disruption and calcium influx. (B) Neurofilament compaction via phosphorylation or sidearm cleavage. (C) Microtubule disassembly and accumulation of axonally transported organelles. (D) Axonal swelling and eventual axotomy. K^+, potassium; Na^+, sodium; Glut, glutamate; $Mg2^+$, magnesium; $Ca2^+$, calcium; NMDA, N-methyl-D-aspartate; AMPA, d-amino-3-hydroxy-5-methyl-4-isoxazole-propionic acid.

Reprinted, by permission, C.C. Giza and D.A. Hovda, 2001, "The neurometabolic cascade of concussion," Journal of Athletic Training 36(3): 228-235.

showed that a marker of oxidative function, cytochrome oxidase, is downregulated after injury in rodent models up to 10 days after mTBI.[58] Certainly, this is disadvantageous for a brain in a hypermetabolic state with already reduced ATP, and it is believed that it exacerbates the cascade of events in acute concussion. Current research is examining the use of energy sources other than glucose as a substrate for energy production. Recent evidence from a study in rats has suggested that ketones may be applicable to this end, as a ketogenic diet improved lesion volume and behavioral outcomes in this model.[6, 117]

Of note, calcium regulation can vary greatly depending on several factors. One of these, the NMDA channel activity, is interesting because it appears to play a specific role in postinjury pathogenesis. The NMDA channel is a tetramer composed of two NMDA receptor-1 (NR1) and two NR2 subunits. In rat brains, it has been shown that there is a shift during development from NR2B (slow channels) to NR2A (fast channels).[24] However, in injury models, the NR2A expression is downregulated from day 2 until day 4 after insult, while NR2B and NR1 levels remain constant.[46] Levels of NR2A return to

Biomechanics, Pathophysiology, and Classification of Concussion • • • **91**

normal by 7 days, indicating that perhaps this is an innate neuroprotective mechanism to minimize calcium influx and its injurious effects. Additionally, NMDA channels have been strongly associated with neurocognitive abilities, specifically learning, long-term potentiation (synaptic basis of learning and memory), and long-term depression, which may help explain some of the symptomatology of concussion.[76, 144]

As mentioned previously, pathologic evidence suggests that concussion does not normally include neuronal death as part of its pathogenesis. Therefore, elevated intracellular calcium may lead to impaired mitochondrial function, but neurons typically survive. This is corroborated by animal models of moderate concussion showing that calcium accumulations peak by day 2 and persist only 4 days out.[39] In contrast, in studies of more severe TBI, calcium levels remain elevated much longer, and it is believed that under these circumstances, neuronal death occurs.[109] In this situation, calcium may trigger apoptosis by a variety of mechanisms, including overactivation of several different cellular enzymes, such as calpains.[37, 63, 121, 148] In turn, this is proposed[45] to cause free radical overproduction,[135] cytoskeletal reorganization,[59] and activation of apoptotic genetic signals.[97]

Axonal Injury

Just as in neuronal cell bodies, mechanical strain on axons results in membrane permeability, depolarization, mitochondrial alterations, and ionic (including calcium) flux for up to 6 hours after injury.[81, 84] Although traumatic axonal injury is best described in more severe models of TBI, it is also thought to play an important role in mTBI.[138] Additionally, neurofilament compaction has been shown to occur as soon as 5 minutes after injury and lasts for approximately 6 hours. It is believed that this is caused by phosphorylation, which leads to instability,[100, 106, 140] or calpain-mediated proteolysis of sidearms, which causes filament collapse, or both.[60] Furthermore, the influx of calcium has been demonstrated to cause microtubule breakdown 6 to 24 hours after the original insult.[60, 114] Ultimately, the ultrastructural alterations of neurofilaments and microtubules cause focal swellings at the site of injury and interference of axonal transport.[83, 128] Eventually, blebbing of the region occurs,

and signs of axonal disconnection have been witnessed as early as 4 hours after injury.[115] It has been reported that this detachment persists for days to weeks in humans.[13]

Though most of the aforementioned discoveries regarding axonal disruption have been made in animal models, advances in neuroimaging technology have allowed us to view in vivo alterations of human axons. Specifically, diffusion tensor imaging (DTI) is a sensitive modality for examining changes in white matter microstructure. The main metric used in studies pertaining to brain trauma is fractional anisotropy (FA), which measures diffusivity of water in a single direction (figure 4.6). This is reviewed in greater detail in the chapter on neuroimaging. In essence, though, elevated FA may represent an inflammatory process, such as axonal swelling or cytotoxic edema.[9, 21] In contrast, decreased FA may indicate axonal degradation and discontinuities with excess water between tracts or in perivascular spaces.[75] In adolescent patients, studies have reported DTI findings consistent with axonal injury that have correlated with postconcussive scores in measures of cognitive, affective, and somatic testing.[105, 155, 158]

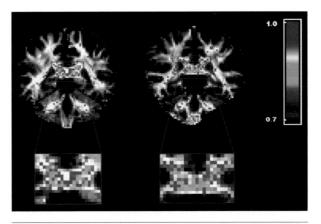

Figure 4.6 Color-coded fractional anisotropy (FA) values in the posterior corpus callosum of a selected control subject (left) and a mild TBI subject (right). The color scheme is NIH color space; higher FA values are red, and lower ones are blue. The color threshold is set to FA 0.7–1.0. Note that the mild TBI subject has more red voxels (higher FA) and the control more blue voxels (lower FA).

Reprinted, by permission, from J.J. Bazarian et al., 2007, "Diffusion tensor imaging detects clinically important axonal damage after mild traumatic brain injury: A pilot study," Journal of Neurotrauma 24: 1447-59. The publisher for this copyrighted material is Mary Ann Liebert, Inc. publishers.

Cerebral Blood Flow Dynamics

When considering postinjury alterations of metabolic state (demand), one must also take into account the ability of the brain to provide blood and therefore nutrients (supply) to damaged neural tissue. Normally, cerebral blood flow (CBF) is a highly regulated physiologic entity with several levels of autoregulation and the ability to rapidly adjust perfusion levels, thus allowing for tight matching of CBF to cellular demands. However, in head injury, we immediately see an uncoupling of these control mechanisms. While an increase in metabolic activity occurs to maintain ionic homeostasis, CBF does not increase in order to fulfill augmented glucose requirements. Instead, it has been shown to decrease immediately after injury.[44, 99] In a rat model of concussion, Yamakami and McIntosh showed that this decreased regional CBF in the perilesional area was present within 15 minutes and persisted for at least 2 hours after injury.[160]

Martin and colleagues first reported on three phases of blood flow dynamics in a study of CBF in 125 severe TBI patients.[80] Phase I, as expected based on animal studies, consists of an acute hypoperfused state and lasts for the first day. Whether this decrease achieves full-fledged ischemia is debated and needs to be examined further.[22, 150] After the first 24 hours, phase II begins, and the brain is hyperemic. The transition to a hypometabolic state (6 hours) should have already occurred, as previously discussed, thereby further demonstrating the mismatch between supply and demand. On day 4, phase III, a vasospasm state commences and can last until postinjury day 15. The characteristics of this phase include low overall CBF with greatly increased blood flow velocities through the middle cerebral artery, which suggest that arterial narrowing is present. Angiographic studies have corroborated vasospasm as a common event in moderate and severe head injury.[143] Though this succinctly characterizes CBF dynamics after moderate and severe TBI, it remains unknown whether congruent changes occur in the setting of concussive or subconcussive head impacts.

Maugans and coauthors recently described CBF alterations after sport-related (mostly American football, but also soccer and wrestling) head injuries in pediatric patients aged 11 to 15 years.[82] They examined 12 players at three time points after injury (within 3 days and at 14 and 30 days or more after concussion), comparing blood flow using phase contrast angiography. Their results showed a significant reduction in blood flow compared to controls at the first time point. In addition, contrary to their hypothesis that CBF would return to control levels within 2 weeks, CBF stayed significantly lower, even at the final time point. In fact, only 27% of the participants had returned to within 10% of control values by the 2-week measurement and only 64% by the final measurement. Additionally, the authors looked for evidence of gross structural injury using DTI, standard magnetic resonance imaging (MRI) sequences, and susceptibility-weighted imaging (SWI). No differences were observed in this cohort of pediatric patients on these imaging sequences. Therefore, the authors concluded that sport-related mTBI in this age group happens to be a more physiologic–metabolic disruption than a structural injury, with CBF diminution playing a vital role in overall pathophysiology.

Blood–Brain Barrier Breakdown

The blood–brain barrier (BBB) is the highly regulated separation between the intravascular and extravascular content of the central nervous system. Not only does it play an integral role in neuronal protection and maintaining normal brain homeostasis; its breakdown has been implicated in a wide variety of diseases, especially neurodegenerative ones such as Alzheimer's disease, amyotrophic lateral sclerosis (Lou Gehrig's disease), and multiple sclerosis.[165] Given the neurodegenerative nature of many postconcussive sequelae (e.g., mild cognitive impairment, chronic traumatic encephalopathy, dementia pugilistica), it is not unreasonable to think that BBB breakdown may also exist in the context of concussive brain injury.

It is well documented in animal models of severe traumatic brain injury[132] and in human pathologic studies[20] that BBB breakdown occurs. Moreover, it has been shown that in animals with mild head injury, focal cortical breakdown is present as well as more profound exacerbations seen with repetitive injuries[71] (figure 4.7). A study of human postconcussion syndrome patients demonstrated that BBB disruption can be seen weeks to months after the original insult.[67] It is believed that the breakdown be may due originally to shearing forces that damage endothelium and lead to increased small vessel

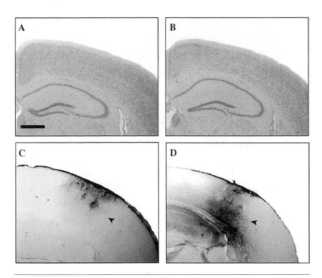

Figure 4.7 Photomicrographs of histopathological specimens following single TBI or repetitive head injury (RHI). Nissl staining revealed no overt histological damage or focal lesions in the cortex or hippocampus in animals subjected to either a single TBI (A) or RHI (B) 56 days after injury. Immunostaining for mouse immunoglobulin G revealed a small area of immunoreactivity restricted to the cortex (arrowhead) in three of five animals subjected to single TBI (C) 48 hours after trauma. Immunoglobulin G immunoreactivity was observed in the cortex, subcortical matter, and hippocampus of four of five animals 1 day after RHI (D, arrowhead). Scale bar = 1 mm.

Reprinted, by permission, from H.L. Laurer et al., 2001, "Mild head injury increasing the brain's vulnerability to a second concussive impact," Journal of Neurosurgery 95: 859-70.

permeability and dysregulation.[134] Damage may result as areas of metabolic imbalance form ischemic zones of tissue hypoxia, potentiating localized BBB destruction. Other mechanisms, such as vasospasm, CBF alterations, irregularities in nitric oxide secretion, and coagulopathy, may also contribute. Further breakdown may occur later, during so-called secondary injury processes that include abnormal brain activity, astrocyte dysfunction, neuroinflammation, and metabolic disturbances as the brain's attempt to repair itself.

There are several implications of BBB breakdown in the context of mTBI. First, increased permeability leads to inevitable fluid exudation that may result in variable amounts of brain edema. An increase in intracranial pressure can occur with sufficient edema accumulation, thereby lowering the perfusion pressure, which may further compromise relative CBF deficiencies. Additionally, loss of ionic flux control allows

extravasation of EAAs, thereby worsening the already present excitotoxicity. Similarly, as other ions and molecules equilibrate in the serum and cerebrospinal fluid, a neuronal microenvironment develops that creates a predisposition for focal seizure activity.[67] Indeed, numerous studies in vitro of isolated brain slices show enhanced cortical excitability, hypersynchronicity, and "epileptiform"-like activity.[5, 124, 129, 131] This provides a possible explanation for the seizure-like activity seen in animal models of mild head trauma[104] and in several reports in humans.[54, 90]

Immunoexcitotoxicity

To this point, discussion on the pathophysiology of concussion has focused on the neurometabolic cascade in neurons and how alterations in blood flow and BBB regulation may compound the results of this problem. Still, it is important to realize that brain tissue is composed of many different cell types, each with specific roles in maintaining normal function and responsibilities when abnormal situations arise. Specifically, when brain injury occurs, a neuroinflammatory response develops. Macrophages and monocytes are the key cells in the initiation of inflammatory events following tissue insult outside the central nervous system; but in the brain, microglia cells assume this position. It is from these cells that we can glean considerable information regarding potential subsequent pathophysiological events following a concussion and perceive how stromal cells interact with neurons in both helpful and harmful ways.

A number of recent studies have implicated microglial activation as an early and primary occurrence after traumatic brain injury.[33, 43, 56] As microglia become agitated, they can release anti- and proinflammatory cytokines, chemokines, nitric oxide, prostaglandins, trophic factors, free radicals, lipid peroxidation products, and three excitatory molecules (glutamate, aspartate, and quinolinic acid) into the extraneuronal space[12, 119] (figure 4.8a). This is especially true if the microglia have been primed by previous disruptions of homeostasis, such as toxic environmental exposures, systemic immune stimulation (from infection or other causes), ischemia-hypoxia, aging, or previous trauma (particularly repetitive TBI).[26, 38, 77] Additionally, some of these chemokines attract peripheral macrophages to the brain to transdifferentiate into microglia and further participate in the cytokine release.[118, 120] It is believed that these molecules are typically released within the first hour after injury, and in most incidences of uncomplicated single concussion, glutamate is removed by intrinsic methods within 24 to 72 hours.[147, 161] Immune factors are also cleared, though after a somewhat longer time period, with retention being reported for up to a month.[69, 123, 136]

Under normal conditions following a single concussion, over time microglia eventually enter a reparative phase, composed of phagocytic activity to repair any debris and damaged cells, and then ultimately return to their resting state[11] (figure 4.8b). However, it is postulated that with repetitive brain injury, microglia enter a constitutively activated state, which can become neurodestructive.[11] It is suspected that with

future research, the role of microglia and other central nervous system cell types may be further elucidated in connection with the neurological sequelae of concussion.

CLASSIFICATION OF CONCUSSION AND GRADING SYSTEMS

When we look at concussion diagnostically, the heterogeneity of clinical presentations makes this a complex disease. This reflects the variations in injury severity and location (as discussed previously in the biomechanics section), as well as differences in a player's sport, age, sex, innate vulnerability to head injury, and other modifying factors. It not only is difficult to assess on the field, but has been traditionally troublesome with

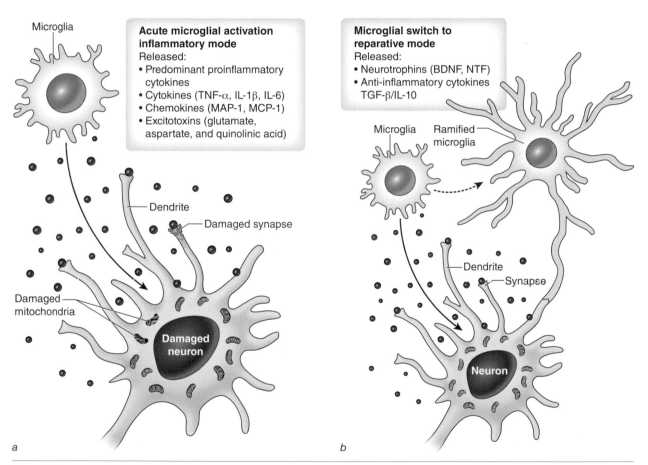

Figure 4.8 (a) Illustration demonstrating the neurotoxic effects of proinflammatory cytokines and chemokines acting in synergy with EAAs. Immunoexcitotoxicity results in damage to neuronal cell membranes, mitochondria, and DNA, as well as dendrites and synapses. (b) Illustration of a microglia in a predominately reparative mode, which will then switch to a resting (ramified) state. In the reparative mode it secretes neurotrophic factors and anti-inflammatory cytokines that shut off the inflammatory reaction.

Adapted from R.L. Blaylock and J. Maroon, 2011, "Immunoexcitotoxicity as a central mechanism is chronic traumatic encephalopathy - a unifying hypothesis," Surgical Neurology International 2: 107. By permission of R.L. Blaylock.

respect to researching outcomes. Grading systems were originally formulated to help diagnose concussion and quantify severity so that return-to-play guidelines could be mainstreamed. Over the years more than 25 grading scales have been developed. Unfortunately, despite their attractiveness, these grading schemes have been largely abandoned due to a lack of solid scientific backing.[61] Still, it is worth examining the various grading scales that have come and gone in order to gain a historical perspective on how the perception and management of concussions in sport have evolved over the last two or three decades.

While concussion symptoms vary greatly, it is interesting to note that most grading systems were traditionally centered on two main symptoms—loss of consciousness and posttraumatic amnesia. Tables 4.1 through 4.3 depict some of the most common and widely adopted grading scales.[1, 18, 66] It can be noted that most concussions graded as mild (Grade 1) represented those

instances in which no loss of consciousness (LOC) and little or no posttraumatic amnesia had occurred. Concussions that were classically considered more serious (Grade III) maintained LOC as a hallmark. We now know and understand that the majority of concussions (>90%) occur without a LOC and that many patients can suffer severe symptoms following a concussion without LOC.[19, 78] It is evident that these scales are antiquated and that they applied a very simplistic approach to a very unpredictable and complicated disease. From a historical standpoint, it is also interesting to note that in Torg's grading system[145] (table 4.4), the term "bell rung" was used to define Grade 1 concussions with only short-term confusion, unsteady gait, dazed appearance, and no amnesia. Even among medical experts of the time (1991), this term was applied widely to concussions. Terms such as "ding" and "bell ringer" have been completely abandoned. Certainly, this type of

Table 4.1 Cantu Grading System for Concussion

Grade level	Concussion symptoms
Grade 1	No loss of consciousness; posttramautic amnesia less than 30 minutes
Grade 2	Loss of consciousness less than 5 minutes in duration or posttraumatic amnesia lasting longer than 30 minutes but less than 24 hours in duration
Grade 3	Loss of consciousness for more than 5 minutes or posttraumatic amnesia for more than 24 hours

Reproduced from "Guidelines for return to contact sports after a cerebral concussion," *Physician Sportsmedicine,* R. C. Cantu, 14(10):75-83, ©1986.

Table 4.2 Colorado Medical Society Grading System for Concussion

Grade level	Concussion symptoms
Grade 1	Confusion without amnesia; no loss of consciousness
Grade 2	Confusion with amnesia; no loss of consciousness
Grade 3	Loss of consciousness

Reprinted from Colorado Medical Society, 1990, *Report of the Sports Medicine Committee: Guidelines for the management of concussion in sports* (Denver, CO: Colorado Medical Society).

Table 4.3 American Academy of Neurology Practice Parameter Grading System for Concussion

Grade level	Concussion symptoms
Grade 1	Transient confusion; no loss of consciousness; concussion symptoms or mental status abnormalities on examination resolve in less than 15 minutes
Grade 2	Transient confusion; no loss of consciousness; concussion symptoms or mental status abnormalities on examination last more than 15 minutes
Grade 3	Any loss of consciousness, either brief (seconds) or prolonged (minutes)

Reprinted from J.P. Kelly and J.H. Rosenberg, 1997, "Diagnosis and management of concussion in sports," *Neurology* 48: 575-80.

Table 4.4 Torg Grading System for Concussion

Grade level	Concussion symptoms
Grade 1	"Bell rung"; short-term concussion; unsteady gait; dazed appearance; no amnesia
Grade 2	Posttraumatic amnesia only; vertigo; no loss of consciousness
Grade 3	Posttraumatic retrograde amnesia; vertigo; no loss of consciousness
Grade 4	Immediate transient loss of consciousness
Grade 5	Paralytic coma; cardiorespiratory arrest
Grade 6	Death

Reprinted from J.S. Torg (ed), 1991, *Athletic injuries to the head, neck and face* (St. Louis, MO: Mosby-Year Book).

language contributed to the dissolution of such grading systems.

In 2004 at the 2nd International Conference on Concussion in Sport in Prague, a new classification system for concussion was attempted. [86] It suggested that simple concussions were those in which symptoms resolved without complication over 7 to 10 days and that could be managed by primary care physicians or certified athletic trainers. Complex concussions, on the other hand, were those in which symptoms persisted, specific sequelae existed (such as concussive convulsions), or prolonged LOC or cognitive impairment occurred. It was thought that these players required more consideration than those on standard return-to-play regimens and should be managed in a multidisciplinary manner by specialists with experience in the field. Even though this "simple versus complex" differentiation has a certain degree of validity, in the majority of cases it does not allow for prediction of injury severity at the time of contact. Therefore, it was suggested that this system also be dropped until further work is performed to elucidate prognostic factors for more severe injuries, and that all forms of concussion be considered a single entity.[79] Likewise, any athlete sustaining a concussion should be evaluated and cared for by a practitioner with specific and up-to-date training in the assessment and management of concussion, regardless of discipline. The most recent International Conference on Concussion in Sport consensus statements echo this belief as well.[88, 89] More attention has focused on modifying factors that might influence outcomes. These modifiers may affect return-to-play advice and prognosis for some players and are discussed in further detail in subsequent chapters.

CONCLUDING THOUGHTS

The science behind concussion continues to evolve at a rapid pace. Concussion grading scales have come and gone—a concussion . . . is a concussion . . . is a concussion. We have come to learn the importance of the various forces at play with head impacts from sports such as American football, boxing, soccer, and hockey. Much of our knowledge regarding molecular processes that occur following a concussion has been derived from models of moderate and severe TBI; however, basic science research in the arena of mild TBI has expanded. As we learn more about the pathophysiology and biophysics underlying concussion, further questions will undoubtedly arise. As this arena of TBI research continues to evolve, it will be imperative that models of concussion replicate injuries in humans as closely as possible. Further elucidation of these pathophysiological mechanisms will allow for the development of translational treatment approaches and answers to questions about how mTBI injury results in the observed spectrum of neurological sequelae.

REFERENCES

1. Colorado Medical Society. Report of the Sports Medicine Committee. Guidelines for the Management of Concussion in Sports. Denver: Colorado Medical Society; 1990.

2. Council on Scientific Affairs. Brain injury in boxing. JAMA 1983;249:254-257.

3. Agel J, Dick R, Nelson B, Marshall SW, Dompier TP. Descriptive epidemiology of collegiate women's ice hockey injuries: National Collegiate Athletic Association Injury Surveillance System, 2000–2001 through 2003–2004. J Athl Train 2007;42:249-254.

4. Andersen TE, Arnason A, Engebretsen L, Bahr R. Mechanisms of head injuries in elite football. Br J Sports Med 2004;38:690-696.

5. Andrew RD. Seizure and acute osmotic change: clinical and neurophysiological aspects. J Neurol Sci 1991;101:7-18.

6. Appelberg KS, Hovda DA, Prins ML. The effects of a ketogenic diet on behavioral outcome after controlled cortical impact injury in the juvenile and adult rat. J Neurotrauma 2009;26:497-506.

7. Atha J, Yeadon MR, Sandover J, Parsons KC. The damaging punch. Br Med J (Clin Res Ed) 1985;291:1756-1757.

8. Barkhoudarian G, Hovda DA, Giza CC. The molecular pathophysiology of concussive brain injury. Clin Sports Med 2011;30:33-48, vii-iii.

9. Bazarian JJ, Zhong J, Blyth B, Zhu T, Kavcic V, Peterson D. Diffusion tensor imaging detects clinically important axonal damage after mild traumatic brain injury: a pilot study. J Neurotrauma 2007;24:1447-1459.

10. Bergsneider M, Hovda DA, Shalmon E, Kelly DF, Vespa PM, Martin NA, et al. Cerebral hyperglycolysis following severe traumatic brain injury in humans: a positron emission tomography study. J Neurosurg 1997;86:241-251.

11. Blaylock RL, Maroon J. Immunoexcitotoxicity as a central mechanism in chronic traumatic encephalopathy—a unifying hypothesis. Surg Neurol Int 2011;2:107.

12. Block ML, Zecca L, Hong J-S. Microglia-mediated neurotoxicity: uncovering the molecular mechanisms. Nat Rev Neurosci 2007;8:57-69.

13. Blumbergs PC, Scott G, Manavis J, Wainwright H, Simpson DA, McLean AJ. Staining of amyloid precursor protein to study axonal damage in mild head injury. Lancet 1994;344:1055-1056.

14. Boden BP, Kirkendall DT, Garrett WE. Concussion incidence in elite college soccer players. Am J Sports Med 1998;26:238-241.

15. Brainard LL, Beckwith JG, Chu JJ, Crisco JJ, McAllister TW, Duhaime A-C, et al. Gender differences in head impacts sustained by collegiate ice hockey players. Med Sci Sports Exerc 2011:297-304.

16. Broglio SP, Eckner JT, Martini D, Sosnoff JJ, Kutcher JS, Randolph C. Cumulative head impact burden in high school football. J Neurotrauma 2011;28:2069-2078.

17. Brust JD, Leonard BJ, Pheley A, Roberts WO. Children's ice hockey injuries. Am J Dis Child 1992;146:741-747.

18. Cantu RC. Guidelines for return to contact sports after a cerebral concussion. Phys Sportsmed 1986;14(10):75-83.

19. Cantu RC. Return to play guidelines after a head injury. Clin Sports Med 1998;17:46-60.

20. Cervós-Navarro J, Lafuente JV. Traumatic brain injuries: structural changes. J Neurol Sci 1991;103 Suppl:S3-14.

21. Chu Z, Wilde EA, Hunter JV, McCauley SR, Bigler ED, Troyanskaya M, et al. Voxel-based analysis of diffusion tensor imaging in mild traumatic brain injury in adolescents. AJNR 2010;31:340-346.

22. Coles JP, Fryer TD, Smielewski P, Chatfield DA, Steiner LA, Johnston AJ, et al. Incidence and mechanisms of cerebral ischemia in early clinical head injury. J Cereb Blood Flow Metab 2004;24:202-211.

23. Crisco JJ, Fiore R, Beckwith JG, Chu JJ, Brolinson PG, Duma S, et al. Frequency and location of head impact exposures in individual collegiate football players. J Athl Train 2010;45:549-559.

24. Cull-Candy S, Brickley S, Farrant M. NMDA receptor subunits: diversity, development and disease. Curr Opin Neurobiol 2001;11:327-335.

25. Daniel RW, Rowson S, Duma SM. Head impact exposure in youth football. Ann Biomed Eng 2012; 40(4): 976-981.

26. Dantzer R, O'Connor JC, Freund GG, Johnson RW, Kelley KW. From inflammation to sickness and depression: when the immune system subjugates the brain. Nat Rev Neurosci 2008;9:46-56.

27. Dashnaw ML, Petraglia AL, Bailes JE. An overview of the basic science of concussion and subconcussion: where we are and where we are going. Neurosurg Focus 2012;33(6):E5: 1-9.

28. Denny-Brown D, Russell WR. Experimental cerebral concussion. Brain 1941;64:93-163.

29. Denny-Brown D, Russell WR. Experimental cerebral concussion. J Physiol 1940;99:153.

30. Duma SM, Manoogian SJ, Bussone WR, Brolinson PG, Goforth MW, Donnenwerth JJ, et al. Analysis of real-time head accelerations in collegiate football players. Clin J Sport Med 2005;15:3-8.

31. Echlin PS, Johnson AM, Riverin S, Tator CH, Cantu RC, Cusimano MD, et al. A prospective study of concussion education in 2 junior ice hockey teams: implications for sports concussion education. Neurosurg Focus 2010;29:E6.

32. Eckner JT, Sabin M, Kutcher JS, Broglio SP. No evidence for a cumulative impact effect on concussion injury threshold. J Neurotrauma 2011;28:2079-2090.

33. Engel S, Wehner HD, Meyermann R. Expression of microglial markers in the human CNS after closed head injury. Acta Neurochir Suppl 1996;66:89-95.

34. Fabricius M, Fuhr S, Willumsen L, Dreier JP, Bhatia R, Boutelle MG, et al. Association of seizures with cortical spreading depression and peri-infarct depolarisations in the acutely injured human brain. Clin Neurophysiol 2008;119:1973-1984.

35. Faden A, Demediuk P, Panter SS, Vink R. The role of excitatory amino acids and NMDA receptors in traumatic brain injury. Science 1989;244:798-800.

36. Farkas O, Lifshitz J, Povlishock JT. Mechanoporation induced by diffuse traumatic brain injury: an irreversible or reversible response to injury? J Neurosci 2006;26(12):3130-3140.

37. Farooqui AA, Horrocks LA. Excitatory amino acid receptors, neural membrane phospholipid metabolism and neurological disorders. Brain Res Rev 1991;16:171-191.

38. Feuerstein GZ, Wang X, Barone FC. The role of cytokines in the neuropathology of stroke and neurotrauma. Neuroimmunomodulation 1998;5:143-159.

39. Fineman I, Hovda DA, Smith M, Yoshino A, Becker DP. Concussive brain injury is associated with a prolonged accumulation of calcium: a 45Ca autoradiographic study. Brain Res 1993;624:94-102.

40. Fuller CW, Junge A, Dvorak J. A six year prospective study of the incidence and causes of head and neck injuries in international football. Br J Sports Med 2005;39 Suppl 1:i3-9.

41. Gerberich SG, Finke R, Madden M, Priest JD, Aamoth G, Murray K. An epidemiological study of high school ice hockey injuries. Childs Nerv Syst 1987;3:59-64.

42. Gessel LM, Fields SK, Collins CL, Dick RW, Comstock RD. Concussions among United States high school and collegiate athletes. J Athl Train 2007;42:495-503.

43. Ghirnikar RS, Lee YL, Eng LF. Inflammation in traumatic brain injury: role of cytokines and chemokines. Neurochem Res 1998;23:329-340.

44. Ginsberg MD, Zhao W, Alonso OF, Loor-Estades JY, Dietrich WD, Busto R. Uncoupling of local cerebral glucose metabolism and blood flow after acute fluid-percussion injury in rats. Am J Physiol 1997;272:H2859-2868.

45. Giza CC, Hovda DA. The neurometabolic cascade of concussion. J Athl Train 2001;36:228-235.

46. Giza CC, Maria NSS, Hovda DA. N-methyl-D-aspartate receptor subunit changes after traumatic injury to the developing brain. J Neurotrauma 2006;23:950-961.

47. Greenwald RM, Gwin JT, Chu JJ, Crisco JJ. Head impact severity measures for evaluating mild traumatic brain injury risk exposure. Neurosurgery 2008;62:789-798.

48. Gurdjian ES. Cerebral contusions: re-evaluation of the mechanism of their development. J Trauma 1976;16:35-51.

49. Gurdjian ES, Lissner HR, Hodgson VR, Patrick LM. Mechanism of head injury. Clin Neurosurg 1964;12:112-128.

50. Guskiewicz KM, Mihalik JP, Shankar V, Marshall SW, Crowell DH, Oliaro SM, et al. Measurement of head impacts in collegiate football players: relationship between head impact biomechanics and acute clinical outcome after concussion. Neurosurgery 2007;61:1244-1253.

51. Guskiewicz KM, Weaver NL, Padua DA, Garrett WE, Hill C, Carolina N. Epidemiology of concussion in collegiate and high school football players. Sports Med 2000;28:643-650.

52. Gwin JT, Chu JJ, McAllister TW, Greenwald RM. In situ measures of head impact acceleration in NCAA Division I men's ice hockey: implications for ASTM F1045 and other ice hockey helmet standards. J ASTM Int 2009;6:1-10.

53. Hartings JA, Strong AJ, Fabricius M, Manning A, Bhatia R, Dreier JP, et al. Spreading depolarizations and late secondary insults after traumatic brain injury. J Neurotrauma 2009;26:1857-1866.

54. Herman ST. Epilepsy after brain insult: targeting epileptogenesis. Neurology 2002;59:S21-26.

55. Hodgson V, Thomas T, Khalil T, eds. The role of impact location in reversible cerebral concussion. Proceedings of the 27th Stapp Car Crash Conference. Warrendale, PA: Society of Automotive Engineers, Inc.; 1983.

56. Homsi S, Piaggio T, Croci N, Noble F, Plotkine M, Marchand-Leroux C, et al. Blockade of acute microglial activation by minocycline promotes neuroprotection and reduces locomotor hyperactivity after closed head injury in mice: a twelve-week follow-up study. J Neurotrauma 2010;27:911-921.

57. Hootman JM, Dick R, Agel J. Epidemiology of collegiate injuries for 15 sports: summary and recommendations for injury prevention initiatives. J Athl Train 2007;42:311-319.

58. Hovda DA, Yoshino A, Kawamata T, Katayama Y, Becker DP. Diffuse prolonged depression of cerebral oxidative metabolism following concussive brain injury in the rat: a cytochrome oxidase histochemistry study. Brain Res 1991;567:1-10.

59. Iwasaki Y, Yamamoto H, Iizuka H, Yamamoto T, Konno H. Suppression of neurofilament degradation by protease inhibitors in experimental spinal cord injury. Brain Res 1987;406:99-104.

60. Johnson GV, Greenwood JA, Costello AC, Troncoso JC. The regulatory role of calmodulin in the proteolysis of individual neurofilament proteins by calpain. Neurochem Res 1991;16:869-873.

61. Johnston KM, McCrory P, Mohtadi NG, Meeuwisse W. Evidence-based review of sport-related concussion: clinical science. Clin J Sport Med 2001;11:150-159.

62. Kalimo H, Rehncrona S, Söderfeldt B. The role of lactic acidosis in the ischemic nerve cell injury. Acta Neuropathol Suppl 1981;7:20-22.

63. Kampfl A, Posmantur RM, Zhao X, Schmutzhard E, Clifton GL, Hayes RL. Mechanisms of calpain proteolysis following traumatic brain injury: implications for pathology and therapy: a review and update. J Neurotrauma 1997;14:121-134.

64. Katayama Y, Becker DP, Tamura T, Hovda DA. Massive increases in extracellular potassium and the indiscriminate release of glutamate following concussive brain injury. J Neurosurg 1990;73:889-900.

65. Kawamata T, Katayama Y, Hovda DA, Yoshino A, Becker DP. Administration of excitatory amino acid antagonists via microdialysis attenuates the increase in glucose utilization seen following concussive brain injury. J Cereb Blood Flow Metab 1992;12:12-24.

66. Kelly JP, Rosenberg JH. Diagnosis and management of concussion in sports. Neurology 1997;48(3):575-580.

67. Korn A, Golan H, Melamed I, Pascual-Marqui R, Friedman A. Focal cortical dysfunction and blood-brain barrier disruption in patients with postconcussion syndrome. J Clin Neurophysiol 2005;22:1-9.

68. Kubota M, Nakamura T, Sunami K, Ozawa Y, Namba H, Yamaura A, et al. Changes of local cerebral glucose utilization, DC potential and extracellular potassium concentration in experimental head injury of varying severity. Neurosurg Rev 1989;12 Suppl 1:393-399.

69. Kumar R, Husain M, Gupta RK, Hasan KM, Haris M, Agarwal AK, et al. Serial changes in the white matter diffusion tensor imaging metrics in moderate traumatic brain injury and correlation with neuro-cognitive function. J Neurotrauma 2009;26:481-495.

70. Lampert PW, Hardman JM. Morphological changes in brains of boxers. JAMA 1984;251:2676-2679.

71. Laurer HL, Bareyre FM, Lee VM, Trojanowski JQ, Longhi L, Hoover R, et al. Mild head injury increasing the brain's vulnerability to a second concussive impact. J Neurosurg 2001;95:859-870.

72. Leao AAP. Further observations on the spreading depression of activity in the cerebral cortex. J Neurophysiol 1947;10:409-414.

73. Lees A, Nolan L. The biomechanics of soccer: a review. J Sports Sci 1998;16:211-234.

74. Lifshitz J, Sullivan PG, Hovda DA, Wieloch T, McIntosh TK. Mitochondrial damage and dysfunction in traumatic brain injury. Mitochondrion 2004;4:705-713.

75. Lipton ML, Gulko E, Zimmerman ME, Friedman BW, Kim M, Gellella E, et al. Diffusion-tensor imaging implicates prefrontal axonal injury in executive function impairment following very mild traumatic brain injury. Radiology 2009;252:816-824.

76. Liu L, Wong TP, Pozza MF, Lingenhoehl K, Wang Y, Sheng M, et al. Role of NMDA receptor subtypes in governing the direction of hippocampal synaptic plasticity. Science 2004;304:1021-1024.

77. Loane DJ, Byrnes KR. Role of microglia in neurotrauma. Neurotherapeutics 2010;7:366-377.

78. Maddocks DL, Dicker GD, Saling MM. The assessment of orientation following concussion in athletes. Clin J Sport Med 1995;5:32-35.

79. Makdissi M. Is the simple versus complex classification of concussion a valid and useful differentiation? Br J Sports Med 2009;43 Suppl 1:i23-27.

80. Martin NA, Patwardhan RV, Alexander MJ, Africk CZ, Lee JH, Shalmon E, et al. Characterization of cerebral hemodynamic phases following severe head trauma: hypoperfusion, hyperemia, and vasospasm. J Neurosurg 1997;87:9-19.

81. Mata M, Staple J, Fink DJ. Changes in intra-axonal calcium distribution following nerve crush. J Neurobiol 1986;17:449-467.

82. Maugans TA, Farley C, Altaye M, Leach J, Cecil KM. Pediatric sports-related concussion produces cerebral blood flow alterations. Pediatrics 2012;129:28-37.

83. Maxwell WL, Graham DI. Loss of axonal microtubules and neurofilaments after stretch-injury to guinea pig optic nerve fibers. J Neurotrauma 1997;14:603-614.

84. Maxwell WL, McCreath BJ, Graham DI, Gennarelli TA. Cytochemical evidence for redistribution of membrane pump calcium-ATPase and ecto-Ca-ATPase activity, and calcium influx in myelinated nerve fibres of the optic nerve after stretch injury. J Neurocytol 1995;24:925-942.

85. Mccaffrey MA, Mihalik JP, Crowell DH, Shields EW, Guskiewicz KM. Measurement of head impacts in collegiate football players: clinical measures of concussion after high- and low-magnitude impacts. Neurosurgery 2007;61:1236-1243.

86. McCrory P, Johnston K, Meeuwisse W, Aubry M, Cantu R, Dvorak J, et al. Summary and agreement statement of the 2nd International Conference on Concussion in Sport, Prague 2004. Br J Sports Med 2005;39:196-204.

87. McCrory P, Johnston KM, Mohtadi NG, Meeuwisse W. Evidence-based review of sport-related concussion: basic science. Clin J Sport Med 2001;11(3):160-165.

88. McCrory P, Meeuwisse W, Johnston K, Dvorak J, Aubry M, Molloy M, et al. Consensus statement on concussion in sport: the 3rd International Conference on Concussion in Sport held in Zurich, November 2008. Br J Sports Med 2009;43 Suppl 1:i76-90.

89. McCrory P, Meeuwisse WH, Aubry M, Cantu B, Dvorak J, Echemendia RJ, et al. Consensus statement on concussion in sport: the 4th International

Conference on Concussion in Sport held in Zurich, November 2012. Br J Sports Med 2013;47(5):250-258.

90. McCrory PR, Berkovic SF. Video analysis of acute motor and convulsive manifestations in sport-related concussion. Neurology 2000;54:1488-1491.

91. Meehan WP, Bachur RG. Sport-related concussion. Pediatrics 2009;123:114-123.

92. Mihalik JP, Bell DR, Ed M, Marshall SW. Measurement of head impacts in collegiate football players: an investigation on positional and event-type differences. Neurosurgery 2007;61:1229-1235.

93. Mihalik JP, Blackburn JT, Greenwald RM, Cantu RC, Marshall SW, Guskiewicz KM. Collision type and player anticipation affect head impact severity among youth ice hockey players. Pediatrics 2010;125:e1394-1401.

94. Mihalik JP, Greenwald RM, Blackburn JT, Cantu RC, Marshall SW, Guskiewicz KM. Effect of infraction type on head impact severity in youth ice hockey. Med Sci Sports Exerc 2010;42:1431-1438.

95. Mihalik JP, Guskiewicz KM, Marshall SW, Blackburn JT, Cantu RC, Greenwald RM. Head impact biomechanics in youth hockey: comparisons across playing position, event types, and impact locations. Ann Biomed Eng 2011;40:141-149.

96. Mihalik JP, Guskiewicz KM, Marshall SW, Greenwald RM, Blackburn JT, Cantu RC. Does cervical muscle strength in youth ice hockey players affect head impact biomechanics? Clin J Sport Med 2011;21:416-421.

97. Morgan JI, Curran T. Role of ion flux in the control of c-fos expression. Nature 1986;322:552-555.

98. Morrison AL, King TM, Korell MA, Smialek JE, Troncoso JC. Acceleration-deceleration injuries to the brain in blunt force trauma. Am J Forensic Med Pathol 1998;19:109-112.

99. Muir JK, Boerschel M, Ellis EF. Continuous monitoring of posttraumatic cerebral blood flow using laser-Doppler flowmetry. J Neurotrauma 1992;9:355-362.

100. Nakamura Y, Takeda M, Angelides KJ, Tanaka T, Tada K, Nishimura T. Effect of phosphorylation on 68 KDa neurofilament subunit protein assembly by the cyclic AMP dependent protein kinase in vitro. Biochem Biophys Res Commun 1990;169:744-750.

101. Naunheim RS, Bayly PV, Standeven J, Neubauer JS, Lewis LM, Genin GM. Linear and angular head accelerations during heading of a soccer ball. Med Sci Sports Exerc 2003;35:1406-1412.

102. Naunheim RS, Standeven J, Richter C, Lewis LM. Comparison of impact data in hockey, football, and soccer. J Trauma 2000;48:938-941.

103. Newman JA, Beusenberg MC, Shewchenko N, Withnall C, Fournier E. Verification of biome-chanical methods employed in a comprehensive study of mild traumatic brain injury and the effectiveness of American football helmets. J Biomech 2005;38:1469-1481.

104. Nilsson P, Ronne-Engström E, Flink R, Ungerstedt U, Carlson H, Hillered L. Epileptic seizure activity in the acute phase following cortical impact trauma in rat. Brain Res 1994;637:227-232.

105. Niogi SN, Mukherjee P, Ghajar J, Johnson CE, Kolster R, Lee H, et al. Structural dissociation of attentional control and memory in adults with and without mild traumatic brain injury. Brain 2008;131:3209-3221.

106. Nixon RA. The regulation of neurofilament protein dynamics by phosphorylation: clues to neurofibrillary pathobiology. Brain Pathol 1993;3:29-38.

107. Ommaya AK. Head injury mechanisms and the concept of preventive management: a review and critical synthesis. J Neurotrauma 1995;12:527-546.

108. Ommaya AK, Gennarelli TA. Cerebral concussion and traumatic unconsciousness. Correlation of experimental and clinical observations of blunt head injuries. Brain 1974;97:633-654.

109. Osteen CL, Moore AH, Prins ML, Hovda DA. Age-dependency of 45calcium accumulation following lateral fluid percussion: acute and delayed patterns. J Neurotrauma 2001;18:141-162.

110. Parkinson D, Jell RM. Concussion. Acceleration limits causing concussion. Surg Neurol 1988;30:102-107.

111. Pellman EJ. Background on the National Football League's research on concussion in professional football. Neurosurgery 2003;53:797-798.

112. Pellman EJ, Viano DC, Tucker AM, Casson IR. Concussion in professional football: location and direction of helmet impacts: part 2. Neurosurgery 2003;53:1328-1341.

113. Pellman EJ, Viano DC, Tucker AM, Casson IR, Waeckerle JF. Concussion in professional football: reconstruction of game impacts and injuries. Neurosurgery 2003;53:799-812.

114. Pettus EH, Povlishock JT. Characterization of a distinct set of intra-axonal ultrastructural changes associated with traumatically induced alteration in axolemmal permeability. Brain Res 1996;722:1-11.

115. Povlishock JT, Christman CW. The pathobiology of traumatically induced axonal injury in animals and humans: a review of current thoughts. J Neurotrauma 1995;12:555-564.

116. Powell JW, Barber-Foss KD. Traumatic brain injury in high school athletes. JAMA 1999;282:958-963.

117. Prins ML, Fujima LS, Hovda DA. Age-dependent reduction of cortical contusion volume by ketones after traumatic brain injury. J Neurosci Res 2005;82:413-420.

118. Rancan M, Otto VI, Hans VH, Gerlach I, Jork R, Trentz O, et al. Upregulation of ICAM-1 and MCP-1 but not of MIP-2 and sensorimotor deficit in response to traumatic axonal injury in rats. J Neurosci Res 2001;63:438-446.

119. Ransohoff RM, Perry VH. Microglial physiology: unique stimuli, specialized responses. Annu Rev Immunol 2009;27:119-145.

120. Rhodes JKJ, Sharkey J, Andrews PJD. The temporal expression, cellular localization, and inhibition of the chemokines MIP-2 and MCP-1 after traumatic brain injury in the rat. J Neurotrauma 2009;26:507-525.

121. Roberts-Lewis JM, Siman R. Spectrin proteolysis in the hippocampus: a biochemical marker for neuronal injury and neuroprotection. Ann N Y Acad Sci 1993;679:78-86.

122. Robertson CL, Saraswati M, Fiskum G. Mitochondrial dysfunction early after traumatic brain injury in immature rats. J Neurochem 2007;101:1248-1257.

123. Rodriguez-Paez AC, Brunschwig JP, Bramlett HM. Light and electron microscopic assessment of progressive atrophy following moderate traumatic brain injury in the rat. Acta Neuropathol 2005;109:603-616.

124. Rosen AS, Andrew RD. Osmotic effects upon excitability in rat neocortical slices. Neuroscience 1990;38:579-590.

125. Rousseau P, Post A, Hoshizaki B. A comparison of peak linear and angular headform accelerations using ice hockey helmets. J ASTM Int 2009;6:1-12.

126. Rowson S, Beckwith JG, Chu JJ, Leonard DS, Greenwald RM, Duma SM. A six degree of freedom head acceleration measurement device for use in football. J Appl Biomech 2011;27:8-14.

127. Rowson S, Brolinson G, Goforth M, Dietter D, Duma S. Linear and angular head acceleration measurements in collegiate football. J Biomech Eng 2009;131:061016.

128. Saatman KE, Abai B, Grosvenor A, Vorwerk CK, Smith DH, Meaney DF. Traumatic axonal injury results in biphasic calpain activation and retrograde transport impairment in mice. J Cereb Blood Flow Metab 2003;23:34-42.

129. Saly V, Andrew RD. CA3 neuron excitation and epileptiform discharge are sensitive to osmolality. J Neurophysiol 1993;69:2200-2208.

130. Schnebel B, Gwin JT, Anderson S, Gatlin R. In vivo study of head impacts in football: a comparison of National Collegiate Athletic Association Division I versus high school impacts. Neurosurgery 2007;60:490-495; discussion 495-496.

131. Schwartzkroin PA, Baraban SC, Hochman DW. Osmolarity, ionic flux, and changes in brain excitability. Epilepsy Res 1998;32:275-285.

132. Shapira Y, Artru A, Shohami E. Blood-brain barrier permeability, cerebral edema, and neurologic function after closed head injury in rats. Anesth Analg 1993:141-148.

133. Shewchenko N, Withnall C, Keown M, Gittens R, Dvorak J. Heading in football. Part 2: biomechanics of ball heading and head response. Br J Sports Med 2005;39 Suppl 1:i26-32.

134. Shlosberg D, Benifla M, Kaufer D, Friedman A. Blood-brain barrier breakdown as a therapeutic target in traumatic brain injury. Nat Rev Neurol 2010;6:393-403.

135. Siesjö BK. Pathophysiology and treatment of focal cerebral ischemia. Part II: mechanisms of damage and treatment. J Neurosurg 1992;77:337-354.

136. Smith DH, Chen XH, Pierce JE, Wolf JA, Trojanowski JQ, Graham DI, et al. Progressive atrophy and neuron death for one year following brain trauma in the rat. J Neurotrauma 1997;14:715-727.

137. Smith DW, Bailes JE, Fisher JA, Robles J, Turner RC, Mills JD. Internal jugular vein compression mitigates traumatic axonal injury in rat model by reducing intracranial slosh effect. Neurosurgery 2011; 70(3):740-746.

138. Spain A, Daumas S, Lifshitz J, Rhodes J, Andrews PJD, Horsburgh K, et al. Mild fluid percussion injury in mice produces evolving selective axonal pathology and cognitive deficits relevant to human brain injury. J Neurotrauma 2010;27:1429-1438.

139. Spiotta AM, Bartsch AJ, Benzel EC. Heading in soccer: dangerous play? Neurosurgery 2012;70:1-11.

140. Sternberger LA, Sternberger NH. Monoclonal antibodies distinguish phosphorylated and non-phosphorylated forms of neurofilaments in situ. Proc Natl Acad Sci U S A 1983;80:6126-6130.

141. Stojsih S, Boitano M, Wilhelm M, Bir C. A prospective study of punch biomechanics and cognitive function for amateur boxers. Br J Sports Med 2010;44:725-730.

142. Strong AJ, Fabricius M, Boutelle MG, Hibbins SJ, Hopwood SE, Jones R, et al. Spreading and synchronous depressions of cortical activity in acutely injured human brain. Stroke 2002;33:2738-2743.

143. Suwanwela C, Suwanwela N. Intracranial arterial narrowing and spasm in acute head injury. J Neurosurg 1972;36:314-323.

144. Tang YP, Wang H, Feng R, Kyin M, Tsien JZ. Differential effects of enrichment on learning and memory function in NR2B transgenic mice. Neuropharmacology 2001;41:779-790.

145. Torg J. Grading system for concussion. In: Torg J, ed. Athletic Injuries to the Head, Neck and Face. St. Louis: Mosby-Year; 1991.

146. Unterharnscheidt F. About boxing: review of historical and medical aspects. Texas Rep Biol Med 1970;28:421-495.

147. van Landeghem FK, Stover JF, Bechmann I, Brück W, Unterberg A, Bührer C, et al. Early expression of glutamate transporter proteins in ramified microglia after controlled cortical impact injury in the rat. Glia 2001;35:167-179.

148. Verity MA. Ca(2+)-dependent processes as mediators of neurotoxicity. Neurotoxicology 1992;13:139-147.

149. Verweij BH, Muizelaar JP, Vinas FC, Peterson PL, Xiong Y, Lee CP. Mitochondrial dysfunction after experimental and human brain injury and its possible reversal with a selective N-type calcium channel antagonist (SNX-111). Neurol Res 1997;19:334-339.

150. Vespa P, Bergsneider M, Hattori N, Wu H-M, Huang S-C, Martin NA, et al. Metabolic crisis without brain ischemia is common after traumatic brain injury: a combined microdialysis and positron emission tomography study. J Cereb Blood Flow Metab 2005;25:763-774.

151. Viano DC, Casson IR, Pellman EJ. Concussion in professional football: biomechanics of the struck player: part 14. Neurosurgery 2007;61:313-327; discussion 327-318.

152. Viano DC, Casson IR, Pellman EJ, Bir CA, Zhang L, Sherman DC, et al. Concussion in professional football: comparison with boxing head impacts: part 10. Neurosurgery 2005;57:1154-1172.

153. Viano DC, Pellman EJ. Concussion in professional football: biomechanics of the striking player: part 8. Neurosurgery 2005;56:266-280.

154. Walilko TJ, Viano DC, Bir CA. Biomechanics of the head for Olympic boxer punches to the face. Br J Sports Med 2005;39:710-719.

155. Wilde EA, McCauley SR, Hunter JV, Bigler ED, Chu Z, Wang ZJ, et al. Diffusion tensor imaging of acute mild traumatic brain injury in adolescents. Neurology 2008;70:948-955.

156. Williamson IJS, Goodman D. Converging evidence for the under-reporting of concussions in youth ice hockey. Br J Sports Med 2006;40:128-132; discussion 128-132.

157. Withnall C, Shewchenko N, Gittens R, Dvorak J. Biomechanical investigation of head impacts in football. Br J Sports Med 2005;39 Suppl 1:i49-57.

158. Wozniak JR, Krach L, Ward E, Mueller BA, Muetzel R, Schnoebelen S, et al. Neurocognitive and neuroimaging correlates of pediatric traumatic brain injury: a diffusion tensor imaging (DTI) study. Arch Clin Neuropsychol 2007;22:555-568.

159. Xiong Y, Gu Q, Peterson PL, Muizelaar JP, Lee CP. Mitochondrial dysfunction and calcium perturbation induced by traumatic brain injury. J Neurotrauma 1997;14:23-34.

160. Yamakami I, McIntosh TK. Effects of traumatic brain injury on regional cerebral blood flow in rats as measured with radiolabeled microspheres. J Cereb Blood Flow Metab 1989;9:117-124.

161. Yi J-H, Hazell AS. Excitotoxic mechanisms and the role of astrocytic glutamate transporters in traumatic brain injury. Neurochem Int 2006;48:394-403.

162. Yoshino A, Hovda DA, Kawamata T, Katayama Y, Becker DP. Dynamic changes in local cerebral glucose utilization following cerebral conclusion in rats: evidence of a hyper- and subsequent hypometabolic state. Brain Res 1991;561:106-119.

163. Zazryn T, Cameron P, McCrory P. A prospective cohort study of injury in amateur and professional boxing. Br J Sports Med 2006;40:670-674.

164. Zhang L, Yang KH, King AI. A proposed injury threshold for mild traumatic brain injury. J Biomech Eng 2004;126:226.

165. Zlokovic BV. The blood-brain barrier in health and chronic neurodegenerative disorders. Neuron 2008;57:178-201.

In the Trenches

Acute Evaluation and Management of Concussion

A concussion is a type of traumatic brain injury (TBI). On the continuum of TBI, it is toward the mild end of the spectrum; however, this certainly does not mean that it is any less important or that the consequences are of less concern. Unfortunately, there is no universally agreed upon definition of concussion. That one statement alone has been reiterated repeatedly over the last decade and should give a sense of how complicated this process is.

Concussion is not a new term. The word is derived from the Latin word concutere ("to shake violently"). There is mention of concussion, later translated to commotio cerebri, in the Hippocratic corpus, a collection of ancient Greek medical works.[77] The text discusses the loss of speech, hearing, and sight that can result from "commotion of the brain."[77] It wasn't until the 16th century, though, that the term concussion really came into use in connection with patients who presented with symptoms of confusion, lethargy, and memory problems following a closed head injury.[77] This concept of disruption of mental function, by the shaking of the brain remained the widely accepted understanding of concussion until the 19th and early 20th centuries.

While no single definition of concussion, minor head injury, or mild traumatic brain injury (mTBI) is universally accepted, a variety of definitions have been offered over the years. One of the first attempts to improve the definition of this condition was made in 1966 by the Congress of Neurological Surgeons.[2] Their proposed consensus definition of concussion, which was subsequently endorsed by the American Medical Association and the International Neurotraumatology Association, stated that concussion is "a clinical syndrome characterized by the immediate and transient posttraumatic impairment of neural function, such as alteration of consciousness, disturbance of vision or equilibrium, etc., due to brain stem involvement."[2, 7] In the past, one of the more commonly used definitions was the one put together in 1993 by the American Congress of Rehabilitation Medicine.[52] The organization defined mild traumatic brain injury as involving an alteration in consciousness (amnesia or confusion), less than 30 minutes of loss of consciousness, or less than 24 hours of posttraumatic amnesia, with focal neurological deficits that "may or may not be transient."[52] Subsequent definitions were presented in 1997 by the American Academy of Neurology[4] and then in 2004 by the World Health Organization Collaborating Task Force on mTBI.[18] Even the Concussion in Sport (CIS) Group has refined its definition over the last decade.[8, 73, 74]

Clearly, the sports medicine definition of concussion is not precisely equivalent to mTBI.[108] Traumatic brain injury is typically graded, from mild to severe, using the Glasgow Coma Scale (GCS). Patients sustaining a head injury can be graded on this neurological scale based on the effects of the injury on their level of consciousness. The GCS score is based on an individual's eye opening, verbal performance, and motor response; and a composite score is given ranging from 3 to 15 (table 5.1). Although the scale demonstrates good validity and is effective for making an objective assessment, it is a crude scale, limited in its applicability in certain cases. A mild TBI based on this scale applies to any patient with a GCS of 13 to 15. This, by definition, may include patients with a focal neurological deficit or even a structural lesion.

Part of the confusion may arise from the fact that concussion is a mild form of traumatic brain injury, hence the inclination to lump it together with mTBI. Indeed, even to this day, many use the terms interchangeably, as noted in the Centers for Disease Control and Prevention (CDC) definition.[1] It has been more recently acknowledged, however, that the terms concussion and mTBI refer to different injury constructs and should not be used interchangeably.[74] The definition of concussion generated from the 3rd International Conference on Concussion in Sport, in Zurich, represents probably the most recent up-to-date consensus definition:

> Concussion is defined as a complex pathophysiological process affecting the brain, induced by traumatic biomechanical forces. . . . 1) Concussion may be caused either

by a direct blow to the head, face or neck, or a blow elsewhere on the body with an impulsive force transmitted to the head. 2) Concussion typically results in the rapid onset of short-lived impairment of neurological function that resolves spontaneously. 3) Concussion may result in neuropathological changes, but the acute clinical symptoms largely reflect a functional disturbance rather than a structural injury. 4) Concussion results in a graded set of clinical symptoms that may or may not involve loss of consciousness. Resolution of the clinical and cognitive symptoms typically follows a sequential course. In a small percentage of cases, however, postconcussive symptoms may be prolonged. 5) No abnormality on standard structural neuroimaging studies is seen in concussion.[74] (p. i76-i77)

The consensus statement from the 4th International Conference on Concussion in Sport was congruent with this definition.[75] An improved definition of concussion in the years to come will help health care professionals identify, diagnose, and manage concussion better, as well as help researchers to develop improved diagnostic and therapeutic approaches. This is the focus of many research efforts currently under way.[15]

Table 5.1   Glasgow Coma Scale (GCS)

Category	Response	Score
Eye opening	Spontaneous	4
	To speech	3
	To pain	2
	None	1
Verbal response	Oriented	5
	Confused	4
	Inappropriate words	3
	Incomprehensible sounds	2
	None	1
Motor response	Follows commands	6
	Localizes to pain	5
	Withdraws to pain	4
	Flexor (decorticate) posturing	3
	Extensor (decerebrate) posturing	2
	None	1

PRESENTATION

Concussion may go undiagnosed or mismanaged because of the variability in type, number, and severity of injury signs and symptoms. The vast majority of patients with a concussion do not exhibit a focal neurological deficit on physical examination.[16] The recognition of signs or symptoms (e.g., decreasing level of consciousness; deterioration in neurological function; decrease or irregularity in heart rate or respirations; signs of a skull fracture; lateralized weakness; sensory deficits; severe headache; vomiting; seizure; or unequal, dilated, or nonreactive pupils) may indicate a more severe form of TBI. Intracranial hemorrhage can occur with even mild forms of TBI and can include subdural or epidural hematomas and cerebral contusions. Thus, it is important that those caring for athletes understand these signs of more severe head injury and transport patients immediately to the nearest emergency medical facility for further workup and management.[42] The diagnosis of acute concussion involves the assessment of a range of domains including clinical symptoms, physical signs, behavior, cognition, and balance.[74]

Signs and Symptoms of Concussion

The signs and symptoms of concussion (table 5.2) can vary from patient to patient and from concussion to concussion, thus highlighting the need for an individualized approach for each athlete suspected of having a concussion. Of the possible signs that one may observe following a concussion, mental status changes and subtle neurocognitive deficits are the most common. Confusion has long been considered a hallmark of concussion.[53, 66] While most people have a general sense of what the term implies, confusion more objectively includes a disturbance of vigilance with heightened distractibility, the inability to maintain a coherent stream of thought, or the inability to carry out a sequence of goal-directed movements.[87] Disorientation may be present during a concussion; however, subtle mental status changes are more common.[54, 62, 71] This is one of the underlying reasons for incorporating more sensitive questions into the mental status examination of an athlete with a suspected concussion,[62] which is discussed in more detail later.

A loss of consciousness (LOC) can also occur with a concussion, although the majority of concussions occur without a LOC, even though an athlete may seem dazed.[17] Loss of consciousness has been reported to occur in 8% to 19% of sport-related concussions.[31, 35, 47, 84, 90, 105] Prolonged LOCs lasting longer than 1 to 2 minutes are much less frequent, with most LOCs lasting less than a minute.[23] Many human concussion studies have documented an array of postconcussive symptoms and neuropsychological deficits following concussion in the absence of a LOC.[23, 107] While the duration of LOC is felt to correlate with outcome in patients with moderate and severe TBI,[50, 74] it has not been noted to be a measure of injury severity in concussion studies.[57, 59]

Posttraumatic amnesia can occur following a concussion, but it is not as common. Several classic studies have documented the presence of amnesia either instantaneously following a

Table 5.2 Example of Signs and Symptoms of a Concussion

Signs observed by staff	Symptoms reported by the athlete
Appears dazed	Headache
Staring, vacant facial expression	Nausea, vomiting
Confusion	Balance problems or dizziness
Disorientation to game, score, and so on	Problems with vision (blurry, "double")
Inappropriate or labile emotions	Photo- or phonophobia
Coordination issues	Feeling "foggy" or "hazy" or "out of it"
Slowness to answer questions	Sleep disturbances
Loss of consciousness	Difficulty with concentration or memory
Change in behavior	Irritability, emotionality, sadness

concussion or delayed by several minutes.[34, 113, 114] Amnesia may be experienced as a loss of memory or an inability to recall the events immediately preceding brain injury (retrograde amnesia) or as a deficit in memory or learning new information following brain injury (anterograde amnesia). Both can occur, or one type can be present in the absence of the other.[70, 71] The duration of amnesia is documented as the time between the occurrence of the injury and the point at which the individual regains normal, continuous memory function. Amnesia may be present as a solid memory gap or as spotty deficits, and usually the duration decreases over time. As with LOC, there is uncertainty as to whether the presence of amnesia carries any prognostic value.[74] Typically, retrograde amnesia varies depending on the time of measurement and thus is felt to be poorly reflective of injury severity[112, 114]; however, the presence of amnesia, in general, does appear predictive of symptoms and neurocognitive deficits following concussion in athletes.[23] The overall clinical postconcussive symptom burden and duration are felt to probably be more important with regard to outcome than the presence of amnesia alone.[57, 58, 76]

While documenting the occurrence and duration of LOC and amnesia may be helpful in characterizing an athlete's head injury, it is critical to remember that the possibility of concussion should not be dismissed if neither of these phenomena are observed or reported.[66] Additionally, it is important to note that a variety of immediate motor phenomena such as tonic posturing or convulsive movements may accompany a concussion.[74] These clinical features are generally benign and require no specific management.[16, 17, 74, 78, 79]

Concussion symptoms can generally be grouped into four different domains: somatic, sleep disturbance, emotional, and cognitive.[3, 74, 83, 92, 94, 101] If any one or more of these components are present, a concussion should be suspected and the appropriate management strategy instituted.[74] That said, there are many conditions in athletes that may cause similar symptoms, such as heat illness, dehydration (in up to 2.5%), exertional migraines, or sleep disorders.[31, 84, 91, 92, 105] Thus when diagnosing a concussion, it is important to try to establish a relationship between an appropriate mechanism of injury and onset or worsening of symptoms.

[92] Although symptoms typically begin immediately following the trauma, some patients may not experience or notice symptoms for several minutes, hours, or sometimes even days after the injury. For example, one study reported a small subset of concussed athletes who did not experience symptom onset until about 15 minutes after injury.[69] There seems to be a link between a greater number of postconcussion symptoms in the first 72 hours and the occurrence of LOC or amnesia.[23] Common symptoms include headaches, fatigue, dizziness, memory issues, irritability, anxiety, poor concentration, or photo- or phonophobia. Postconcussion symptoms can occur alone or in combination; and the presentation, with regard to severity and duration, varies widely among concussed athletes, as well as from concussion to concussion in the same individual. Some symptoms, though, are reported more often than others. Headache has been reported in 83% to 86% of concussions, whereas dizziness and confusion appear in 65% and 57% of concussed patients, respectively.[44, 46, 76, 90] Even subtle symptoms like "feeling mentally foggy" are important to note, though, as studies have highlighted that concussed athletes exhibiting fogginess had worse performance on memory, reaction time, and processing speed measures as well as an overall higher total symptom score.[49] It cannot be stressed enough how critical it is to pay attention to all symptoms following a potential concussion.

Natural History

The factors that play into an individual's recovery or postconcussive course are poorly defined. Most (80-90%) concussions resolve spontaneously within 7 to 10 days, although this recovery period varies from athlete to athlete.[74] Children and adolescents in particular may have a longer recovery period.[33, 47, 74, 84, 85] Those with a prior history of concussion may also have a more protracted, albeit normal, recovery course.[44] A small percentage of patients have symptoms that persist beyond a normal recovery period, consistent with a postconcussion syndrome picture.[94] Cognitive function likely recovers independently from concussion symptoms; however, a complex dynamic certainly exists between the two.

Several studies have investigated the relationship between concussion symptoms and the severity of postinjury neuropsychological performance and symptom presentation in an athlete-specific population.[22, 23, 49, 55, 56] In one multicenter case–control study, a total of 78 high school athletes sustaining sport-related concussion were selected for study.[23] On-field presence of disorientation, posttraumatic amnesia, retrograde amnesia, and LOC were reviewed. ImPACT, a computerized neuropsychological test battery, was administered preseason and, on average, 2 days postinjury. In this study, a good postinjury presentation was defined as no measurable change relative to baseline in terms of both ImPACT memory and symptom composite scores. A poor presentation was defined as a 10-point increase in symptom reporting and a 10-point decrease in memory functioning (exceeding the 80% confidence interval for measurement error on ImPACT).[23] Odds ratios revealed that athletes demonstrating poor presentation at 2 days postinjury were over 10 times more likely (p value < 0.001) to have exhibited retrograde amnesia following concussive injury than athletes exhibiting good presentation. Similarly, athletes with poor presentation were over four times more likely (p value < 0.013) to have exhibited posttraumatic amnesia and at least 5 minutes of mental status change. Conversely, there were no differences between good and poor presentation groups in terms of on-field LOC. Thus, the authors concluded that the presence of amnesia, not LOC, appears predictive of symptom and neurocognitive deficits following concussion in athletes.[23]

Iverson and colleagues examined the relationship between the subjective report of feeling foggy at 1 week postconcussion and acute neuropsychological outcome.[49] Participants were 110 high school students who sustained a sport-related concussion and were evaluated on average 5 to 10 days postinjury. The majority of athletes were football players (63.6%); however, other represented sports included basketball (12.7%), soccer (11.8%), hockey (3.6%), lacrosse (2.7%), softball (1.8%), track (0.9%), volleyball (0.9%), and wrestling (0.9%). Nearly half of the subjects (50.9%) reported at least one prior concussion, and 33.6% reported that this was their first concussion. Athletes were divided into two groups on the basis of self-reported fogginess. The first group reported no fogginess (n = 91), whereas the second group reported experiencing some degree of fogginess (n = 19)

on a 6-point symptom scale. The authors found that the athletes with persistent fogginess experienced a large number of other postconcussion symptoms compared to those with no reported fogginess. In addition, the athletes with persistent fogginess had significantly slower reaction times, reduced memory performance, and slower processing speed on computerized neuropsychological testing.[49]

Recent findings suggest that a delayed return to sport could be associated with an initially greater symptom load, prolonged headache, or subjective concentration deficits.[63] The authors of this study found that a headache lasting more than 60 hours, fatigue, tiredness, fogginess, or more than three symptoms at presentation correlated with a prolonged recovery.

While prior studies have shown that neurocognitive testing and symptom clusters postinjury may predict protracted recovery in concussed athletes, only recently have on-field signs and symptoms been examined empirically as possible predictors of protracted recovery. A recent study was undertaken to determine which on-field signs and symptoms were predictive of a protracted (greater than or equal to 21 days) versus rapid (less than or equal to 7 days) recovery after a sport-related concussion.[56] On-field signs and symptoms included confusion, LOC, posttraumatic amnesia, retrograde amnesia, imbalance, dizziness, visual problems, personality changes, fatigue, sensitivity to light or noise, numbness, and vomiting. This was a cohort study that included 107 male high school football athletes who completed computerized neurocognitive testing within an average 2.4 days after injury, and who were followed until return to play. Athletes were grouped into rapid (n = 62) or protracted (n = 36) recovery time groups. The researchers found that dizziness at the time of injury was associated with a 6.34 odds ratio of a protracted recovery from concussion.[56] Surprisingly, the remaining on-field signs and symptoms were not associated with an increased risk of protracted recovery in this study.

There were several limitations to this study (as with any study), and even though the findings qualified only as level 2 evidence, they did demonstrate that the presence of on-field dizziness was a robust predictor of protracted recovery from sport-related concussions. The results also indicate that perhaps we should consider using separate and specific tests for dizziness (e.g., questionnaires) in addition to traditional postural–balance tests (e.g., Balance Error Scoring System [BESS]) rather than relying on postural–balance tests as indicators of dizziness, as this specific symptom may potentially help identify high school athletes at risk for a protracted recovery. Such on-field identification of dizziness could lead to earlier implementation of vestibular rehabilitation and other modalities to treat dizziness, which could potentially expedite recovery from concussion.

Effect of Age on Concussion

The age of the athlete is an important consideration in concussion. For starters, there are differences between adolescent, preadolescent, and adult athletes with regard to the role that sport participation plays in their lives, the amount of knowledge they are expected to acquire on a daily basis, and the frequency with which their cognitive function is assessed or tested.[86] There is also basic science and clinical evidence to suggest that TBI in the youth and adolescent population differs from that in adults.

From a pathophysiological standpoint, many studies in animal models of TBI have provided a foundation for our understanding of age-related effects in concussion and have suggested a more pronounced response to brain injury in younger animals with regard to motor and cognitive deficits as well as pathophysiological markers of injury.[21, 37, 41, 51] Juvenile animals also have been found to be more vulnerable to repetitive brain injury than aged animals.[98]

Studies in moderate to severe TBI have suggested that developmental physiological differences may underlie age effects. The most significant maturation of the brain occurs between birth and age 5; however, the brain continues to mature well into adolescence. Overall differences in brain water content, cerebral blood volume, myelination, skull geometry, and suture elasticity may account for a differential response to brain injury. Throughout childhood and adolescence, the brain undergoes a significant structural remodeling process, which includes a substantial increase in white matter, as well as an overall decrease in gray matter attributable to the activity-dependent process of synaptic pruning. Synaptic pruning is a neuronal regulatory process necessary for normal brain development.

It results in the elimination of approximately half of the neurons originally present at birth. It is through this mechanism that excess neurons and synapses in the immature central nervous system are eliminated throughout development, leaving more efficient synaptic circuitry in the adult brain. Injury can affect this process. These changes directly influence the levels and distributions of several neurotransmitters in the brain. These widespread changes involve areas known to be involved in emotion and high-order cognitive processes, including planning, executive control, and decision making. These dynamic regions of the brain may be particularly vulnerable to injury.

After injury, more widespread and prolonged cerebral swelling may occur in children than in adults.[5, 13, 95] Although the exact reasons for this severity of swelling are not known, differences in the expression of glutamate receptors or of aquaporin-4 by microglia may play a role.[11] The developing brain is also thought to be 60 times more sensitive to glutamate, N-methyl-d-aspartate (NMDA), and excitotoxic brain injury.[80]

From a biomechanics standpoint, the importance of rotational acceleration in concussion has been reviewed. It has been postulated that increasing both the cervical muscle strength and tone at the time of impact can reduce the risk of concussion by increasing the effective mass of the head, which becomes more of a unit with the rest of the body as the neck muscles strengthen.[86] This would presumably then buffer the blow for any given force. This idea has been supported at the clinical level.[88] Young children and adolescents have been shown to have weaker neck strength and decreased head segment mass.[89] Therefore, younger athletes might be at increased risk for concussion when hit with the same magnitude of force due to their relatively weak cervical muscle strength compared with their older counterparts. This makes sense when one takes into consideration that a greater force is required to cause similar concussive injury in smaller brains than in larger brains with greater mass.[38, 72, 86, 89] So, while it may seem inconceivable that a youth athlete could generate such large forces, it may be that a lesser force is required to generate the same effect because of the decreased support from weaker neck musculature.

Clinical studies in concussion have suggested that younger age may portend a greater risk for slow recovery or poor outcome following concussion. When time to recover was analyzed based on symptom resolution and memory performance, collegiate athletes were found to recover more rapidly than high school athletes. During neurocognitive testing of high school students, the average times to normalization back to preconcussion baselines were reported as 10 to 14 days compared with 5 to 7 days in collegiate athletes and 2 to 5 days in professionals.[33, 39, 93] In high school athletes, neurocognitive deficits may persist well after self-reported symptoms of concussion have resolved.[58, 65, 111] One study detected ongoing verbal memory deficits at 14 days after the injury despite resolution of clinical symptoms.[65] Another study reported that nearly 14% of children aged 6 to 18 years who experienced concussion remained symptomatic 3 months after the date of injury.[9] Approximately 2.3% of children aged 0 to 18 years were symptomatic at 1 year in that same study.[9] Altogether, the current literature seems to suggest a longer recovery time from concussion for youth athletes and to indicate that this may be due to the differences in anatomy, physiology, and biomechanics of injury. Future studies are needed in this population of athletes to help elucidate some of the underlying reasons for these observations.

Effect of Sex on Concussion

While many studies have documented the frequent occurrence of concussion in males,[19] a growing body of evidence suggests that female athletes may be at greater risk of concussion.[28] In a 3-year study of collegiate athletes across several sports, women were at an increased risk for sustaining a concussion during games (9.5%) when compared to men (6.5%).[28] Female athletes had a greater incidence of concussion per 1,000 athletic exposures than their male counterparts across most sports, with women's soccer carrying one of the highest concussion rates. A similar trend was observed in a more recent study carried out over a 16-year period in collegiate athletes.[48]

Such sex differences are also observed in recovery from concussion. Several researchers have suggested that female athletes present with more acute symptoms and take a longer period to recover from concussions.[25, 27] A meta-analysis exploring the effect of sex differences on outcome following TBI found that women performed worse than men on 85% of measured variables.

[32] Primarily these variables included symptoms such as headache, dizziness, anxiety, fatigue, and poor memory and concentration. These findings have been corroborated by similar reports of women tending to present with a significantly greater number of acute symptoms postinjury.[60, 82, 96, 97] Another study found that a sample of high school and collegiate women demonstrated significantly worse reaction times, processing speed, and symptom scores than their male counterparts.[12] In that same study, when controlling for sports that require the use of a helmet (e.g., football), the authors found that women were twice as likely as men to exhibit cognitive impairments.[12] Covassin and colleagues used a prospective dependent-sample cohort design to compare baseline and postconcussion neuropsychological test scores and endorsed symptoms as functions of serial postconcussion assessment with respect to time and sex.[27] Female concussed athletes had significantly lower scores on visual memory than male concussed athletes. Along the same lines, a recent study of collegiate soccer players found that concussed females showed significantly slower reaction times and higher total symptom scores than concussed males.[25]

Some possible explanations have been offered to explain these sex differences. As has been suggested in youth athletes, women tend to have decreased head–neck segment mass when compared to male athletes. In one study, sex differences existed in head–neck segment dynamic stabilization during head angular acceleration.[109] Females exhibited significantly greater head–neck segment peak angular acceleration (50%) and displacement (39%) than males despite initiating muscle activity significantly earlier.[109] Female athletes exhibited significantly less isometric strength (49%), neck girth (30%), and head mass (43%), resulting in lower levels of head–neck segment stiffness (29%).[109] It is felt that this could result in greater angular acceleration to the head after a head impact, making the female athlete more susceptible to sustaining a concussion. In addition to neck musculature, differences in the reporting of postconcussion symptoms between male and female athletes have also been attributed to other neuroanatomical factors such as variability in cerebral organization and hormonal differences.[12, 26] The role that estrogen, the primary female sex hormone, plays in these differences is uncertain. The evidence is equivocal, as some studies have demonstrated a neuroprotective effect and others have found the hormone to be detrimental in the setting of brain injury. Most of these studies have been in animal models.

Sport environment and social differences between the sexes may help explain the different response to concussion. It is the nature of the male sport environment, especially in contact and collision sports, to play through pain in efforts to demonstrate toughness and masculinity. Male athletes are often even praised for their courage and rewarded when playing through pain and injury. Some studies have suggested that female athletes may be more concerned about their future health than male athletes. Women tend to report more concern about the impact of injury on their health.[40]

Other Influencing Factors

There are modifying factors that may predict the potential for prolonged or persistent symptoms[74] (table 5.3). The presence of any one of these factors may influence the overall assessment and management strategies; thus these are important to tease out in a detailed history as best as possible. Patients who score lower on IQ testing have been found to be more likely to experience per-

sistent postconcussive symptoms and to fall into the postconcussion syndrome category following brain injury.[61, 82] Athletes with a self-reported diagnosed learning disability were shown in one study to perform more poorly on baseline testing than did those with a history of multiple concussions without a diagnosis of a learning disability. [74] Some studies have suggested that specific premorbid emotional and personality characteristics potentially place some people at an increased risk for a poor outcome following concussion.[64, 103] Postconcussive symptoms may be mediated by an interaction of neurological and psychological factors after a TBI. Psychiatric disease preceding or following brain injury, including acute stress disorder, posttraumatic stress disorder (PTSD), depression, and anxiety, has been linked to an increased risk of poor outcome following concussion.[14, 61, 82]

ACUTE EVALUATION

Identification of concussions has always been a challenge for the sports medicine practitioner. Kevin Guskiewicz stated it best when he said, "Perhaps the most challenging aspect of managing sports related concussion is recognizing the injury, especially in athletes with no obvious signs

Table 5.3 Modifying Factors for Concussion

Factors	Modifier
Symptoms	Number Duration (>10 days) Severity
Signs	Prolonged loss of consciousness (>1 min), amnesia
Sequelae	Concussive convulsions
Temporal	Frequency—repeated concussions over time Timing—injuries close together in time "Recency"—recent concussion or traumatic brain injury
Threshold	Repeated concussions occurring with progressively less impact force or slower recovery after each successive concussion
Age	Child and adolescent (<18 years old)
Co- and premorbidities	Migraine, depression or other mental health disorders, attention deficit hyperactivity disorder, learning disabilities, sleep disorders
Medication	Psychoactive drugs, anticoagulants
Behavior	Dangerous style of play
Sport	High-risk activity, contact and collision sport, high sporting level

Reproduce from "Consensus statement on concussion in sport: the 4th International Conference on Concussion in Sport held in Zurich, November 2012," *British Journal of Sports Medicine*, 47(5): 250-258, ©2013, with permission from BMJ Publishing Group Ltd.

that a concussion has actually occurred" (p. 283).[43] The highly variable nature of concussion calls for an organized and individualized approach to injury management.[8, 42, 73, 74] Having preseason baseline evaluations and scores also provides tremendous benefit to the assessment of an athlete should an injury occur. Baseline assessments should include measures of concussion-related symptoms, balance, and neuropsychological function.[43] Such premorbid data can be used to objectively identify postinjury changes of concern. This also underscores the importance of knowing the athletes and their preinjury dispositions.[42] Any athlete suspected of having experienced a concussion should be immediately removed from play and evaluated by appropriately trained staff. Any initial condition involving severe or progressively worsening headache, positive findings on neurological examination, vomiting, or a rapidly deteriorating mental status may indicate a more severe underlying injury and warrants immediate transfer to the nearest designated emergency medical facility for further evaluation and management. Once the primary survey has been completed and cervical spine injury ruled out, a standardized approach to the acute evaluation of athletes with suspected concussion involves the use of a seven-step process that includes history, observation and palpation, special tests, range of motion, and strength testing as well as functional tests.[42]

History

In some instances, sports medicine practitioners have a unique perspective that most clinicians do not, in that they get to see the injury occur. When this is not the case, gathering history from as many sources as possible, including the player, coaches, other personnel, or teammates, is crucial. Mental status and the presence of any amnesia (retrograde or posttraumatic) can typically be ascertained quickly through detailed questioning. To assess retrograde amnesia, questions should begin at the point of concussion and work backward: for example, "Do you remember getting hit?," "Do you recall the play you were running?," "What was the score of the game?," "How did you get to the game?," and "What did you have for breakfast?"[42] Conversely, anterograde or posttraumatic amnesia can be ascertained by questioning beginning at the point

of injury and proceeding forward: for example, "Who was the first person you saw on the field?" or "Who brought you to the sideline?"[42] Three- or five-word immediate and delayed recall (10 minutes) can also be a useful way to assess ongoing memory issues. The concussion history should also include a determination of any prior history of injury, the symptoms that occurred, the duration of symptoms, and the length of time out of activity. In addition, it should include any special testing obtained as well as the temporal relationship of prior injuries.

Symptom Scales

The sideline history evaluation should then be followed systematically by a series of questions addressing the presence or absence and qualitative nature of concussion-related symptoms. Complicating the picture is the fact that some signs and symptoms of concussion may not be present immediately but rather evolve over several hours to days following a brain injury. This highlights the necessity for close observation of an athlete after a suspected concussion. Many standardized concussion symptom scales have been developed with the goal of aiding the sports medicine practitioner in objectively detecting and characterizing an individual athlete's concussion. Most scales have evolved from the neuropsychology literature pertaining to head-injured populations.[81] These symptom scales vary in the symptoms they include and the rating methods. Some excellent critical reviews of the relevant literature regarding the various scales have been published recently.[6, 30, 81]

As described in these reviews, there are six core symptoms scales, along with additional variants that have been developed. The majority of these scales use a 7-point Likert scale for symptom severity ranging from 0 (not present) to 6 (severe).[30] Many of the scales more or less incorporate the same basic symptoms, but they vary considerably in the number of items included. Many can be readily used on the sidelines for assessment of the concussed athlete, although a few are computer based and are incorporated into some of the computerized neuropsychological testing modalities. The reviews indicate that very few of these checklists were created in a systematic manner consistent with scale development processes and have published psychometric properties.[81]

Nonetheless, a standardized symptom checklist is preferable to open-ended questions such as "How are you?" or "Are you okay?"; these are likely to underdiagnose injury.[99]

The six core common checklists include the Pittsburgh Steelers Post-Concussion Scale, Post-Concussion Symptom Assessment Questionnaire (PCSQ), Concussion Resolution Index (CRI) postconcussion questionnaire, Signs and Symptoms Checklist (SSC), Sport Concussion Assessment Tool–Post-Concussion Symptom Scale (SCAT-PCSS), and the Concussion Symptom Inventory (CSI). Other scales include the Post-Concussion Scale (PCS), ImPACT Post-Concussion Symptom Scale (ImPACT-PCSS), Vienna Post-Concussion Symptom Scale (PCSS), Graded Symptom Checklist/Scale (GSC/GSS), Head Injury Scale (HIS), McGill Abbreviated Concussion Evaluation–Post-Concussion Symptom Scale, and CogState-Sport Symptom Checklist. These are all variants of the Pittsburgh Steelers Post-Concussion Scale.

Of the various checklists and scales, the CSI is the most empirically derived symptom scale for use in sport concussion detection and management to date.[30] To develop the scale, data encompassing 27 concussion symptoms (assessed with a 7-point Likert scale) were combined from three studies.[100] A total of 16,350 high school and collegiate athletes were included, and of those, 641 had sustained a concussion. A sensitivity analysis of the 27 concussion symptoms was conducted, and that ultimately resulted in the CSI's being reduced to 12 symptoms: headache, nausea, balance problems/dizziness, fatigue, drowsiness, feeling "in a fog," difficulty concentrating, difficulty remembering, sensitivity to light, sensitivity to noise, blurred vision, and feeling "slowed down." The scale is also based on a 7-point Likert rating. The study demonstrated that the 12-item scale performed nearly identically to the 27-item scale.[100] The shortened scale is convenient in that it reduces the time required for use. All of the scales would benefit from further investigation of their psychometric properties in well-designed, prospective studies.

Additionally, many of these scales focus primarily on high school- and college-aged athletes, and there is a need for the development and implementation of scales appropriate for use in the pediatric population, as a large proportion of sport-related concussions occur in younger athletes. A recent review looked at some of the postconcussion symptom scales that are available and appropriate for use in the pediatric athlete.[36] These scales include the GSC/GSS, Acute Concussion Evaluation (ACE), Rivermead Post-Concussion Symptom Questionnaire (RPCSQ), Health and Behavioral Inventory (HBI), Post-Concussion Symptom Inventory (PCSI), PCS, Post-Injury Symptom Checklist, and 7 Measures. Some of these scales were not designed to be used as a sideline tool or even in athletes, but they nonetheless can be helpful in assessing and managing a difficult pediatric patient population.

Neurological Examination

The neurological examination should begin with an assessment of the level of consciousness. The GCS, as discussed previously, allows for a quantifiable rating of a patient's level of consciousness but was really designed for use in more moderate and severe forms of TBI. The practitioner should be attentive to the athlete's speech pattern and any deviation from the athlete's normal speech, word-finding difficulty, use of inappropriate words, or slurring. A thorough examination of the 12 cranial nerves should be conducted. Attention should be paid to pupil size, position, and reactivity to light. Full extraocular movements should be assessed in all directions and any nystagmus noted. Visual acuity, facial movements, facial sensation, hearing, and tongue movement should be inspected. A brief assessment of coordination, sensation, and motor function can also be completed in an expeditious manner on the sidelines. It is also important to get a basic assessment of the athlete's vital signs including blood pressure and pulse. A clinical examination that reveals abnormalities in any of these areas suggests that there may be a more significant underlying injury than a concussion, and immediate transport to a medical facility for a more detailed neurological examination and evaluation is warranted. The cervical spine and facial bones should also be palpated and examined to rule out fractures or other trauma to these areas, which can be associated with high-acceleration impacts to the head.[42]

Sideline Assessment Tools

Most concussions lead to subtle changes that can make the evaluation process challenging. Thus, a multifaceted approach to the assessment of an athlete with a suspected concussion is paramount to efficient and effective care. Sideline tools for evaluating sport-related concussion that are useful to the athletic trainer and team physician include the Standardized Assessment of Concussion (SAC),[67, 70, 71] the Sport Concussion Assessment Tool (SCAT),[73] and the Sport Concussion Assessment Tool-2 (SCAT2).[74] These tools are abbreviated sideline batteries and are not designed to take the place of more comprehensive evaluation or neuropsychological testing.

The Standardized Assessment of Concussion was developed as a quick and reliable mental status examination for use on the sidelines.[67, 70, 71] The SAC can be given in approximately 6 to 8 minutes and does not require specific training in neuropsychology to administer or interpret. [42] The test consists of five sections that evaluate areas of orientation, immediate memory, concentration, and delayed recall. A brief screening is incorporated to rule out more overt neurological deficits. Performance is scored on the five sections assessing cognitive functioning and summed for a total possible score of 30. It is helpful and more accurate to compare to a preinjury baseline assessment if available. There are multiple versions of the SAC to help to reduce the potential practice effects associated with multiple test administrations. The test has been validated as a sideline tool for athletes junior high school aged and older; and an emergency department version has been validated for use in adults. A decrease in the score by only 1 point or more is consistent with impaired cognitive functioning; and when the test is administered immediately following injury, it has a 94% sensitivity and 76% specificity with the 1-point decrement used as a cutoff. [10] Similar sensitivity (80%) and specificity (91%) were found in a subsequent study.[68]

The SCAT was the by-product of the 2nd International Conference on Concussion in Sport and was revised into the SCAT2 following the 3rd International Conference on Concussion in Sport. The SCAT2 combines aspects of several different concussion tools into eight main components. The assessment tools incorporated into the SCAT2 include a symptom checklist, Maddock's questions (concentration and memory), the SAC, Balance Error Scoring System (BESS), and GCS. These components are designed to assess concussion symptoms, cognition, and some neurological

signs. The SCAT2 includes a "score card" portion and has been designed for use serially following a concussion to track performance over time. The Maddock's score portion of the SCAT2, however, pertains to the initial sideline diagnosis only. The SCAT2 may take a little longer to administer than the SAC. The length could limit its use on the sideline and make it more appropriate for use in a controlled situation like the locker or training room, which is not necessarily a bad thing either. Both the SCAT and the SCAT2 are limited by their undefined psychometric properties and a lack of scientific studies validating their utility for concussion diagnosis and recovery. However, SCAT2 remains a promising, sophisticated sideline tool. [99] The SCAT2 has also since been modified at the most recent Conference on Concussion in Sport to the new SCAT3 version.[75]

There have been several reports regarding the variability in baseline testing as well as test reliability. One recent study reported baseline values for 260 collegiate athletes on the original SCAT.[106] In this patient cohort, 58.8% reported the presence of at least one symptom at baseline, and the overall mean PCSS was 4.29.[106] Nearly 96% of the athletes had a SAC immediate recall score of 5; however, only 36.9% had a delayed recall score of 5. Ninety-one percent were able to recite the months in reverse order, and only 51% of the athletes were able to complete strings of six digits in reverse order. Sex differences were observed in the study, and a history of concussion in athletes also accounted for some differences in baseline scores. A recent study investigated representative baseline values on the SCAT2.[110] The authors evaluated 1,134 adolescent athletes and found that baseline values on the SCAT2 in their group of participants varied by sex, grade in school, and history of a prior concussion. Supporting this trend of variability in baseline scores, another study demonstrated trial and sex effects in finger-to-nose testing, as measured on the SCAT2, in a sample of 172 healthy men and women between the ages of 16 and 37 years. [104] The choice to use SAC versus SCAT versus SCAT2 as a sideline concussion assessment tool is probably less important than just picking one and standardizing the approach to the sideline assessment. The results of the previously mentioned studies of baseline scores highlight how important it is to obtain preinjury scores on athletes in order to individualize concussion management and take each injury in the context of an athlete's own baseline.

Postural Stability and Balance Testing

An objective balance assessment is an important component of the physical examination to include at baseline and during postinjury evaluations, especially in the setting of vestibulomotor symptoms. Balance testing has been found to be a sensitive component of the evaluation in detecting concussion, particularly in the first few days.[20, 45, 102] A variety of balance testing options are available, including the Sensory Organization Test on the NeuroCom Smart Balance Master System, balance testing using the Nintendo Wii, and the Balance Error Scoring System (BESS). A modified BESS was included as part of the SCAT2 as noted previously. A large body of literature supports the use of balance testing in the assessment of athletes with a suspected concussion,[29] and this is reviewed in further detail in a subsequent chapter.

Range of Motion and Strength Testing

The examiner should then continue with a more detailed evaluation of cervical range of motion (ROM). Range of motion tests should examine flexion, extension, and rotation in all directions, both actively and passively.[42] A more formal assessment of motor strength testing in all muscle groups should then be conducted. If any limitations are noted in either ROM or muscle strength testing, the athlete should be withheld from participation (even in the absence of deficits on previous portions of the concussion assessment) for further evaluation, because limitations in these areas may place athletes at risk for further injury by restricting their ability to protect their head and anticipate impacts from oncoming opponents.[42]

Functional Testing

Functional testing marks the final step in the concussion evaluation. This is not something to be used to make "same-day return-to-play" decisions. Any athlete who is suspected to have had a concussion is to sit out. This type of testing is to be completed only if the athlete has performed at or above baseline on all other aspects of the assessment (i.e., no overt symptoms, normal exam, normal scores with sideline assessment tools, normal balance testing). The goal is to elicit symptoms that may present themselves under the physical and cognitive demands that athletes face should they return to play.[42]

The approach is a progressive one that almost serves as an expedited, "mini-sideline version" of the more graduated return-to-play protocol used to return athletes to activity following a concussion. With each step, the practitioner should ask the athlete if any concussion-related symptoms have been elicited before progressing to an increase in activity level. Simple tasks like a Valsalva maneuver, push-ups, and sit-ups should be performed first.[42] One can then advance activity by having the athlete jog, followed by increased aerobic activity such as sideline sprints. The progression culminates with a complete series of sport-specific activities (e.g., throwing and catching a football, shooting a puck, dribbling a basketball, passing drills with a soccer ball), at an intensity level necessary for a safe return to play. [42] If an athlete at any time reports symptoms that result from the exertion, the player should not be returned to participation (or progressed to the next step). If no symptoms are elicited through these functional tests and all other assessments demonstrate normal findings, then the athlete has not likely sustained a concussion and may be considered for a return to play.

CONCLUDING THOUGHTS

A single definition of concussion has remained elusive through the years. Simply put, concussion can be viewed as a disturbance of neurological function resulting from acceleration–deceleration forces imparted to the head, neck, or elsewhere on the body. The symptoms can vary from one injury to another as well as from athlete to athlete. While myriad symptoms are possible, headache is one of the most common complaints. It is important that all athletes be removed from play and evaluated. Athletes should be observed closely in the acute period to ensure that no deterioration occurs. Several tools have been developed to aid the practitioner in identifying head injury in sport. Ultimately, it is imperative that instructions regarding concussion be communicated to the athlete and family, including the symptoms and signs that should prompt referral to a physician or a hospital for further evaluation. Effective care of the athlete with a concussion starts in the trenches and requires a complete and thorough examination.

REFERENCES

1. Centers for Disease Control and Prevention: National Center for Injury Prevention and Control. Heads up: brain injury in your practice. 2007. Available from: www.cdc.gov/concussion/headsup/pdf/Facts_for_Physicians_booklet-a.pdf.

2. Committee on Head Injury Nomenclature of the Congress of Neurological Surgeons. Glossary of head injury, including some definitions of injury to the cervical spine. Clin Neurosurg 1966;12:386-394.

3. Concussion (mild traumatic brain injury) and the team physician: a consensus statement. Med Sci Sports Exerc 2006;38(2):395-399.

4. Practice parameter: the management of concussion in sports (summary statement). Report of the Quality Standards Subcommittee. Neurology 1997;48(3):581-585.

5. Aldrich EF, Eisenberg HM, Saydjari C, Luerssen TG, Foulkes MA, Jane JA, et al. Diffuse brain swelling in severely head-injured children. A report from the NIH Traumatic Coma Data Bank. J Neurosurg 1992;76(3):450-454.

6. Alla S, Sullivan SJ, Hale L, McCrory P. Self-report scales/checklists for the measurement of concussion symptoms: a systematic review. Br J Sports Med 2009;43 Suppl 1:i3-12.

7. AMA. Subcommittee on Classification of Sports Injuries. Standard Nomenclature of Athletic Injuries. Chicago: American Medical Association; 1966.

8. Aubry M, Cantu R, Dvorak J, Graf-Baumann T, Johnston K, Kelly J, et al. Summary and agreement statement of the First International Conference on Concussion in Sport, Vienna 2001. Recommendations for the improvement of safety and health of athletes who may suffer concussive injuries. Br J Sports Med 2002;36(1):6-10.

9. Barlow KM, Crawford S, Stevenson A, Sandhu SS, Belanger F, Dewey D. Epidemiology of postconcussion syndrome in pediatric mild traumatic brain injury. Pediatrics 2010;126(2):e374-381.

10. Barr WB, McCrea M. Sensitivity and specificity of standardized neurocognitive testing immediately following sports concussion. J Int Neuropsychol Soc 2001;7:693-702.

11. Bauer R, Fritz H. Pathophysiology of traumatic injury in the developing brain: an introduction and short update. Exp Toxicol Pathol 2004;56(1-2):65-73.

12. Broshek DK, Kaushik T, Freeman JR, Erlanger D, Webbe F, Barth JT. Sex differences in outcome following sports-related concussion. J Neurosurg 2005;102(5):856-863.

13. Bruce DA, Alavi A, Bilaniuk L, Dolinskas C, Obrist W, Uzzell B. Diffuse cerebral swelling following head injuries in children: the syndrome of "malignant brain edema." J Neurosurg 1981;54(2):170-178.

14. Bryant RA, Harvey AG. Postconcussive symptoms and posttraumatic stress disorder after mild traumatic brain injury. J Nerv Ment Dis 1999;187(5):302-305.

15. BTF. Press Release: Brain Trauma Foundation awarded DOD Contract to Define Concussion. New York: Brain Trauma Foundation; 2012. Available from: www.braintrauma.org/pdf/concussion_press_release.pdf.

16. Cantu RC. Athletic head injuries. Clin Sports Med 1997;16(3):531-542.

17. Cantu RC. Head injuries in sport. Br J Sports Med 1996;30(4):289-296.

18. Carroll LJ, Cassidy JD, Holm L, Kraus J, Coronado VG. Methodological issues and research recommendations for mild traumatic brain injury: the WHO Collaborating Centre Task Force on Mild Traumatic Brain Injury. J Rehabil Med 2004(43 Suppl):113-125.

19. Cassidy JD, Carroll LJ, Peloso PM, Borg J, von Holst H, Holm L, et al. Incidence, risk factors and prevention of mild traumatic brain injury: results of the WHO Collaborating Centre Task Force on Mild Traumatic Brain Injury. J Rehabil Med 2004(43 Suppl):28-60.

20. Cavanaugh JT, Guskiewicz KM, Giuliani C, Marshall S, Mercer V, Stergiou N. Detecting altered postural control after cerebral concussion in athletes with normal postural stability. Br J Sports Med 2005;39(11):805-811.

21. Cernak I, Chang T, Ahmed FA, Cruz MI, Vink R, Stoica B, et al. Pathophysiological response to experimental diffuse brain trauma differs as a function of developmental age. Dev Neurosci 2010;32(5-6):442-453.

22. Collins MW, Field M, Lovell MR, Iverson G, Johnston KM, Maroon J, et al. Relationship between postconcussion headache and neuropsychological test performance in high school athletes. Am J Sports Med 2003;31(2):168-173.

23. Collins MW, Iverson GL, Lovell MR, McKeag DB, Norwig J, Maroon J. On-field predictors of neuropsychological and symptom deficit following sports-related concussion. Clin J Sport Med 2003;13(4):222-229.

24. Collins MW, Lovell MR, McKeag DB. Current issues in managing sports-related concussion. JAMA 1999;282(24):2283-2285.

25. Colvin AC, Mullen J, Lovell MR, West RV, Collins MW, Groh M. The role of concussion history and gender in recovery from soccer-related concussion. Am J Sports Med 2009;37(9):1699-1704.

26. Covassin T, Elbin RJ. The female athlete: the role of gender in the assessment and management of sport-related concussion. Clin Sports Med 2011;30(1):125-131, x.

27. Covassin T, Schatz P, Swanik CB. Sex differences in neuropsychological function and post-concussion symptoms of concussed collegiate athletes. Neurosurgery 2007;61(2):345-350; discussion 350-341.

28. Covassin T, Swanik CB, Sachs ML. Sex differences and the incidence of concussions among collegiate athletes. J Athl Train 2003;38(3):238-244.

29. Davis GA, Iverson GL, Guskiewicz KM, Ptito A, Johnston KM. Contributions of neuroimaging, balance testing, electrophysiology and blood markers to the assessment of sport-related concussion. Br J Sports Med 2009;43 Suppl 1:i36-45.

30. Eckner JT, Kutcher JS. Concussion symptom scales and sideline assessment tools: a critical literature update. Curr Sports Med Rep 2010;9(1):8-15.

31. Ellemberg D, Henry LC, Macciocchi SN, Guskiewicz KM, Broglio SP. Advances in sport concussion assessment: from behavioral to brain imaging measures. J Neurotrauma 2009;26(12):2365-2382.

32. Farace E, Alves WM. Do women fare worse: a meta-analysis of gender differences in traumatic brain injury outcome. J Neurosurg 2000;93(4):539-545.

33. Field M, Collins MW, Lovell MR, Maroon J. Does age play a role in recovery from sports-related concussion? A comparison of high school and collegiate athletes. J Pediatr 2003;142(5):546-553.

34. Fisher CM. Concussion amnesia. Neurology 1966;16:826-830.

35. Gessel LM, Fields SK, Collins CL, Dick RW, Comstock RD. Concussions among United States high school and collegiate athletes. J Athl Train 2007;42(4):495-503.

36. Gioia GA, Schneider JC, Vaughan CG, Isquith PK. Which symptom assessments and approaches are uniquely appropriate for paediatric concussion? Br J Sports Med 2009;43 Suppl 1:i13-22.

37. Giza CC, Griesbach GS, Hovda DA. Experience-dependent behavioral plasticity is disturbed following traumatic injury to the immature brain. Behav Brain Res 2005;157(1):11-22.

38. Goldsmith W, Plunkett J. A biomechanical analysis of the causes of traumatic brain injury in infants and children. Am J Forensic Med Pathol 2004;25(2):89-100.

39. Grady MF. Concussion in the adolescent athlete. Curr Probl Pediatr Adolesc Health Care 2010;40(7):154-169.

40. Granite V, Carroll J. Psychological response to athletic injury: sex differences. J Sport Behav 2002;25:243-259.

41. Gurkoff GG, Giza CC, Hovda DA. Lateral fluid percussion injury in the developing rat causes an acute, mild behavioral dysfunction in the absence of significant cell death. Brain Res 2006;1077(1):24-36.

42. Guskiewicz KM, Broglio SP. Sport-related concussion: on-field and sideline assessment. Phys Med Rehabil Clin N Am 2011;22(4):603-617, vii.

43. Guskiewicz KM, Bruce SL, Cantu RC, Ferrara MS, Kelly JP, McCrea M, et al. National Athletic Trainers' Association position statement: management of sport-related concussion. J Athl Train 2004;39(3):280-297.

44. Guskiewicz KM, McCrea M, Marshall SW, Cantu RC, Randolph C, Barr W, et al. Cumulative effects associated with recurrent concussion in collegiate football players: the NCAA Concussion Study. JAMA 2003;290(19):2549-2555.

45. Guskiewicz KM, Ross SE, Marshall SW. Postural stability and neuropsychological deficits after concussion in collegiate athletes. J Athl Train 2001;36(3):263-273.

46. Guskiewicz KM, Weaver NL, Padua DA, Garrett WE Jr. Epidemiology of concussion in collegiate and high school football players. Am J Sports Med 2000;28(5):643-650.

47. Halstead ME, Walter KD. American Academy of Pediatrics. Clinical report—sport-related concussion in children and adolescents. Pediatrics 2010;126(3):597-615.

48. Hootman JM, Dick R, Agel J. Epidemiology of collegiate injuries for 15 sports: summary and recommendations for injury prevention initiatives. J Athl Train 2007;42(2):311-319.

49. Iverson GL, Gaetz M, Lovell MR, Collins MW. Relation between subjective fogginess and neuropsychological testing following concussion. J Int Neuropsychol Soc 2004;10(6):904-906.

50. Jennett B, Bond M. Assessment of outcome after severe brain damage. Lancet 1975;1(7905):480-484.

51. Karlin AM. Concussion in the pediatric and adolescent population: "different population, different concerns." PM R 2011;3(10 Suppl 2):S369-379.

52. Kay T, Harrington DE, Adams R, Anderson T, Berrol S, Cicerone K, et al. Report of the Mild Traumatic Brain Injury Committee of the Head Injury Interdisciplinary Special Interest Group of the American Congress of Rehabilitation Medicine. Definition of mild traumatic brain injury. J Head Trauma Rehabil 1993;8:86-87.

53. Kelly JP, Nichols JS, Filley CM, Lillehei KO, Rubinstein D, Kleinschmidt-DeMasters BK. Concussion in sports. Guidelines for the prevention of catastrophic outcome. JAMA 1991;266(20):2867-2869.

54. Kelly JP, Rosenberg JH. Diagnosis and management of concussion in sports. Neurology 1997;48(3):575-580.

55. Lau B, Lovell MR, Collins MW, Pardini J. Neurocognitive and symptom predictors of recovery in high school athletes. Clin J Sport Med 2009;19(3):216-221.

56. Lau BC, Kontos AP, Collins MW, Mucha A, Lovell MR. Which on-field signs/symptoms predict protracted recovery from sport-related concussion among high school football players? Am J Sports Med 2011;39(11):2311-2318.

57. Leininger BE, Gramling SE, Farrell AD, Kreutzer JS, Peck EA III. Neuropsychological deficits in symptomatic minor head injury patients after concussion and mild concussion. J Neurol Neurosurg Psychiatry 1990;53(4):293-296.

58. Lovell MR, Collins MW, Iverson GL, Field M, Maroon JC, Cantu R, et al. Recovery from mild concussion in high school athletes. J Neurosurg 2003;98(2):296-301.

59. Lovell MR, Iverson GL, Collins MW, McKeag D, Maroon JC. Does loss of consciousness predict neuropsychological decrements after concussion? Clin J Sport Med 1999;9(4):193-198.

60. Lovell MR, Iverson GL, Collins MW, Podell K, Johnston KM, Pardini D, et al. Measurement of symptoms following sports-related concussion: reliability and normative data for the post-concussion scale. Appl Neuropsychol 2006;13(3):166-174.

61. Luis CA, Vanderploeg RD, Curtiss G. Predictors of postconcussion symptom complex in community dwelling male veterans. J Int Neuropsychol Soc 2003;9(7):1001-1015.

62. Maddocks D, Saling M. Neuropsychological deficits following concussion. Brain Inj 1996;10(2):99-103.

63. Makdissi M, Darby D, Maruff P, Ugoni A, Brukner P, McCrory PR. Natural history of concussion in sport: markers of severity and implications for management. Am J Sports Med 2010;38(3):464-471.

64. McCauley SR, Boake C, Levin HS, Contant CF, Song JX. Postconcussional disorder following mild to moderate traumatic brain injury: anxiety, depression, and social support as risk factors and comorbidities. J Clin Exp Neuropsychol 2001;23(6):792-808.

65. McClincy MP, Lovell MR, Pardini J, Collins MW, Spore MK. Recovery from sports concussion in high school and collegiate athletes. Brain Inj 2006;20(1):33-39.

66. McCrea M. Sideline assessment of concussion. In: Bailes JE, Day AL, eds. Neurological Sports Medicine: A Guide for Physicians and Trainers. Rolling Meadows, IL: American Association of Neurological Surgeons; 2001:109-122.

67. McCrea M. Standardized mental status assessment of sports concussion. Clin J Sport Med 2001;11(3):176-181.

68. McCrea M, Barr WB, Guskiewicz K, Randolph C, Marshall SW, Cantu R, et al. Standard regression-based methods for measuring recovery after sport-related concussion. J Int Neuropsychol Soc 2005;11(1):58-69.

69. McCrea M, Guskiewicz KM, Marshall SW, Barr W, Randolph C, Cantu RC, et al. Acute effects and recovery time following concussion in collegiate football players: the NCAA Concussion Study. JAMA 2003;290(19):2556-2563.

70. McCrea M, Kelly JP, Kluge J, Ackley B, Randolph C. Standardized assessment of concussion in football players. Neurology 1997;48(3):586-588.

71. McCrea M, Kelly JP, Randolph C, Kluge J, Bartolic E, Finn G, et al. Standardized assessment of concussion (SAC): on-site mental status evaluation of the athlete. J Head Trauma Rehabil 1998;13(2):27-35.

72. McCrory P, Collie A, Anderson V, Davis G. Can we manage sport related concussion in children the same as in adults? Br J Sports Med 2004;38(5):516-519.

73. McCrory P, Johnston K, Meeuwisse W, Aubry M, Cantu R, Dvorak J, et al. Summary and agreement statement of the 2nd International Conference on Concussion in Sport, Prague 2004. Br J Sports Med 2005;39(4):196-204.

74. McCrory P, Meeuwisse W, Johnston K, Dvorak J, Aubry M, Molloy M, et al. Consensus statement on concussion in sport: the 3rd International Conference on Concussion in Sport held in Zurich, November 2008. Br J Sports Med 2009;43 Suppl 1:i76-90.

75. McCrory P, Meeuwisse WH, Aubry M, Cantu B, Dvorak J, Echemendia RJ, et al. Consensus statement on concussion in sport: the 4th International Conference on Concussion in Sport held in Zurich, November 2012. Br J Sports Med 2013;47(5):250-258.

76. McCrory PR, Ariens T, Berkovic SF. The nature and duration of acute concussive symptoms in Australian football. Clin J Sport Med 2000;10(4):235-238.

77. McCrory PR, Berkovic SF. Concussion: the history of clinical and pathophysiological concepts and misconceptions. Neurology 2001;57(12):2283-2289.

78. McCrory PR, Berkovic SF. Video analysis of acute motor and convulsive manifestations in

sport-related concussion. Neurology 2000; 54(7):1488-1491.

79. McCrory PR, Bladin PF, Berkovic SF. Retrospective study of concussive convulsions in elite Australian rules and rugby league footballers: phenomenology, aetiology, and outcome. BMJ 1997;314(7075):171-174.

80. McDonald JW, Johnston MV. Physiological and pathophysiological roles of excitatory amino acids during central nervous system development. Brain Res Brain Res Rev 1990;15(1):41-70.

81. McLeod TC, Leach C. Psychometric properties of self-report concussion scales and checklists. J Athl Train 2012;47(2):221-223.

82. Meares S, Shores EA, Taylor AJ, Batchelor J, Bryant RA, Baguley IJ, et al. Mild traumatic brain injury does not predict acute postconcussion syndrome. J Neurol Neurosurg Psychiatry 2008;79(3):300-306.

83. Meehan WP III. Medical therapies for concussion. Clin Sports Med 2011;30(1):115-124, ix.

84. Meehan WP III, Bachur RG. Sport-related concussion. Pediatrics 2009;123(1):114-123.

85. Meehan WP III, d'Hemecourt P, Comstock RD. High school concussions in the 2008-2009 academic year: mechanism, symptoms, and management. Am J Sports Med 2010;38(12):2405-2409.

86. Meehan WP III, Taylor AM, Proctor M. The pediatric athlete: younger athletes with sport-related concussion. Clin Sports Med 2011;30(1):133-144, x.

87. Mesulam MM. Principles of Behavioral Neurology. Philadelphia: Davis; 1985.

88. Mihalik JP, Blackburn JT, Greenwald RM, Cantu RC, Marshall SW, Guskiewicz KM. Collision type and player anticipation affect head impact severity among youth ice hockey players. Pediatrics 2010;125(6):e1394-1401.

89. Ommaya AK, Goldsmith W, Thibault L. Biomechanics and neuropathology of adult and paediatric head injury. Br J Neurosurg 2002;16(3):220-242.

90. Pardini J, Bailes JE, Maroon JC. Mild traumatic brain injury in adults and concussion in sports. In: Winn HR, ed. Youmans Neurological Surgery. 6th ed. Philadelphia: Saunders; 2011:3380-3389.

91. Patel AV, Mihalik JP, Notebaert AJ, Guskiewicz KM, Prentice WE. Neuropsychological performance, postural stability, and symptoms after dehydration. J Athl Train 2007;42(1):66-75.

92. Patel DR, Reddy V. Sport-related concussion in adolescents. Pediatr Clin North Am 2010;57(3):649-670.

93. Pellman EJ, Lovell MR, Viano DC, Casson IR. Concussion in professional football: recovery of NFL and high school athletes assessed by computerized neuropsychological testing--part 12. Neurosurgery 2006;58(2):263-274; discussion 263-274.

94. Petraglia AL, Maroon JC, Bailes JE. From the field of play to the field of combat: a review of the pharmacological management of concussion. Neurosurgery 2012; 70(6):1520-1533.

95. Pickles W. Acute general edema of the brain in children with head injuries. New Engl J Med 1950;242(16):607-611.

96. Ponsford J, Willmott C, Rothwell A, Cameron P, Kelly AM, Nelms R, et al. Factors influencing outcome following mild traumatic brain injury in adults. J Int Neuropsychol Soc 2000;6(5):568-579.

97. Preiss-Farzanegan SJ, Chapman B, Wong TM, Wu J, Bazarian JJ. The relationship between gender and postconcussion symptoms after sport-related mild traumatic brain injury. PM R 2009;1(3):245-253.

98. Prins ML, Hales A, Reger M, Giza CC, Hovda DA. Repeat traumatic brain injury in the juvenile rat is associated with increased axonal injury and cognitive impairments. Dev Neurosci 2010;32(5-6):510-518.

99. Putukian M. The acute symptoms of sport-related concussion: diagnosis and on-field management. Clin Sports Med 2011;30(1):49-61, viii.

100. Randolph C, Millis S, Barr WB, McCrea M, Guskiewicz KM, Hammeke TA, et al. Concussion symptom inventory: an empirically derived scale for monitoring resolution of symptoms following sport-related concussion. Arch Clin Neuropsychol 2009;24(3):219-229.

101. Reddy C. A treatment paradigm for sports concussion. Brain Injury Professional 2004;4:24-25.

102. Riemann BL, Guskiewicz KM. Effects of mild head injury on postural stability as measured through clinical balance testing. J Athl Train 2000;35(1):19-25.

103. Ruff RM, Camenzuli L, Mueller J. Miserable minority: emotional risk factors that influence the outcome of a mild traumatic brain injury. Brain Inj 1996;10(8):551-565.

104. Schneiders AG, Sullivan SJ, Gray AR, Hammond-Tooke GD, McCrory PR. Normative values for three clinical measures of motor performance used in the neurological assessment of sports concussion. J Sci Med Sport 2010;13(2):196-201.

105. Scorza KA, Raleigh MF, O'Connor FG. Current concepts in concussion: evaluation and management. Am Fam Physician 2012;85(2):123-132.

106. Shehata N, Wiley JP, Richea S, Benson BW, Duits L, Meeuwisse WH. Sport concussion assessment tool: baseline values for varsity collision sport athletes. Br J Sports Med 2009;43(10):730-734.

107. Strugar J, Sass KJ, Buchanan CP, Spencer DD, Lowe DK. Long-term consequences of minimal brain injury: loss of consciousness does not predict memory impairment. J Trauma 1993;34(4):555-558; discussion 558-559.

108. Tator CH. Let's standardize the definition of concussion and get reliable incidence data. Can J Neurol Sci 2009;36(4):405-406.

109. Tierney RT, Sitler MR, Swanik CB, Swanik KA, Higgins M, Torg J. Gender differences in head-neck segment dynamic stabilization during head acceleration. Med Sci Sports Exerc 2005;37(2):272-279.

110. Valovich McLeod TC, Bay RC, Lam KC, Chhabra A. Representative baseline values on the Sport Concussion Assessment Tool 2 (SCAT2) in adolescent athletes vary by gender, grade, and concussion history. Am J Sports Med 2012;40(4):927-933.

111. Van Kampen DA, Lovell MR, Pardini JE, Collins MW, Fu FH. The "value added" of neurocognitive testing after sports-related concussion. Am J Sports Med 2006;34(10):1630-1635.

112. Yarnell PR, Lynch S. The "ding": amnestic states in football trauma. Neurology 1973;23(2):196-197.

113. Yarnell PR, Lynch S. Progressive retrograde amnesia in concussed football players: observation shortly postimpact. Neurology 1970;20(4):416-417.

114. Yarnell PR, Lynch S. Retrograde memory immediately after concussion. Lancet 1970;1(7652):863-864.

Neuroimaging and Neurophysiological Studies in the Head–Injured Athlete

The role of neuroimaging in concussion has been a progressive one. As noted in the definition of concussion derived from the 3rd International Conference on Concussion in Sport, "no abnormality on standard structural neuroimaging studies is seen in concussion" (p. i77).[83] While the acute symptoms in concussion may be largely due to a functional disturbance, neuropathological injury does occur at the microscopic and ultrastructural level. Imaging studies have been evaluated as a tool with the potential to objectively assess damage resulting from traumatic brain injury (TBI) and aid in the development of individual-specific recovery plans.[103] In this sense, the high incidence of concussion has increased attention regarding assessment and prognosis, and newer techniques have been investigated for their potential role in the head-injured athlete. Some of these techniques are readily used in other clinical realms of neurological medicine, while others are used in research but may have clinical relevance. Further well-designed studies are needed across the board to demonstrate a clear benefit in concussion management.

STANDARD NEUROIMAGING

Shear strain and tissue deformation caused by rotational acceleration after a closed head injury can result in diffuse axonal damage, and concussion can be viewed as residing at the mild end of the diffuse axonal injury (DAI) spectrum.[11, 68, 80] Typically, DAI presents histologically with microscopic axonal damage including myelin loss, axonal degeneration, or axonal swellings or some combination of these; however, these changes (much as with concussion) are difficult to detect with traditional neuroimaging techniques.[1, 39, 80, 98, 102, 113] Nonetheless, standard neuroimaging techniques like computed tomography (CT) and magnetic resonance imaging (MRI) still play a role in the workup of the head-injured athlete.

Computed Tomography

It is well recognized that the advent of CT in the 1970s revolutionized the management of neurotrauma.[21, 36, 57, 62, 76, 81, 116, 127-129] Modern ultrafast, multislice CT scanners can complete imaging in seconds, and for that reason, CT is still the modality of choice in emergency departments to look for macroscopic abnormalities associated with acute brain trauma.[103] Computed tomography is widely available, and from an imaging modality standpoint, a noncontrast CT of the head is exquisite in its ability to detect fractures, intracranial hemorrhage, and contusions[25, 68, 85, 132] (figure 6.1). While structural abnormalities such as contusions and extra-axial hematomas are generally absent in sport-related concussions, this is not always the case. The decision to obtain a CT scan needs to be made on an individual basis for each athlete.

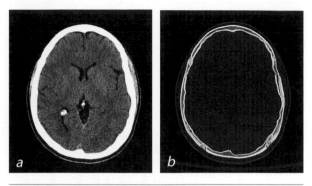

Figure 6.1 Normal computed tomography of the head with (a) brain and (b) bone windows.

Although infrequently, athletes can have a mild TBI, as defined by their Glasgow Coma Scale (GCS), with a normal neurological examination, and still have an underlying hemorrhage or contusion.[23] In one study, 209 of 1,538 patients with normal neurological examinations were found to have abnormalities on CT, with 58 of those patients even requiring neurosurgery.[122] Computed tomography has important limitations, as it is poor at detecting DAI[3, 90]; and as mentioned previously, images often are normal for concussion patients.[104] Studies of boxers with repetitive concussions have demonstrated that the majority of the time there are no significant findings on CT.[58, 91, 106] Thus, the role of CT scanning in the present-day acute management of concussion is to identify and rule out more serious pathologies. In the acute period, no other imaging study of the brain is typically indicated.

Predicting who is likely to have abnormalities on imaging and at the same time avoiding unnecessary scans has proven to be difficult.[105] Some groups have advocated for scanning all patients with concussion in order not to miss an underlying abnormality; this approach would lead to a predominance of negative scans that were not likely needed in the first place. To refine the criteria for CT scanning, several groups have developed clinical rules to aid in the decision making. Two of the better-known sets of rules are the New Orleans Criteria[45] and the Canadian CT Head Rule.[124]

New Orleans Criteria (NOC) for Determining the Need for CT Following Mild TBI

Computed tomography is required for patients with minor head injury with any one of the following findings. The criteria apply only to patients who also have a Glasgow Coma Scale score of 15.

- Headache
- Vomiting
- Older than 60 years
- Drug or alcohol intoxication
- Persistent anterograde amnesia (deficits in short-term memory)
- Visible trauma above the clavicle
- Seizure

Adapted from Haydel et al. 2000.

The Canadian CT Head Rule

Computed tomography is required only for patients with minor head injury who present with any one of the following findings: Glasgow Coma Scale score of 13 to 15 after witnessed loss of consciousness, amnesia, or confusion.

High Risk for Neurosurgical Intervention

- Glasgow Coma Scale score lower than 15 at 2 hours after injury
- Suspected open or depressed skull fracture
- Any sign of basal skull fracture†
- Two or more episodes of vomiting
- 65 years or older

Medium Risk for Brain Injury Detection by CT Imaging

- Retrograde amnesia of 30 or more minutes
- Dangerous mechanism‡

Note: The rule is not applicable if the patient did not experience a trauma, has a Glasgow Coma Scale score lower than 13, is younger than 16 years, is taking warfarin or has a bleeding disorder, or has an obvious open skull fracture.

† Signs of basal skull fracture include hemotympanum, raccoon eyes, cerebrospinal fluid, otorrhea or rhinorrhea, and Battle's sign.

‡ Dangerous mechanism includes a pedestrian struck by a motor vehicle, an occupant ejected from a motor vehicle, or a fall from an elevation of 3 or more feet (>0.9 m) or five stairs.

Adapted from Stiell et al. 2001.

Each of these clinical decision rules has been validated prospectively, and both include seven criteria, although the only ones they have in common are older age and vomiting. The efficacy of relying on the presence of any of the clinical features in deciding whether to order a CT was studied in two large prospective validation trials.[114, 123] The sensitivity and specificity of the New Orleans Criteria were 99% and 5%, respectively, for detecting any lesion or clinically important CT abnormality.[45, 114, 124] The sensitivity and specificity for detecting lesions requiring neurosurgery were 100% and 5%, respectively. The studies defined clinically important lesions not requiring immediate surgery as contusions, subarachnoid blood, small subdural hematomas, and skull fractures as well as parenchymal and intraventricular hemorrhages. The sensitivity and specificity of the Canadian CT Head Rule criteria for detecting clinically important CT lesions was found to be 87% and 39%, respectively; the sensitivity and specificity for detecting lesions requiring neurosurgery was 100% and 38%, respectively.[114, 123, 124] Patients 15 years and younger were excluded from one of the original studies[124] and from both validation studies[114, 123]; therefore, the applicability of these rules to that age group is uncertain. The CHALICE criteria and rule was derived from a prospective multicenter cohort study in an attempt to provide a rule for selection of high-risk children with head injury for CT scanning.[29] The study included children with head injury of any severity. The criteria were found to have a sensitivity of 98% and a specificity of 87% for the prediction of clinically significant head injury and resulted in a CT scan rate of 14%.[29]

The CHALICE Rule: The Children's Head Injury Algorithm for the Prediction of Important Clinical Events Rule

A CT scan is required if any of the following criteria are present.

History

- Witnessed loss of consciousness of >5 minutes duration
- History of amnesia (either anterograde or retrograde) of >5 minutes duration
- Abnormal drowsiness (defined as drowsiness in excess of that expected by the examining doctor)
- Three or more vomits after head injury (a vomit is defined as a single discrete episode of vomiting)
- Suspicion of nonaccidental injury (NAI) (defined as any suspicion of NAI by the examining doctor)

- Seizure after head injury in a patient who has no history of epilepsy

Examination

- Glasgow Coma Scale <14 or GCS <15 if <1 year old
- Suspicion of penetrating or depressed skull injury or tense fontanelle
- Sign of basal skull fracture (defined as evidence of blood or cerebrospinal fluid leakage from the ear or nose, panda eyes, Battle's sign, hemotympanum, facial crepitus, or serious facial injury)
- Positive focal neurology (defined as any focal neurology, including motor, sensory, coordination, or reflex abnormality)
- Presence of bruise, swelling, or laceration >5 cm if <1 year old

Mechanism

- High-speed road traffic accident as either a pedestrian, cyclist, or occupant (defined as accident with speed >40 miles per hour [64 km/h])
- Fall of >3 m in height
- High-speed injury from a projectile or an object

No clinically based rule for obtaining a CT scan is likely to be universally accurate. In using these rules, the physician should consider the level of acceptable risk for overlooking any intracranial lesion as opposed to missing lesions that require monitoring or immediate neurosurgical intervention.[105] Some cost-effectiveness studies have argued that although the incidence of intracranial lesions, especially those that require surgery, is low in mild TBI, the consequences of delayed diagnosis are forbidding; and the adverse outcome of an intracranial hematoma is so costly that it more than balances the expense of CT scans.[118-120] Additionally, it is important to remember that the absence of CT abnormalities is not a guarantee of good outcome, nor does the presence of CT abnormalities reflect long-term impairment.[57, 93] In general, with concussion, most agree that a CT should be performed in the presence of loss of consciousness (LOC); a severe or prolonged alteration in level of consciousness; disorientation, posttraumatic amnesia, severe headache, or vomiting; or any focal neurological deficit.[75, 119, 121, 122, 137]

Magnetic Resonance Imaging

Magnetic resonance imaging (MRI) has greater detail resolution than CT, is more sensitive and specific (particularly in the evaluation of mild TBI), and can detect structural abnormalities earlier than CT.[39, 41, 44, 57, 59, 60, 99, 117] Until recently, it had not been used in the acute setting as frequently because of its susceptibility to metal- and motion-related artifact, as well as long scan times and decreased sensitivity in detecting skull fractures; however, these limitations have been addressed in the past decade.[103] Magnetic resonance imaging also has the advantage of providing multiplanar imaging, absence of bone artifact, high level of contrast between brain and cerebrospinal fluid (CSF), and the ability to easily differentiate gray from white matter.[57] Also, the scans do not expose patients to radiation as occurs with CT scanning. An MRI of the brain generally consists of routine T1 and T2 spin-echo sequences, a fluid attenuation inversion recovery (FLAIR) sequence, and a gradient-echo (GRE) sequence (figure 6.2).

Conventional MRI sequences such as T1-weighted and T2-weighted provide exquisite detail of intracranial and cerebral structure and can identify occult lesions not typically visualized on CT scans.[26, 50] Diffuse axonal injury on MRI images appear as numerous, small, deeply situated lesions that typically spare the overlying cortex. The vast majority of these lesions are nonhemorrhagic (80%), and the rest contain small central areas of petechial hemorrhage.[57, 88] One study examining the prevalence of MRI evidence of DAI in patients with mild head injury and normal CT findings demonstrated that there are lesions compatible with hemorrhagic and nonhemorrhagic DAI in approximately 30% of cases of mild TBI with normal head CT scans.[90] Still, even though MRI outperforms CT in detecting DAI, injuries are difficult to detect with conventional sequences.[80]

Fluid attenuation inversion recovery sequences offer another form of soft tissue contrast. The sequence is considered extremely sensitive in detecting traumatic lesions.[50, 60] The sequence essentially provides a T2-weighted image without the CSF signal by running a 180-degree inversion pulse. The resultant image provides superior discrimination between the CSF and underlying cerebral cortex, improving the detection of cortical trauma.[5] Gradient-echo (GRE) sequences are better at detecting hemorrhagic change. The sequence has incredible magnetic susceptibility, which aids in detecting small areas of hemorrhage. The technique is most often useful after time has elapsed since the initial injury, when only remnants of extracellular hemosiderin persist.[57, 85]

Although a number of published studies have evaluated the sensitivity of MRI in mild TBI,[26, 48, 50, 70, 134] no study has addressed the role of MRI in the management of sport-related concussion. This may partly explain the absence of guidelines for the use of MRI as a routine tool in the investigation of concussion.[23] Additionally, the overall availability of MRI machines and costs may limit

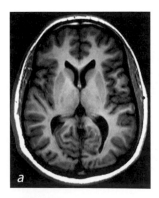 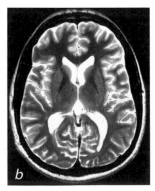 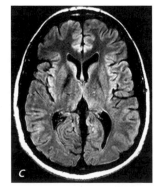 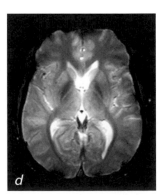

Figure 6.2　Axial magnetic resonance images of a healthy brain at basal ganglia level acquired with high spatial resolution on a 3T. (a) T1-weighted image, (b) T2-weighted image, (c) FLAIR, (d) gradient-echo MRI.

its routine use. Another important point of consideration that has been raised in several recent reviews[80, 85] is that standard structural MRI imaging, like CT scans, does not correlate well with the number of self-reported postconcussive symptoms, performance on neuropsychological tests, or long-term outcome.[50, 69, 94, 110]

ADVANCED STRUCTURAL TECHNIQUES

While many of the previously mentioned MRI sequences have been designed to evaluate for structural damage at the macroscopic level, recently developed advanced sequences have the potential to increase the sensitivity of MRI to detect both structural and functional abnormalities associated with concussion, both in the acute setting and subsequently in the subacute and chronic phase of recovery. These newer structural techniques include susceptibility-weighted imaging (SWI), diffusion-weighted imaging (DWI) with apparent diffusion coefficient (ADC) mapping, quantitative MRI techniques (i.e., voxel-based morphometry [VBM], brain segmentation), diffusion tensor imaging (DTI), and high-density fiber tracking (HDFT). The use of these new techniques is especially relevant in cases in which conventional CT and MRI sequences are unable to detect macroscopic structural abnormalities.[103]

Susceptibility–Weighted Imaging

Improvements in gradient-echo imaging techniques have increased our ability to detect the susceptibility-related effects of shear-related hemorrhagic injury.[103] Susceptibility-weighted imaging (SWI) uses rapid spin dephasing to accentuate signal dropout and increase the visibility of microhemorrhages (figure 6.3). The method is extremely sensitive to paramagnetic properties of iron and blood products and detects microhemorrhages where conventional MRI fails.[103]

Susceptibility-weighted imaging is best used at higher field strengths, as the TE (time to echo) is much longer at low fields and acquisitions need to be longer.[8, 42, 89] In addition, higher field strengths allow isotropic in-plane resolution to be obtained, increase the signal-to-noise ratio

(SNR), and increase the resolution.[8, 42, 89] Additionally, SWI goes beyond GRE sequences in its ability to differentiate between hemorrhage and calcium and visualize vessel connectivity and microbleed location in relation to the vasculature and other structures in the brain.[8, 141, 143]

Despite its ability to detect intraparenchymal injury, the exact role that microhemorrhages detected by SWI plays in determining prognosis is not completely clear, especially in concussion.[103] Some studies have reported that the number and volume of SWI hemorrhagic lesions measured using automated methods in the head-injured patient may correlate with specific neuropsychological deficits on long-term follow-up.[7, 103] Conversely, a recent study failed to demonstrate prognostic value in SWI-detected lesions.[16] The study sought to identify which modality and anatomic model best predicted outcome in 38 adults with TBI over a 3-year study period. The authors found that T2-weighted and FLAIR imaging most consistently discriminated between good and poor outcomes by median total lesion volume, median volume per lesion, median number of lesions, and zonal distribution.[16] While SWI rarely discriminated by outcome, it was very sensitive to intraparenchymal injury.

Foci of microhemorrhages in TBI patients likely do not correlate directly with neurological

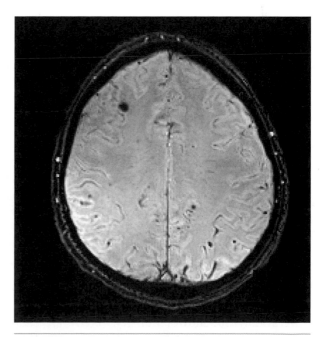

Figure 6.3 Susceptibility-weighted image (SWI) identifying multiple punctate hypointense microhemorrhages in central semiovale and gray–white matter junctions.

impairment but rather are markers of a more severe injury and may indicate a more significant amount of DAI. There is clearly room for improvement in the technical aspects of acquiring the SWI sequence, such as standardizing across scanner manufacturers, reducing acquisition times, and decreasing artifact around the skull base.[103] Further well-designed, prospective studies are needed, and only time will tell whether or not SWI could add to the diagnostic workup of patients with concussion.

Diffusion–Weighted Imaging With Apparent Diffusion Coefficient

Diffusion-weighted imaging (DWI) has been shown to identify shearing injuries not evident on T2-weighted, FLAIR, or gradient-echo sequences, thus making it valuable in evaluating closed head injuries.[6, 52, 72, 135, 136] Diffusion-weighted imaging can be performed with the same hardware that is concurrently used with conventional MRI images and does not require contrast injection. More commonly known as an imaging tool in stroke,[72, 135, 136] DWI provides the ability to detect subtle alterations in the cellular microenvironment or Brownian motion of water molecules. Recent studies have indicated that the addition of DWI to standard MRI imaging sequences increased the prevalence of signal abnormalities in athletes with concussion from 20% to 33%.[57, 74] One study demonstrated that the volume of lesions on DWI imaging provided the strongest correlation with score on a modified Rankin scale at discharge when compared to other standard MRI modalities.[109] An additional strength of DWI, with its associated apparent diffusion coefficient (ADC) mapping, is the ability to distinguish recent from old injury, which can often be difficult on routine T2 and FLAIR imaging[57, 79] (figure 6.4). The intracellular accumulation of water that occurs in cytotoxic edema is expressed as a reduction in the ADC.[103]

Quantitative MRI Techniques

Advances in quantitative morphometric MRI analyses allow measurement of differences in gray and white matter density or volume that may identify regional structural damage possibly too subtle for standard clinical interpretation.[4, 104] Two types of quantitative techniques include

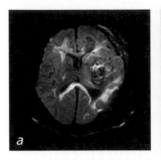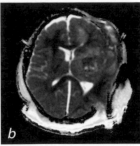

Figure 6.4 Magnetic resonance imaging of the head following severe traumatic brain injury with (a) diffusion-weighted imaging and (b) apparent diffusion coefficient imaging sequences. Note the left intracerebral hemorrhage and the bilateral hyperintense regions on the DWI sequence (corresponding dark areas on ADC map) representing restricted diffusion consistent with significant white matter tract injury, particularly in the corpus callosum and subcortical white matter.

brain segmentation and voxel-based morphometry (VBM). The differences in the MRI signal intensity of the gray and white matter allow for segmentation of the brain parenchyma into two separate compartments. Likewise, the extra-axial spaces and CSF-filled ventricles can be separated. This segmentation enables volume calculation of the three different compartments because the slice thickness of the scan and the distance between slices are known.[14, 103] Qualitative and quantitative volumetric changes in specific brain areas can be accurately determined following mild to moderate trauma.[48, 78] One of the measures studied in patients following TBI is the ventricle-to-brain ratio (VBR). This ratio represents the total volume of the ventricles divided by the total brain volume, with increased VBR values indicating increasing atrophy. The ratio is directly related to the severity of injury.[103] While VBR measurements are less likely to be useful in acute cases of concussion, future studies should explore their utility in identifying changes associated with repetitive concussive and subconcussive impacts.

Voxel-based morphometry is a method of voxel-by-voxel analysis of 3-D MRI data. In subjects following TBI, VBM has been used to key in on sites where major differences are thought to occur in patients with TBI. These measurements can then be compared to those for uninjured, age-matched control patients. Voxel density in the gray and white matter is plotted on a standard 3-D surface plot of the brain.[125, 138] While studies using VBM have identified differences in frontal and temporal regions following moderate and severe TBI, it still remains primarily a research tool, and its benefit in concussion is uncertain. [38, 103]

Diffusion Tensor Imaging

Over the last decade, diffusion tensor imaging (DTI) has emerged as a valuable additional technique to investigate traumatic axonal injury in mild to severe TBI.[15, 23, 27, 28, 80, 103, 104, 107, 108] Diffusion tensor imaging is an MRI modality that is capable of providing exquisite quantitative characterization of tissue microstructure and microdynamics.[10, 80] The technique provides information regarding white matter microstructure and fiber tract integrity by measuring the degree and direction of water diffusion.[3, 9, 22, 51] It takes advantage of the Brownian motion of water molecules in the brain.[56, 67] Myelin sheaths and the cell membranes of white matter tracts restrict the movement of water molecules; therefore, while water molecules can diffuse into various directions in the brain, they often travel along the length of axons. This enables DTI to derive the directional characteristics of the neural tracts from the imaging data, using at least six diffusion gradient directions. This is sufficient to compute the diffusion tensor and create images of axons (figure 6.5).

Axonal tract integrity is assessed using a calculation of fractional anisotropy (FA), which quantifies the degree of a preferred diffusion direction in each voxel.[61, 100, 103] Fractional anisotropy is a scalar value between 0 and 1 that describes the degree of anisotropy of a diffusion process. A value of 0 indicates that diffusion is isotropic, meaning that free diffusion occurs in all directions (expected to be associated with disrupted tracts). A value of 1 indicates that diffusion occurs only along one axis and is fully restricted along all other directions (expected to be associated with normal intact white matter tracts). Therefore, FA is a measure used in DTI that is thought to reflect fiber density and integrity, axonal diameter, and myelination in white matter.[103] Overall diffusion in a tissue is characterized by mean diffusivity (MD), which is calculated as the mean of the three eigenvalues of the diffusion tensor. [22] Mean diffusivity thus measures the overall, nondirectional mobility of water molecules in

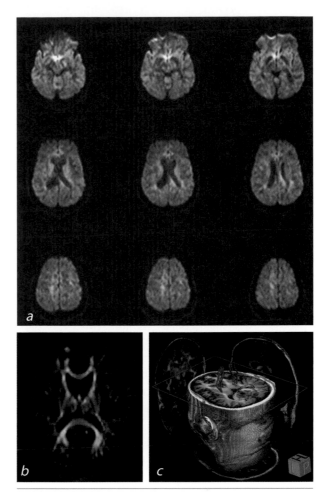

Figure 6.5 (a) Diffusion tensor images (DTI), (b) directional color fractional anisotropy (FA) map derived from DTI images, (c) FA directional color maps fused with reformatted sagittal and coronal MR images and overlaid to a 3-D rendering for spatial reference. Note that the pyramidal and callosal tractography were generated to illustrate the white matter fiber architecture in vivo. Color code: Red fibers represent left-to-right direction; green represents anterior-to-posterior direction; and blue represents superior-to-inferior direction.

the brain tissue. The modality is more sensitive to focal ischemic lesions and to diffuse axonal damage than most other imaging techniques.[22, 49] Interestingly, DTI can also provide important information regarding gray matter integrity, particularly as it relates to gliosis and necrosis, which may be of particular value in TBI.[92]

Several DTI studies have demonstrated that mild TBI is associated with widespread structural changes in cortical white matter tracts.[3, 12, 13, 22, 46, 51, 64, 73, 82, 86, 94, 96, 107, 108, 115, 139] Most DTI studies in mild TBI have focused on subjects with GCS scores ranging from 13 to 15 and have not been limited to sport-related concussion. Some studies assessed only FA in these patients,[94, 95, 107, 108] while others have assessed both FA and MD.[3, 53, 73, 82, 86, 139] This is important because a recent study suggested that MD may be a more sensitive measure than FA at detecting small structural white matter abnormalities.[22] These results were corroborated by another study that reported increased MD and no FA changes in individuals with mild TBI and persistent neurobehavioral impairment.[86] Collectively, these studies have reported abnormalities in a variety of brain regions, including the corona radiata, uncinate fasciculus, corpus callosum, inferior longitudinal fasciculus, superior longitudinal fasciculus, inferior fronto-occipital fasciculus, cingulum bundle, and internal capsule, as well as the posterior thalamic and acoustic radiations.[22]

There are some conflicting studies in the literature regarding DTI imaging in TBI. Some studies performed in the days following injury report decreased FA or increased MD or both,[3, 53, 87] while others have demonstrated increased FA or decreased MD or both.[12, 82, 139] Some studies have reported decreased FA[94] and increased MD[73] in patients with persistent cognitive impairment months following their injury. Many investigations have shown that DTI can correlate injury severity with symptoms[115] and functional deficits measured by neuropsychological tests and other behavioral measures.[63, 73, 94, 95] One study, assessing white matter integrity measured through FA in normal control subjects and mild TBI patients, revealed significant correlations between attention control and FA within the left anterior corona radiata, as well as memory performance and FA within the uncinate fasciculus.[95] Increased reaction time at 3 months postinjury has also correlated with abnormalities on DTI.[96] Another recent study did not find correlation between DTI imaging findings and postconcussion symptoms 2 months following mild TBI.[65] The authors examined the relationship between DTI imaging of the corpus callosum and postconcussion symptom reporting at 6 to 8 weeks postinjury, and there were no differences between groups on all DTI measures. Restricting analysis to just the corpus callosum in this study, though, may have resulted in the lack of clinical correlation.

Others have investigated the effects of sport concussion on white matter in both the acute and chronic phases using three different DTI measures (FA, MD, and axial diffusivity [AD]) and a voxel-based approach (VBA).[46] Henry and colleagues compared a group of 10 nonconcussed athletes with a group of 18 concussed athletes, all matched for age and education, in both the acute and chronic postinjury phases. All concussed athletes were scanned 1 to 6 days postconcussion and again 6 months later. There was a main group effect of FA, which was increased in dorsal regions of both corticospinal tracts (CST) and in the corpus callosum in concussed athletes at both time points.[46] There was a main group effect of AD in the right CST, where concussed athletes showed elevated values relative to controls at both time points.[46] Mean diffusivity values were decreased in concussed athletes, in whom analyses revealed significant group differences in the CST and corpus callosum at both time points.[46] It is key to note, though, that the use of VBA in this study limited the analyses to large tracts, and thus there are clinical limitations with regard to individual analyses.

Only a few studies have looked at the use of DTI in adolescents. In a study of children aged 10 to 18 years with mild and moderate TBI, changes in FA were identified 6 to 12 months postinjury.[140] Another study assessed adolescents aged 14 to 17 years with mild TBI and normal CT and conventional MRI scans and found altered FA on DTI within 6 days of injury, which they attributed to cytotoxic edema.[139] No studies have looked at DTI in children younger than age 10, and these findings cannot be extrapolated to that patient population. As mentioned previously, one of the other problems in interpreting many of the DTI studies has been the heterogeneous population studied with regard to severity of "mild TBI." Only a few studies have investigated purely sport-related concussion.[22, 145] One of these compared student-athletes who had sustained a recent sport-related concussion with age-matched, healthy controls using both functional MRI and DTI.[145] Concussed athletes showed an abnormal, more widespread brain activation pattern with increased blood oxygen level–dependent (BOLD) signal in the left dorsolateral prefrontal cortex (DLPC) during a spatial working memory task compared with controls. Interestingly, no significant alterations in whole-brain or region of interest (ROI) FA were observed, although there a was larger variability of FA in the genu and body of the corpus callosum in concussed athletes.[145] Decreased diffusivity, as reflected in left and right DLPC ADC maps, correlated significantly with percent change of functional MRI BOLD signal in concussed athletes but not in healthy control subjects.[145]

Although DTI is being used more commonly, its use as a regular tool in the diagnosis and management of concussion in adults and children remains to be seen. The studies thus far have suggested that DTI could be used in future research to evaluate treatment efficacy, given its enhanced sensitivity to alterations in the brain.[111] Future studies may demonstrate that DTI could potentially direct rehabilitation after concussion and possibly aid in the decision regarding when it is safe for an athlete to return to play;[84] there is no evidence at the present time to support those conclusions.

High-Density Fiber Tracking

High-density fiber tracking (HDFT) uses MRI-based DWI to produce high-resolution images of fiber tracts. This cutting edge technology is a novel combination of processing, reconstruction, and tractography methods that can track white matter fibers from cortex through complex fiber crossings to cortical and subcortical targets with subvoxel resolution[33-35, 112, 133] (figure 6.6). High-density fiber tracking can also show the shape morphology of the contact surface of the cortex, show clear gyral patterns, and allow quantification of the tract volume and integrity.

This novel approach has been reported in a few cases to successfully detect, visualize, and quan-

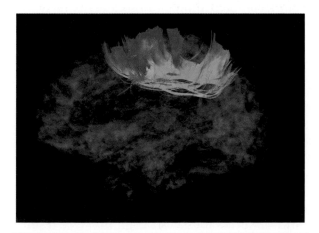

Figure 6.6 High density fiber tracking showing the fiber tracks running through the cortical and subcortical layers of the brain.

Photo courtesy of Walter Schneider Lab. Website http://hdft.info

tify damage when previous methods (CT, structural MRI, and DTI) did not provide these details. In a recent study, HDFT was used to identify a specific lesion of the corticospinal pathway in the corona radiata that was directly associated with the functional deficits in a TBI patient.[112] Fiber loss estimates at 4 months postinjury accurately predicted the nature of the motor deficits (severe, focal left-hand weakness) in this patient when other standard clinical imaging modalities did not; and a repeat scan at 10 months postinjury, when edema and hemorrhage had subsided, replicated the fiber loss.[112] The resolution is exquisite. In another case report, the authors were able to demonstrate that HDFT could identify the location of surgical cuts through individual fibers in a postoperative patient.[33]

There are some limitations to even DTI-based estimates of voxel FA, which is similarly used to assess fiber tract integrity. Diffusion tensor imaging measures have limited spatial resolution at the level of an individual voxel, their values are difficult to interpret, and they cannot identify the specificity of the cortical origins of damaged fibers.[34, 112] It is thought that DTI may have a limited ability to resolve the crossing of fibers within a voxel.[43] Additionally, DTI FA measurement may be compromised by the presence of interstitial fluid; thus the DTI measurement becomes ambiguous in the presence of hemorrhage and edema (i.e., FA decreases when there is an increase in interstitial fluid or loss of axons).[43, 55, 112, 142, 144] The HDFT imaging is thought to overcome some of these shortcomings because its analysis uses diffusion spectrum imaging, which has a high angular resolution that allows tractography to navigate complex fiber crossings accurately.[112] Thus, HDFT provides high-resolution details of axonal pathways and projection fields that allow detection of specific location and degree of damage.[34, 112] The results emerging from initial studies using this new modality are just preliminary and need to be validated in larger studies; however, the emerging data are encouraging.

ADVANCED FUNCTIONAL TECHNIQUES

Functional imaging can possibly supplement behavioral and structural imaging techniques by aiding in the evaluation of the pathophysiological and functional sequelae of concussion.[80] These methods include functional MRI, magnetic resonance spectroscopy, single-photon emission computed tomography, and positron emission tomography. Some of the algorithms reported have shown promise in objectively assessing changes and also have the potential to increase our understanding of changes in the microstructure and electrochemical alterations in the brain parenchyma following TBI, particularly concussion.

Functional Magnetic Resonance Imaging

Functional MRI (fMRI) is an imaging modality that provides information regarding neural function during task performance.[17, 31, 54] Rather than imaging brain activity, fMRI is based on the detection of changes in various physiological correlates of neuronal activation such as cerebral blood volume, cerebral blood flow, and blood oxygenation (figure 6.7). The most common approach is based on blood oxygenation changes, and the signal contrast thus generated has been termed BOLD (for blood oxygen level dependent).[57] The BOLD signal is an indirect measure of neural activity. Functional MRI uses blood oxygenation as a measure of activation of particular areas of the brain. The methodology relies on the

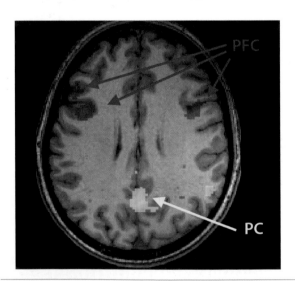

Figure 6.7 Abnormal fMRI activation by a concussion patient during memory recall. Unlike a normal-functioning group of subjects (red), a concussion patient fails to activate prefrontal cortex (PFC) during memory recall but shows compensatory activation in the posterior cingulate gyrus (PC, yellow).

premise that when a particular cerebral area is active, the local increase in oxygen-rich blood is greater than the amount of oxygen that can be extracted by the brain tissue, thus leading to the relatively greater proportion of oxygenated blood to deoxygenated blood changes in that local region.[19] The difference between the magnetic properties of the oxygen-rich blood in the vein and the deoxygenated blood in the surrounding brain tissue can be detected as an increased signal. [19] The advantages of fMRI include its improved spatial and temporal resolution, the absence of exposure to radiation, and its ability to allow for multiple scans for individuals. Tasks can be tailored to obtain information regarding specific neurological functions.

Several fMRI studies have been carried out in the setting of sport concussion, and these have been discussed thoroughly in recent reviews.[23, 40, 57, 61, 85, 103, 104] One study of college American football players compared individual brain activation patterns before and after concussive injury. [54] Brain activation was more widespread following concussion compared to both preinjury levels and levels in uninjured subjects during the performance of various memory and sensorimotor tasks. Working memory has also been evaluated in adult athletes who had sustained a concussion over the 1 to 14 months before the study and were experiencing persistent postconcussive symptoms.[17] When compared to controls, concussed athletes had less task-related activation in the mid-dorsolateral prefrontal cortex (DLPC), which is important for working memory. There also seemed to be an inverse correlation between right DLPC activation and the severity of symptoms. Interestingly, none of the symptomatic athletes had evidence of axonal injury on structural MRI.[17] Thus, this study demonstrated that functional impairment could exist in the absence of abnormalities on clinical imaging. In one of the patients, a follow-up showed that resolution of symptoms was accompanied by normalization of the observed widespread activation pattern.

Along the same lines, many studies have explored the role of fMRI in detecting recovery and compensatory patterns in serial follow-up investigations. Some researchers have correlated fMRI abnormalities with cognitive test results. One investigation looked at fMRI in 28 concussed athletes.[77] The authors performed a measure of working memory (N-back task) using fMRI soon after concussion, and then repeated the fMRI following clinical and neuropsychological recovery. They found that those athletes with hyperactivation on fMRI at the time of their first scan had a more prolonged clinical recovery than those who did not have hyperactivation.[77]

At present, fMRI (as with most of these advanced imaging modalities) is used primarily as a research tool in the area of concussion and TBI in general. Analysis of the scans requires considerable expertise, both in the reconstruction and in the interpretation of the data. There is a need for standardization of the activation tasks used, as the tasks vary from one study to another.

Additionally, the utility of fMRI in children is uncertain, and further studies are needed in this patient population.

Magnetic Resonance Spectroscopy

Magnetic resonance spectroscopy (MRS) has long been used as a noninvasive method to measure concentrations of various compounds in the brain within a sampled region.[103] The use of higher field strengths has increased the ability to accurately determine concentrations of a broader range of metabolites including neurotransmitters

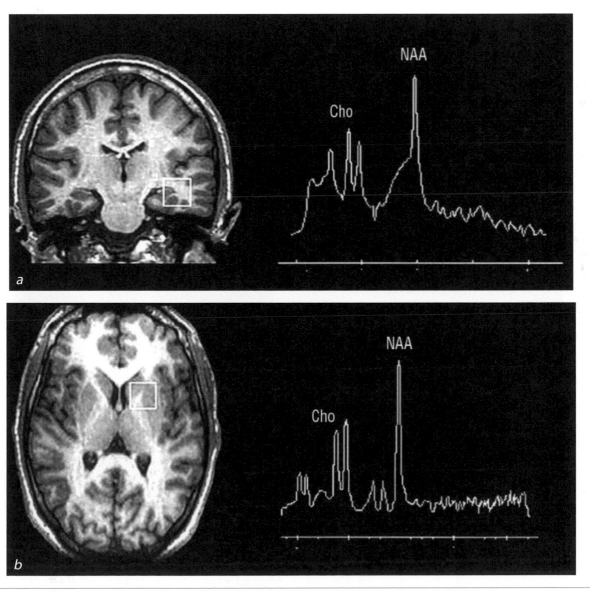

Figure 6.8 Coronal and axial proton magnetic resonance spectroscopic images show placement of the volume of interest in the left midtemporal region (a) and the left basal ganglia region (b).

Reprinted, by permission, from M.S. Mar Ariza et al., 2004, "Neuropsychological correlates of basal ganglia and medial temporal lobe NAA/Cho reductions in traumatic brain injury," Archive of Neurology 61(4): 541-544. Copyright ©2004 American Medical Association. All rights reserved.

like glutamate, glutamine, gamma-amino butyric acid (GABA), and glycine (figure 6.8). The more common metabolites measured in TBI are N-acetyl aspartate (NAA), a marker of neuronal integrity; choline, a marker of membrane damage and turnover; creatine, a cellular energy marker for adensoine triphosphate (ATP) resynthesis; lactate, an indirect marker for ischemia and hypoxia; and myoinositol, a glial marker.[23, 25, 32, 61]

The technique has been used to assess focal brain biochemistry in the context of sport concussion injury in several studies. One MRS study investigated 14 individuals who sustained a sport-related concussion.[131] The researchers performed MRS in patients at 3 or 4, 15, and 30 days postinjury. Decreased NAA/Creatine (Cr) ratios were observed at 3 days following concussion, with modest recovery at 15 days postinjury, and normalization of the NAA/Cr ratio by 30 days postinjury.[131] Interestingly, on average, the concussed athletes reported postconcussion symptom resolution by day 3 following injury despite abnormal MRS findings.[131] One individual experienced a second concussion before the day 15 MRS time point and was observed to have a further decrease in NAA/Cr, and complete metabolic recovery was delayed in this patient until 45 days postconcussion. The intriguing results from this study suggest differences in recovery as determined by symptom reporting versus metabolic recording; and more importantly, a second concussion before recovery from a first concussion was noted to result in further metabolic compromise and to delay the metabolic recovery period. A similar reduction in NAA was observed in a separate MRS study in athletes with mild TBI.[20]

Yet another investigation showed a significant decrease in NAA/Cr in prefrontal and primary motor cortices but not in the hippocampal regions in concussed athletes compared with nonconcussed athletes.[47] Additionally, decreased glutamate/Cr ratios were observed in primary motor cortices, but not in DLPC. In contrast, though, to the results in the aforementioned study,[131] the neurometabolic changes correlated temporally with resolution of self-reported postconcussive symptoms in these patients.[47]

Despite the encouraging preliminary results, the evidence for MRS does not yet support its use in routine clinical practice in all patients undergoing MRI for evaluation of TBI, and it thus remains largely a research tool. Magnetic resonance spectroscopy should be studied further, particularly in the follow-up of athletes with concussion and those who continue to have persistent symptoms consistent with a postconcussion syndrome or prolonged postconcussion syndrome.

Single–Photon Emission Computed Tomography

Single-photon emission computed tomography (SPECT) is an invasive test that involves the intravenous injection of a radioisotope (e.g., technetium-99m), followed by acquisition of brain images from a scintillation gamma camera. [23] The technique gives a measure of regional cerebral blood flow by imaging the extent and location of the radioisotope as it moves through brain vasculature[104] (figure 6.9). Its utility is limited because of the procedural complexity and the risk of radiation exposure to otherwise healthy subjects. Also, SPECT is less helpful in assessing diffuse injury (e.g., TBI) than focal injuries (e.g., cerebrovascular accident, brain tumor).[104] The reason is that SPECT analyses are typically done

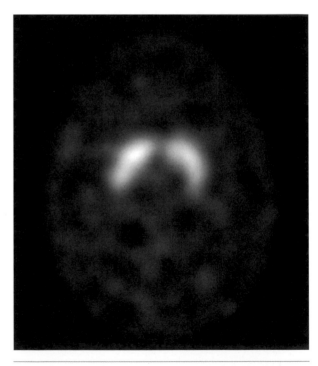

Figure 6.9 SPECT Dopamine transporter (DaT) image of a healthy brain. Note the two symmetric comma-shaped areas of normal dopamine uptake in bilateral striatal areas.

via comparing a ROI in the brain to another part that is assumed to be normal, which in the case of TBI may be an incorrect assumption if the injury is diffuse.

Some preliminary work in adults with non–sport-related mild TBI identified SPECT abnormalities in the medial temporal lobe.[130] Another study, on children ranging from 2 to 18 years of age with non–sport-related mild TBI, suggested that medial temporal hypoperfusion on SPECT imaging was associated with persistent post-concussion syndrome.[2] This study was limited, though, by poor study design, small patient numbers, and lack of neuropsychological assessment.[23] No study to date has investigated purely sport-related concussion or TBI with SPECT imaging. For this reason and many of the aforementioned limitations, SPECT is not routinely used in the evaluation of patients with concussion.

Positron Emission Tomography

Positron emission tomography (PET) is an invasive test, like SPECT, that uses radionuclides. The technique is used to measure aspects of cerebral metabolism, including blood flow and the cerebral metabolic rate of oxygen. Radionuclides such as 2-(F-18)fluoro-2-deoxyglucose (FDG), injected intravenously, cross the blood–brain barrier and are then taken up into cells. Of note, such radionuclides are produced from a cyclotron and have very short half-lives.[23] The patient is then imaged within the PET scanner, and the images display details regarding cerebral metabolism (figure 6.10).

No studies to date have used PET in the investigation of sport-related concussion, but it has been used with other causes of mild TBI. One study in adults with mild TBI and persistent postconcussive symptoms demonstrated areas of medial temporal hypometabolism.[130] Another looked at five adults with mild TBI and persistent symptoms, both at rest and during a spatial working memory task.[18] The authors found normal regional cerebral FDG uptake at rest; however, there were notable differences in cerebral metabolism during the visual–spatial working memory task. Similar to SPECT, this technique has many limitations including exposure to radiolabeled tracers, overall expense, and time necessary to use the technology, and as such remains primarily a research tool at this time.

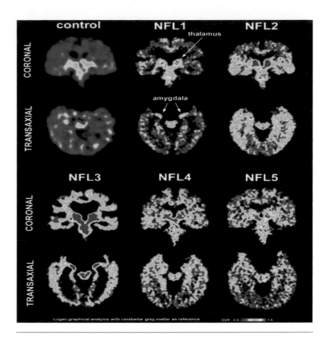

Figure 6.10 Figure Legend: FDDNP-PET scan results for NFL players and a control. Coronal and transaxial FDDNP-PET scans of the retired NFL players include: NFL1: 59-year-old linebacker with MCI, who experienced momentary loss of consciousness after each of two concussions; NFL2: 64-year-old quarterback with age-consistent memory impairment, who experienced momentary loss of consciousness and 24-hour amnesia following one concussion; NFL3: 73-year-old guard with dementia and depression, who suffered brief loss of consciousness after 20 concussions, and a 12-hour coma following 1 concussion; NFL4: 50-year-old defensive lineman with MCI and depression, who suffered two concussions and loss of consciousness for 10 minutes following one of them; NFL5: 45-year-old center with MCI, who suffered 10 concussions and complained of light sensitivity, irritability, and decreased concentration after the last two. The players' scans show consistently high signals in the amygdala and subcortical regions and a range of cortical binding from extensive to limited, whereas the control subject shows limited binding in these regions. Red and yellow areas indicate high FDDNP binding signals.

Reprinted from *American Journal of Geriatric Psychiatry*, Vol. 21(2), G.W. Small et al., "PET scanning of brain tau in retired National Football League players: Preliminary findings," pgs. 138-44, copyright 2013, with permission from Elsevier.

NEUROPHYSIOLOGICAL TECHNIQUES

Forms of neurophysiological measurement have been investigated in mild TBI and are aimed at representing direct measurements of the brain's cellular activity. These techniques include electroencephalography, evoked potentials, event-related potentials, and magnetoencephalography.

Electrophysiology

Electroencephalography (EEG) involves placing electrodes on the scalp to record the electrical properties of neurons. Although EEG has revealed abnormalities postconcussion, its clinical significance is still not clear.[23] One study evaluated 12 male athletes between the ages of 18 and 25 years who had sustained a mild TBI on average 89.4 days before.[126] The researchers examined EEG testing with the patient seated and eyes open, seated and eyes closed, standing and eyes open, and standing with eyes closed. They found under each condition an overall decrease in EEG amplitude, especially during standing postures, and postural instability was greatest when eyes were closed.[126] Other studies have revealed abnormalities; however, the significance of these changes is uncertain.[37, 101]

Evoked potentials (EPs) and event-related potentials (ERPs) represent the averaged EEG signal in response to a given stimulus, with EP thought to represent processing in the primary sensory pathways and ERP being associated with cognitive processes.[23, 85] Studies using EPs and ERPs in the evaluation of mild TBI have yielded promising results. From a laboratory standpoint, EP studies have consistently found the cortical waveform to be briefly extinguished immediately following a concussion in animal models.[97] Brain stem auditory evoked potentials (BAEPs) have been the type of EP primarily used, as the BAEP is a marker of brain stem function.[85] Studies have yielded conflicting results, with some reporting change in BAEP latency following concussion and others reporting no change.[37, 97]

The results from studies using ERPs in concussion have been more encouraging.[24, 30, 37, 40, 66] It is important to keep in mind that although ERPs have good temporal resolution, the technique has poor spatial resolution, making it difficult to localize the brain region generating the abnormal activity. One group examined ERPs following concussion in college athletes.[30] They found a significant decrease in the waveform around 300

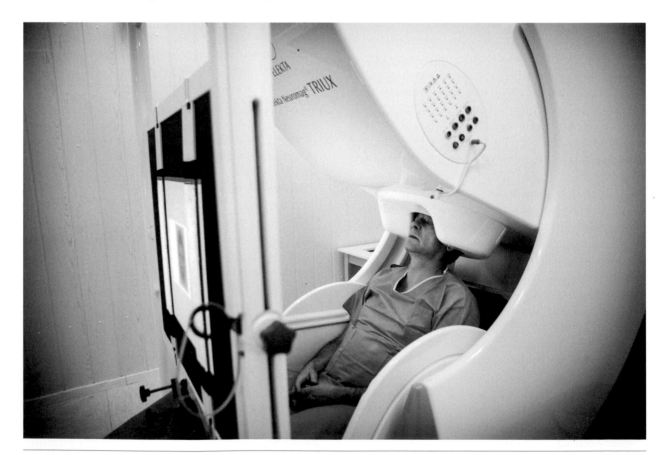

Figure 6.11 A magnetoencephalography scanner may be able to identify traumatic brain injury in patients.
AMELIE-BENOIST / BSIP/age fotostock

ms (P300), which was related to the severity of postconcussive symptoms. Another study compared the effects of concussion on attention and ERPs in athletes with postconcussion symptoms. [66] The authors demonstrated that symptomatic athletes exhibited longer reaction times and that there was an inverse relationship between the severity of postconcussion symptoms and P300 amplitude. So, although the clinical significance of the P300 differences shown by the symptomatic athletes is still uncertain, the results indicated that symptom severity may be a crucial indicator of functional impairments following concussion. [66]

Magnetoencephalography

Magnetoencephalography (MEG) is a noninvasive modality used to measure the neuromagnetic fields generated by the activation of neurons[103] (figure 6.11). It measures the neuromagnetic field of the dendrites organized parallel to the skull surface, whereas EEG measures the potential gradients of dendrites perpendicular to the skull surface.[85] The magnetic fields can be measured outside the head using supercooled sensors connected to superconducting quantum interference devices, generating data similar to those with standard EEG but with fewer artifacts and better spatial resolution. A retrospective study evaluated 30 adults with greater than 1 year of symptoms following non–sport-related mild TBI using MEG, standard structural MRI, and SPECT imaging.[70] Magnetoencephalography demonstrated abnormal activity in 19 of the 30 patients. None of the imaging methods produced findings statistically associated with postconcussive psychiatric symptoms; however, for patients with cognitive complaints, abnormalities were more likely to be detected by MEG (86%) than by either SPECT (40%) or MRI (18%).[70] Magnetoencephalography also revealed significant associations between temporal lobe dipolar slow wave activity (DSWA) and memory problems, parietal DSWA and attention problems, and frontal DSWA and problems in executive function.[70]

Magnetic source imaging (MSI) integrates anatomic and structural data from MRI with electrophysiology data from MEG. One study compared MRI and resting EEG with resting MSI in postconcussion and control patients.[71] The study showed that MSI detected more patients with postconcussion symptoms than either EEG or MRI alone. There are currently no published studies evaluating MSI in sport-related concussion. The use of MEG, in general, is limited because it is expensive and requires installation in magnetic-shielded rooms. Presently, MEG is available in only a few centers across the world because of its relatively high cost, and it remains mainly a research tool at this time.

CONCLUDING THOUGHTS

The increased interest in concussion has led to attempts at understanding the role that imaging can play in assessment and prognosis. Traditional neuroimaging seems to be limited in its role in concussion management; however, it is important in ruling out more moderate and severe levels of sport-related head injury. While advanced neuroimaging techniques have the potential to identify brain abnormalities related to concussion that are not appreciated with traditional clinical neuroimaging, their use in the regular management of the majority of mild traumatic brain injury is not yet practical. The extent to which these techniques may become useful in guiding clinicians in the clinical management of sport concussion is unknown.

We need to continue to explore and understand the true clinical implications of neuroimaging results in concussion. If imaging normalizes, does this indicate safe return to play? Conversely, if the patient is asymptomatic but has neuroimaging abnormalities, what is the significance acutely? What is it chronically? There will likely be an increased emphasis on understanding the functional changes in the brain that may explain the long-term effects of concussion. With time, we will come to have a better understanding of how more advanced neuroimaging findings correlate with neurophysiology and how these data can be used in combination with other variables to guide management of the athlete with a head injury.

REFERENCES

1. Adams JH, Doyle D, Ford I, Gennarelli TA, Graham DI, McLellan DR. Diffuse axonal injury in head injury: definition, diagnosis and grading. Histopathology 1989;15(1):49-59.

2. Agrawal D, Gowda NK, Bal CS, Pant M, Mahapatra AK. Is medial temporal injury responsible for pediatric postconcussion syndrome? A prospective controlled study with single-photon

emission computerized tomography. J Neurosurg 2005;102(2 Suppl):167-171.

3. Arfanakis K, Haughton VM, Carew JD, Rogers BP, Dempsey RJ, Meyerand ME. Diffusion tensor MR imaging in diffuse axonal injury. AJNR 2002;23(5):794-802.

4. Ashburner J, Friston KJ. Voxel-based morphometry—the methods. NeuroImage 2000;11(6 Pt 1):805-821.

5. Ashikaga R, Araki Y, Ishida O. MRI of head injury using FLAIR. Neuroradiology 1997;39(4):239-242.

6. Assaf Y, Beit-Yannai E, Shohami E, Berman E, Cohen Y. Diffusion- and T2-weighted MRI of closed-head injury in rats: a time course study and correlation with histology. Magn Reson Imaging 1997;15(1):77-85.

7. Babikian T, Freier MC, Tong KA, Nickerson JP, Wall CJ, Holshouser BA, et al. Susceptibility weighted imaging: neuropsychologic outcome and pediatric head injury. Pediatr Neurol 2005;33(3):184-194.

8. Barnes SR, Haacke EM. Susceptibility-weighted imaging: clinical angiographic applications. Magn Reson Imaging Clin N Am 2009;17(1):47-61.

9. Basser PJ, Jones DK. Diffusion-tensor MRI: theory, experimental design and data analysis - a technical review. NMR Biomed 2002;15(7-8):456-467.

10. Basser PJ, Pierpaoli C. Microstructural and physiological features of tissues elucidated by quantitative-diffusion-tensor MRI. J Magn Reson B 1996;111(3):209-219.

11. Bayly PV, Cohen TS, Leister EP, Ajo D, Leuthardt EC, Genin GM. Deformation of the human brain induced by mild acceleration. J Neurotrauma 2005;22(8):845-856.

12. Bazarian JJ, Zhong J, Blyth B, Zhu T, Kavcic V, Peterson D. Diffusion tensor imaging detects clinically important axonal damage after mild traumatic brain injury: a pilot study. J Neurotrauma 2007;24(9):1447-1459.

13. Bazarian JJ, Zhu T, Blyth B, Borrino A, Zhong J. Subject-specific changes in brain white matter on diffusion tensor imaging after sports-related concussion. Magn Reson Imaging 2012;30(2):171-180.

14. Bigler ED. Quantitative magnetic resonance imaging in traumatic brain injury. J Head Trauma Rehabil 2001;16(2):117-134.

15. Bigler ED, Bazarian JJ. Diffusion tensor imaging: a biomarker for mild traumatic brain injury? Neurology 2010;74(8):626-627.

16. Chastain CA, Oyoyo UE, Zipperman M, Joo E, Ashwal S, Shutter LA, et al. Predicting outcomes of traumatic brain injury by imaging modality and injury distribution. J Neurotrauma 2009;26(8):1183-1196.

17. Chen JK, Johnston KM, Frey S, Petrides M, Worsley K, Ptito A. Functional abnormalities in symptomatic concussed athletes: an fMRI study. NeuroImage 2004;22(1):68-82.

18. Chen SH, Kareken DA, Fastenau PS, Trexler LE, Hutchins GD. A study of persistent post-concussion symptoms in mild head trauma using positron emission tomography. J Neurol Neurosurg Psychiatry 2003;74(3):326-332.

19. Cheng K. Recent progress in high-resolution functional MRI. Curr Opin Neurol 2011;24(4):401-408.

20. Cimatti M. Assessment of metabolic cerebral damage using proton magnetic resonance spectroscopy in mild traumatic brain injury. J Neurosurg Sci 2006;50(4):83-88.

21. Cooper PR, Maravilla K, Moody S, Clark WK. Serial computerized tomographic scanning and the prognosis of severe head injury. Neurosurgery 1979;5(5):566-569.

22. Cubon VA, Putukian M, Boyer C, Dettwiler A. A diffusion tensor imaging study on the white matter skeleton in individuals with sports-related concussion. J Neurotrauma 2011;28(2):189-201.

23. Davis GA, Iverson GL, Guskiewicz KM, Ptito A, Johnston KM. Contributions of neuroimaging, balance testing, electrophysiology and blood markers to the assessment of sport-related concussion. Br J Sports Med 2009;43 Suppl 1:i36-45.

24. De Beaumont L, Brisson B, Lassonde M, Jolicoeur P. Long-term electrophysiological changes in athletes with a history of multiple concussions. Brain Inj 2007;21(6):631-644.

25. DiFiori JP, Giza CC. New techniques in concussion imaging. Curr Sports Med Rep 2010;9(1):35-39.

26. Doezema D, King JN, Tandberg D, Espinosa MC, Orrison WW. Magnetic resonance imaging in minor head injury. Ann Emerg Med 1991;20(12):1281-1285.

27. Ducreux D, Huynh I, Fillard P, Renoux J, Petit-Lacour MC, Marsot-Dupuch K, et al. Brain MR diffusion tensor imaging and fibre tracking to differentiate between two diffuse axonal injuries. Neuroradiology 2005;47(8):604-608.

28. Ducreux D, Nasser G, Lacroix C, Adams D, Lasjaunias P. MR diffusion tensor imaging, fiber tracking, and single-voxel spectroscopy findings in an unusual MELAS case. AJNR 2005;26(7):1840-1844.

29. Dunning J, Daly JP, Lomas JP, Lecky F, Batchelor J, Mackway-Jones K. Derivation of the children's head injury algorithm for the prediction of important clinical events decision rule for head injury in children. Arch Dis Child 2006;91(11):885-891.

30. Dupuis F, Johnston KM, Lavoie M, Lepore F, Lassonde M. Concussions in athletes produce brain dysfunction as revealed by event-related potentials. Neuroreport 2000;11(18):4087-4092.

31. Easdon C, Levine B, O'Connor C, Tisserand D, Hevenor S. Neural activity associated with response inhibition following traumatic brain injury: an event-related fMRI investigation. Brain Cogn 2004;54(2):136-138.

32. Ellemberg D, Henry LC, Macciocchi SN, Guskiewicz KM, Broglio SP. Advances in sport concus-

sion assessment: from behavioral to brain imaging measures. J Neurotrauma 2009;26(12):2365-2382.

33. Fernandez-Miranda JC, Engh JA, Pathak SK, Madhok R, Boada FE, Schneider W, et al. High-definition fiber tracking guidance for intraparenchymal endoscopic port surgery. J Neurosurg 2010;113(5):990-999.

34. Fernandez-Miranda JC, Pathak S, Engh J, Jarbo K, Verstynen T, Yeh F, et al. High-definition fiber tractography of the human brain: neuroanatomical validation and neurosurgical applications. Neurosurgery 2012; 71(2):430-453.

35. Fernandez-Miranda JC, Pathak S, Schneider W. High-definition fiber tractography and language. J Neurosurg 2010;113(1):156-157; author reply 157-158.

36. French BN, Dublin AB. The value of computerized tomography in the management of 1000 consecutive head injuries. Surg Neurol 1977;7(4):171-183.

37. Gaetz M, Bernstein DM. The current status of electrophysiologic procedures for the assessment of mild traumatic brain injury. J Head Trauma Rehabil 2001;16(4):386-405.

38. Gale SD, Baxter L, Roundy N, Johnson SC. Traumatic brain injury and grey matter concentration: a preliminary voxel based morphometry study. J Neurol Neurosurg Psychiatry 2005;76(7):984-988.

39. Gentry LR, Godersky JC, Thompson B. MR imaging of head trauma: review of the distribution and radiopathologic features of traumatic lesions. AJR 1988;150(3):663-672.

40. Gosselin N, Saluja RS, Chen JK, Bottari C, Johnston K, Ptito A. Brain functions after sports-related concussion: insights from event-related potentials and functional MRI. Phys Sportsmed 2010;38(3):27-37.

41. Groswasser Z, Reider-Groswasser I, Soroker N, Machtey Y. Magnetic resonance imaging in head injured patients with normal late computed tomography scans. Surg Neurol 1987;27(4):331-337.

42. Haacke EM, Mittal S, Wu Z, Ncclavalli J, Cheng YC. Susceptibility-weighted imaging: technical aspects and clinical applications, part 1. AJNR 2009;30(1):19-30.

43. Hagmann P, Jonasson L, Maeder P, Thiran JP, Wedeen VJ, Meuli R. Understanding diffusion MR imaging techniques: from scalar diffusion-weighted imaging to diffusion tensor imaging and beyond. Radiographics 2006;26 Suppl 1:S205-223.

44. Han JS, Kaufman B, Alfidi RJ, Yeung HN, Benson JE, Haaga JR, et al. Head trauma evaluated by magnetic resonance and computed tomography: a comparison. Radiology 1984;150(1):71-77.

45. Haydel MJ, Preston CA, Mills TJ, Luber S, Blaudeau E, DeBlieux PM. Indications for computed tomography in patients with minor head injury. New Engl J Med 2000;343(2):100-105.

46. Henry LC, Tremblay J, Tremblay S, Lee A, Brun C, Lepore N, et al. Acute and chronic changes in diffusivity measures after sports concussion. J Neurotrauma 2011;28(10):2049-2059.

47. Henry LC, Tremblay S, Boulanger Y, Ellemberg D, Lassonde M. Neurometabolic changes in the acute phase after sports concussions correlate with symptom severity. J Neurotrauma 2010;27(1):65-76.

48. Hofman PA, Stapert SZ, van Kroonenburgh MJ, Jolles J, de Kruijk J, Wilmink JT. MR imaging, single-photon emission CT, and neurocognitive performance after mild traumatic brain injury. AJNR 2001;22(3):441-449.

49. Horsfield MA, Larsson HB, Jones DK, Gass A. Diffusion magnetic resonance imaging in multiple sclerosis. J Neurol Neurosurg Psychiatry 1998;64 Suppl 1:S80-84.

50. Hughes DG, Jackson A, Mason DL, Berry E, Hollis S, Yates DW. Abnormalities on magnetic resonance imaging seen acutely following mild traumatic brain injury: correlation with neuropsychological tests and delayed recovery. Neuroradiology 2004;46(7):550-558.

51. Huisman TA, Schwamm LH, Schaefer PW, Koroshetz WJ, Shetty-Alva N, Ozsunar Y, et al. Diffusion tensor imaging as potential biomarker of white matter injury in diffuse axonal injury. AJNR 2004;25(3):370-376.

52. Huisman TA, Sorensen AG, Hergan K, Gonzalez RG, Schaefer PW. Diffusion-weighted imaging for the evaluation of diffuse axonal injury in closed head injury. J Comput Assist Tomogr 2003;27(1):5-11.

53. Inglese M, Makani S, Johnson G, Cohen BA, Silver JA, Gonen O, et al. Diffuse axonal injury in mild traumatic brain injury: a diffusion tensor imaging study. J Neurosurg 2005;103(2):298-303.

54. Jantzen KJ, Anderson B, Steinberg FL, Kelso JA. A prospective functional MR imaging study of mild traumatic brain injury in college football players. AJNR 2004;25(5):738-745.

55. Jbabdi S, Johansen-Berg H. Tractography: where do we go from here? Brain Connect 2011;1(3):169-183.

56. Johansen-Berg H, Rushworth MF. Using diffusion imaging to study human connectional anatomy. Ann Rev Neurosci 2009;32:75-94.

57. Johnston KM, Ptito A, Chankowsky J, Chen JK. New frontiers in diagnostic imaging in concussive head injury. Clin J Sport Med 2001;11(3):166-175.

58. Jordan BD, Jahre C, Hauser WA, Zimmerman RD, Zarrelli M, Lipsitz EC, et al. CT of 338 active professional boxers. Radiology 1992;185(2):509-512.

59. Jordan BD, Zimmerman RD. Computed tomography and magnetic resonance imaging comparisons in boxers. JAMA 1990;263(12):1670-1674.

60. Kelly AB, Zimmerman RD, Snow RB, Gandy SE, Heier LA, Deck MD. Head trauma: comparison of MR and CT—experience in 100 patients. AJNR 1988;9(4):699-708.

61. Khurana VG, Kaye AH. An overview of concussion in sport. J Clin Neurosci 2012;19(1):1-11.

62. Koo AH, LaRoque RL. Evaluation of head trauma by computed tomography. Radiology 1977;123(2):345-350.

63. Kraus MF, Susmaras T, Caughlin BP, Walker CJ, Sweeney JA, Little DM. White matter integrity and cognition in chronic traumatic brain injury: a diffusion tensor imaging study. Brain 2007;130(Pt 10):2508-2519.

64. Krishna R, Grinn M, Giordano N, Thirunavukkarasu M, Tadi P, Das S. Diagnostic confirmation of mild traumatic brain injury by diffusion tensor imaging: a case report. J Med Case Rep 2012;6(1):66.

65. Lange RT, Iverson GL, Brubacher JR, Madler B, Heran MK. Diffusion tensor imaging findings are not strongly associated with postconcussional disorder 2 months following mild traumatic brain injury. J Head Trauma Rehabil 2012; 27(3):188-198.

66. Lavoie ME, Dupuis F, Johnston KM, Leclerc S, Lassonde M. Visual p300 effects beyond symptoms in concussed college athletes. J Clin Exp Neuropsychol 2004;26(1):55-73.

67. Le Bihan D, Mangin JF, Poupon C, Clark CA, Pappata S, Molko N, et al. Diffusion tensor imaging: concepts and applications. J Magn Reson Imaging 2001;13(4):534-546.

68. Le TH, Gean AD. Neuroimaging of traumatic brain injury. Mt Sinai J Med 2009;76(2):145-162.

69. Lee H, Wintermark M, Gean AD, Ghajar J, Manley GT, Mukherjee P. Focal lesions in acute mild traumatic brain injury and neurocognitive outcome: CT versus 3T MRI. J Neurotrauma 2008;25(9):1049-1056.

70. Lewine JD, Davis JT, Bigler ED, Thoma R, Hill D, Funke M, et al. Objective documentation of traumatic brain injury subsequent to mild head trauma: multimodal brain imaging with MEG, SPECT, and MRI. J Head Trauma Rehabil 2007;22(3):141-155.

71. Lewine JD, Davis JT, Sloan JH, Kodituwakku PW, Orrison WW Jr. Neuromagnetic assessment of pathophysiologic brain activity induced by minor head trauma. AJNR 1999;20(5):857-866.

72. Li TQ, Chen ZG, Hindmarsh T. Diffusion-weighted MR imaging of acute cerebral ischemia. Acta Radiol 1998;39(5):460-473.

73. Lipton ML, Gellella E, Lo C, Gold T, Ardekani BA, Shifteh K, et al. Multifocal white matter ultrastructural abnormalities in mild traumatic brain injury with cognitive disability: a voxel-wise analysis of diffusion tensor imaging. J Neurotrauma 2008;25(11):1335-1342.

74. Liu AY, Maldjian JA, Bagley LJ, Sinson GP, Grossman RI. Traumatic brain injury: diffusion-weighted MR imaging findings. AJNR 1999;20(9):1636-1641.

75. Livingston DH, Lavery RF, Passannante MR, Skurnick JH, Baker S, Fabian TC, et al. Emergency department discharge of patients with a negative cranial computed tomography scan after minimal head injury. Ann Surg 2000;232(1):126-132.

76. Lobato RD, Cordobes F, Rivas JJ, de la Fuente M, Montero A, Barcena A, et al. Outcome from severe head injury related to the type of intracranial lesion. A computerized tomography study. J Neurosurg 1983;59(5):762-774.

77. Lovell MR, Pardini JE, Welling J, Collins MW, Bakal J, Lazar N, et al. Functional brain abnormalities are related to clinical recovery and time to return-to-play in athletes. Neurosurgery 2007;61(2):352-359; discussion 359-360.

78. MacKenzie JD, Siddiqi F, Babb JS, Bagley LJ, Mannon LJ, Sinson GP, et al. Brain atrophy in mild or moderate traumatic brain injury: a longitudinal quantitative analysis. AJNR 2002;23(9):1509-1515.

79. Marks MP, de Crespigny A, Lentz D, Enzmann DR, Albers GW, Moseley ME. Acute and chronic stroke: navigated spin-echo diffusion-weighted MR imaging. Radiology 1996;199(2):403-408.

80. Maruta J, Lee SW, Jacobs EF, Ghajar J. A unified science of concussion. Ann N Y Acad Sci 2010;1208:58-66.

81. Mauersberger W, Lanksch W, Kazner E, Grumme T. [Computerized tomography in head injuries (author's transl)]. Zentralbl Chir 1978;103(8):501-511.

82. Mayer AR, Ling J, Mannell MV, Gasparovic C, Phillips JP, Doezema D, et al. A prospective diffusion tensor imaging study in mild traumatic brain injury. Neurology 2010;74(8):643-650.

83. McCrory P, Meeuwisse W, Johnston K, Dvorak J, Aubry M, Molloy M, et al. Consensus statement on concussion in sport: the 3rd International Conference on Concussion in Sport held in Zurich, November 2008. Br J Sports Med 2009;43 Suppl 1:i76-90.

84. McCullough BJ, Jarvik JG. Diagnosis of concussion: the role of imaging now and in the future. Phys Med Rehabil Clin North Am 2011;22(4):635-652, viii.

85. Mendez CV, Hurley RA, Lassonde M, Zhang L, Taber KH. Mild traumatic brain injury: neuroimaging of sports-related concussion. J Neuropsychiatry Clin Neurosci 2005;17(3):297-303.

86. Messe A, Caplain S, Paradot G, Garrigue D, Mineo JF, Soto Ares G, et al. Diffusion tensor imaging and white matter lesions at the subacute stage in mild traumatic brain injury with persistent neurobehavioral impairment. Hum Brain Mapp 2011;32(6):999-1011.

87. Miles L, Grossman RI, Johnson G, Babb JS, Diller L, Inglese M. Short-term DTI predictors of cognitive dysfunction in mild traumatic brain injury. Brain Inj 2008;22(2):115-122.

88. Minderhoud JM, Boelens ME, Huizenga J, Saan RJ. Treatment of minor head injuries. Clin Neurol Neurosurg 1980;82(2):127-140.

89. Mittal S, Wu Z, Neelavalli J, Haacke EM. Susceptibility-weighted imaging: technical aspects and clinical applications, part 2. AJNR 2009;30(2):232-252.

90. Mittl RL, Grossman RI, Hiehle JF, Hurst RW, Kauder DR, Gennarelli TA, et al. Prevalence of MR evidence of diffuse axonal injury in patients with mild head injury and normal head CT findings. AJNR 1994;15(8):1583-1589.

91. Moseley IF. The neuroimaging evidence for chronic brain damage due to boxing. Neuroradiology 2000;42(1):1-8.

92. Mukherjee P, Miller JH, Shimony JS, Philip JV, Nehra D, Snyder AZ, et al. Diffusion-tensor MR imaging of gray and white matter development during normal human brain maturation. AJNR 2002;23(9):1445-1456.

93. Newton MR, Greenwood RJ, Britton KE, Charlesworth M, Nimmon CC, Carroll MJ, et al. A study comparing SPECT with CT and MRI after closed head injury. J Neurol Neurosurg Psychiatry 1992;55(2):92-94.

94. Niogi SN, Mukherjee P, Ghajar J, Johnson C, Kolster RA, Sarkar R, et al. Extent of microstructural white matter injury in postconcussive syndrome correlates with impaired cognitive reaction time: a 3T diffusion tensor imaging study of mild traumatic brain injury. AJNR 2008;29(5):967-973.

95. Niogi SN, Mukherjee P, Ghajar J, Johnson CE, Kolster R, Lee H, et al. Structural dissociation of attentional control and memory in adults with and without mild traumatic brain injury. Brain 2008;131(Pt 12):3209-3221.

96. Niogi SN, Mukherjee P, McCandliss BD. Diffusion tensor imaging segmentation of white matter structures using a Reproducible Objective Quantification Scheme (ROQS). NeuroImage 2007;35(1):166-174.

97. Noseworthy JH, Miller J, Murray TJ, Regan D. Auditory brainstem responses in postconcussion syndrome. Arch Neurol 1981;38(5):275-278.

98. Oppenheimer DR. Microscopic lesions in the brain following head injury. J Neurol Neurosurg Psychiatry 1968;31(4):299-306.

99. Orrison WW, Gentry LR, Stimac GK, Tarrel RM, Espinosa MC, Cobb LC. Blinded comparison of cranial CT and MR in closed head injury evaluation. AJNR 1994;15(2):351-356.

100. Pierpaoli C, Jezzard P, Basser PJ, Barnett A, Di Chiro G. Diffusion tensor MR imaging of the human brain. Radiology 1996;201(3):637-648.

101. Pointinger H, Sarahrudi K, Poeschl G, Munk P. Electroencephalography in primary diagnosis of mild head trauma. Brain Inj 2002;16(9):799-805.

102. Povlishock JT, Becker DP, Cheng CL, Vaughan GW. Axonal change in minor head injury. J Neuropathol Exp Neurol 1983;42(3):225-242.

103. Prabhu SP. The role of neuroimaging in sport-related concussion. Clin Sports Med 2011;30(1):103-114, ix.

104. Pulsipher DT, Campbell RA, Thoma R, King JH. A critical review of neuroimaging applications in sports concussion. Curr Sports Med Rep 2011;10(1):14-20.

105. Ropper AH, Gorson KC. Clinical practice. Concussion. New Engl J Med 2007;356(2):166-172.

106. Ross RJ, Casson IR, Siegel O, Cole M. Boxing injuries: neurologic, radiologic, and neuropsychologic evaluation. Clin Sports Med 1987;6(1):41-51.

107. Rutgers DR, Fillard P, Paradot G, Tadie M, Lasjaunias P, Ducreux D. Diffusion tensor imaging characteristics of the corpus callosum in mild, moderate, and severe traumatic brain injury. AJNR 2008;29(9):1730-1735.

108. Rutgers DR, Toulgoat F, Cazejust J, Fillard P, Lasjaunias P, Ducreux D. White matter abnormalities in mild traumatic brain injury: a diffusion tensor imaging study. AJNR 2008;29(3):514-519.

109. Schaefer PW, Huisman TA, Sorensen AG, Gonzalez RG, Schwamm LH. Diffusion-weighted MR imaging in closed head injury: high correlation with initial glasgow coma scale score and score on modified Rankin scale at discharge. Radiology 2004;233(1):58-66.

110. Scheid R, Walther K, Guthke T, Preul C, von Cramon DY. Cognitive sequelae of diffuse axonal injury. Arch Neurol 2006;63(3):418-424.

111. Shenton ME, Hamoda HM, Schneiderman JS, Bouix S, Pasternak O, Rathi Y, et al. A review of magnetic resonance imaging and diffusion tensor imaging findings in mild traumatic brain injury. Brain Imaging Behav 2012.

112. Shin SS, Verstynen T, Pathak S, Jarbo K, Hricik AJ, Maserati M, et al. High-definition fiber tracking for assessment of neurological deficit in a case of traumatic brain injury: finding, visualizing, and interpreting small sites of damage. J Neurosurg 2012;116(5):1062-1069.

113. Smith DH, Meaney DF, Shull WH. Diffuse axonal injury in head trauma. J Head Trauma Rehabil 2003;18(4):307-316.

114. Smits M, Dippel DW, de Haan GG, Dekker HM, Vos PE, Kool DR, et al. External validation of the Canadian CT Head Rule and the New Orleans Criteria for CT scanning in patients with minor head injury. JAMA 2005;294(12):1519-1525.

115. Smits M, Houston GC, Dippel DW, Wielopolski PA, Vernooij MW, Koudstaal PJ, et al. Microstructural brain injury in post-concussion syndrome after minor head injury. Neuroradiology 2011;53(8):553-563.

116. Snoek J, Jennett B, Adams JH, Graham DI, Doyle D. Computerised tomography after recent severe head injury in patients without acute intracranial haematoma. J Neurol Neurosurg Psychiatry 1979;42(3):215-225.

117. Snow RB, Zimmerman RD, Gandy SE, Deck MD. Comparison of magnetic resonance imaging and computed tomography in the evaluation of head injury. Neurosurgery 1986;18(1):45-52.

118. Stein SC, Burnett MG, Glick HA. Indications for CT scanning in mild traumatic brain injury: a cost-effectiveness study. J Trauma 2006;61(3):558-566.

119. Stein SC, Fabbri A, Servadei F. Routine serial computed tomographic scans in mild traumatic brain injury: when are they cost-effective? J Trauma 2008;65(1):66-72.

120. Stein SC, O'Malley KF, Ross SE. Is routine computed tomography scanning too expensive for mild head injury? Ann Emerg Med 1991;20(12):1286-1289.

121. Stein SC, Ross SE. Clinical predictors of abnormality disclosed by computed tomography after mild head trauma. Neurosurgery 1993;33(2):339-340.

122. Stein SC, Ross SE. Mild head injury: a plea for routine early CT scanning. J Trauma 1992;33(1):11-13.

123. Stiell IG, Clement CM, Rowe BH, Schull MJ, Brison R, Cass D, et al. Comparison of the Canadian CT Head Rule and the New Orleans Criteria in patients with minor head injury. JAMA 2005;294(12):1511-1518.

124. Stiell IG, Wells GA, Vandemheen K, Clement C, Lesiuk H, Laupacis A, et al. The Canadian CT Head Rule for patients with minor head injury. Lancet 2001;357(9266):1391-1396.

125. Tardif CL, Collins DL, Pike GB. Regional impact of field strength on voxel-based morphometry results. Hum Brain Mapp 2010;31(7):943-957.

126. Thompson J, Sebastianelli W, Slobounov S. EEG and postural correlates of mild traumatic brain injury in athletes. Neurosci Lett 2005;377(3):158-163.

127. Tsai FY, Huprich JE, Gardner FC, Segall HD, Teal JS. Diagnostic and prognostic implications of computed tomography of head trauma. J Comput Assist Tomogr 1978;2(3):323-331.

128. Tsai FY, Teal JS, Itabashi HH, Huprich JE, Hieshima GB, Segall HD. Computed tomography of posterior fossa trauma. J Comput Assisted Tomogr 1980;4(3):291-305.

129. Tsai FY, Teal JS, Quinn MF, Itabashi HH, Huprich JE, Ahmadi J, et al. CT of brainstem injury. AJR 1980;134(4):717-723.

130. Umile EM, Sandel ME, Alavi A, Terry CM, Plotkin RC. Dynamic imaging in mild traumatic brain injury: support for the theory of medial temporal vulnerability. Arch Phys Med Rehabil 2002;83(11):1506-1513.

131. Vagnozzi R, Signoretti S, Tavazzi B, Floris R, Ludovici A, Marziali S, et al. Temporal window of metabolic brain vulnerability to concussion: a pilot 1H-magnetic resonance spectroscopic study in concussed athletes—part III. Neurosurgery 2008;62(6):1286-1295; discussion 1295-1286.

132. Van Boven RW, Harrington GS, Hackney DB, Ebel A, Gauger G, Bremner JD, et al. Advances in neuroimaging of traumatic brain injury and posttraumatic stress disorder. J Rehabil Res Dev 2009;46(6):717-757.

133. Verstynen T, Jarbo K, Pathak S, Schneider W. In vivo mapping of microstructural somatotopies in the human corticospinal pathways. J Neurophysiol 2011;105(1):336-346.

134. Voller B, Benke T, Benedetto K, Schnider P, Auff E, Aichner F. Neuropsychological, MRI and EEG findings after very mild traumatic brain injury. Brain Inj 1999;13(10):821-827.

135. Warach S, Gaa J, Siewert B, Wielopolski P, Edelman RR. Acute human stroke studied by whole brain echo planar diffusion-weighted magnetic resonance imaging. Ann Neurol 1995;37(2):231-241.

136. Warach S, Mosley M, Sorensen AG, Koroshetz W. Time course of diffusion imaging abnormalities in human stroke. Stroke 1996;27(7):1254-1256.

137. Warren WL Jr, Bailes JE. On the field evaluation of athletic head injuries. Clin Sports Med 1998;17(1):13-26.

138. Whitwell JL. Voxel-based morphometry: an automated technique for assessing structural changes in the brain. J Neurosci 2009;29(31):9661-9664.

139. Wilde EA, McCauley SR, Hunter JV, Bigler ED, Chu Z, Wang ZJ, et al. Diffusion tensor imaging of acute mild traumatic brain injury in adolescents. Neurology 2008;70(12):948-955.

140. Wozniak JR, Krach L, Ward E, Mueller BA, Muetzel R, Schnoebelen S, et al. Neurocognitive and neuroimaging correlates of pediatric traumatic brain injury: a diffusion tensor imaging (DTI) study. Arch Clin Neuropsychol 2007;22(5):555-568.

141. Wu Z, Mittal S, Kish K, Yu Y, Hu J, Haacke EM. Identification of calcification with MRI using susceptibility-weighted imaging: a case study. J Magn Reson Imaging 2009;29(1):177-182.

142. Yamada K, Kizu O, Mori S, Ito H, Nakamura H, Yuen S, et al. Brain fiber tracking with clinically feasible diffusion-tensor MR imaging: initial experience. Radiology 2003;227(1):295-301.

143. Yang Q, Liu J, Barnes SR, Wu Z, Li K, Neelavalli J, et al. Imaging the vessel wall in major peripheral arteries using susceptibility-weighted imaging. JMRI 2009;30(2):357-365.

144. Yokoyama K, Matsuki M, Shimano H, Sumioka S, Ikenaga T, Hanabusa K, et al. Diffusion tensor imaging in chronic subdural hematoma: correlation between clinical signs and fractional anisotropy in the pyramidal tract. AJNR 2008;29(6):1159-1163.

145. Zhang K, Johnson B, Pennell D, Ray W, Sebastianelli W, Slobounov S. Are functional deficits in concussed individuals consistent with white matter structural alterations: combined FMRI & DTI study. Exp Brain Res 2010;204(1):57-70.

Neuropsychological Assessment in Concussion

In collaboration with
Elizabeth M. Pieroth, PsyD, ABPP

Researchers and clinicians have been examining both the pathophysiology of concussion and the physical and cognitive sequelae of these injuries for many years. For more than 30 years, neuropsychologists have been assessing the cognitive and emotional symptoms associated with concussion. Neuropsychologists employ pencil-and-paper and computerized measures to examine cognitive functions such as memory, attention, visual abilities, language, and executive functioning (i.e., problem solving, reasoning, and cognitive flexibility), as well as affective functioning.

In the 1970s, Gronwall and Wrightson used neuropsychological measures to assess cognitive impairment in mild traumatic brain-injured (mTBI) patients.[55] Ten years later, research began to appear on the cognitive symptoms associated with boxing and soccer. However, there was a more significant growth in interest in concussive injuries in collegiate sports, particularly American football, during this same period. Barth and colleagues were among the first to systematically examine the collegiate athlete. [6] Their initial study comprised 2,350 collegiate football players from 10 universities over a 4-year period. This study was the first to show the benefit of using neuropsychological assessment with concussed athletes. The authors developed the Sports as a Laboratory Assessment Model (SLAM), which relied on preseason baseline testing and postinjury assessment to examine the cognitive deficits associated with concussion and the natural recovery of these injuries. This work led to the development of various return-to-play protocols and contributed to research focusing on mTBI outside of sport, which included research on American veterans who have suffered blast injuries.

During the 1990s, attention turned to the American professional athlete. Mark Lovell and Joseph Maroon were the first to use neuropsychological evaluations with the Pittsburgh Steelers. Building on the work of Barth and the SLAM model, paper–pencil neuropsychological batteries were developed for the professional football and hockey player.[90, 91] From this work, the National Football League (NFL) Neuropsychology Program was developed in 1993, and this program now includes all 32 NFL teams. In 1997, the National Hockey League (NHL) began its concussion program, which mandated preseason baseline and postinjury neuropsychological testing of all NHL players.

Currently, the major professional sport leagues, including the NFL, NHL, Major League Baseball (MLB), Major League Soccer (MLS), and the National Basketball Association (NBA), use neuropsychological tests in their return-to-play protocols with concussed athletes. The test instruments used and methods of evaluation vary between leagues, but all use neuropsychological tests to obtain an objective measure of cognitive functioning and subjective complaints of concussed athletes. The use of both computerized and paper–pencil testing with concussed athletes is now embraced in college and high school sport programs, as well.[92] Concussion education and cognitive testing that targets younger athletes are also expanding.

More recently, abbreviated sideline assessments have been developed by neuropsychologists to aid in the on-the-field evaluation of athletes. The Standardized Assessment of Concussion (SAC) is a 5-minute test that assesses orientation, attention, and verbal memory.[101] It has been shown to be sensitive to cognitive impairment after concussion.[5, 99] A structured interview tool (Acute Concussion Evaluation; ACE) developed by neuropsychologist and used with pediatric patients has also been validated.[53]

Another common assessment tool, designed by neuropsychologists and a panel of international experts, is the Sport Concussion Assessment Tool-2 (SCAT2).[104] It consists of components of various measures, including the SAC, to assess cognition, balance, and subjective symptoms. It has been used with adult, adolescent, and pediatric athletes. However, it was not designed specifically for youth athletes. Thus, users should be cautious when assessing pediatric athletes and should understand the developmental differences in pediatric athletes when using the SCAT.[137]

USE OF SYMPTOM CHECKLISTS

Lovell and Collins first formalized the assessment of a patient's subjective complaints following a concussion (both physical and cognitive).[92] This checklist was subsequently incorporated into the Immediate Post-Concussion Assessment and Cognitive Testing (ImPACT) computerized test battery (discussed in detail later in this chapter).[93] Rather than a simple yes/no format, Lovell and Collin's checklist uses a 0 to 6 Likert rating scale to document both the type and severity of the patient's symptoms.

There has been a significant growth in the development of checklists that assess the concussed patient's symptoms. However, it is well known that athletes can underreport their symptoms for a variety of reasons, including lack of appreciation that they suffered a concussion, not

believing that their injury was severe enough to warrant medical attention, and not wanting to be kept out of the game.[100]

The reliance on symptom checklists alone could thus potentially result in athletes' returning to play before they have fully healed from a concussion. Fazio and colleagues found that concussed athletes who reported being symptom free still demonstrated evidence of impairment on cognitive testing.[47] This was supported by Makdissi and coauthors, who reported that computerized cognitive testing showed greater sensitivity to impairment, stating that reliance on symptom assessment alone "may underestimate time to complete recovery (p. 464)."[94] Other studies have confirmed the lack of relationship, in athletes, between self-reported symptoms and objective findings on tests of both postural stability and cognitive functioning.[13] The authors noted, "Ultimately, the cognitive tests produce a higher sensitivity to concussion's deleterious effects than the balance assessments implemented here and elsewhere (p. 380)." Their results indicated that 10% of athletes diagnosed with a concussion underreported their cognitive symptoms or were unaware of their cognitive changes.

One recent study found that the use of symptom reporting and neurocognitive test results together resulted in a 29% improvement in detecting unresolved deficits in concussed athletes compared to relying on symptom reporting alone.[151] Broglio and colleagues reported that 38% of concussed athletes who said they were asymptomatic still showed evidence of cognitive impairment on computerized testing.[11] This was evident in 35% of the athletes who had suffered a "simple" concussion (defined in this study as no loss of consciousness and resolution of subjective symptoms within 10 days). The authors concluded that neurocognitive testing should be employed in all instances when postconcussive return-to-play decisions are to be made because some athletes with seemingly minor concussive injuries may continue to demonstrate cognitive impairment after symptom resolution. Lau and colleagues found a net increase in sensitivity of predicting protracted recovery (defined as greater than 14 days postinjury) of 24.41% when using cognitive testing versus symptom checklist alone.[86]

Team physicians, coaches, and parents often comment that they "know their players" so they can accurately assess cognitive changes and recovery from a concussion. However, a study has shown that there is little association between clinician-assessed cognitive abilities via interview and psychometric data from neuropsychological tests.[111] In that study, 20% to 40% of the subjects were judged by physicians to have normal memory but were found to have significant impairment on objective cognitive testing. In a recent position statement, the American Medical Society of Sports Medicine noted, "Neuropsychological tests are an objective measure of brain-behavior relationships and are more sensitive to subtle cognitive impairment than the clinical exam (p. 2)."[61]

Another interesting study examined athletes' perception of recovery from concussion and found that adolescent athletes based their recovery primarily on somatic symptoms.[129] In other words, when reporting that they had recovered from their injuries they focused on their previous physical complaints (e.g., headaches, nausea) and did not appreciate lingering cognitive deficits that may indicate incomplete recovery. Some symptoms, such as mental fogginess or slowed reaction time, are harder for athletes, as well as those around them, to appreciate.

VALUE OF NEUROPSYCHOLOGICAL ASSESSMENT OF CONCUSSION

Numerous studies have demonstrated the utility of neuropsychological assessment with concussed patients.[9, 13, 24, 47, 75, 151] The use of neuropsychological testing in concussion management is derived from the fact that cerebral concussion can affect cognitive functioning. In particular, deficits in attention, processing speed, and reaction time, as well as learning and memory are well known sequelae of concussion.[8, 73, 76] Administration of comprehensive batteries is unnecessary in most cases of concussion; however, there are times when more extensive cognitive and psychological testing is appropriate.

The first International Conference on Concussion in Sport in Vienna[3] called neuropsychological assessment the "cornerstone" of any concussion program, and this was reaffirmed during the 2nd International Conference in Prague.

[102] During the 3rd International Conference in Zurich,[104] the utility of neuropsychological assessment was once again acknowledged:

The application of neuropsychological (NP) testing has been shown to be of clinical value and continues to contribute significant information in concussion evaluation. Although in most cases cognitive recovery largely overlaps with the time course of symptom recovery, it has been demonstrated that cognitive recovery may occasionally precede or more commonly follow clinical symptom resolution suggesting that the assessment of cognitive function should be an important component in any return–to–play protocol. It must be emphasized, however, that NP assessment should not be the sole basis of management decisions; rather, it should be seen as an aid to the clinical decision-making process in conjunction with a range of clinical domains and investigational results. (p. 187)

A position statement by the National Academy of Neuropsychology recommended neuropsychological testing to assess and manage concussed patients.[112] The American Academy of Pediatrics also endorsed the use of neuropsychological testing in children and adolescents.[60] A 2009 review noted that "accumulating evidence indicates that cognitive testing should be viewed as one of several complementary tools necessary for a comprehensive assessment of concussion (p. 2365)."[41] A consensus statement for team physicians recommended that team physicians "work in collaboration with the neuropsychologist to interpret neuropsychological testing (p. 2415)."[63] There is also widespread agreement that any cognitive assessment is to be done in conjunction with a thorough examination by a physician. Cognitive testing is not a stand-alone measure but one part of a comprehensive evaluation of the concussed athlete.

A recent review comprehensively examined the role of neuropsychologists in sport-related concussion.[39] This interorganization manuscript reviews current literature supporting the value of neuropsychological assessment in concussions and briefly explains the specialized training of neuropsychologists. Iverson has discussed the evidence-based nature of neuropsychology and the unique expertise of neuropsychologists in concussion assessment,[71] and Echemendia and colleagues have discussed the value of neuropsychologists in interpretation of cognitive data.[38]

New Uses for Neuropsychological Testing of Concussed Patients

One of the exciting developments in concussion assessment and management is the use of neurocognitive test data in the prediction of recovery after concussion. A number of new studies have examined clusters of cognitive and physical symptoms and their relationship to recovery patterns. This line of research is in its infancy and over time will likely contribute new avenues to clinical management of concussed patients.

Collins and colleagues first noted that athletes with amnesia surrounding their injury, not loss of consciousness, tended to report more symptoms and were more likely to endorse impaired memory functioning.[26, 28] Iverson noted that athletes with impaired performance on three of four composite scores on ImPACT were 94.6% more likely to have a complicated recovery (defined in the study as greater than 10 days).[70] Lau and colleagues determined that the use of neurocognitive test data, in conjunction with symptom clusters, resulted in a 24.41% increase in sensitivity in predicting lengthier recovery (defined in the study as longer than 14 days).[86]

Another study showed that athletes who took longer to recover from concussion (defined as longer than 10 days) had more migraine headache symptoms and substantially lower reaction time composite scores on ImPACT.[88] An investigation of subjective symptom reporting found only on-field dizziness to be a risk factor for protracted recovery (defined as longer than 21 days).[87] Lau and colleagues found further support for the use of specific cognitive and symptom clusters to predict recovery.[85] In that study, the self-reported "migraine symptom cluster" (headache, visual problems, dizziness, noise/light sensitivity, balance problems, numbness/tingling), "cognitive symptom cluster" (fatigue, fogginess, drowsiness, difficulty concentrating/remembering, and cognitive slowing), and objective test data (ImPACT visual memory and processing speed score) improved sensitivity to predict protracted recovery. All of these studies used ImPACT and high school athletes, and the

generalizability of the results to other cognitive instruments and other age groups is not known.

Paper–Pencil Testing

Traditional paper–pencil cognitive tests are frequently used in concussion assessment, and there are a number of measures that evaluate the cognitive deficits demonstrated after concussion. One of the problems with the use of these tests is the lack of equivalent, alternate versions for repeat testing. Serial testing may be required to monitor cognitive recovery in concussed patients. The test–retest reliability of many paper–pencil tests may not be satisfactory, and repeated use in the same patient may result in an improvement in scores simply due to exposure to the test (i.e., practice effects).[4, 23] An increase in a score can then be inadvertently misinterpreted as recovery. One suggestion for combating this problem is the use of change scores.[125] Some literature suggests that standard neuropsychological paper–pencil tests are not sensitive to the cognitive changes seen in concussion. For example, standard paper–pencil tests lack the sensitivity to detect subtle changes in reaction time.[96] Additionally, many of the commonly used paper–pencil tests have not been validated for the pediatric patient.

The administration and interpretation of neuropsychological testing is best completed by well-trained neuropsychologists with specific experience in assessing the concussed individual. As noted by Echemendia, Herring, and Bailes, "Neuropsychologists possess the training and skill sets necessary to provide unique expertise in the assessment of cognitive functioning and post-injury neurocognitive and psychological assessment (p. i32)."[38] Unfortunately, access to neuropsychologists within a reasonable time after injury is severely limited in many parts of the country. A 2006 study surveyed primary care providers in Maine and found that only 43% had neuropsychological testing available to them locally and only 16% could arrange this testing within a week of the injury.[120]

Given the limited number of neuropsychologists (particularly those trained in the assessment of concussion) compared to the number of individuals playing organized sports, the widespread use of paper–pencil tests for baseline or postinjury testing is not practical. Additionally, many paper–pencil tests cannot be administered in a group setting as is typically required for baseline testing of teams of athletes.

Computerized Testing Batteries

Due to the increasing focus on assessing cognitive impairment after concussion, a number of computerized measures have been developed and have been widely adapted.[116] Computer-administered tests have several advantages over standard paper–pencil measures. They are quick to administer (20-45 minutes depending on the test), which allows widespread use for both baseline and postinjury assessment. The tests are typically designed with multiple alternative forms so that serial assessment is possible, which is often required in concussion assessment. The computerized test batteries have the advantage of more precise measurements than standard tests that employ the use of a stopwatch, which is susceptible to human error, creating variability in measurement. This is of particular importance in assessing functions such as reaction time.[102, 103]

Computerized Cognitive Tests for Assessment of Concussion

ImPACT	www.impacttest.com
ANAM	www.armymedicine.army.mil/r2d/anam.html
CogSport	www.axonsports.com
HeadMinder	www.headminder.com
Concussion Vital Signs	www.concussionvitalsigns.com

Recent studies have shown that the use of computerized testing is widespread, even at the high school level. Guerriero and colleagues found that among high schools that employ at least one athletic trainer, approximately 40% use computerized neurocognitive assessment with their athletes.[57] There is evidence that this practice has positively affected the return-to-play decisions. When neuropsychological testing was used, concussed athletes were less likely to return to play within 7 to 10 days of their injury.[108-110] Given what we now know about the importance of not returning a newly concussed athlete to play, the data obtained from neuropsychological testing are beneficial in youth athletes.

A number of computerized instruments are commercially available. Each has its own strengths and weaknesses in the assessment of concussed patients. The following subsections discuss the five most commonly used tests. A detailed examination of the psychometric properties of these measures is outside the scope of this chapter; rather, we provide more general reviews.

ImPACT

The Immediate Post-Concussion Assessment and Cognitive Testing (ImPACT) was developed in the early 1990s by Mark Lovell and Joseph Maroon.[69, 93] This computerized test battery takes approximately 20 to 25 minutes to complete and measures verbal and visual memory, information processing time, and reaction time. The patient's test scores can be viewed with or without normative data (i.e., the examinee's scores are compared relative to those of age- and sex-matched peers, and this information is provided in percentiles). There is also a 20-question symptom checklist that requires patients to rate their subjective physical and cognitive symptoms. ImPACT has built-in validity measures that alert the test administrator to a possible invalid test, and the test manual provides additional comparisons for review. The ImPACT website also provides normative data for other comparisons, for example with students who have attention deficit disorder.

The test can be administered postinjury even if a baseline test has not been given. Normative data are then applied. For athletes who have taken a baseline ImPACT test, their scores on a postinjury test are compared to their baseline scores. Any change in performance that is in excess of normal variance (using reliable change indices) is then highlighted on the test printout. One of the criticisms of ImPACT is that the end user (often an athletic trainer) uses only these reliable change scores to indicate impairment. In other words, scores that are not highlighted are viewed as not indicating impairment, while highlighted scores are judged to be indicative of cognitive impairment. While this may be correct in many cases, a review of the raw data may point toward a different assessment of the athlete's abilities. In other words, the raw data may suggest that the athlete is still demonstrating residual cognitive impairment even if there is not a statistically significant change from baseline on the composite scores. Conversely, a close review of the raw scores may indicate intact functioning even though there is change from a baseline. The ability, then, to closely examine the results of ImPACT or any neurocognitive measure requires the appropriate training in statistics and neurologic functioning.

ImPACT is now administered to athletes in all major professional sports in the United States, as well as Olympic and international sport associations. The test is used in many colleges and high schools as well. A recent study found that of the high school programs that use computerized neurocognitive testing with their concussed athletes, 93% use the ImPACT program.[108] A pediatric version of ImPACT is in development. The pediatric version is designed for children aged 5 to 12 years and consists of seven subtests that assess episodic learning, verbal and visual memory, working memory, reaction time, and processing speed.[54]

Various studies have demonstrated the utility of ImPACT in concussion.[40, 74, 75, 86, 93, 130, 133-135] In a recent study, Schatz and Sandel concluded that the online version of ImPACT (the older version was a desktop test) is a valid measure with high levels of sensitivity and specificity in the acute stages of concussion, even when an athlete is denying symptoms.[135] However, other studies have shown low reliability scores. One investigation found low reliability scores on both ImPACT and paper–pencil tests.[128] That study demonstrated that even with alternative forms, practice effects can be seen on ImPACT, particularly with processing speed scores.

A 2007 study by Broglio and colleagues is often cited as evidence of the lack of test–retest reliability of three computerized tests (ImPACT, CogSport, and HeadMinder).[10] This study was limited, however, as there was little consistency regarding the number of days between administration of the test, and the subjects were required to complete all three computerized tests on the same day. The increased variability in performance may be attributed to error from having participants complete similar tasks, measuring nearly identical constructs, over a considerably demanding testing session.[130, 132, 134] Additionally, 34% of the subjects were excluded due to poor effort. This is in stark contrast to the typical number of invalid scores typically seen in clinical

practice. Other studies have demonstrated invalidity rates of 8.7% in a high school sample[132] and 6% in collegiate athletes.[135]

Automated Neuropsychological Assessment Metrics (ANAM)

This computerized battery was originally developed by the Department of Defense for use with the military[126] and is the most commonly used measure in service personnel in theater.[17] The test comprises seven subtests that assess simple reaction time, verbal and visual memory, sustained attention, processing speed, and working memory and visual matching. The test takes 15 to 20 minutes to complete. It also uses the baseline and postinjury assessment model.

Not as many studies have examined the validity and reliability of ANAM. Segalowitz and colleagues found that retest reliability "was good" overall but lower for individual subtests, particularly those assessing speed of information processing.[138] Kaminski and colleagues found sufficient stability of the ANAM across two baseline tests.[78] However, other research has been critical of the test.[22, 77] Coldren and colleagues examined the validity of ANAM in the combat environment and concluded, "The ANAM appears to have no utility as an individual diagnostic or population screening tool for detection of neurocognitive dysfunction from a single, uncomplicated concussion when administered 10 or more days following injury" (p. 179).[22]

CogSport

The CogSport test is a larger battery that evaluates visuomotor function, processing speed, visual attention/vigilance, attention/working memory, verbal memory, executive functioning, and social cognition.[21] CogState Sport (now commercially available in North America under the name Axon Sports; www.axonsports.com) is a briefer battery designed to assess the cognitive changes after concussion. It uses a playing card model and requires 8 to 10 minutes to administer. It assesses processing speed, visual recognition memory, attention/working memory, and accuracy. It is administered baseline and postinjury to assess change after concussive injury.

A number of studies have examined the validity of CogState Sport.[25, 46, 94, 97] The test designer

---

reports that the playing card design reduces the language demands of this test, but further research is needed to examine this claim.

HeadMinder

HeadMinder is an Internet-administered test (www.headminder.com) that requires 20 to 25 minutes to complete and evaluates processing speed, reaction time (simple and complex), and memory.[44] Like the other computerized tests, HeadMinder is completed by the athlete at baseline and then postinjury. Many of the published studies with HeadMinder have examined medical conditions, including cardiac disease,[150] multiple sclerosis,[148] and cancer.[153] Some studies have used HeadMinder with concussed athletes.[43, 45] This test was found to be sensitive to concussion (78.6%) in one study.[12]

Concussion Vital Signs

The newest computerized test to hit the market is Concussion Vital Signs (www.concussionvital-signs.com). The test is administered at baseline and postinjury with concussed patients and includes a subjective symptom checklist. The test can also be used to gather sideline assessment information, which can be transferred to the printout. It can take up to 45 minutes to complete. Concussion Vital Signs measures verbal and visual memory, psychomotor speed, cognitive flexibility, reaction time, complex attention, and subjective symptom reporting. Research is available regarding the reliability of the Concussion Vital Signs computerized test,[56] but nothing is currently available regarding the Concussion Vital Signs test specifically.

ISSUES WITH COMPUTERIZED ASSESSMENTS

While use of computerized instruments in concussion has become widely accepted, it is not without its problems and legitimate criticisms. The American Academy of Clinical Neuropsychology and the National Academy of Neuropsychology recently published a joint position paper addressing the use of computerized neuropsychological assessment devices (CNADs).[7] While this paper did not highlight any one particular test used in the assessment of concussion, it did generally address the most commonly used concussion instruments. Many of the issues discussed next are also not specific to computerized testing but are relevant to neuropsychological instruments.

The authors outlined eight key issues pertaining to the development and use of CNADs:

> (a) device marketing and performance claims made by developers of CNADs; (b) issues involved in appropriate end-use for administration and interpretation of CNADs; (c) technical hardware/software/firmware issues; (d) privacy, data security, identity verification, and testing environment; (e) psychometric development issues, especially reliability and validity; (f) cultural, experiential, and disability factors affecting examinee interaction with CNADs; (g) use of computerized testing and reporting services; (h) the need for checks on response validity and effort in the CNAD environment.[7]

An earlier paper reviewed the sources of possible error in computerized neuropsychological assessment.[18] This paper also did not address concussion assessment specifically but rather the use of computerized tests in general. Concerns were raised regarding the various hardware and software platforms used, particularly when a test relies on the accurate measurement of reaction time. Other factors, such as the resolution of the computer display, variability between available computer peripherals (i.e., keyboard and mouse), and the Internet connection speed were all reviewed. The authors concluded that neuropsychologists should continue to use appropriate computerized instruments but also educate themselves on the computer systems used in their practices. The paper also provided a useful checklist of computer issues to address.

Baseline Versus Normative Comparisons

Baseline testing in athletes is now widely used for high school, college, and professional athletes. The National Collegiate Athletic Association (NCAA) protocol recommends baseline testing for collegiate athletes.[115] A 2011 team physician consensus statement asserted that "post-injury NP [i.e., neuropsychological] test data are more useful if compared to the athlete's pre-injury baseline (p. 2415)."[63] The use of an athlete's own preinjury baseline data has its advantages. A clinician can compare the preinjury functioning to postinjury scores to note any changes suggestive of impairment. This can be particularly helpful with individuals who have preexisting conditions, such as a learning disability or attention deficit disorder. Additionally, accurate baseline testing is beneficial in patients with abilities that are higher or lower than average. Bright students may have baseline functioning in the above-average range, so average scores on their postinjury testing may reflect change (due to the injury or other causes). Without baseline testing, these athletes may be incorrectly classified as intact. Similarly, individuals functioning in the low average range before their injury may have low average postinjury scores incorrectly identified as indicating impairment.

There is expert consensus that baseline and postinjury testing are important in the assessment of concussed patients.[104] Legitimate questions are being raised about baseline testing, though. Some have questioned whether it is cost-effective. Others have wondered whether administration of individual or group baseline testing aids in the care of athletes after they have suffered a concussion. Randolph argues that it does not,[124] positing that the incidence of death or permanent disability in American football is very low and that baseline testing does not alter these numbers. While it is not likely that any concussion management program can prevent the tragic occurrence of severe brain trauma in contact sports, assessment of concussed athletes (with the use of baseline and postinjury cognitive testing) is performed solely to provide individualized treatment protocols. As Shuttleworth-Edwards commented in her rebuttal to the Randolph article, "the value of baseline testing lies in its availability for **comparative** purposes with subsequent follow-up testing, all of which need to be contextualized further in the overall clinical evaluation process (p. 391)."[141]

Randolph also questioned whether the use of repeated testing (baseline and postinjury) introduces greater error variability into the assessment.

This is a valid question that warrants further examination, particularly when those without the appropriate training in statistical analysis of change are interpreting the test results. Another recent study questioned the broad use of baseline testing with athletes. Echemendia and coauthors used two separate reliable change methods to examine postinjury scores of collegiate athletes on ImPACT.[37] They found that the method used by ImPACT to determine reliable change between baseline and postinjury testing may misclassify a number of injured athletes as cognitively intact. The authors concluded that athletes with "clinically meaningful postconcussion cognitive decline can be identified without baseline data (p. 1087)." However, they also acknowledged that postinjury cognitive decline "may be difficult to identify without the use of baseline data" for athletes with "histories of learning disabilities, Attention Deficit Hyperactivity Disorder, multiple previous concussions, linguistic differences, or high or low levels of intelligence (p. 1087)." This study also used collegiate athletes and the ImPACT test, so the results may not generalize to other populations and other concussion assessment measures.

Schmidt and coauthors performed a study using the ANAM test, along with a symptom checklist and a postural control measure.[136] They found that the use of normative data (vs. baseline data) was adequate in assessing cognitive functioning postinjury in collegiate students. A separate study examined the use of reliable change indices (RCI) after concussion with paper–pencil cognitive tests.[65] The authors concluded that RCI models are not equivalent and can lead to different decisions about whether an athlete is demonstrating impairment after a concussive injury relative to baseline.

Finally, Schatz and Putz examined the concurrent validity of three computerized measures (CogSport, ImPACT, and HeadMinder). [134] These tests were also compared to standard paper–pencil cognitive tests. The authors found that the three computerized tests shared similar properties, particularly on measures of reaction time and processing, but varied with regard to assessment of memory. They warned that clinicians, therefore, should not use the baseline results of one test as a comparison to postinjury results on another computerized test.

"Sandbagging" of Baseline Testing

In order for any neurocognitive test results to be useful, adequate effort is required on the part of the examinee. There are many reasons people may not put forth their optimal effort on testing. "Sandbagging" occurs when athletes purposefully perform below their abilities on baseline testing. The athlete intentionally chooses the incorrect answer to lower the baseline scores. The belief is that any low postinjury scores would then be consistent with the preinjury or baseline performance and result in the athlete's being cleared to return to play. This concept is in contrast to malingering of cognitive deficits after an injury, which is discussed later in the chapter.

Most of the computerized tests have built-in validity indicators that will "flag" a baseline test as likely invalid. Many athletes believe they can make enough errors to lower their baseline scores without making enough errors to invalidate their tests. However, a study by Erdal showed that sandbagging a baseline test without detection is more difficult than would be expected.[42] The ImPACT test was administered to undergraduate athletes with instructions to perform poorly on the test but not reach a level that would be detected by the validity indicators. Only 11% of the subjects were successfully able to do so, suggesting that it is "difficult for athletes to intentionally perform poorly on the ImPACT without reaching threshold on the 'red flags' of validity indicators (p. 477)." Other research has also shown that individuals who are purposefully attempting to lower their scores on cognitive tests tend to have longer reaction times, likely due to the need to think about how many questions they need to answer incorrectly.[157]

Researchers have looked at the frequency of invalid test scores on baseline cognitive testing. It should be noted that all invalid scores are not due solely to "sandbagging" (e.g., a patient may simply be unmotivated to take the test or misunderstand the test directions). Hunt and colleagues found that 11% of their sample (high school athletes) had invalid baseline testing.[68] Similarly, Schatz and colleagues revealed that 9% of the high school athletes they examined had invalid baseline tests.[130] In a separate study of collegiate athletes, 6% of the baseline test results were excluded for invalidity.[135] In 2008, Solomon and Haase demonstrated that 6% of players in the NFL had invalid baseline test scores.[145]

Individualized Versus Group Administration

One of the appealing attributes of computerized testing is the ability to administer the test in a group setting. It is often impractical and cost-prohibitive to administer a neurocognitive test on an individualized basis when there are a large number of athletes to assess; however, there are special considerations with respect to group administration, including the testing environment. Attention should be given to ensure that the room is as free from distractions as possible. This means both internal and external noise (e.g., voices easily heard in an adjoining hallway) and commotion (e.g., a window that allows people passing by to see inside the testing room). An authority figure should also be available as a proctor to ensure that the examinees do not disrupt each other during the administration of the test.

Moser and colleagues examined the effect of group testing on computerized testing results versus individual testing.[113] Athletes who completed baseline testing in a group scored significantly lower on memory, motor processing speed, and reaction time indices. There was also a higher rate of invalid baseline tests, but there was no difference in symptom reporting. Further research is needed to determine the optimal number of athletes that should be tested in a group setting.

When to Test After an Injury

When concussion protocols were first developed, the initial recommendation for postinjury testing was to have the athlete retested 24 to 48 hours after a documented concussion. This was useful both in assessing the athletes' subjective reporting of their symptoms and in documenting the degree of any cognitive deficits, particularly relative to their baseline. There are questions about the appropriateness of this recommendation for a few important reasons.

The most consistent recommendation given to athletes immediately postinjury is to rest and to reduce the amount of stimulation during the next few days. However, when athletes are told that they will be tested 1 or 2 days postinjury, they may be returning to school or to their practice facilities while still significantly symptomatic. Additionally, the demands of taking a computerized test can worsen their symptoms. It would seem more beneficial to have the concussed athlete remain at home and away from the highly stimulating environment of a school. Athletes who are reporting physical or cognitive symptoms of concussion are not going to be cleared for play in any case, so cognitive testing will not assist in that decision. In most cases, therefore, athletes are not tested cognitively until they are fully asymptomatic.

Still, in some cases, completion of a cognitive assessment while the patient is still symptomatic can provide valuable information. This may include documentation to a school of cognitive impairment so that absences can be excused or to validate that temporary academic accommodations should be allowed. It may also offer objective data of cognitive deficits to the athlete, parent, or coach who is minimizing the injury or is resistant to treatment recommendations. Finally, as previously discussed, cognitive data may indicate which athletes will have a more protracted recovery, although again, further research is needed in this area.

On a separate but related note, the time of cognitive testing and exercise is also to be considered. Covassin and coauthors found that athletes who completed a maximal treadmill exercise test demonstrated lower verbal memory composite scores on ImPACT.[34] No differences were seen on other composite scores. Thus, the authors suggested that neurocognitive testing should not be conducted immediately after a game or practice.

OTHER CONSIDERATIONS

Clinicians working with concussed patients must also understand the emerging research on the myriad other factors that can affect the recovery process. These issues, including age, sex, ethnicity, prior medical history, previous concussions, and preexisting learning disability or affective disorders, may influence recovery or alter the results of neurocognitive testing. Therefore, one needs to take these characteristics into consideration when interpreting test results.

The age of the patient may result in different patterns of recovery. Several studies have shown that high school athletes take longer to recover than collegiate athletes[48, 158] and professional athletes.[119] Sim and colleagues stated that high school athletes demonstrated slower recovery of memory functioning than college-aged athletes.[143] Register-Mihalik and coauthors reported better reaction time scores in college-aged versus high school athletes.[128] Covassin and colleagues also found that high school athletes took longer to recover from concussion than collegiate athletes.[31, 32] Differences were even noted during the 4 years of high school. Hunt and Ferrara found differences among high school–aged athletes on various paper–pencil tests, with 11th- and 12th-grade athletes performing better on measures of information processing speed, attention, and motor dexterity than 9th and 10th graders.[67]

Recent research has examined pathophysiological changes after concussion in the young, developing brain and raised concerns about the increased vulnerability to repeated injuries in youth athletes.[140] A recent review of the pediatric literature reported that there is still less research on sport-related concussion in the pediatric population but noted that most authors recommend a more conservative approach with return-to-play decisions in younger athletes.[149]

There are divergent opinions on the role of sex in concussions. Some research has shown that collegiate and high school–aged female athletes sustain a higher percentage of concussions than their male counterparts.[33, 52, 66, 95] As discussed in chapter 5, theories behind these findings involve a greater willingness of females to report their symptoms; hormonal differences affecting vulnerability to concussion; and less neck musculature or strength, allowing greater movement of the female head with contact.

Some have investigated whether male or female sex plays a role in recovery. One literature review of research pertaining to sex and concussions concluded that there was some evidence of sex differences in outcomes of traumatic brain injury and concussions.[35] The authors also noted that these were based on self-reporting of symptoms and might reflect a greater willingness on the part of females to report their symptoms. Mounce and colleagues found that women with persistent postconcussion symptoms reported more severe symptoms than men.[114] Colvin and colleagues noted that concussed female soccer players performed more poorly on neurocognitive testing than male soccer players.[30] Broshek and colleagues showed that female college-aged athletes were more impaired on simple and complex reaction times than their male counterparts, even after adjustment for the use of helmets in many male sports.[14] Another recent study reported that female athletes performed worse than male athletes on the ImPACT visual memory index and reported more symptoms.[31] All of this being said, Frommer and coauthors found that concussed female (high school) athletes reported different types of symptoms than male athletes but did not report more symptoms or take longer to recover from concussion.[49] Zuckerman and coauthors also did not find sex-specific differences in cognitive deficits or symptom reporting in concussed high school soccer players.[159]

Other research has shown that athletes with a history of a learning disability perform more poorly than others on neurocognitive testing.[27] Solomon and Haase examined NFL football players and reported that those athletes with a history of a learning disability or attention deficit disorder scored lower on measures of verbal and visual memory but not on reaction time or processing speed.[145]

Ethnic and cultural differences are also being explored. Kontos and colleagues examined differences in baseline and postinjury testing with ImPACT between African American and Caucasian high school and collegiate athletes.[83] No significant differences in baseline and post-concussion verbal and visual memory, reaction time, or total symptoms were reported. However, African American athletes were 2.4 times more likely to show a clinically significant decline on the postinjury processing speed measure. Further research was recommended to understand the reason for this finding. Shuttleworth-Edwards and her colleagues examined the equivalency of the ImPACT test between South African rugby players and U.S. football players.[142] The conclusion was that the U.S. normative data were appropriate for use with the South African athletes but that cultural differences did affect symptom reporting.

Some investigators have studied whether postconcussive symptoms themselves alter cognitive performance in patients. Register-Mihalik and coauthors examined the effects of preseason

headaches and posttraumatic headaches on neurocognitive functioning.[127] Concussed athletes who reported moderate to severe posttraumatic headaches performed more poorly on mental processing and reaction time tasks. An earlier study by Collins and coauthors also found that athletes with posttraumatic headaches demonstrated lower performance on reaction time and memory and that they were more likely to have reported on-field anterograde amnesia.[26] Solomon and Haase, too, found differences on neurocognitive testing in NFL players with physician-treated headaches versus those with nontreated headaches.[145]

A great deal of ongoing research is examining the effects of multiple concussions. Much of the research and media focus has been on the professional athlete,[58, 117, 118] but the collegiate[59, 79] and high school athlete[29, 131] have been examined, as well. While no definitive conclusion has been reached, the research suggests that athletes with a history of previous concussion are at an increased risk of suffering another concussion and may recover more slowly than athletes without that history.

Finally, preexisting psychological conditions, such as depression, may also affect cognitive performance. Covassin and colleagues reported that nonconcussed athletes with severe depression (assessed by a self-report questionnaire) performed worse on baseline visual memory tests and reported a greater number of symptoms (somatic, cognitive, emotional, and sleep) than nondepressed subjects.[32] They recommended that baseline assessment include a measure of affective functioning.

OTHER ISSUES ADDRESSED BY NEUROPSYCHOLOGISTS IN ASSESSING CONCUSSED PATIENTS

The discussion about the role of neuropsychologists in concussion assessment typically focuses on cognitive testing. Even within this chapter, the majority of the information presented addresses neurocognitive evaluation. However, there is less focus on the contribution of neuropsychologists beyond testing. Neuropsychologists also examine many other factors that contribute to the functioning of individuals who have suffered a concussion.

Psychological Disorders Warranting Exploration in Patients With Prolonged Concussion Symptoms

- Anxiety disorders
- Depressive disorders
- Somatoform disorder
- Factitious disorder
- Malingering

Psychological Factors

One of the most complex tasks for a clinician assessing a concussed patient is to sort out the contributions of psychological factors to persistent symptoms after concussion. The physical (e.g., headache, fatigue), cognitive (e.g., impaired attention and memory), and emotional symptoms (e.g., sad or anxious affect) following a concussion are certainly not pathognomonic to concussion but rather are experienced in numerous conditions. They are commonplace in healthy community-based individuals[50, 51, 152] and non-concussed students.[155] This is also true among military veterans,[89, 156] trauma patients,[107, 122] orthopedic patients,[114] chronic pain patients,[144] and those suffering from depression.[72, 74]

As discussed later in the book, several studies have suggested that persistent subjective symptoms may be in part due to psychological factors rather than solely the result of the initial concussion or mTBI. A recent study showed that postconcussion syndrome symptoms are reported in a number of psychiatric groups, including somatization disorder, posttraumatic stress disorder (PTSD), generalized anxiety disorder, and major depressive disorder.[36] In fact, the data indicate that the reported postconcussion symptoms are more likely due to PTSD and depression than the mTBI. Suhr and Gunstad concluded that reported cognitive complaints after concussion were accounted for more by depression than by head injury.[146] Garden and colleagues used psychological tests to assess the influence of personality traits on the persistence of postconcussion symptoms.[51] They noted that factors including depression, dysthymia, and anxiety, as well as

negativistic, sadistic, dependent, and borderline personality traits, all played a contributing role in the persistent postconcussion syndrome.

Somatoform Disorder

Individuals are diagnosed with a somatoform disorder when they have physical symptoms that "suggest a medical condition and are not fully explained by a general medical condition, by the direct effects of a substance, or by another mental disorder (p. 445)."[2] In this condition, the symptoms are not purposely produced and must significantly affect a person's functioning in order to be diagnosed. This is in contrast to factitious disorder, which is characterized by "physical or psychological symptoms that are intentionally produced or feigned in order to assume the sick role, (p. 471)"[2] or malingering (discussed next). The diagnostic differentiation between somatoform disorder, factitious disorder, malingering, and legitimate cognitive impairment requires expertise in both the sequelae of brain injury and psychological functioning. The psychological contribution to the development of postconcussion syndrome is reviewed in a later chapter.

Effort and Malingering

The utility of neurocognitive test data is reliant on the examinee's adequate effort. If the person does not put forth adequate effort on a test, lower scores may be misperceived as evidence of cognitive impairment. However, there are multiple reasons a person may behave in this way. These include fatigue or illness, oppositional nature, dislike of the examiner or test situation, lack of understanding of the reason for the assessment, factitious disorder, or malingering. Malingering is defined as the "intentional production of false or grossly exaggerated physical or psychological symptoms, motivated by external incentives (p. 683)" such as monetary gain or avoidance of criminal prosecution.[2] Individuals who feign or exaggerate their symptoms may be awarded financial compensation that they were not entitled to, use limited resources that should be available for legitimately injured patients, or wrongly avoid legal or military responsibilities.

Neuropsychologists are trained specifically in the examination of malingered cognitive and psychological dysfunction, and the role of neuropsychologists in assessment of effort and response bias has been widely recognized. The National Academy of Neuropsychology published a position paper on the assessment of effort in neuropsychological testing,[15] and the American Academy of Clinical Neuropsychology also produced a consensus statement.[62] These papers were not specific to concussion or mTBI; however, a new book is dedicated entirely to symptom validity and malingering in mTBI.[16]

The frequency of malingered responding has been long examined in the neuropsychological literature. In his review, Larrabee reported an overall base rate of malingering in 40% of individuals who undergo a neuropsychological evaluation.[84] Symptom-validity test failure has been found to be as high as 42% to 50% in disability examinations.[19, 20] It should be noted that Iverson and colleagues reviewed the literature and concluded that **exaggeration** of postconcussion complaints is much more common that complete feigning of symptoms.[73, 76]

Even in a pediatric mTBI sample, malingered effort is prevalent. Kirkwood and Kirk found that 17% of their patients with concussion, aged 8 to 17 years, exerted suboptimal effort. [80, 81] The authors also noted that the incentive for poor effort is not always known and that the use of specific measures of symptom validity is warranted.

Necessity of Academic and Employment Accommodations

The cognitive and physical symptoms of concussion can result in significant difficulties in the classroom and on the job. Neuropsychological testing provides objective data on the exact nature of the patient's deficits following a brain injury. This information allows for individualized recommendations for academic accommodations or accommodations in the workplace.

The focus on concussion assessment in athletes has long been on return-to-play decisions; there has not been as much emphasis on returning the concussed athlete to the classroom. This "return-to-learn" emphasis is needed, as most athletes return to the classroom long before they return to the field of play.[98] One of the current trends in the school setting is the application of the standard academic accommodations to all concussed students. This is a mistake, as some students do not require any accommodations while others require extensive changes to their school environment and routine. Students without cognitive impairment should not have accommodations similar to those for students with clear cognitive deficits from concussion.

Academic accommodations can be as simple as not requiring concussed students to take tests or quizzes during the acute recovery period because of their impaired attention and memory. In some cases, though, accommodations are made to address the specific needs of a particular student (e.g., individuals with vestibular dysfunction postinjury can become overstimulated in the chaotic environment of a school hallway, so they are allowed to leave class a few minutes early to travel in hallways unobstructed).

Some schools have policies stating that concussed athletes must remain out of school or cannot complete any classroom work until they are entirely symptom free. This can result in significant stress for students, as many become quite anxious about getting behind in their classes. Such a policy also does not address the severity of symptoms. Some athletes may have persistent but tolerable headaches that would not prevent them from attending school. This all-or-nothing approach to accommodations also does not address the particular activities that may be the cause of the student's symptoms. There are students who perform adequately on most schoolwork but struggle with using the computer. These students should be allowed to complete schoolwork that does not aggravate their symptoms and given accommodations to reduce the use of the computer. Alternatively, a student may falsely claim cognitive deficits from a concussion to avoid school responsibilities. The objective data provided by a cognitive assessment can help make these distinctions. There have been some excellent recent reviews of academic accommodations for the concussed student.[98, 105]

Most of the research addressing vocational return focuses on more severe traumatic brain injury.[106, 139, 154] There is significantly less research on return to work after a concussion. The problem then becomes the misapplication of recommendations for moderate-severe brain injury to those who have suffered a concussion. A neuropsychological assessment after a concussion can assist the employer or case manager with job-specific and injury-specific recommendations to assist in transitioning the patient back to work.

Education to Patients and Family Members

The increased media focus on concussion has had both positive and negative outcomes. Athletes, both amateur and professional, are significantly better educated on the signs and symptoms of concussion, which has resulted in an increase in diagnosis of these injuries. There has also been a concomitant increase in the anxiety about concussions in both patients and their family members. Parents commonly complain that they were not given adequate information from the emergency department (ED) or clinician on how to manage a concussion. Meehan and Mannix found that nearly one-third of pediatric patients were discharged from the ED without any specific instructions to follow up with their primary health care provider for additional treatment.[110] This study was based on the years 2002 through 2006, so it is quite plausible that more current ED policies include proper instructions for follow-up care.

It has become increasingly difficult for a parent to wade through the information on concussion available on the Internet. Sullivan and colleagues found extensive information and personal stories about concussions posted on Twitter.[147] It is not possible for the average parent to find the most appropriate and up-to-date information among countless sites. The quality of the information provided by websites also varies greatly.[1] Additionally, the parent may not have the educational background to understand much of the available research literature that is written for the medical professional.

Many parents then rely on word-of-mouth information from friends or family members, which may be scientifically inaccurate, or media reports, which may be hyperbolic or biased. One of the benefits of consultation with a neuropsychologist trained in concussion management is the opportunity to review and explain the current state of the science. The neuropsychologist can also help assess how a patient's or parent's anxiety surrounding these injuries is affecting the recovery.

One study found that adults who were given an information booklet on concussions and coping strategies reported fewer symptoms and were "significantly less stressed" at 3 months postinjury.[123] Ponsford noted that both children and adults who were provided with information about concussions early after their injuries reported reduced symptoms.[121] Another study, though, found no effect on reports of psychological distress in those provided with early educational intervention; however, this study included "minimal, mild and moderate head injury," so the effect on mTBI or concussion patients specifically was not examined.[64]

Comprehensive Neuropsychological Testing

Most of the research on neuropsychological assessment in concussion focuses on brief batteries. A single concussive injury does not typically result in long-lasting impairment, so extensive testing is not generally warranted. However, more extensive neuropsychological assessment may be appropriate in some situations. Such is the case when there is a need to determine what other factors may be associated with poor recovery, such as premorbid learning issues (e.g., a learning disability or attention deficit disorder) or emotional disorders.[54] In a pediatric patient, the evaluation may also involve interviews with use of questionnaires by parents and teachers.

Assessment of a wider range of cognitive abilities and psychological functioning may also be necessary to distinguish between legitimate complaints of cognitive impairment and other noninjury-related factors. These diagnostic differentials require more in-depth questioning during the clinical interview and the use of specialized psychological and cognitive measures. Additionally, the use of more comprehensive neuropsychological testing may be appropriate for individuals with prolonged symptoms (i.e., greater than 3 months) or those with multiple concussive injuries. As noted by Kirkwood and colleagues, more comprehensive neuropsychological testing may be warranted months after an injury to assist in indentifying factors that may be producing problems, to ensure that accurate diagnostic decisions are made, and to help develop an appropriate clinical management plan.[82]

Brief cognitive assessments are also not recommended in any case that involves litigation (e.g., motor vehicle accidents) or cases in which monetary compensation depends on claims of cognitive loss secondary to a concussion (e.g., workers' compensation cases). The use of comprehensive testing, including symptom-validity measures, is particularly important in these evaluations. Finally, premorbid histories that may affect cognitive abilities, such as substance abuse or other neurologic conditions, also warrant more thorough cognitive assessments.

CONCLUDING THOUGHTS

The expertise of neuropsychologists has been long recognized in the evaluation and treatment of individuals with concussive injuries, and neuropsychologists have contributed greatly to our knowledge of the effects of concussion on cognition and emotional functioning. The burgeoning research in this area will likely increase our understanding of how concussion affects cognitive and emotional functioning and help develop improved treatment protocols for concussed patients. The use of traditional paper–pencil neuropsychological tests, as well as computerized measures, has become standard practice in concussion management, particularly among athletes. While the reliability and validity of currently available tests are being appropriately examined and legitimate concerns about computerized tests have been raised, the use of neuropsychological measures continues to expand. Neuropsychologists can contribute not only in the cognitive assessment of athletes, but also in making difficult distinctions between true cognitive impairment secondary to a concussion and other factors and conditions that present after a concussion.

REFERENCES

1. Ahmed OH, Sullivan SJ, Schneiders AG, McCrory PR. Concussion information online: evaluation of information quality, content, and readability of concussion-related websites. Br J Sports Med 2012;46:675-683.

2. American Psychological Association. Diagnostic and Statistical Manual of Mental Disorders. 4th ed. Washington, DC: American Psychiatric Association; 1994.

3. Aubry M, Cantu R, Dvorak J. Summary and agreement statement of the first International Conference on Concussion in Sport, Vienna 2001: recommendations for the improvement and safety and health of athletes who may suffer concussive injuries. Br J Sports Med 2002:6-10.

4. Barr WB. Neuropsychological testing of high school athletes: preliminary norms and test-retest indices. Arch Clin Neuropsychol 2003;18:91-101.

5. Barr WB, McCrea M. Sensitivity and specificity of standardized neurocognitive testing immediately following sports concussion. J Int Neuropsychol Soc 2001;7:693-702.

6. Barth JT, Alves WM, Ryan TV, et al. Mild head injury in sports: neuropsychological sequelae and recovery of function. In: Levin HS, Eisenberg HM, Benton AL, eds. Mild Head Injury. New York, NY: Oxford University Press; 1989:257-275.

7. Bauer RM, Iverson GL, Cernich AN, Binder LM, Ruff RM, Naugle RI. Computerized neuropsychological assessment devices: joint position paper of the American Academy of Clinical Neuropsychology and the National Academy of Neuropsychology. Clin Neuropsychol 2012;26:177-196.

8. Belanger HG, Curtis G, Demery JA, Lebowitz BK, Vanderploeg RD. Factors moderating neuropsychological outcomes following mild traumatic brain injury: a meta-analysis. J Int Neuropsychol Soc 2005;11(3):215-217.

9. Belanger HG, Vanderploeg RD. The neuropsychological impact of sports-related concussion: a meta-analysis. J Int Neuropsychol Soc 2005;11(4):345-347.

10. Broglio SP, Ferrara MS, Macciocchi SN, Baumgartner TA, Elliott R. Test-retest reliability of computerized concussion assessment programs. J Athl Train 2007;42(4):509-514.

11. Broglio SP, Macciocchi SN, Ferrara MS. Neurocognitive performance of concussed athletes when symptom free. J Athl Train 2007;42(4):504-508.

12. Sensitivity of the concussion assessment battery [database on the Internet]. 2007.

13. Broglio SP, Sosnoff JJ, Ferrara MS. The relationship of athlete-reported concussion symptoms and objective measures of neurocognitive function and postural control. Clin J Sport Med 2009;19(5):377-382.

14. Broshek DK, Kaushik T, Freeman JR, Erlanger D, Webbe F, Barth JT. Sex differences in outcome following sports-related concussion. J Neurosurg 2005;102(5):856-863.

15. Bush SS, Ruff RM, Troster AI, Barth JT, Koffler SP, Pliskin NH, et al. Symptom validity assessment: practice issues and medical necessity NAN policy and planning committee. Arch Clin Neuropsychol 2005;20(4):419-426.

16. Carone DA, Bush SS. Mild Traumatic Brain Injury: Symptom Validity and Malingering. New York: Springer; 2013.

17. Cernich A, Reeves D, Sun W, Bleiberg J. Automated neuropsychological assessment metrics sports medicine battery. Arch Clin Neuropsychol 2007;22(S):S101-S114.

18. Cernich AN, Brennana DM, Barker LM, Bleiberg J. Sources of error in computerized neuropsychological assessment. Arch Clinical Neuropsychol 2007;22(Suppl 1):39-48.

19. Chafetz M. The psychological consultative examination for social security disability. Psychol Inj Law 2011;4(3-4):235-244.

20. Chafetz M, Prenthowski E, Rao A. To work or not to work: motivation (not low IQ) determines SVT findings. Arch Clin Neuropsychol 2011;26:306-313.

21. CogState. CogSport. Parkville, Victoria, Australia: CogState; 1999.

22. Coldren RL, Russell ML, Parish PV, Dretsch M, Kelly MP. The ANAM lacks utility as a diagnostic or screening tool for concussion more than 10 days following injury. Mil Med 2012;177(2):179-183.

23. Collie A, Darby D, Maruff P. Computerized cognitive assessment of athletes with sports related head injury. Br J Sports Med 2001;35:297-302.

24. Collie A, Makdissi M, Maruff P, Bennell K, McCrory P. Cognition in the days following concussion: comparison of symptomatic versus asymptomatic athletes. J Neurol Neurosurg Psychiatry 2006;77(2):241-245.

25. Collie A, Maruff P, Makdissi M, McCrory P, McStephen M, Darby D. CogSport: reliability and correlation with conventional cognitive tests used in postconcussion medical evaluations. Clin J Sport Med 2003;13(1):28-32.

26. Collins MW, Field M, Lovell MR, Iverson G, Johnston KM, Maroon J, et al. Relationship between postconcussion headache and neuropsychological test performance in high school athletes. Am J Sports Med 2003;31(2):168-173.

27. Collins MW, Grindel SH, Lovell MR, Dede DE, Moser DJ, Phalin BR, et al. Relationship between concussion and neuropsychological performance in college football players. JAMA 1999;282(10):964-970.

28. Collins MW, Iverson GL, Lovell MR, McKeag DB, Norwig J, Maroon J. On-field predictors of neuropsychological and symptom deficit following sports-related concussion. Clin J Sport Med 2003;13(4):222-229.

29. Collins MW, Lovell MR, Iverson GL, Cantu RC, Maroon JC, Field M. Cumulative effects of concussion in high school athletes. Neurosurgery 2002;51:1175-1179.

30. Colvin AC, Mullen J, Lovell MR, West RV, Collins MW, Groh M. The role of concussion history and gender in recovery from soccer-related concussion. Am J Sports Med 2009;37(9):1699-1704.

31. Covassin T, Elbin RJ, Harris W, Parker T, Kontos AP. The role of age and sex in symptoms, neurocognitive performance, and postural stability in athletes after concussion. Am J Sports Med 2012;40(6):1303-1312.

32. Covassin T, Elbin RJ, Larson E, Kontos AP. Sex and age differences in depression and baseline sport-related concussion neurocognitive performance and symptoms. Clin J Sport Med 2012;22(2):98-104.

33. Covassin T, Swanik CB, Sachs ML. Sex differences and the incidences of concussion among collegiate athletes. J Athl Train 2003;38(3):238-244.

34. Covassin T, Weiss L, Powell J, Womack C. Effects of a maximal exercise test on neurocognitive function. Br J Sports Med 2007;41(6):370-374.

35. Dick RW. Is there a gender difference in concussion incidence and outcome? J Sports Med 2009;43(Suppl 1):i46-50.

36. Donnell AJ, Kim MS, Silva MA, Vanderploeg RD. Incidence of postconcussion symptoms in psychiatric diagnostic groups, mild traumatic brain injury and comorbid conditions. Clin Neuropsychol 2012;26(7):1092-1101.

37. Echemendia RJ, Bruce JM, Baily CM, Sanders JF, Arnett P, Vargas G. The utility of post-concussion neuropsychological data in identifying cognitive change following sports-related MTBI in the absence of baseline data. Clin Neuropsychol 2012;26(7):1077-1091.

38. Echemendia RJ, Herring S, Bailes J. Who should conduct and interpret the neuropsychological assessment in sports-related concussion? Br J Sports Med 2009;43(i32-35).

39. Echemendia RJ, Iverson GL, McCrea M, Broshek DK, Gioia G, Sautter SW, et al. Role of neuropsychologists in the evaluation and management of sport-related concussion: an inter-organization position statement. Archives of Clinical Neuropsychology 2012;27:119-122.

40. Elbin RJ, Schatz P, Covassin T. One-year test-retest reliability of the online version of ImPACT in high school athletes. Am J Sports Med 2011;39(11):2319-2324.

41. Ellemberg D, Henry LC, Macciocchi SN, Guskiewicz KM, Broglio SP. Advances in sports concussion assessment from behavioral to brain imaging measures. Neurotrauma 2009;26(12):2365-2382.

42. Erdal K. Neuropsychological testing for sports-related concussion: how athletes can sandbag their baseline testing without detection. Arch Clin Neuropsychol 2012;27(5):473-479.

43. Erlanger D, Kaushik T, Cantu R, Barth JT, Broshek DK, Freeman JR, et al. Symptom-based assessment of concussion severity. J Neurosurg 2003;98:477-484.

44. Erlanger DM, Feldman DJ, Kutner K. Concussion Resolution Index. New York: HeadMinder; 1999.

45. Erlanger DM, Kaushik K, Broshek D, Freeman J, Feldman D, Festa J. Development and validation of a web-based screening tool for monitoring cognitive status. J Head Trauma Rehabil 2002;17(5):458-476.

46. Falleti M, Maruff P, Collie A, Darby D. Practice effects associated with the repeated assessment of cognitive function using the CogState Battery at 10-minute, one weekend, one month test-retest intervals. J Clin Exp Neuropsychol 2006;28:1095-1112.

47. Fazio VC, Lovell MR, Pardini JE, Collins MW. The relation between post concussion symptoms and neurocognitive performance in concussed athletes. NeuroRehabilitation 2007;22(3):207-216.

48. Field M, Collins MW, Lovell MR, Maroon JC. Does age play a role in recovery from sports-related concussion? A comparison of high school and collegiate athletes. J Pediatr 2003;142(5):546-553.

49. Frommer LJ, Gurka KK, Cross KM, Ingersoll CD, Comstock RD, Saliba SA. Sex differences in concussion symptoms of high school athletes. J Athl Train 2011;46(1):76-84.

50. Garden N, Sullivan K. An examination of the base rates of post-concussion symptoms: the influence of demographics and depression. Appl Neuropsychol 2010;17(1):1-7.

51. Garden N, Sullivan KA, Lange RT. The relationship between personality characteristics and postconcussion symptoms in a nonclinical sample. Neuropsychology 2010;24(2):168-175.

52. Gessel LM, Fields SK, Collins CL, Dick RW, Comstock RD. Concussions among United States high school and collegiate athletes. J Athl Train 2007;42(4):495-503.

53. Gioia GA, Collins M, Isquith PK. Improving identification and diagnosis of mild traumatic brain injury with evidence: psychometric support for the acute concussion evaluation. J Head Trauma Rehabil 2008;23(4):230-242.

54. Gioia GA, Isquith PK, Schneider JC, Vaughan CG. New approaches to assessment and monitoring of concussion in children. Top Lang Disord 2009;29(3):266-281.

55. Gronwall D, Wrighttson P. Delayed recovery of intellectual function after mild head injury. Lancet 1974;2(7881):605-609.

56. Gualtieri CT, Johnson LG. Reliability and validity of a computerized neurocognitive test battery, CNS Vital Signs. Arch Clin Neuropsychol 2006;21(7):623-643.

57. Guerriero RM, Proctor MR, Mannix R, Meehan WP. Epidemiology, trends, assessment and management of sport-related concussion in United States high schools. Curr Opin Pediatr 2012;24(6):696-701.

58. Guskiewicz KM, Marshall SW, Bailes JE, McCrea M, Cantu R, Randolph C, et al. Association between recurrent concussion and late-life cognitive impairment in retired professional football players. Neurosurgery 2005;57(4):719-726.

59. Guskiewicz KM, McCrea M, Marshall SW, Cantu RC, Randolph C, Barr W, et al. Cumulative effects associated with recurrent concussion in collegiate football players: the NCAA Concussion Study. JAMA 2003;290(19):2549-2555.

60. Halstead ME, Walter KD. American Academy of Pediatrics. Clinical report—sport-related concussion in children and adolescents. Pediatrics 2010;126(3):597-615.

61. Harmon KG, Drezner JA, Gammons M, Guskiewicz KM, Halstead M, Herring SA, et al. American Medical Society for Sports Medicine position statement: concussion in sport. Br J Sports Med 2013;47:15-26.

62. Heilbronner RL, Sweet JJ, Morgan JE, Larrabee GJ, Millis SR. American Academy of Clinical Neuropsychology consensus conference statement on the neuropsychological assessment of effort, response bias, and malingering. Clin Neuropsychol 2009;23:1093-1129.

63. Herring SA, Cantu RC, Guskiewicz KM, Putukian M, Kibler WB, Bergfeld JA, et al. Concussion (mild traumatic brain injury) and the team physician: a consensus statement—2011 update. Med Sci Sports Exerc 2011;43(12):2412-2422.

64. Heskestad B, Waterloo K, Baardsen R, Helseth E, Romner B, Ingebrigtsen T. No impact of early intervention on late outcome after minimal, mild and moderate head injury. Scand J Trauma Resusc Emerg Med 2010;18:1-5.

65. Hinton-Bayre AD. Choice of reliable change model can alter decisions regarding neuropsychological impairment after sports-related concussion. Clin J Sport Med 2012;22(2):105-108.

66. Hootman JM, Dick R, Agel J. Epidemiology of collegiate injuries for 15 sports: summary and recommendations for injury prevention initiatives. J Athl Train 2007;42:311-319.

67. Hunt TN, Ferrara MS. Age-related differences in neuropsychological testing among high school athletes. J Athl Train 2009;44(4):405-409.

68. Hunt TN, Ferrara MS, Miller LS, Macciocchi S. The effect of effort on baseline neuropsychological test scores in high school football athletes. Arch Clin Neuropsychol 2007;22(5):615-621.

69. ImPACT Applications, Inc. ImPACT 6.0. ImPACT Applications, Inc.: Pittsburgh; 2007.

70. Iverson G. Predicting slow recovery from sport-related concussion: the next simple-complex distinction. Clin J Sport Med 2007;17(1):31-37.

71. Iverson GL. Evidence-based neuropsychological assessment in sport-related concussion. In: Webbe FM, ed. Handbook of Sport Neuropsychology. New York: Springer; 2011.

72. Iverson GL. Misdiagnosis of the persistent post-concussion syndrome in patients with depression. Arch Clin Neuropsychol 2006;21:303-310.

73. Iverson GL, Brooks BL, Collins MW, Lovell MR. Tracking neuropsychological recovery following concussion in sport. Brain Inj 2006;20(3):245-252.

74. Iverson GL, Lange RT. Examination of "post-concussion-like" symptoms in a healthy sample. Appl Neuropsychol 2003;21:303-310.

75. Iverson GL, Lovell MR, Collins MW. Validity of ImPACT for measuring processing speed following sports-related concussion. J Clin Exp Neuropsychol 2005;27(6):683-689.

76. Iverson GL, Zasler NF, Lange RT. Post-concussion disorder. In: Zasler ND, Katz DI, Zafonte RZ, eds. Brain Injury Medicine: Principles and Practice. New York: Demos Medical; 2006.

77. Ivins BJ, Kane R, Schwab KA. Performance on the automated neuropsychological assessment metrics in a nonclinical sample of soldiers screened for mild TIB after returning from Iraq and Afghanistan: a descriptive analysis. J Head Trauma Rehabil 2009;24:24-31.

78. Kaminski TW, Groff RM, Glutting JJ. Examining the stability of Automated Neuropsychological Assessment Metric (ANAM) baseline test scores. J Clin Exp Neuropsychol 2009;31(6):689-697.

79. Killam C, Cautin RL, Santucci AC. Assessing the enduring residual neuropsychological effects of head trauma in college athletes who participate in contact sports. Arch Clin Neuropsychol 2005;20(5):599-611.

80. Kirkwood MW, Kirk JW. The base rate of suboptimal effort in a pediatric mild TBI sample: performance on the Medical Symptom Validity Test. Clin Neuropsychol 2010;24(5):860-872.

81. Kirkwood MW, Kirk JW, Blaha RZ, Wilson P. Non-credible effort during pediatric neuropsychological exam: a case series and literature review. Child Neuropsychol 2010;16(6):604-618.

82. Kirkwood MW, Yeates KO, Taylor HG, Randolph C, McCrea M, Anderson VA. Management of pediatric mild traumatic brain injury: a neuropsychological review from injury through recovery. Clin Neuropsychol 2008;22(5):769-800.

83. Kontos AP, Elbin RJ, Covassin T, Larson E. Exploring differences in computerized neurocognitive concussion testing between African American and White athletes. Arch Clin Neuropsychol 2010;25(8):734-744.

84. Larrabee GJ. Detection of malingering using atypical performance patterns on standard neuropsychological tests. Clin Neuropsychol 2003;17:395-401.

85. Lau BC, Collins MW, Lovell MR. Cutoff scores in neurocognitive testing and symptom clusters that predict protracted recovery from concussions in high school athletes. Neurology 2012;70(2):371-3799; discussion 379.

86. Lau BC, Collins MW, Lovell MR. Sensitivity and specificity of subacute computerized neurocognitive testing and symptom evaluation in predicting outcomes after sport-related concussion. Am J Sports Med 2011;39(6):1209-1216.

87. Lau BC, Kontos AP, Collins MW, Much A, Lovell MR. Which on-field signs/symptoms predict protracted recovery from sport-related concussion among high school football players? Am J Sports Med 2011;39(11):2311-2318.

88. Lau BC, Lovell MR, Collins MW, Pardini J. Neurocognitive and symptom predictors of recovery in high school athletes. Clin J Sport Med 2009;19(3):216-221.

89. Lippa SM, Pastorek NJ, Benge JF, Thornton GM. Postconcussive symptoms after blast and nonblast-related mild traumatic brain injuries in Afghanistan and Iraq war veterans. J Int Neuropsychol Soc 2010;16(5):856-866.

90. Lovell MR. Evaluation of the professional athlete. In: Bailes JE, Lovell MR, Maroon JC, Eds. Sports Related Concussion. St. Louis, Mo: Quality Medical Publishing Inc; 1999:200-214.

91. Lovell MR, Burke CW. Concussion in Ice Hockey. In R Cantu, Ed. Neurologic injuries of the head and spine. Oxford Press, 2000.

92. Lovell MR, Collins MW. Neuropsychological assessment of the college football player. J Head Trauma Rehabil 1998;13(2):9-26.

93. Lovell MR, Collins MW, Podell K, Powell K, Maroon JC. ImPACT: Immediate Post-Concussion Assessment and Cognitive Testing. Pittsburgh: NeuroHealth Systems; 2000.

94. Makdissi M, Darby D, Maruff P, Ugoni A, Brukner P, McCrory PR. Natural history of concussion in sport: markers of severity and implications for management. Am J Sports Med 2010;38(3):464-471.

95. Marar M, McIlvain NM, Fields SK, Comstock ED. Epidemiology of concussions among United States high school athletes in 20 sports. Am J Sports Med 2012;40(4):747-755.

96. Maroon JC, Lovell MR, Norwig J, Podell K, Powell JW, Hartl R. Cerebral concussion in athletes: evaluation and neuropsychological testing. Neurosurgery 2000;47(3):659-669.

97. Maruff P, Thomas E, Cysique L, Brew B, Collie A, Snyder P, et al. Validity of the CogState Brief Battery: relationship to standardized tests and sensitivity to cognitive impairment in mild traumatic brain injury, schizophrenia, and AIDS dementia complex. Arch Clin Neuropsychol 2009;24(2):165-178.

98. Master CL, Gioia GL, Leddy JJ, Grady MF. Importance of "return-to-learn" in pediatric and adolescent concussion. Pediatr Ann 2012;41(9):1-6.

99. McCrea M, Barr WB, Guskiewicz KM, Randolph C, Marshall SW, Cantu R, et al. Standard regression-based methods for measuring recovery after sports-related concussion. J Int Neuropsychol Soc 2005;11(1):58-69.

100. McCrea M, Hammeke T, Olsen G, Leo P, Guskiewicz KM. Unreported concussion in high school football players. Clin J Sport Med 2004;14:13-17.

101. McCrea M, Kelly JP, Randolph C. Standardized Assessment of Concussion (SAC): Manual for Administration, Scoring and Interpretation. 3rd ed. Waukesha, WI: CNS; 2000.

102. McCrory P, Johnston P, Meeuwisse W, Aubry M, Cantu R, Dvorak J, et al. Summary and agreement statement of the 2nd International Conference on Concussion in Sport, Prague 2004. Br J Sports Med 2005;43(Suppl 1):i76-i84.

103. McCrory P, Makdissi M, Davis G, Collie A. Value of neuropsychological testing after head injuries in football. Br J Sports Med 2005;39:i58-i63.

104. McCrory P, Meeuwisse W, Johnston K, Dvorak J, Aubry M, Molloy M, et al. Consensus statement on concussion in sport: the 3rd International Conference on Concussion in Sport held in Zurich, November 2008. Clin J Sport Med 2009;19(3):185-193.

105. McGrath N. Supporting the student-athlete's return to the classroom after a sport-related concussion. J Athl Train 2010;45(5):492-498.

106. McNamee S, Walker W, Cifu DX, Wehman H. Minimizing the effect of TBI-related physical sequelae of vocational return. J Rehabil Res Dev 2009;46(6):893-908.

107. Meares S, Shores EA, Taylor AJ, Batchelor J, Bryant RA, Baguley IJ, et al. The prospective course of postconcussion syndrome: the role of mild traumatic brain injury. Neuropsychology 2011;25(4):454-465.

108. Meehan WP, d'Hemecourt P, Collins CL, Taylor AM, Comstock RD. Computerized neurocognitive testing for the management of sport-related concussions. Pediatrics 2012;129(1):38-44.

109. Meehan WP, d'Hemocourt P, Comstock RD. High school concussions in the 2008-2009 academic year: mechanisms, symptoms and management. Am J Sports Med 2010;38(12):2405-2409.

110. Meehan WP, Mannix R. Pediatric concussion in United States emergency departments in the years 2002-2006. J Pediatr 2010;157(6):889-893.

111. Moritz S, Ferahli S, Naber D. Memory and attention performance in psychiatric patients: lack of correspondence between clinician-rated and patient-rated functioning with neuropsychological test results. J Int Neuropsychol Soc 2004;10:623-633.

112. Moser RS, Iverson GL, Echemendia RJ, Lovell MR, Schatz P, Webbe FM, et al. Neuropsychological evaluation in the diagnosis and management of sports-related concussion. Arch Clin Neuropsychol 2007;22(8):909-916.

113. Moser RS, Schatz P, Neidzwski K, Ott SD. Group versus individual administration affects baseline neurocognitive test performance. Am J Sports Med 2011;39(11):2325-2330.

114. Mounce LT, Williams WH, Jones JM, Harris A, Haslam SA, Jetten J. Neurogenic and psychogenic acute post-concussion symptoms can be identified after mild traumatic brain injury. J Head Trauma Rehabil 2012; 28(5):397-405.

115. NCAA. 2011-2012 Sports Medicine Handbook. Indianapolis: National Collegiate Athletic Association; 2011.

116. Notebaert AJ, Guskiewicz KM. Current trends in athletic training practice for concussion assessment and management. J Athl Train 2005;40(4):320-325.

117. Omalu BI, DeKosky ST, Minister RL, Kamboh MI, Hamilton RL, Cyril H. Chronic traumatic encephalopathy in a National Football League Player. Neurosurgery 2005;57(1):128-134.

118. Omalu BI, Hamilton RL, Kabmoh MI, DeKosky ST, Bailes JE. Chronic traumatic encephalopathy (CTE) in a national football league player: case report and emerging medicolegal practice questions. J Forensic Nurs 2010;6(3):130-136.

119. Pellman EJ, Lovell MR, Viano DC, Casson IR. Concussion in professional football: recovery of NFL and high school athletes assessed by computerized neuropsychological testing- part 12. Neurosurgery 2006;58(2):263-274.

120. Pleacher MD, Dexter WW. Concussion management by primary care providers. Br J Sports Med 2006;40(1):1-2.

121. Ponsford J. Rehabilitation interventions after mild head injury. Curr Opin Neurol 2005;18(6):692-697.

122. Ponsford J, Cameron P, Fitzgerald M, Grant M, Mikocka-Walus A, Schonberger M. Predictors of postconcussive symptoms 3 months after mild traumatic brain injury. Neuropsychology 2012;26(3):304-313.

123. Ponsford J, Willmott C, Rothwell A, Cameron P, Kelly AM, Nelms R, et al. Impact of early intervention on outcome following mild head injury in adults. J Neurol Neurosurg Psychiatry 2002;73(3):330-332.

124. Randolph C. Baseline neuropsychological testing in managing sport-elated concussion: does it modify risk? Curr Sports Med Rep 2011;10(1):21-26.

125. Randolph C, McCrea M, Barr WB. Is neuropsychological testing useful in the management of sports-related concussion? J Athl Train 2005;40:139-152.

126. Reeves D, Thorne R, Winter S, Hegge F. Cognitive performance assessment battery (UTC-PAB). 1989; Report 89-1. San Diego, CA: Naval

Aerospace Medical Research Laboratory and Walter Reed Army Institute of Research.

127. Register-Mihalik J, Guskiewicz KM, Mann JD, Shields EW. The effects of headache on clinical measures of neurocognitive function. Clin J Sport Med 2007;17(4):282-288.

128. Register-Mihalik JK, Kontos DL, Guskiewicz KM, Mihali JP, Conder R, Shields EW. Age-related differences and reliability on computerized and paper-pencil neurocognitive assessment batteries. J Athl Train 2012;47(3):297-305.

129. Sandell NK, Lovell MR, Kegel NE, Collins MW, Kontos AP. The relationship of symptoms and neurocognitive performance to perceived recovery from sports-related concussion amongst adolescent athletes. Applied Neuropsychol Child 2013;2(1):64-9.

130. Schatz P. Long-term test-retest reliability of baseline cognitive assessments using ImPACT. Am J Sports Med 2010;38(1):47-53.

131. Schatz P, Moser RS, Covassin T, Karpf R. Early indicators of enduring symptoms in high school athletes with multiple previous concussions. Neurosurgery 2011;68(6):1562-1567.

132. Schatz P, Neidzwski K, Moser RS, Karpf R. Relationship between subjective test feedback provided by high-school athletes during computer-based assessment of baseline cognitive functioning and self-reported symptoms. Arch Clin Neuropsychol 2010;25(4):285-292.

133. Sensitivity and specificity of the ImPACT test battery for concussion in athletes. [database on the Internet]. Elsevier. 2006. Available from: http://proxy.lib.umich.edu/login?url=http://search.proquest.com.proxy.lib.umich.edu/docview/64556895?accountid=14667.

134. Schatz P, Putz BO. Cross-validation of measures used for computer-based assessment of concussion. Appl Neuropsychol 2006;13(3):151-159.

135. Schatz P, Sandel N. Sensitivity and specificity of the online version of ImPACT in high school and collegiate athletes. Am J Sports Med 2012;9.

136. Schmidt JD, Register-Mihalik JK, Mihalik JP, Kerr ZY, Guskiewic KM. Identifying impairment after concussion: normative data versus individualized baselines. Med Sci Sports Exerc 2012;44(9):1621-1628.

137. Schneider KJ, Emery CA, Kang J, Schneider GM, Meeuwisse WH. Examining sport concussion assessment tool ratings for male and female youth hockey players with and without a history of concussion. Br J Sports Med 2010;44(15):1112-1117.

138. Segalowitz SJ, Mahaney P, Santesso DL, MacGregor L, Dywan J, Willer B. Retest reliability in adolescents of a computerized neuropsychological battery used to assess recovery from concussion. NeuroRehabilitation 2007;22(3):243-251.

139. Shames J, Treger I, Ring H, Giaquinto S. Return to work following traumatic brain injury: trends and challenges. Disabil Rehabil 2007;29(17):1387-1395.

140. Shrey DW, Griesbach GS, Giza CC. The pathophysiology of concussions in youth. Phys Med Rehabil Clin N Am 2011;22(4):577-602.

141. Shuttleworth-Edwards AB. Response to the article on baseline neuropsychological testing: throwing away clinical gold with the statistical bathwater. Curr Sports Med Rep 2011;10(6):391-392.

142. Shuttleworth-Edwards AB. Computerized neuropsychological profiles of South African versus US athletes: a basis for commentary on cross-cultural norming issues in the sports concussion arena. Phys Sportsmed 2009;37(4):45-52.

143. Sim A, Terryberry-Spohr L, Wilson KR. Prolonged recovery of memory functioning after mild traumatic brain injury in adolescent athletes. J Neurosurg 2008;108(3):511-516.

144. Smith-Seemiller L, Fow NR, Kant R, Franzen MD. Presence of post-concussion symptoms in patients with chronic pain vs mild traumatic brain injury. Brain Inj 2003;17(3):199-206.

145. Solomon GS, Haase RF. Biopsychosocial characteristics and neurocognitive test performance in National Football League players: an initial assessment. Arch Clin Neuropsychol 2008;23(5):563-577.

146. Suhr JA, Gunstad K. Postconcussive symptom report: the relative influence of head injury and depression. J Clin Exp Neuropsychol 2002;24:981-993.

147. Sullivan SJ, Schneiders AG, Cheang C, Kitto E, Lee H, Redhead J, et al. What's happening? A content analysis of concussion-related traffic on Twitter. Br J Sports Med 2012;46(4):258-263.

148. Sumowski JF, Chiarvalloti N, Erlanger D, Kaushik T, Benedict R, DeLuca J. L-amphetamine improves memory in MS patients with objective memory impairment. Multiple Sclerosis J 2011;17(9):1141-1145.

149. Taylor AM. Neuropsychological evaluation and management of sport-related concussion. Curr Opin Pediatr 2012;24(6):717-723.

150. Uysal S, Massefi M, Lin H, Fischer GW, Griepp RB, Adams D, et al. Internet-based assessment of post-operative neurocognitive function in cardiac and thoracic aortic surgery patients. J Thoracic Cardiovasc Surg 2011;141(3):777-781.

151. Van Kampen DA, Lovell MR, Pardini JE, Collins MW, Fu FH. The "value added" of neurocognitive testing after sports-related concussion. Am J Sports Med 2006;34(10):1630-1635.

152. Vanderploeg RD, Curtiss G, Luis CA, Salazar AM. Long-term morbidities following self-reported mild traumatic brain injury. J Clin Exp Neuropsychol 2007;29(6):585-598.

153. Vardy J, Wong K, Yi QL, Park A, Maruff P, Wanger L, et al. Assessing cognitive function in cancer patients. Support Care Cancer 2006;14(11):1111-1118.

154. Walker WC, Marwitz JH, Kreutzer JS, Hart T, Novack TA. Occupational categories and return to work after traumatic brain injury: a multicenter study. Arch Phys Med Rehabil 2006;87(12):1576-1582.

155. Wang Y, Chan RC, Deng Y. Examination of post-concussion-like symptoms in healthy university students: relationship to subjective and objective neuropsychological function performance. Arch Clin Neuropsychol 2006;21(4):339-347.

156. Wilk JE, Thomas JL, McGurk DM, Riviere LA, Castro CA, Hoge CW. Mild traumatic brain injury (concussion) during combat: lack of association of blast mechanism with persistent postconcussive symptoms. J Head Trauma Rehabil 2010;25(1):41-52.

157. Willison J, Tombaugh T. Detecting simulation of attention deficits using reaction time tests. Arch Neuropsychol 2006;21:41-52.

158. Zuckerman SL, Lee YM, Odom MJ, Solomon GS, Forbes JA, Sills AK. Recovery from sports-related concussion: days to return to neurocognitive baseline in adolescents versus young adults. Surg Neurol Int 2012;3:130.

159. Zuckerman SL, Solomon GS, Forbes JA, Haase RF, Sills AK, Lovell MR. Response to acute concussive injury in soccer players: is gender a modifying factor? J Neurosurg Pediatr 2012; Dec;10(6):504-10.

Role of Balance Testing and Other Adjunct Measures in Concussion

Concussion presents with varying symptomatology; and as discussed thus far, given the complexity of the injury, it should be evaluated using a multifactorial approach. Given that athletes may underreport concussions, having several objective measures of assessment aids in the diagnosis and management of concussion. The evaluation of an athlete with a suspected concussion should be conducted in a systematic manner, whether on the field or in the clinical setting. As noted in previous chapters, a thorough history and examination, sideline assessment tools, imaging, and neuropsychological testing all are invaluable in concussion management, especially when administered as part of a comprehensive assessment battery.[41-43, 60, 62, 63, 73] Balance is defined as the process of maintaining the center of gravity within the body's base of support.[39] An objective balance assessment should be considered a reliable and valid addition to the workup of athletes suffering from concussion, particularly where signs or symptoms indicate a balance component.[6, 18, 19, 38, 39, 74, 78] Dr. Kevin Guskiewicz has pioneered much of the research regarding balance in the setting of concussion. Here we review the role of balance testing in concussion and also discuss some future adjunct measures of assessment.

BALANCE ASSESSMENT IN CONCUSSION

Balance assessment, whether through the use of a force plate or a clinical balance test, is useful in identifying neurological impairment in athletes following concussion.[39] In order to understand the role of balance testing in concussion, it is essential to understand the central nervous system mechanism for maintaining postural equilibrium.

Postural Equilibrium and the Central Nervous System

Maintaining equilibrium requires the central nervous system (CNS) to process and integrate afferent information from the visual, somatosensory (proprioceptive), and vestibular systems to execute appropriate and coordinated musculoskeletal responses.[39, 52] Following a concussion, athletes may have difficultly integrating information from these three components of the balance mechanism. Despite what may seem like an intact somatosensory component, integration between the visual and vestibular components may not function properly.

One of the primary purposes of the vestibular system is to maintain the eyes fixed on a stationary target in the presence of head–body movement. In order to maintain the eyes on a stationary object during movement, the semicircular canals of the vestibular labyrinth sense angular acceleration of the head and rapidly convert it to velocity information. This information is then relayed through the vestibulo-ocular reflex pathways to the ocular muscles. Linear acceleration information (including gravity) is transmitted from the utricles and saccules of the inner ear and via the vestibulospinal spinal tract to the spinal and lower extremity muscles. Balance is also maintained by the vestibular system in conjunction with additional information from visual and somatosensory inputs via central integration of vestibular, visual, and somatosensory orientation information.

The CNS mechanisms underlying balance control involve a complex network of neural connections and centers that are related by peripheral and central feedback mechanisms. The cerebral cortex, cerebellum, basal ganglia, brain stem, and spinal cord are all integrated to control voluntary movements.[39, 40, 47] Areas of the brain responsible for attention, concentration, and memory, as well as limbic structures and association cortex, are all implicated in postural equilibrium control, as well. On the whole, the cerebellum is likely the most important structure for coordinating and controlling balance. The afferent sensory arc of the postural reflex originates in the eyes, the vestibular apparatus, and the proprioceptors. The efferent pathways of the postural reflex involve the alpha motor neurons to the skeletal muscles. The overarching coordination–integration center resides in the brain stem and spinal cord.

The process of maintaining upright posture can be divided into two components. The first component involves sensory organization. The term sensory organization refers to those processes that determine timing, direction, and amplitude of corrective postural actions based on information obtained from the vestibular, visual, and somatosensory inputs.[39] It is important to point out that despite the availability of multiple sensory inputs, the CNS generally relies on only one sense at a time for orientation information.[39] In healthy adults, the preferred sense for balance control originates from somatosensory information, such as feet in contact with the ground or

playing surface.[68] Muscle coordination is the second component. It involves processes that determine the temporal sequencing and distribution of contractile activity among the muscles of the legs and trunk that generate supportive reactions for maintaining balance.[39]

Postural Equilibrium and Traumatic Brain Injury

Disruption of static and dynamic balance has been described thoroughly in patients with moderate to severe traumatic brain injury (TBI).[14, 36, 37, 53, 55, 57, 76, 97] Communication between the three essential sensory systems in balance control is lost or impaired in many of these individuals, causing moderate to severe postural instability in the anterior–posterior direction, medial–lateral direction, or both. In many of these circumstances, patients report associated visual or vestibular symptoms, dizziness, vertigo, tinnitus, lightheadedness, blurred vision, or photophobia.[14, 36, 37, 53, 55, 57, 76, 97]

In 2000, Guskiewicz and colleagues studied 1,003 high school– and collegiate sport–related concussions and found that balance problems were present 30% of the time following concussive injury.[48] Balance issues trailed only headache, dizziness, confusion, disorientation, and blurred vision in frequency of occurrence among a list of 18 symptoms. Other studies have since corroborated the not-so-uncommon presence of balance deficits following concussion.[8, 18, 21, 24, 35, 61, 74] These postural deficits may be due to both functional and microscopic ultrastructural neurophysiologic changes in the cortex and the brain stem's reticular formation.

Like many of the other concussion symptoms, balance deficits in this brain injury population are in most cases transient and should resolve quickly. Several longitudinal studies in athletes have demonstrated most balance deficits to resolve within 3 to 10 days following injury, although some patients may continue to have persistent balance deficits.[18, 19, 39, 40, 45, 46, 62, 66, 72, 75] A variety of balance assessment tools have been validated for assessing the initial deficits and tracking recovery following concussive injury. The two most commonly used postural assessments are the NeuroCom Sensory Organization Test (SOT) and the Balance Error Scoring System (BESS).

Sensory Organization Test

The Clinical Test of Sensory Interaction and Balance (CTSIB) was originally designed and used to isolate and clarify which sensory inputs are most involved with regulating posture and how the interaction among these inputs affects postural control. The technique was used to systematically remove or conflict sensory input from one or more of three senses. One of the earliest studies assessing balance deficits in concussed athletes used a modified CTSIB on a force plate to systematically remove or conflict sensory inputs.[45] The authors recorded two indices of center of pressure displacement about a fixed, central reference point to quantify impairments in postural stability in college and high school athletes with concussion.[45] They found that concussed athletes demonstrated decreased postural stability compared with their own baseline scores and those of healthy, matched controls during the initial 3 days after injury. Additionally, the degree of balance impairment in the concussed patients increased with increasing task demands, for example when the visual, vestibular, or somatosensory feedback was altered during the trial.[45]

A similar form of postural assessment, the Sensory Organization Test (SOT), has been used more recently to assess balance following concussion. The SOT within the NeuroCom Smart Balance Master uses a force plate that has the ability to measure angles and forces being generated at the ankle, knee, and hip[52] (figure 8.1). The force plate system is designed to systematically disrupt the sensory selection process by altering the orientation information available to the somatosensory or visual inputs while at the same time measuring the patient's ability to maintain a quiet stance.[39] Sway referencing is used throughout the test because the movement of the platform beneath the patient's feet and the environment surrounding the patient move in response to the anterior–posterior sway.[39, 52] The SOT uses six different conditions, with each condition performed three times to assess balance (figure 8.2). These three 20-second trials occur under three different visual conditions (eyes open, eyes closed, sway referenced) and two different surface conditions (fixed, sway referenced). Patients are asked to stand as motionless as possible for each of the 20-second trials in a normal stance with the feet shoulder-width apart. An

overall composite equilibrium score describing a person's overall level of performance during all of the trials in the SOT is calculated, with higher scores indicative of better balance performance. The composite score is the average of 14 scores.

Several studies have used the SOT to study sport-related concussions and have demonstrated sensory interaction and balance deficits that generally resolve within 3 to 5 days following concussion.[39, 46, 47, 66, 72, 75] Other studies have found that when approximate entropy techniques are applied to the SOT data, athletes' balance deficits can be shown to persist longer than 3 or 4 days.[18, 19] Collectively, studies with SOT have suggested that the sensory system most often affected following concussion is the vestibular system. Guskiewicz has noted that there are two possible mechanisms for vestibular dysfunction following cerebral concussion.[39] The first mechanism involves the peripheral receptors themselves becoming damaged and therefore providing inaccurate senses of motion. In the alternative mechanism, the brain centers responsible for central integration of vestibular, visual, and somatosensory information may be impaired. It is more likely that various combinations of peripheral and central deficits are the cause of balance deficits in athletes with concussion. Interestingly, it has been proposed that concentration and attention impairments identified on day 1 after injury could also be a factor contributing to decreased postural stability.[15, 17, 39, 47, 95]

While the SOT may be the ultimate test for postural stability, it is not portable and is very expensive. The test requires a sophisticated force plate system that provides a way to challenge and alter information sent to the various sensory systems. Thus, the test may not be very practical or accessible for the sports medicine clinician evaluating many athletes for concussion. For this reason, more clinical balance assessment tests have been used for the assessment of sport-related concussion.

Balance Error Scoring System

In an attempt to provide a more cost-effective, objective, and quantifiable method of assessing balance in athletes, the Balance Error Scoring System (BESS) was developed by researchers at the University of North Carolina at Chapel Hill.[39] The test requires minimal cost and training

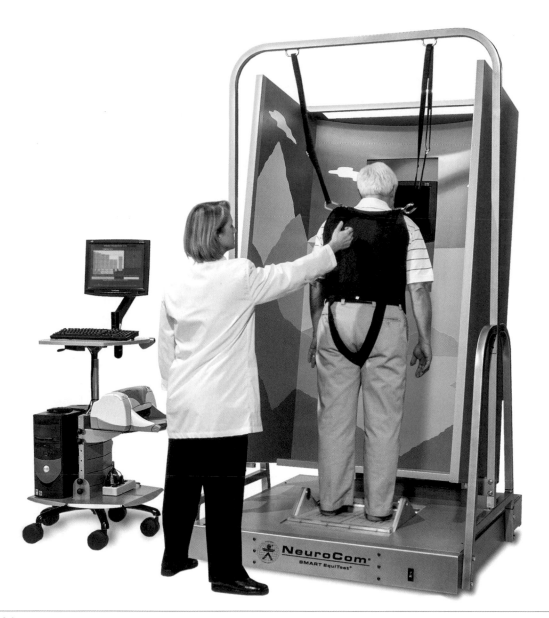

Figure 8.1 The NeuroCom Smart Balance Master has the ability to measure angles and forces and can be utilized as an effective adjunct tool to assess balance disturbance in the post-concussion setting.

Image courtesy of Natus Medical Incorporated.

for the evaluation of postural stability. The BESS can be performed on the sideline, with the use of only a stopwatch and a piece of medium-density foam. Testing involves three different stances (double, single, and tandem) completed twice, once on a firm surface and once on the medium-density foam, for a total of six trials[39] (figure 8.3). Athletes place their hands on the iliac crests, and upon eye closure, the 20-second test begins; the athlete is to remain as motionless as possible. During the single-leg stances, the athletes are asked to stand on the nondominant foot and to maintain the contralateral limb in approximately 20 to 30 degrees of hip flexion and 40 to 50 degrees of knee flexion. In the tandem stance tests, the athlete is to place the nondominant foot toward the rear. Patients are instructed that on losing their balance, they are to make any necessary adjustments and return to the testing position as quickly as possible. Performance is scored by adding 1 error point for each error committed. Trials are considered

| Normal vision | Eyes closed | Sway-referenced vision |

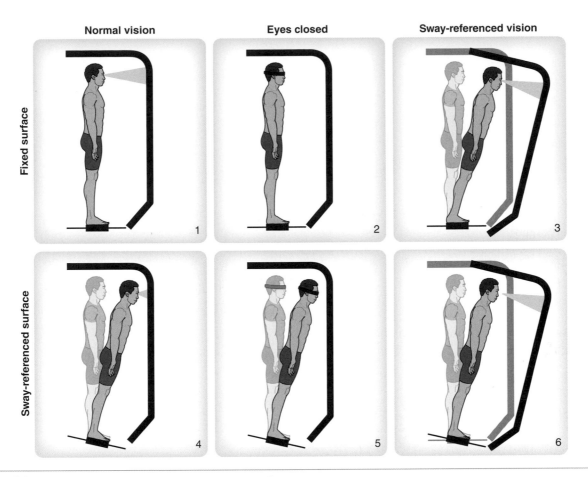

Figure 8.2 Sensory Organization Test (SOT)—six conditions.
Image courtesy of Natus Medical Incorporated.

incomplete if the athlete is unable to sustain the stance position for longer than 5 seconds during the entire 20-second testing period, and these trials are assigned a standard maximum error score of 10.

Like the SOT, the BESS has been used in several studies of sport-related concussion to identify balance deficits; the BESS is quicker and easier to administer, as well as less expensive.[12, 47, 60, 62, 75, 89] Collegiate athletes with a concussion have shown deficits in postural stability using the BESS for up to 5 days postinjury, with recovery to preinjury baseline levels usually occurring within 3 to 7 days after injury.[62] Impairment on the BESS was seen in 36% of injured subjects immediately following concussion, compared with 5% of the control group.[62] A total of 24% of injured subjects remained impaired on the BESS at 2 days after injury, compared with 9% by day 7 after injury.[60, 62] Sensitivity values for the BESS were highest at the time of injury (34%), and specific-

ity values for this assessment test ranged from 91% to 96% across postinjury days 1 to 7.[60, 62]

Some have reported that BESS performance can be influenced by a number of factors, including the type of sport played, a history of ankle injuries or ankle instability, exertion, and fatigue.[10, 25, 87, 96] Healthy athletes typically demonstrate a subtle practice effect on the BESS when it is administered over brief retest intervals, which one should consider when interpreting postinjury results during serial testing; a practice effect should be factored in if the test is being administered multiple times over a short period.[39, 92, 93]

Concussion assessment tools are recommended in combination to obtain the most complete information regarding deficits postconcussion. The BESS is sensitive to the effects of concussion with and without the use of other brief screening instruments; however, when used in combination with a graded symptom checklist and the Standardized Assessment of Concussion

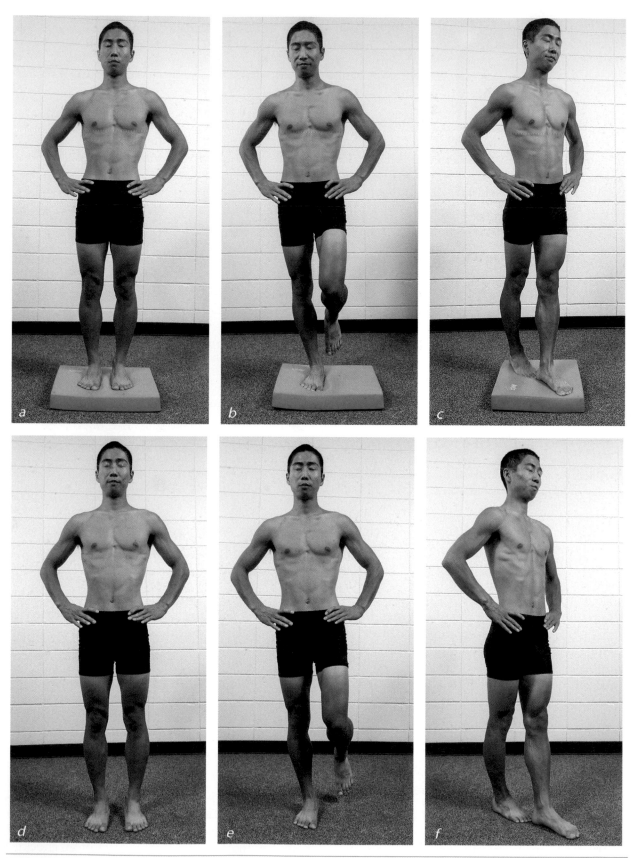

Figure 8.3 Postural stability assessments, such as the Balance Error Scoring System (BESS), are objective measures of testing balance.

(SAC), the BESS is more sensitive and specific for accurately classifying injured and noninjured athletes during the acute postinjury phase.[60, 62] Included as part of the Sport Concussion Assessment Tool (SCAT2) is a systematic balance assessment similar to that of the BESS. The only difference is that in the SCAT2, the balance test component uses the first three trials (firm conditions) of the BESS and not the foam trials. It is still generally recommended that whenever possible, the BESS be completed in its entirety (including the foam conditions) for assessing clinical balance of concussed athletes.[39] Deficits can be highly variable after a concussion. A multifaceted approach to concussion provides information regarding as many deficit areas as possible. Obtaining the most information possible enables clinicians to offer quality care and management and make good, reliable, and safe return-to-play decisions.[39, 41]

EMERGING TECHNOLOGY AND FUTURE DIRECTIONS FOR ADJUNCT MEASURES OF ASSESSMENT IN CONCUSSION

Research continues to evolve at a rapid pace, and there has been increased attention to developing adjunct diagnostic measures of assessment in concussion. In this section, we discuss some of the literature on the use of helmet accelerometers, virtual reality, visual diagnostic tools, and tests of reaction time. Additionally, although they are currently more of a research tool, we review the concept of biomarkers of injury.

Helmet Accelerometers

One of the more recent adjuncts of assessment in sport has been the use of helmet accelerometers to record head impact data. The helmets are equipped with sensors that receive impact data that are continuously and wirelessly transmitted to a sideline laptop, where medical staff can monitor them. One such technology is the Head Impact Telemetry System (HITS; Simbex LLC, Lebanon, NH), a six-accelerometer array integrated into existing football and ice hockey helmets (figure 8.4). This system is capable of measuring both linear and angular head accelerations in each plane, as well as impact location and number.[79]

Biophysics data gathered through football helmet accelerometer studies have shown that youth, high school, and college players may experience a wide range of head impacts, from 100 to over 1,000 during the course of a season. Compared to location and magnitude of forces, it may likely be that the cumulative number of head impacts best correlates with the potential for concussion occurrence or chronic effects. It is uncertain if head impacts have a threshold for magnitude or number or both, which could result in a cumulative risk for detrimental effects on brain structures or physiological function. Our understanding of the issue is further clouded by the marked variability between the thresholds for clinically diagnosed concussion in terms of linear acceleration, rotational acceleration, and location and number of impacts.[5, 9, 11, 23, 44, 49, 65, 71, 80, 81, 88] With ongoing research efforts, the HITS system and other similar devices may one day become a sideline tool capable of alerting medical staff to athletes who have sustained high-magnitude head impacts and warrant additional evaluation.

Virtual Reality and Dual Task Assessment

Virtual reality is another interesting high-tech tool that has been used recently (figure 8.5). Recent research has demonstrated that this modality can be used for balance assessment to assist the sports medicine practitioner in concussion assessment.[50, 64, 82-84] One study concluded that the mass of the head-mounted display did not adversely affect performance on balance assessment and that such displays are not contraindicated for use in virtual reality environments in concussion research.[64] This same group and other researchers have experimented with virtual environments for assessing an athlete's ability to react and respond to environmental stimuli.[64, 83] One study tested balance in concussed athletes at 3, 10, and 30 days after injury, and athletes were exposed to a virtual reality image of the room moving.[83] The authors demonstrated that standard balance testing scores recovered by day 10 in athletes; but interestingly, responses to visual field motion remained abnormal at 30 days postconcussion despite subjective symptoms and neuropsychological testing returning to baseline levels in these subjects. A follow-up study by the same group identified residual postural abnormalities in subjects recovering from mild TBI.[82] In this study, virtual time-to-contact measures were investigated; these essentially assess the dynamic properties of postural control in a three-dimensional space. The authors concluded that residual deficits of balance become more prominent when concussed individuals are exposed to more demanding conflicting visual scenes.[82]

In addition to a virtual environment, other approaches for identifying postural instability and movement dysfunction following brain injury have focused on gait and balance assessment during conditions of divided attention. This paradigm has been referred to as a dual-task assessment and may perhaps be more of a

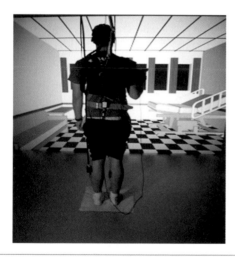

Figure 8.5 Image from the Kinesiology Virtual Reality (VR) Lab and the Traumatic Brain Injury (TBI) Lab at Pennsylvania State University. The VR labs support human subject research relating to task performance, posture, and balance, particularly in individuals who have suffered concussion or similar TBI. The labs include 3-D stereoscopic VR displays combined with data collection from motion analysis and brain imaging techniques. Subjects are instrumented with a motion tracking system, a force plate, and electroencephalogram measurement to monitor posture-related response during the performance of navigation or similar tasks.

Photo courtesy of Center for Sports Concussion Research and Service. Penn State University.

functional assessment compared to others. Some studies have used the SOT to assess balance with attention divided; a cognitive task is given either verbally or visually as the patient takes the SOT. [13, 77] These assessment methods may have utility in the sports medicine setting but must first be validated using concussed athletes.[39] These methods may even someday have utility as a means of rehabilitation for athletes recovering from postconcussion syndrome.[39]

Other studies have examined a dual-task paradigm in concussion while focusing more on gait analysis as a means to identify motor dysfunctions.[16, 69] One such study examined college athletes who had sustained concussion using neuropsychological and gait stability testing.[69] Gait was assessed as a single task, and then during completion of a simple mental task. A persistent, significant difference was noted in the dual-task gait assessment at day 28, although not in the single-task or isolated neuropsychological assessment. A similar study found that walking with a concurrent verbal cognitive task was able to distinguish between individuals with concussion and those without concussion.[16]

Visual Tracking and Saccades

One possible measure of assessment in concussion that has been considered is saccadic reaction time or latency. Latency reflects the operation of cerebral decision mechanisms and is strongly influenced by many agents that impair cortical function.[70] One study used a portable, microminiature saccadometer to record the eye movements of amateur boxers before and after competitive bouts.[70] Individual latency distributions were significantly affected after blows to the head, though the effects seemed to be reversible, with recovery over a few days. The authors concluded that the technique should perhaps be investigated more widely for its potential in monitoring the effects of sport-related concussion and head impacts.

More recently some researchers have investigated the role of visual tracking in mild TBI assessment.[58, 59] Frequent lapses in attention are not uncommon in TBI.[85, 86] Anti-saccade tasks rely on discrete stimulus–response sets and are sensitive to frontal lobe dysfunction.[67] Antisaccade tasks may be useful once subjects have perceived postconcussion symptoms; however, this paradigm may not be sensitive enough for acute concussion diagnosis.[22, 51, 58] Attention varies over time, though, and a relatively continuous measure of performance may be needed to detect moment-to-moment fluctuations in attention within individuals. This point serves as the foundation for the work of Ghajar, Maruta, and colleagues on visual tracking performance of a moving target as a supplement to conventional behavioral assessments of concussion patients[58, 59] (figure 8.6). Using video-oculography, eye movement can be monitored easily, precisely, and continuously. Visual tracking of a moving target (much like a dual-task paradigm) requires the integration of multiple sensory inputs and motor efforts. Visual tracking also requires cognitive processes including target selection, sustaining of

attention, spatiotemporal memory, and expectation.[2, 3, 20, 56, 58, 59]

Maruta and colleagues have quantified visual tracking performance in mild TBI using a circular target trajectory,[58, 59] as studies have done in other patient populations.[91, 94] The authors quantified visual tracking gaze error variability by the standard deviation of the error distribution and compared this parameter to diffusion tensor imaging (DTI) fractional anisotropy (FA) values. Large gaze error variability was associated with low mean FA values in the right anterior corona radiata, the left superior cerebellar peduncle, and the genu of the corpus callosum.[58, 59] The anterior corona radiata and superior cerebellar peduncle are tracts known to support the sustaining of attention and spatial processing; and additionally, the anterior corona radiata and genu of the corpus callosum include fibers that connect to

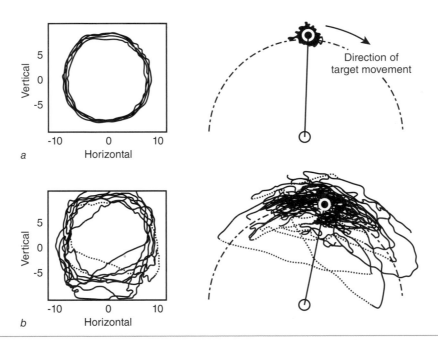

Figure 8.6   Visual tracking of a target moving in a circular trajectory of 8.5-degree radius at 0.4 Hz. (a) Example of a good performance (visual tracking) by a normal subject, characterized by overall tight clustering of the gaze positions around the target. (b) Example of a poor performance by a subject with chronic postconcussive symptoms, characterized by a wide distribution of the gaze along the circular path, which indicates spatiotemporal dyssynchrony with the stimulus. Right panel: Two-dimensional trajectory of the gaze superimposed over nine cycles. Left panel: Scattergram of gaze positions relative to the target fixed at the 12 o'clock position. The white circle indicates the average gaze position. The dot–dashed curve indicates the circular path.

Reprinted, by permission, from J. Maruta et al., 2010, "A unified science of concussion," Annals of the New York Academy of Sciences 1208(1): 58-66.

the dorsolateral prefrontal cortex. The prefrontal cortex is considered an important substrate for both attention and working memory, and these cognitive functions are often compromised in concussion patients.[58, 59] Thus the authors conclude that predictive visual tracking may be an important metric of assessment for concussion patients. Further work is needed to examine the diagnostic potential of this method and whether it may be used as a means of monitoring recovery and aiding in return-to-play decisions following concussion.

Reaction Time

Reaction time attenuation is a common consequence of concussion. Currently most reaction time assessment methods rely on computers running specialized software.[26] Some believe that this may limit the applicability of reaction time assessment on the sideline and in athletes whose teams do not have access to such computer programs. Some investigators have recently worked on developing a computer-independent clinical test of reaction time (RT[clin]) for use in sport concussion assessment and management on the sideline.[27-33] The test is modified from a simple school experiment in which a student catches a vertical ruler that is suddenly released.[26] Pilot reliability and validity data in participants from a population of healthy adult volunteers demonstrated that recognition RT(clin) is feasible to measure and appears to represent a portable, computer-independent measure of cognitive processing speed and inhibitory capacity.[32] Initial work in National Collegiate Athletic Association (NCAA) football players has been promising and has demonstrated a positive correlation with other computerized measures of reaction time. [29, 30]

In a recent study, Eckner and colleagues sought to determine the effect of concussion on RT(clin) and its sensitivity and specificity for concussion. [27] In the study, 28 concussed athletes and 28 nonconcussed control teammates completed RT(clin) assessments at baseline and within 48 hours of injury. The RT(clin) differed significantly between groups (p < 0.001) such that there was significant prolongation from baseline to postinjury in the concussed group (p = 0.003). [27] Sensitivity and specificity were maximized when any increase in RT(clin) from baseline was interpreted as abnormal, which corresponded to a sensitivity of 75%, a specificity of 68%, and a 65% reliable change confidence level.[27] The authors concluded that RT(clin) appeared to be sensitive to the effects of concussion and was able to distinguish concussed and nonconcussed athletes with sensitivity and specificity similar to those of other commonly used concussion assessment tools. Given its simplicity, low cost, and minimal time requirement, RT(clin) should be further studied as a potential adjunct measure of assessment in concussion.

Biomarkers

The National Institutes of Health defines biomarker as a characteristic that is objectively measured and evaluated as an indicator of normal biologic processes, pathogenic processes, or pharmacologic responses to a therapeutic intervention.[1, 4] In the case of a pathogenic process such as concussion, an appropriate biomarker would detect a particular aspect of the process that begins with stretch injury to axons and ends with disrupted brain function.[4] Biomarkers of concussion would be used in an attempt to detect different aspects of the injury including structural changes to cellular elements, leakage of brain-related proteins into the peripheral circulation, and subtle changes in neurological function.

Structural changes may be identified in the future with increasingly sensitive forms of imaging including susceptibility-weighted imaging (SWI), DTI, high-density fiber tracking (HDFT), and magnetic resonance spectroscopic (MRS) imaging, as discussed in the earlier chapter on neuroimaging.[4, 7] These advanced neuroimaging modalities may be able to detect white matter injury, shear injury to small blood vessels (with resultant microhemorrhages), and abnormal metabolites resulting from mitochondrial failure. Neurological function can also be assessed with advanced functional magnetic resonance imaging (fMRI) techniques. Recently some researchers have introduced a new concept for the discovery of biomarkers (termed symptophenotypes) to predict common and unique symptoms of concussion—also markers of neurological function. [54] Several studies have investigated the ability to detect leakage of brain-related proteins into the peripheral circulation and cerebrospinal fluid following TBI, including S100-B, neuron-specific enolase (NSE), and cleaved tau, to name a few. [4, 34, 54, 90] These markers and others (see list titled "Putative Biomarkers of Mild Traumatic Brain Injury") still require further research in the realm of sport-related concussion. This burgeoning area of research will hopefully produce, in the future, an adjunct measure that could aid in the diagnosis, prognosis, and management of sport-related concussion; however, currently these tools are all research based and require further elucidation.

Putative Biomarkers of Mild Traumatic Brain Injury

S100B

Neuron specific enolase (NSE)

Protein breakdown products (BDPs)

Glial fibrillary acidic protein (GFAP)

Ubiquitin carboxyl-terminal esterase L1 (UCHL-1)

Myelin basic protein (MBP)

Cleaved tau

Micro RNA (miRNA)

Metabolites

Symptophenotype

N-acetylaspartate (NAA): creatine (Cr) ratio

Genetic polymorphisms

Advanced neuroimaging (DTI, fMRI, SWI, HDFT, MRS)

Epigenetics

CONCLUDING THOUGHTS

Balance assessment is useful in identifying neurological impairment in athletes following sport-related head injuries. Testing can be accomplished through the use of a force plate or clinical balance testing (BESS). Balance testing has also been incorporated into many of the standardized sideline assessment tools. In many cases, vestibular–balance impairment lasts only transiently after injury; however, in a small number of cases vestibular deficits can linger significantly longer. In such cases, balance–vestibular training may be indicated.

Balance testing is only one part of the workup and management of concussion. Other adjunct measures of assessment are being developed or are currently being used as research tools. As the technology improves, virtual reality testing may become more commonplace and assist in making complex return-to-play decisions. Visual tracking may also aid in the diagnosis of concussion early on, particularly when patients are not terribly symptomatic. Reaction time is a quintessential part of participating in any athletic endeavor. Already incorporated into computerized neuropsychological testing paradigms, its use on the sideline or in the clinic separately from the computerized testing may prove to be a cost-effective and efficient way to diagnose and track patients with a concussion. Future research will continue to identify biomarkers for concussion. An ideal scenario would be to have a sensitive and specific serum biomarker (akin to troponin testing for heart attacks) such that a small device could be developed to test a small sample of blood on any athlete in the field to diagnose concussion, much as a glucometer device is used to measure glucose levels for diabetics. Such science and technology are far away and will require years of rigorous, well-designed research.

REFERENCES

1. Biomarkers and surrogate endpoints: preferred definitions and conceptual framework. Clin Pharmacol Ther 2001;69(3):89-95.

2. Barnes GR. Cognitive processes involved in smooth pursuit eye movements. Brain Cogn 2008;68(3):309-326.

3. Barnes GR, Collins CJ. Internally generated smooth eye movement: its dynamic characteristics and role in randomised and predictable pursuit. Prog Brain Res 2008;171:441-449.

4. Bazarian JJ. Diagnosing mild traumatic brain injury after a concussion. J Head Trauma Rehabil 2010;25(4):225-227.

5. Bazarian JJ, Zhu T, Blyth B, Borrino A, Zhong J. Subject-specific changes in brain white matter on diffusion tensor imaging after sports-related concussion. Magn Reson Imaging 2012;30(2):171-180.

6. Bell DR, Guskiewicz KM, Clark MA, Padua DA. Systematic review of the balance error scoring system. Sports Health 2011;3(3):287-295.

7. Bigler ED, Bazarian JJ. Diffusion tensor imaging: a biomarker for mild traumatic brain injury? Neurology 2010;74(8):626-627.

8. Blume HK, Lucas S, Bell KR. Subacute concussion-related symptoms in youth. Phys Med Rehabil Clin N Am 2011;22(4):665-681, viii-ix.

9. Breedlove EL, Robinson M, Talavage TM, Morigaki KE, Yoruk U, O'Keefe K, et al. Biomechanical correlates of symptomatic and asymptomatic neurophysiological impairment in high school football. J Biomech 2012;45(7):1265-1272.

10. Bressel E, Yonker JC, Kras J, Heath EM. Comparison of static and dynamic balance in female collegiate soccer, basketball, and gymnastics athletes. J Athl Train 2007;42(1):42-46.

11. Broglio SP, Eckner JT, Martini D, Sosnoff JJ, Kutcher JS, Randolph C. Cumulative head impact burden in high school football. J Neurotrauma 2011;28(10):2069-2078.

12. Broglio SP, Puetz TW. The effect of sport concussion on neurocognitive function, self-report symptoms and postural control: a meta-analysis. Sports Med 2008;38(1):53-67.

13. Broglio SP, Tomporowski PD, Ferrara MS. Balance performance with a cognitive task: a dual-task testing paradigm. Med Sci Sports Exerc 2005;37(4):689-695.

14. Campbell M, Parry A. Balance disorder and traumatic brain injury: preliminary findings of a multi-factorial observational study. Brain Inj 2005;19(13):1095-1104.

15. Catena RD, van Donkelaar P, Chou LS. Altered balance control following concussion is better detected with an attention test during gait. Gait Posture 2007;25(3):406-411.

16. Catena RD, van Donkelaar P, Chou LS. Different gait tasks distinguish immediate vs. long-term effects of concussion on balance control. J Neuroeng Rehabil 2009;6:25.

17. Catena RD, van Donkelaar P, Chou LS. The effects of attention capacity on dynamic balance control following concussion. J Neuroeng Rehabil 2011;8:8.

18. Cavanaugh JT, Guskiewicz KM, Giuliani C, Marshall S, Mercer V, Stergiou N. Detecting altered postural control after cerebral concussion in athletes with normal postural stability. Br J Sports Med 2005;39(11):805-811.

19. Cavanaugh JT, Guskiewicz KM, Stergiou N. A nonlinear dynamic approach for evaluating postural control: new directions for the management of sport-related cerebral concussion. Sports Med 2005;35(11):935-950.

20. Chen Y, Holzman PS, Nakayama K. Visual and cognitive control of attention in smooth pursuit. Prog Brain Res 2002;140:255-265.

21. Covassin T, Elbin RJ, Harris W, Parker T, Kontos A. The role of age and sex in symptoms, neurocognitive performance, and postural stability in athletes after concussion. Am J Sports Med 2012;40(6):1303-1312.

22. Crevits L, Hanse MC, Tummers P, Van Maele G. Antisaccades and remembered saccades in mild traumatic brain injury. J Neurol 2000;247(3):179-182.

23. Crisco JJ, Fiore R, Beckwith JG, Chu JJ, Brolinson PG, Duma S, et al. Frequency and location of head impact exposures in individual collegiate football players. J Athl Train 2010;45(6):549-559.

24. De Beaumont L, Mongeon D, Tremblay S, Messier J, Prince F, Leclerc S, et al. Persistent motor system abnormalities in formerly concussed athletes. J Athl Train 2011;46(3):234-240.

25. Docherty CL, Valovich McLeod TC, Shultz SJ. Postural control deficits in participants with functional ankle instability as measured by the balance error scoring system. Clin J Sport Med 2006;16(3):203-208.

26. Eckner JT, Kutcher JS. Concussion symptom scales and sideline assessment tools: a critical literature update. Curr Sports Med Rep 2010;9(1):8-15.

27. Eckner JT, Kutcher JS, Broglio SP, Richardson JK. Effect of sport-related concussion on clinically measured simple reaction time. Br J Sports Med 2014; 48(2):112-118.

28. Eckner JT, Kutcher JS, Richardson JK. Between-seasons test-retest reliability of clinically measured reaction time in National Collegiate Athletic Association Division I athletes. J Athl Train 2011;46(4):409-414.

29. Eckner JT, Kutcher JS, Richardson JK. Effect of concussion on clinically measured reaction time in 9 NCAA division I collegiate athletes: a preliminary study. PM R 2011;3(3):212-218.

30. Eckner JT, Kutcher JS, Richardson JK. Pilot evaluation of a novel clinical test of reaction time in national collegiate athletic association division I football players. J Athl Train 2010;45(4):327-332.

31. Eckner JT, Lipps DB, Kim H, Richardson JK, Ashton-Miller JA. Can a clinical test of reaction time predict a functional head-protective response? Med Sci Sports Exerc 2011;43(3):382-387.

32. Eckner JT, Richardson JK, Kim H, Lipps DB, Ashton-Miller JA. A novel clinical test of recognition reaction time in healthy adults. Psychol Assess 2012;24(1):249-254.

33. Eckner JT, Whitacre RD, Kirsch NL, Richardson JK. Evaluating a clinical measure of reaction time: an observational study. Percept Mot Skills 2009;108(3):717-720.

34. Finnoff JT, Jelsing EJ, Smith J. Biomarkers, genetics, and risk factors for concussion. PM R 2011;3(10 Suppl 2):S452-459.

35. Gagnon I, Forget R, Sullivan SJ, Friedman D. Motor performance following a mild traumatic brain injury in children: an exploratory study. Brain Inj 1998;12(10):843-853.

36. Geurts AC, Ribbers GM, Knoop JA, van Limbeek J. Identification of static and dynamic postural instability following traumatic brain injury. Arch Phys Med Rehabil 1996;77(7):639-644.

37. Greenwald BD, Cifu DX, Marwitz JH, Enders LJ, Brown AW, Englander JS, et al. Factors associated with balance deficits on admission

to rehabilitation after traumatic brain injury: a multicenter analysis. J Head Trauma Rehabil 2001;16(3):238-252.

38. Guskiewicz KM. Assessment of postural stability following sport-related concussion. Curr Sports Med Rep 2003;2(1):24-30.

39. Guskiewicz KM. Balance assessment in the management of sport-related concussion. Clin Sports Med 2011;30(1):89-102, ix.

40. Guskiewicz KM. Postural stability assessment following concussion: one piece of the puzzle. Clin J Sport Med 2001;11(3):182-189.

41. Guskiewicz KM, Broglio SP. Sport-related concussion: on-field and sideline assessment. Phys Med Rehabil Clin North Am 2011;22(4):603-617, vii.

42. Guskiewicz KM, Bruce SL, Cantu RC, Ferrara MS, Kelly JP, McCrea M, et al. Recommendations on management of sport-related concussion: summary of the National Athletic Trainers' Association position statement. Neurosurgery 2004;55(4):891-895; discussion 896.

43. Guskiewicz KM, Bruce SL, Cantu RC, Ferrara MS, Kelly JP, McCrea M, et al. National Athletic Trainers' Association position statement: management of sport-related concussion. J Athl Train 2004;39(3):280-297.

44. Guskiewicz KM, Mihalik JP, Shankar V, Marshall SW, Crowell DH, Oliaro SM, et al. Measurement of head impacts in collegiate football players: relationship between head impact biomechanics and acute clinical outcome after concussion. Neurosurgery 2007;61(6):1244-1252; discussion 1252-1243.

45. Guskiewicz KM, Perrin DH, Gansneder BM. Effect of mild head injury on postural stability in athletes. J Athl Train 1996;31(4):300-306.

46. Guskiewicz KM, Riemann BL, Perrin DH, Nashner LM. Alternative approaches to the assessment of mild head injury in athletes. Med Sci Sports Exerc 1997;29(7 Suppl):S213-221.

47. Guskiewicz KM, Ross SE, Marshall SW. Postural stability and neuropsychological deficits after concussion in collegiate athletes. J Athl Train 2001;36(3):263-273.

48. Guskiewicz KM, Weaver NL, Padua DA, Garrett WE Jr. Epidemiology of concussion in collegiate and high school football players. Am J Sports Med 2000;28(5):643-650.

49. Gysland SM, Mihalik JP, Register-Mihalik JK, Trulock SC, Shields EW, Guskiewicz KM. The relationship between subconcussive impacts and concussion history on clinical measures of neurologic function in collegiate football players. Ann Biomed Eng 2012;40(1):14-22.

50. Haibach PS, Slobounov SM, Slobounova ES, Newell KM. Virtual time-to-contact of postural stability boundaries as a function of support surface compliance. Exp Brain Res 2007;177(4):471-482.

51. Heitger MH, Jones RD, Macleod AD, Snell DL, Frampton CM, Anderson TJ. Impaired eye movements in post-concussion syndrome indicate suboptimal brain function beyond the influence of depression, malingering or intellectual ability. Brain 2009;132(Pt 10):2850-2870.

52. Hunt T, Asplund C. Concussion assessment and management. Clin Sports Med 2010;29(1):5-17; table of contents.

53. Ingersoll CD, Armstrong CW. The effects of closed-head injury on postural sway. Med Sci Sports Exerc 1992;24(7):739-743.

54. Jeter CB, Hergenroeder GW, Hylin MJ, Redell JB, Moore AN, Dash PK. Biomarkers for the diagnosis and prognosis of mild traumatic brain injury/concussion. J Neurotrauma 2013; 30(8):657-670.

55. Kaufman KR, Brey RH, Chou LS, Rabatin A, Brown AW, Basford JR. Comparison of subjective and objective measurements of balance disorders following traumatic brain injury. Med Eng Physics 2006;28(3):234-239.

56. Krauzlis RJ. The control of voluntary eye movements: new perspectives. Neuroscientist 2005;11(2):124-137.

57. Mallinson AI, Longridge NS. Dizziness from whiplash and head injury: differences between whiplash and head injury. Am J Otol 1998;19(6):814-818.

58. Maruta J, Lee SW, Jacobs EF, Ghajar J. A unified science of concussion. Ann N Y Acad Sci 2010;1208:58-66.

59. Maruta J, Suh M, Niogi SN, Mukherjee P, Ghajar J. Visual tracking synchronization as a metric for concussion screening. J Head Trauma Rehabil 2010;25(4):293-305.

60. McCrea M, Barr WB, Guskiewicz K, Randolph C, Marshall SW, Cantu R, et al. Standard regression-based methods for measuring recovery after sport-related concussion. J Int Neuropsychol Soc 2005;11(1):58-69.

61. McCrea M, Guskiewicz K, Randolph C, Barr WB, Hammeke TA, Marshall SW, et al. Incidence, clinical course, and predictors of prolonged recovery time following sport-related concussion in high school and college athletes. J Int Neuropsychol Soc 2013;19(1):22-33.

62. McCrea M, Guskiewicz KM, Marshall SW, Barr W, Randolph C, Cantu RC, et al. Acute effects and recovery time following concussion in collegiate football players: the NCAA Concussion Study. JAMA 2003;290(19):2556-2563.

63. McCrory P, Meeuwisse W, Johnston K, Dvorak J, Aubry M, Molloy M, et al. Consensus statement on concussion in sport: the 3rd International Conference on Concussion in Sport held in Zurich, November 2008. Clin J Sport Med 2009;19(3):185-200.

64. Mihalik JP, Kohli L, Whitton MC. Do the physical characteristics of a virtual reality device

contraindicate its use for balance assessment? J Sport Rehabil 2008;17(1):38-49.

65. Miller JR, Adamson GJ, Pink MM, Sweet JC. Comparison of preseason, midseason, and postseason neurocognitive scores in uninjured collegiate football players. Am J Sports Med 2007;35(8):1284-1288.

66. Mrazik M, Ferrara MS, Peterson CL, Elliott RF, Courson RW, Clanton MD, et al. Injury severity and neuropsychological and balance outcomes of four college athletes. Brain Inj 2000;14(10):921-931.

67. Munoz DP, Everling S. Look away: the antisaccade task and the voluntary control of eye movement. Nat Rev Neurosci 2004;5(3):218-228.

68. Nashner LM, Black FO, Wall C III. Adaptation to altered support and visual conditions during stance: patients with vestibular deficits. J Neurosci 1982;2(5):536-544.

69. Parker TM, Osternig LR, van Donkelaar P, Chou LS. Recovery of cognitive and dynamic motor function following concussion. Br J Sports Med 2007;41(12):868-873; discussion 873.

70. Pearson BC, Armitage KR, Horner CW, Carpenter RH. Saccadometry: the possible application of latency distribution measurement for monitoring concussion. Br J Sports Med 2007;41(9):610-612.

71. Pellman EJ, Viano DC, Tucker AM, Casson IR, Waeckerle JF. Concussion in professional football: reconstruction of game impacts and injuries. Neurosurgery 2003;53:799-812.

72. Peterson CL, Ferrara MS, Mrazik M, Piland S, Elliott R. Evaluation of neuropsychological domain scores and postural stability following cerebral concussion in sports. Clin J Sport Med 2003;13(4):230-237.

73. Register-Mihalik JK, Guskiewicz KM, Mihalik JP, Schmidt JD, Kerr ZY, McCrea MA. Reliable change, sensitivity, and specificity of a multidimensional concussion assessment battery: implications for caution in clinical practice. J Head Trauma Rehabil 2012; 28(4):274-283.

74. Register-Mihalik JK, Mihalik JP, Guskiewicz KM. Balance deficits after sports-related concussion in individuals reporting posttraumatic headache. Neurosurgery 2008;63(1):76-80; discussion 80-72.

75. Riemann BL, Guskiewicz KM. Effects of mild head injury on postural stability as measured through clinical balance testing. J Athl Train 2000;35(1):19-25.

76. Rinne MB, Pasanen ME, Vartiainen MV, Lehto TM, Sarajuuri JM, Alaranta HT. Motor performance in physically well-recovered men with traumatic brain injury. J Rehabil Med 2006;38(4):224-229.

77. Ross LM, Register-Mihalik JK, Mihalik JP, McCulloch KL, Prentice WE, Shields EW, et al. Effects of a single-task versus a dual-task paradigm on cognition and balance in healthy subjects. J Sport Rehabil 2011;20(3):296-310.

78. Ross SE, Guskiewicz KM. Examination of static and dynamic postural stability in individuals with functionally stable and unstable ankles. Clin J Sport Med 2004;14(6):332-338.

79. Rowson S, Brolinson G, Goforth M, Dietter D, Duma S. Linear and angular head acceleration measurements in collegiate football. J Biomech Eng 2009;131(6):061016.

80. Rowson S, Duma SM, Beckwith JG, Chu JJ, Greenwald RM, Crisco JJ, et al. Rotational head kinematics in football impacts: an injury risk function for concussion. Ann Biomed Eng 2012;40(1):1-13.

81. Schnebel B, Gwin JT, Anderson S, Gatlin R. In vivo study of head impacts in football: a comparison of National Collegiate Athletic Association Division I versus high school impacts. Neurosurgery 2007;60(3):490-495; discussion 495-496.

82. Slobounov S, Cao C, Sebastianelli W, Slobounov E, Newell K. Residual deficits from concussion as revealed by virtual time-to-contact measures of postural stability. Clin Neurophysiol 2008;119(2):281-289.

83. Slobounov S, Slobounov E, Newell K. Application of virtual reality graphics in assessment of concussion. Cyberpsychol Behav 2006;9(2):188-191.

84. Slobounov S, Tutwiler R, Sebastianelli W, Slobounov E. Alteration of postural responses to visual field motion in mild traumatic brain injury. Neurosurgery 2006;59(1):134-139; discussion 134-139.

85. Stuss DT, Stethem LL, Hugenholtz H, Picton T, Pivik J, Richard MT. Reaction time after head injury: fatigue, divided and focused attention, and consistency of performance. J Neurol Neurosurg Psychiatry 1989;52(6):742-748.

86. Stuss DT, Stethem LL, Picton TW, Leech EE, Pelchat G. Traumatic brain injury, aging and reaction time. Can J Neurolog Sci 1989;16(2):161-167.

87. Susco TM, Valovich McLeod TC, Gansneder BM, Shultz SJ. Balance recovers within 20 minutes after exertion as measured by the balance error scoring system. J Athl Train 2004;39(3):241-246.

88. Talavage TM, Nauman E, Breedlove EL, Yoruk U, Dye AE, Morigaki K, et al. Functionally-detected cognitive impairment in high school football players without clinically-diagnosed concussion. J Neurotrauma 2014; 31(4):327-338.

89. Thompson J, Sebastianelli W, Slobounov S. EEG and postural correlates of mild traumatic brain injury in athletes. Neurosci Lett 2005;377(3):158-163.

90. Topolovec-Vranic J, Pollmann-Mudryj MA, Ouchterlony D, Klein D, Spence J, Romaschin A, et al. The value of serum biomarkers in prediction models of outcome after mild traumatic brain injury. J Trauma 2011;71(5 Suppl 1):S478-486.

91. Umeda Y, Sakata E. The circular eye-tracking test. I. Simultaneous recording of the horizontal and vertical component of eye movement in the eye-tracking test. ORL 1975;37(5):290-298.

92. Valovich McLeod TC, Perrin DH, Guskiewicz KM, Shultz SJ, Diamond R, Gansneder BM. Serial administration of clinical concussion assessments and learning effects in healthy young athletes. Clin J Sport Med 2004;14(5):287-295.

93. Valovich TC, Perrin DH, Gansneder BM. Repeat administration elicits a practice effect with the balance error scoring system but not with the standardized assessment of concussion in high school athletes. J Athl Train 2003;38(1):51-56.

94. van der Steen J, Tamminga EP, Collewijn H. A comparison of oculomotor pursuit of a target in circular real, beta or sigma motion. Vision Res 1983;23(12):1655-1661.

95. van Donkelaar P, Osternig L, Chou LS. Attentional and biomechanical deficits interact after mild traumatic brain injury. Exerc Sport Sci Rev 2006;34(2):77-82.

96. Wilkins JC, Valovich McLeod TC, Perrin DH, Gansneder BM. Performance on the Balance Error Scoring System decreases after fatigue. J Athl Train 2004;39(2):156-161.

97. Wober C, Oder W, Kollegger H, Prayer L, Baumgartner C, Wober-Bingol C, et al. Posturographic measurement of body sway in survivors of severe closed head injury. Arch Phys Med Rehabil 1993;74(11):1151-1156.

Postconcussion Syndrome

Concussion and its postconcussive symptoms were first described by physicians more than a century ago; however, since that time the identification and management of concussive injury has undergone a dramatic "paradigm shift."[57] Postconcussion syndrome (PCS), the term most commonly used to refer to the collection of symptoms that occur after a concussion, remains as controversial today as it was when it was first described. Although most patients recover spontaneously from the initial injury, a significant proportion of concussion patients are at risk of developing persistent physical, cognitive, and emotional symptoms. Different schools of thought have arisen regarding the pathophysiology of this condition; some propose that the symptoms associated with PCS are a direct consequence of brain injury, while others feel that the symptoms are functional and represent the psychological or emotional sequelae of the brain injury.[7, 8, 27] While the relative contribution of these two mechanisms remains unclear, what is certain is that mild traumatic brain injury is associated with high health care costs and substantial ongoing disability and distress for patients; thus an understanding of the basis for this phenomenon is essential for the sports medicine practitioner.

WHAT'S IN A DEFINITION

A syndrome is a collection of symptoms that, when taken together, characterize an underlying condition.[57] Some have argued that the collection of symptoms identified as PCS are so nonspecific that they do not fulfill the requirements of this definition.[57, 65] There is some uncertainty about the definition of PCS, in part because it is diagnosed according to clinical criteria and the diagnosis may differ depending on the classification scheme used. The most widely recognized and cited definitions of PCS are from the **Diagnostic and Statistical Manual of Mental Diseases**, 4th edition (DSM-IV),[3] and the World Health Organization's **International Classification of Diseases**, 10th edition (ICD-10).[74] These two classification schemes differ in their language and diagnostic criteria. Postconcussion syndrome is defined by the DSM-IV as (1) cognitive deficits in attention or memory and (2) at least three or more of the following symptoms: fatigue, sleep disturbance, headache, dizziness, irritability, affective disturbance, apathy, or personality change.[3] Some feel that these criteria are conservative and that a broader definition is represented by the ICD-10.[36] The World Health Organization's ICD-10 defines PCS as three or more of the following symptoms: headache, dizziness, fatigue, irritability, insomnia, concentration difficulty, or memory difficulty.

Diagnostic Criteria for Postconcussional Disorder (DSM-IV) and Postconcussional Syndrome (ICD-10)

DSM-IV Criteria: Postconcussional Disorder

a. History of head trauma that has caused significant cerebral concussion

b. Difficulty in attention (concentrating, shifting of focus, performing simultaneous tasks) or memory (learning or recalling information) based on neuropsychological testing

c. Three or more of the following occur shortly after the trauma and last for at least 3 months:

1. Becoming fatigued easily
2. Disordered sleep
3. Headache
4. Vertigo or dizziness
5. Irritability or aggression on little or no provocation
6. Anxiety, depression, or affective ability
7. Changes in personality
8. Apathy or lack of spontaneity

d. The symptoms in criteria B and C have their onset after head trauma or else represent a substantial worsening of preexisting symptoms spontaneously.

e. The disturbance causes significant impairment in social or occupational functioning and represents a significant decline from a previous level of functioning.

f. The symptoms do not meet criteria for dementia due to head trauma and are not better accounted for by another mental disorder.

ICD-10 Clinical Criteria: Postconcussional Syndrome

The syndrome occurs after head trauma (usually sufficient to result in a loss of consciousness).

At least three of the following features should be present. Objective evidence to substantiate the symptoms is often negative.

- Headache
- Dizziness (not necessarily true vertigo)
- Fatigue
- Irritability
- Difficulty in concentrating and performing mental tasks
- Impairment of memory
- Insomnia
- Reduced tolerance to stress, emotional excitement, or alcohol. Symptoms may be accompanied by feelings of depression or anxiety resulting from loss of self-esteem or fear of permanent brain damage; such feelings enhance the original symptoms, and a vicious cycle results; some patients become hypochondriacal and may adopt a permanent sick role.

The inconsistent criteria applied to PCS result in considerable inconsistencies in diagnosis and subsequent treatment for patients with PCS. One prospective study of patients with concussion 3 months after injury reported that when the DSM-IV criteria were used, the diagnosis rate of PCS was 11%, compared with a diagnosis rate of 64% when the ICD-10 criteria for PCS were used.[10] Additionally, the study identified that neither the DSM-IV nor the ICD-10 criteria are specific in differentiating patients with PCS from those with extracranial trauma. This finding highlights another aspect of PCS that fuels considerable controversy. The symptoms of PCS are nonspecific and not unique to concussion. Similar "PCS-like" symptoms have been reported in uninjured normal control subjects and personal injury claimants.[25, 37, 57] The diagnostic criteria for major depressive disorder, anxiety disorders, acute stress disorder, posttraumatic stress disorder (PTSD), and PCS all reveal considerable overlap with one another.[64] The differential diagnosis also can include somatization, chronic fatigue and pain, cervical injury, vestibular dysfunction, visual dysfunction, or some combination of these conditions.[2, 36]

DSM-IV, Diagnostic and Statistical Manual of Mental Disorders, 4th edition; ICD-10, International Classification of Diseases, 10th edition.

Reprinted PM&R, Vol. 3(10): Suppl 2, C.C. Reddy, "Postconcussion syndrome: A physiatrist's approach," pgs. S396-405, copyright 2011, with permission of Elsevier.

SCOPE OF THE PROBLEM

Most patients who sustain a concussion have a spontaneous, sequential resolution of their symptoms within a period of 7 to 10 days.[17, 19, 23, 45, 52, 72] It is important to remember that children and adolescents require more time to recover than do collegiate or professional athletes.[5, 43, 45] Some patients have a prolonged recovery and display signs and symptoms of concussion past the usual period. The accepted time frame for recovery is not scientifically established and is influenced by factors such as age, sex, and history of prior concussions.[19, 24, 36, 42, 45] Postconcussion syndrome may be underreported in sports, although relatively few studies have followed sporting populations for significant lengths of time.[7, 27, 38, 39, 64] The percentage of patients who experience persistent symptoms has varied in the literature, although typically it ranges from 10% to 30% of patients who sustain a concussion.[30, 52, 59, 73] Some reports have estimated that approximately 10% of athletes will have persistent signs and symptoms of concussion beyond 2 weeks.[72] In non–sport-related concussion, most individuals recover completely within the first 3 months; however, it has been reported that up to 33% of patients may exhibit symptoms beyond that.[7, 9, 36, 58] Other prospective studies in non-athlete populations have widely varied, reporting a prevalence of symptoms of 6% to 80% at 3 months after injury.[22, 34, 53, 57, 63, 67] Symptoms are generally grouped into four categories[45, 49, 56]: somatic, sleep disturbance, emotional, and cognitive.

Different time points have been suggested in the literature as to when a patient can be considered to exhibit PCS. The DSM-IV criteria suggest that symptoms persisting for 3 months are required for the diagnosis, whereas the ICD-10 criteria do not identify such a time frame. For some, a diagnosis of PCS may be made when symptoms resulting from concussion last for more than 3 months after the injury.[46] Postconcussion syndrome has also been described in the literature as symptoms lasting more than 10 days.[61] A small minority of patients have symptoms lasting longer than 6 months, and this is referred to as prolonged postconcussion syndrome (PPCS).[15] Still, discrepancy exists in the literature regarding the timing of this phenomenon, as PPCS has been identified by other standards as symptoms lasting longer than 3 months.[6] The authors of this book consider the persistence of symptoms between 6 weeks and 3 months consistent with PCS and regard any symptoms lasting longer than 3 months as indicative of PPCS.[52, 62]

A NEUROANATOMICAL SUBSTRATE FOR PROLONGED SYMPTOMS

The clinical challenge with concussion patients is to determine whether prolonged symptoms reflect a version of the concussion pathophysiology versus a manifestation of a secondary process, such as premorbid clinical depression, anxiety, or migraine headaches.[35, 36] Over 20 years ago, Lishman proposed that organic factors are chiefly relevant in the earlier stages, whereas long-continued symptoms are perpetuated by "secondary neurotic developments."[39] He felt that acute PCS symptoms were firmly organic in origin at the outset, but that over the many weeks and months following concussion there was a shifting balance whereby neurobiological factors subside and psychological factors emerge to maintain PCS.[39] He did acknowledge that symptomatic and functional recovery could be hampered by psychological problems. In a more modern framework, Leddy and colleagues, as well as others, have stated that if symptoms experienced early after the injury are exacerbated with exertion but improve with rest, then the original concussion pathophysiology is likely persisting.[35, 36] Ongoing symptoms that are exacerbated by even minimal activity and no longer respond to rest may ultimately be a representation of psychological symptoms related to prolonged inactivity and frustration with inability to return to usual activities.[35, 36]

Data from advanced neuroimaging studies suggest that at least some patients with PCS have measurable pathophysiology. For example, concussed athletes with prolonged depressive symptoms showed reduced functional magnetic resonance imaging activation in the dorsolateral prefrontal cortex and striatum and attenuated deactivation in medial frontal and temporal regions accompanied by gray matter loss in these areas.[13] Some PCS patients have persistent abnormalities of brain blood flow on single-photon emission computed tomography scan (SPECT).[1] In another study, quantitative electroencephalography (EEG) and SPECT showed focal cortical dysfunction in conjunction with persistent blood–brain barrier disruption and reduced global and regional cerebral blood flow in patients with PCS for more than a month postinjury.[33] Other studies have suggested a neurometabolic[17, 36, 52, 70] and electrophysiologic[4, 16, 26] basis for impairment in PCS patients.

It is possible that mild traumatic brain injury could cause both emotional–psychological and PCS symptoms. Initial neurometabolic changes in the brain could evolve and include perturbations in endogenous neurotransmitter systems that could theoretically precipitate a depressive disorder.[64] Brain injury may possibly make people less resilient and adaptable to personal and environmental stressors, which in combination could precipitate the development of psychological symptoms; however, the underlying cause or causes of depression following injury of any severity are complex and not well elucidated.

Having said all that, the severity of a brain injury or concussion does not appear to be strongly associated with either PCS or emotional symptoms. Predictors of PCS are not known with certainty, but some clinical variables appear to increase the risk; these include a history of prior concussions,[18, 19, 54] female sex,[54, 55] younger age,[40, 54] history of cognitive dysfunction,[36] and affective disorders such as anxiety and depression.[12, 41, 42] Again, no study has identified injury severity as a factor contributing to the development of PCS.

PSYCHOGENESIS OF PCS AND PPCS

As mentioned previously, some believe that psychological factors may play into patients presenting with PCS, more so than any organic causes. There is literature to suggest that psychological distress is common after mild traumatic brain injury and is related to concurrent PCS symptoms.[47, 64, 66] Psychological factors play into the acute presentation of symptoms following a concussion in some people, particularly during the first week postinjury. It is less clear, though, whether psychological distress increases over time in patients who do not recover. Research-

ers have noted that patients who remain highly symptomatic in the chronic phase, on average, reported similar symptom severity in the acute phase.[28, 44] Group studies such as these seem to suggest that people with considerable psychological distress chronically also showed psychological distress acutely; however, the longitudinal course of symptoms at the individual level cannot be discerned from these group data.[64] There is also insufficient evidence to determine whether the relationship between psychological distress and PCS increases over time. Several prospective longitudinal studies, however, have demonstrated good evidence to suggest that early psychological distress predicts later PCS. The evidence to date regarding psychosocial factors in the development of PCS indicates that premorbid psychopathology, comorbidity of anxiety and depression, negative illness perceptions, expectation, and compensation or litigation are all potential risk factors.[11, 21, 29-32, 39, 47, 48, 50, 51, 66, 68, 69, 71]

In 1996, King reported on outcome data at 3 months postinjury.[29] Univariate correlations between the psychological measures shortly after injury and PCS symptoms at follow-up were very similar to the correlations between these two measures in the acute phase. Simply put, the relationship between psychological distress and PCS symptoms was the same concurrently and prospectively. The study demonstrated that only the anxiety subscale of the Hospital Anxiety and Depression Scale was a significant predictor, possibly due to multicollinearity between the psychological measures.[29] Interestingly, duration of posttraumatic amnesia and neuropsychological testing had negligible univariate associations with PCS symptom severity. A few years later, King and colleagues attempted to replicate these findings with a new sample of patients.[31] While a few key differences were noted in this group of patients (they were less severely injured; the follow-up time point was 6 months; and most of the neuropsychological tests were dropped from the assessment battery), acute postinjury anxiety was again a strong predictor of PCS symptoms at follow-up.[31]

Stulemeijer and colleagues conducted comprehensive assessments and attempted to define favorable outcomes at 6 months postinjury.[68] In their univariate analysis with low PCS symptoms as the outcome, high education (odds ratio [OR] = 5.4), absence of comorbid physical injury (OR =

5.5), initial low PCS symptom severity (OR = 6.3), and low levels of posttraumatic stress on Impact of Events Scale (OR = 16.1) were significant.[68] Multivariate analyses with backward stepwise regression revealed that posttraumatic stress had the strongest predictive power (OR = 10.0) of any variable.[68] With that said, when return to work was the final outcome assessed, posttraumatic stress was nonsignificant and not associated with a decreased likelihood of returning to work.

In another study, Meares and colleagues examined mild traumatic brain injury patients and trauma controls over 3 months.[48] In a multivariate analysis with acute postinjury predictors and PCS status at follow-up as the dependent variable, Acute Stress Disorder scores (OR = 1.05) and a preinjury history of psychiatric diagnosis (OR = 2.99) emerged as the significant factors-predictors.[48] Pain, neuropsychological performance, injury type, and duration of posttraumatic amnesia were not associated with PCS at follow-up.

Several studies have documented that early postconcussive symptom severity predicts PCS status at follow-up.[28, 71] One study examined the prognostic value of different early PCS symptom clusters and found that emotional symptoms (anxiety, depression, irritability, or some combination of these) within 3 to 10 days postinjury were the strongest predictors of 3-month PCS status, associated with an 8.4-fold risk.[14] In this study, anxiety was the strongest single symptom predictor, but only in women.

A MODERN CONCEPTUAL FRAMEWORK FOR PCS AND PPCS

A biopsychosocial conceptualization is a more modern and appropriate framework regarding the development and maintenance of PCS. Biological, psychological, and social factors can all contribute to PCS throughout its course, and there are likely considerable individual differences in their relative contributions.[59, 64] Neuroanatomic and psychosocial factors both provide substrate for the development of this phenomenon.[39, 60, 64, 73] The neurobiological effects of concussion appear to be, for most, time limited; and the neurocognitive and neurobehavioral consequences of structural damage improve, at least partially, over time.[40, 43, 44] The pathophysi-ology following concussion occurs on a spectrum from completely reversible to permanent micro- or ultrastructural damage or both.

It is important to appreciate that each person enters an injury event with a diverse range of individualized genetic, developmental, social, psychological, and biological resilience and vulnerability factors that contribute to both good and poor outcome.[64, 73] Studies have shown that negative cognitive responses to mild traumatic brain injury are present early in the development of PCS.[21, 47] Factors such as the role of negative illness perception have been identified. One study found that patients' early negative beliefs about their head injury were a significant independent predictor of PCS at 6 months postinjury.[21] This study was also the first to show that an all-or-nothing behavior response to the acute injury predicted the onset of PCS. This is seen in patients who overdo things when they believe symptoms are abating and then spend prolonged periods recovering when symptoms reappear. These findings are consistent with previous studies and theories[39, 71, 73] according to which patients who were at heightened risk of developing PCS tended to believe that their brain injury symptoms would last a long time and have a negative impact on their life. These patients were also more likely to associate their head injury with a number of symptoms and to feel that they had little control over these symptoms.[71]

As has been noted, when conceptualizing PCS it is important to remember that these symptoms are nonspecific. Postconcussion syndrome symptoms can arise from other conditions, singly or in combination, such as chronic headaches, chronic bodily pain, depression, or PTSD. These symptoms are also common in the general population and in people with medical problems other than head injury. The nature and extent of symptoms reported by individual patients can be readily influenced by psychological distress, preinjury personality characteristics, and social psychological factors. One example of a social psychological factor is the "good-old-days bias." This refers to the tendency for an individual to view himself as having been healthier in the past and to focus on current problems while underestimating past problems.[64] This bias, combined with an expectation of certain symptoms, can significantly affect symptom reporting. Another example is the "nocebo effect."[20] This refers to causation of sickness via the expectation of sickness and via associated emotional states. In this situation, concussion patients would have persistent postconcussive symptoms in essence because of the expectation of symptoms. In summary, maintaining a biopsychosocial appreciation and considering all contributing factors for the etiology of PCS and PPCS have important implications for early intervention, treatment, and rehabilitation. Ultimately, further research is needed that focuses on early predictors of PCS development, and future interventions may then be fashioned to curtail the development of this troubling chronic condition.

Examples of Personality Characteristics and Social Psychological Factors

• **Diagnosis threat:** Specifically, if people are told that the reason for neuropsychological testing is that they might have problems due to a past head trauma, they might perform more poorly than if given a more benign explanation for the purpose of testing.

• **Expectation as etiology:** Following an injury, people's anticipation or expectation of certain symptoms might cause them to misattribute future normal, everyday symptoms to the remote injury—or fail to appreciate the relation between more proximal factors (e.g., life stress, poor sleep, and mild depression) and their symptoms.

• **Good-old-days bias:** This refers to the tendency to view oneself as healthier in the past and to underestimate past problems. This response bias, combined with an expectation of certain symptoms following mild traumatic brain injury, can have a potent impact on symptom reporting.

• **Neuroticism:** This is a personality trait characterized by a strong tendency to experience negative emotions such as anxiety, depression, anger, and self-consciousness. Individuals with this trait have considerable difficulty coping with stress.

• **Nocebo effect:** The nocebo effect is the causation of sickness by the expectation of sickness and by associated emotional states. That is, the sickness is essentially caused by expectation of sickness.

• **Reinforced illness behavior:** Some patients with chronic pain conditions and somatoform disorders develop entrenched rein-

forced illness behaviors and evolve in such a way that they describe their symptoms and problems in a dramatic or exaggerated manner. That is, their behavior and interpersonal style change over time, through environmental factors and social reinforcement, to include verbal and nonverbal illness behaviors.

Adapted from: Silverberg ND, Iverson GL. Etiology of the post-concussion syndrome: Physiogenesis and Psychogenesis revisited. NeuroRehabilitation. 2011;29(4):317-29.

CONCLUDING THOUGHTS

A percentage of concussion patients are at risk of developing persistent physical, cognitive, and emotional symptoms. The overall clinical picture is a combination of organic pathophysiology and psychological factors. Biological, psychological, and social factors can all contribute to PCS or PPCS throughout its course, and there are likely considerable individual differences in their relative contributions from person to person. Distilling out these factors on a case-by-case basis may assist in the management of these patients, which can often be challenging.

REFERENCES

1. Agrawal D, Gowda NK, Bal CS, Pant M, Mahapatra AK. Is medial temporal injury responsible for pediatric postconcussion syndrome? A prospective controlled study with single-photon emission computerized tomography. J Neurosurg 2005;102(2 Suppl):167-171.

2. Al Sayegh A, Sandford D, Carson AJ. Psychological approaches to treatment of postconcussion syndrome: a systematic review. J Neurol Neurosurg Psychiatry 2010;81(10):1128-1134.

3. American Psychiatric Association. Diagnostic and Statistical Manual of Mental Disorders. 4th ed. Washington, DC: American Psychiatric Association; 2000.

4. Arciniegas DB, Topkoff JL. Applications of the P50 evoked response to the evaluation of cognitive impairments after traumatic brain injury. Phys Med Rehabil Clin North Am 2004;15(1):177-203, viii.

5. Belanger HG, Vanderploeg RD. The neuropsychological impact of sports-related concussion: a meta-analysis. J Int Neuropsychol Soc 2005;11(4):345-357.

6. Bigler ED. Neuropsychology and clinical neuroscience of persistent post-concussive syndrome. J Int Neuropsychol Soc 2008;14(1):1-22.

7. Binder LM. Persisting symptoms after mild head injury: a review of the postconcussive syndrome. J Clin Exp Neuropsychol 1986;8(4):323-346.

8. Binder LM, Rohling ML. Money matters: a meta-analytic review of the effects of financial incentives on recovery after closed-head injury. Am J Psychiatry 1996;153(1):7-10.

9. Binder LM, Rohling ML, Larrabee GJ. A review of mild head trauma. Part I: meta-analytic review of neuropsychological studies. J Clin Exp Neuropsychol 1997;19(3):421-431.

10. Boake C, McCauley SR, Levin HS, Pedroza C, Contant CF, Song JX, et al. Diagnostic criteria for postconcussional syndrome after mild to moderate traumatic brain injury. J Neuropsychiatry Clin Neurosci 2005;17(3):350-356.

11. Bryant RA, Harvey AG. Relationship between acute stress disorder and posttraumatic stress disorder following mild traumatic brain injury. Am J Psychiatry 1998;155(5):625-629.

12. Chamelian L, Feinstein A. The effect of major depression on subjective and objective cognitive deficits in mild to moderate traumatic brain injury. J Neuropsychiatry Clin Neurosci 2006;18(1):33-38.

13. Chen JK, Johnston KM, Petrides M, Ptito A. Neural substrates of symptoms of depression following concussion in male athletes with persisting postconcussion symptoms. Arch Gen Psychiatry 2008;65(1):81-89.

14. Dischinger PC, Ryb GE, Kufera JA, Auman KM. Early predictors of postconcussive syndrome in a population of trauma patients with mild traumatic brain injury. J Trauma 2009;66(2):289-296; discussion 296-287.

15. Evans RW. Post-traumatic headaches. Neurol Clin 2004;22(1):237-249, viii.

16. Gaetz M, Weinberg H. Electrophysiological indices of persistent post-concussion symptoms. Brain Inj 2000;14(9):815-832.

17. Giza CC, Hovda DA. The neurometabolic cascade of concussion. J Athl Train 2001;36(3):228-235.

18. Guskiewicz KM, Marshall SW, Bailes J, McCrea M, Harding HP Jr, Matthews A, et al. Recurrent concussion and risk of depression in retired professional football players. Med Sci Sports Exerc 2007;39(6):903-909.

19. Guskiewicz KM, McCrea M, Marshall SW, Cantu RC, Randolph C, Barr W, et al. Cumulative effects associated with recurrent concussion in collegiate football players: the NCAA Concussion Study. JAMA 2003;290(19):2549-2555.

20. Hahn RA. The nocebo phenomenon: concept, evidence, and implications for public health. Prev Med 1997;26(5 Pt 1):607-611.

21. Hou R, Moss-Morris R, Peveler R, Mogg K, Bradley BP, Belli A. When a minor head injury results in enduring symptoms: a prospective investigation of risk factors for postconcussional syndrome after mild traumatic brain injury. J Neurol Neurosurg Psychiatry 2012;83(2):217-223.

22. Ingebrigtsen T, Waterloo K, Marup-Jensen S, Attner E, Romner B. Quantification of postconcussion symptoms 3 months after minor head injury in 100 consecutive patients. J Neurol 1998;245(9):609-612.

23. Iverson GL, Brooks BL, Collins MW, Lovell MR. Tracking neuropsychological recovery following concussion in sport. Brain Inj 2006;20(3):245-252.

24. Iverson GL, Gaetz M, Lovell MR, Collins MW. Cumulative effects of concussion in amateur athletes. Brain Inj 2004;18(5):433-443.

25. Iverson GL, McCracken LM. "Postconcussive" symptoms in persons with chronic pain. Brain Inj 1997;11(11):783-790.

26. Jantzen KJ. Functional magnetic resonance imaging of mild traumatic brain injury. J Head Trauma Rehabil 2010;25(4):256-266.

27. Johnston KM, McCrory P, Mohtadi NG, Meeuwisse W. Evidence-based review of sport-related concussion: clinical science. Clin J Sport Med 2001;11(3):150-159.

28. Kashluba S, Paniak C, Casey JE. Persistent symptoms associated with factors identified by the WHO Task Force on Mild Traumatic Brain Injury. Clin Neuropsychol 2008;22(2):195-208.

29. King NS. Emotional, neuropsychological, and organic factors: their use in the prediction of persisting postconcussion symptoms after moderate and mild head injuries. J Neurol Neurosurg Psychiatry 1996;61(1):75-81.

30. King NS. Post-concussion syndrome: clarity amid the controversy? Br J Psychiatry 2003;183:276-278.

31. King NS, Crawford S, Wenden FJ, Caldwell FE, Wade DT. Early prediction of persisting postconcussion symptoms following mild and moderate head injuries. Br J Clin Psychol 1999;38 (Pt 1):15-25.

32. King NS, Kirwilliam S. Permanent post-concussion symptoms after mild head injury. Brain Inj 2011;25(5):462-470.

33. Korn A, Golan H, Melamed I, Pascual-Marqui R, Friedman A. Focal cortical dysfunction and blood-brain barrier disruption in patients with postconcussion syndrome. J Clin Neurophysiol Soc 2005;22(1):1-9.

34. Kraus J, Schaffer K, Ayers K, Stenehjem J, Shen H, Afifi AA. Physical complaints, medical service use, and social and employment changes following mild traumatic brain injury: a 6-month longitudinal study. J Head Trauma Rehabil 2005;20(3):239-256.

35. Kutcher JS, Eckner JT. At-risk populations in sports-related concussion. Curr Sports Med Rep 2010;9(1):16-20.

36. Leddy JJ, Sandhu H, Sodhi V, Baker JG, Willer B. Rehabilitation of concussion and post-concussion syndrome. Sports Health 2012;4(2):147-154.

37. Lees-Haley PR, Brown RS. Neuropsychological complaint base rates of 170 personal injury claimants. Arch Clin Neuropsychol 1993;8(3):203-209.

38. Levin HS, Mattis S, Ruff RM, Eisenberg HM, Marshall LF, Tabaddor K, et al. Neurobehavioral outcome following minor head injury: a three-center study. J Neurosurg 1987;66(2):234-243.

39. Lishman WA. Physiogenesis and psychogenesis in the "post-concussional syndrome." Br J Psychiatry 1988;153:460-469.

40. Lovell MR, Collins MW, Iverson GL, Field M, Maroon JC, Cantu R, et al. Recovery from mild concussion in high school athletes. J Neurosurg 2003;98(2):296-301.

41. Luis CA, Vanderploeg RD, Curtiss G. Predictors of postconcussion symptom complex in community dwelling male veterans. J Int Neuropsychol Soc 2003;9(7):1001-1015.

42. McCauley SR, Boake C, Levin HS, Contant CF, Song JX. Postconcussional disorder following mild to moderate traumatic brain injury: anxiety, depression, and social support as risk factors and comorbidities. J Clin Exp Neuropsychol 2001;23(6):792-808.

43. McCrea M, Guskiewicz KM, Marshall SW, Barr W, Randolph C, Cantu RC, et al. Acute effects and recovery time following concussion in collegiate football players: the NCAA Concussion Study. JAMA 2003;290(19):2556-2563.

44. McCrea M, Iverson GL, McAllister TW, Hammeke TA, Powell MR, Barr WB, et al. An integrated review of recovery after mild traumatic brain injury (MTBI): implications for clinical management. Clin Neuropsychol 2009;23(8):1368-1390.

45. McCrory P, Meeuwisse W, Johnston K, Dvorak J, Aubry M, Molloy M, et al. Consensus statement on concussion in sport: the 3rd International Conference on Concussion in Sport held in Zurich, November 2008. Br J Sports Med 2009;43 Suppl 1:i76-90.

46. McHugh T, Laforce R Jr, Gallagher P, Quinn S, Diggle P, Buchanan L. Natural history of the long-term cognitive, affective, and physical sequelae of mild traumatic brain injury. Brain Cogn 2006;60(2):209-211.

47. Meares S, Shores EA, Batchelor J, Baguley IJ, Chapman J, Gurka J, et al. The relationship of psychological and cognitive factors and opioids in the development of the postconcussion syndrome in general trauma patients with mild traumatic brain injury. J Int Neuropsychol Soc 2006;12(6):792-801.

48. Meares S, Shores EA, Taylor AJ, Batchelor J, Bryant RA, Baguley IJ, et al. The prospective course of postconcussion syndrome: the role of mild traumatic brain injury. Neuropsychology 2011;25(4):454-465.

49. Meehan WP III. Medical therapies for concussion. Clin Sports Med 2011;30(1):115-124, ix.

50. Moore EL, Terryberry-Spohr L, Hope DA. Mild traumatic brain injury and anxiety sequelae: a review of the literature. Brain Inj 2006;20(2):117-132.

51. Mulhern S, McMillan TM. Knowledge and expectation of postconcussion symptoms in the general population. J Psychosom Res 2006;61(4):439-445.

52. Petraglia AL, Maroon JC, Bailes JE. From the field of play to the field of combat: a review of the pharmacological management of concussion. Neurosurgery 2012;70(6):1520-1533; discussion 1533.

53. Ponsford J, Willmott C, Rothwell A, Cameron P, Kelly AM, Nelms R, et al. Impact of early intervention on outcome following mild head injury in adults. J Neurol Neurosurg Psychiatry 2002;73(3):330-332.

54. Ponsford J, Willmott C, Rothwell A, Cameron P, Kelly AM, Nelms R, et al. Factors influencing outcome following mild traumatic brain injury in adults. J Int Neuropsychol Soc 2000;6(5):568-579.

55. Preiss-Farzanegan SJ, Chapman B, Wong TM, Wu J, Bazarian JJ. The relationship between gender and postconcussion symptoms after sport-related mild traumatic brain injury. PM R 2009;1(3):245-253.

56. Reddy C. A treatment paradigm for sports concussion. Brain Injury Professional 2004;4:24-25.

57. Reddy CC. Postconcussion syndrome: a physiatrist's approach. PM R 2011;3(10 Suppl 2):S396-405.

58. Rimel RW, Giordani B, Barth JT, Boll TJ, Jane JA. Disability caused by minor head injury. Neurosurgery 1981;9(3):221-228.

59. Ruff RM. Mild traumatic brain injury and neural recovery: rethinking the debate. NeuroRehabilitation 2011;28(3):167-180.

60. Sandy Macleod AD. Post concussion syndrome: the attraction of the psychological by the organic. Med Hypotheses 2010;74(6):1033-1035.

61. Schnadower D, Vazquez H, Lee J, Dayan P, Roskind CG. Controversies in the evaluation and management of minor blunt head trauma in children. Curr Opin Pediatr 2007;19(3):258-264.

62. Sedney CL, Orphanos J, Bailes JE. When to consider retiring an athlete after sports-related concussion. Clin Sports Med 2011;30(1):189-200, xi.

63. Sigurdardottir S, Andelic N, Roe C, Jerstad T, Schanke AK. Post-concussion symptoms after traumatic brain injury at 3 and 12 months post-injury: a prospective study. Brain Inj 2009;23(6):489-497.

64. Silverberg ND, Iverson GL. Etiology of the post-concussion syndrome: physiogenesis and psychogenesis revisited. NeuroRehabilitation 2011;29(4):317-329.

65. Smith DH. Postconcussional symptoms not a syndrome. Psychosomatics 2006;47(3):271-272; author reply 272.

66. Snell DL, Siegert RJ, Hay-Smith EJ, Surgenor LJ. Associations between illness perceptions, coping styles and outcome after mild traumatic brain injury: preliminary results from a cohort study. Brain Inj 2011;25(11):1126-1138.

67. Spinos P, Sakellaropoulos G, Georgiopoulos M, Stavridi K, Apostolopoulou K, Ellul J, et al. Postconcussion syndrome after mild traumatic brain injury in Western Greece. J Trauma 2010;69(4):789-794.

68. Stulemeijer M, van der Werf S, Borm GF, Vos PE. Early prediction of favourable recovery 6 months after mild traumatic brain injury. J Neurol Neurosurg Psychiatry 2008;79(8):936-942.

69. Tsanadis J, Montoya E, Hanks RA, Millis SR, Fichtenberg NL, Axelrod BN. Brain injury severity, litigation status, and self-report of postconcussive symptoms. Clin Neuropsychol 2008;22(6):1080-1092.

70. Vagnozzi R, Signoretti S, Cristofori L, Alessandrini F, Floris R, Isgro E, et al. Assessment of metabolic brain damage and recovery following mild traumatic brain injury: a multicentre, proton magnetic resonance spectroscopic study in concussed patients. Brain 2010;133(11):3232-3242.

71. Whittaker R, Kemp S, House A. Illness perceptions and outcome in mild head injury: a longitudinal study. J Neurol Neurosurg Psychiatry 2007;78(6):644-646.

72. Willer B, Leddy JJ. Management of concussion and post-concussion syndrome. Curr Treat Options Neurol 2006;8(5):415-426.

73. Wood RL. Understanding the "miserable minority": a diasthesis-stress paradigm for post-concussional syndrome. Brain Inj 2004;18(11):1135-1153.

74. World Health Organization. International Statistical Classification of Diseases and Related Health Problems, 10th rev. 2010 ed. Geneva: World Health Organization; 2011.

Neuropathology of Chronic Traumatic Encephalopathy

In collaboration with
Bennet I. Omalu, MD, MBA, MPH • Jennifer Hammers, DO

Mike Webster is regarded as one of the greatest players in National Football League (NFL) history.[98] When he died suddenly in 2002, examination of his brain revealed neuropathological evidence of brain damage and neurodegeneration. In 2005, his case was published and reported as chronic traumatic encephalopathy (CTE), or Mike Webster's disease (MWD), in a deceased professional football player, a unique disease entity with a distinctive neuropathology,[103] causally associated with repetitive blows to the head, subconcussions, and concussions.

Chronic traumatic encephalopathy occurs as sequelae of all types of brain trauma in survivors of brain trauma, from a single episode of traumatic brain injury to repeated episodes of traumatic brain injuries in and outside sporting and military activities and in all walks of life, including in victims of repeated physical abuse and repeated karate kicks.[9, 130] The most highly publicized subtype of CTE has been dementia pugilistica (DP) in boxers, which was described as "punch drunk" in 1928 by Dr. Harrison Martland, the chief medical examiner of Essex County, Newark, New Jersey.[76] Over 70 years later, beginning in 2002, another medical examiner, Dr. Bennet Omalu,[98, 99, 101-105] an associate medical examiner in Allegheny County, Pittsburgh, Pennsylvania, performed the autopsy on Mike Webster and described CTE in other professional football players and professional wrestlers.[99, 104] Dr. Martland's and Dr. Omalu's work underscores the indispensable role the autopsy will continue to play in 21st-century medical sciences.[99, 101]

DEFINITION OF CHRONIC TRAUMATIC ENCEPHALOPATHY

Chronic traumatic encephalopathy is defined as a progressive neurodegenerative syndrome that can be caused by single, episodic, or repetitive blunt force impacts to the head and transfer of acceleration–deceleration forces to the brain. It presents clinically after a prolonged latent period as a composite syndrome of mood disorders and neuropsychiatric and cognitive impairment, with or without sensorimotor impairment. Definitive and confirmatory diagnoses of CTE remain direct tissue histochemical and immunohistochemical analyses, which reveal topographically multifocal or diffuse cortical and subcortical taupathy, in the form of neurofibrillary tangles and neuritic–neuropil threads; this is accompanied by topographical low- to high-grade subcortical white matter rarefaction, isomorphic fibrillary astrogliosis, microglial activation, and perivascular and neuropil histiocytic infiltration. Amyloidopathy may or may not be present in the form of cortical and subcortical diffuse or neuritic amyloid plaques. Other secondary proteinopathies like ubiquitinopathy and transactive response DNA binding protein 43 (TDP-43) proteinopathy may or may not be present. Chronic traumatic encephalopathy usually presents clinically after a prolonged latency period; however, some patients with CTE may not exhibit the classic prolonged latency period before clinical symptoms begin.[99]

Omalu and his colleagues[98-105] identified a constellation of progressive multidomain neurobehavioral, neuropsychiatric, and neurocognitive symptomatology, which is common to CTE sufferers, using postmortem surrogate forensic interviews and interrogations of next of kin of deceased CTE sufferers. In the early 20th century, Osnato and Giliberti[110] described a similar constellation of multidomain symptomatology in persons with CTE, which they termed postconcussion neurosis-traumatic encephalitis (table 10.1).

Omalu's Constellation of CTE Symptomatology Common to His CTE Cohort

1. Long latent period between initial exposure to repeated blows to the head and manifestation of noticeable symptoms impairing activities of daily living

2. Progressive deterioration in socioeconomic and cognitive functioning
   a. Loss of memory and memory disturbances
   b. Loss of previously acquired language and incoherence
   c. Loss of executive functioning
   d. Dismal business–investment performance
   e. Dismal money management
   f. Progressive deterioration in job performance and inability to maintain intellectually high-performance jobs
   g. Deterioration in socioeconomic status
   h. Bankruptcy

3. Paranoid ideations
   a. Social phobias

4. Exaggerated responses to life stressors
   a. Bouts of anger, worry, and agitation over minor issues of daily living

5. Rampant fluctuations in mood (highs and lows; happy and sullen)

6. Breakdown of intimate and family relationships
   a. Spousal separation and divorces

7. Insomnia

8. Hyperactivity, restlessness, high energy level, high-performance drive levels
   a. Poor attainment of set goals
   b. Dismal achievement levels in set tasks

9. Major depression
   a. Suicidal ideations and thoughts
   b. Suicide attempts, completed suicides

10. Disinhibition and manifestation of poor judgment
    a. Criminal and violent tendencies and behavior
    b. Abuse of alcohol, prescription and illicit drugs
    c. Social indiscretions, sexual indiscretions, and sexual improprieties
    d. Increasing religiosity

11. Headaches, generalized body aches and pain

Historically, physicians and researchers have referred to CTE by a variety of names and terms. The underlying commonality of all these terms is the causal association of CTE with brain trauma. Some of these terms are as follows:[1-3, 9, 16, 17, 19, 20, 22, 23, 26-31, 33-35, 38, 39, 43, 44, 50, 53, 54, 56-58, 60-62, 66-68, 70, 74-76, 78-81, 85-89, 97, 106-111, 114, 115, 119, 123, 125, 134, 136-138, 141, 142, 144-146, 150, 151, 154-162, 167-169, 171-173]

Cerebral neurasthenia

Chronic traumatic brain injury, chronic brain injury

Compensation hysteria

Concussion neurosis

DSM-IV, Diagnostic and Statistical Manual of Mental Disorders, 4th edition; ICD-10, International Classification of Diseases, 10th edition.

Table 10.1   Osnato and Giliberti's Postconcussion Neurosis Symptoms and Prevalence of Symptoms

Symptom	Percentage of cases manifesting symptom
Dizziness	51%
Giddiness	6%
Tinnitus	19%
Visual disturbances	
Dimness	0%
Blurred	16%
Double	0%
Subjective scotoma	3%
Optic atrophy	2%
Headache	69%
Pain in eyeballs	7%
Nervous fears	11%
Drowsiness	8%
Hypersensitivities, especially to noises	16%
Delirium	11%
Restlessness	22%
Depression	8%
Disturbance of sleep	
Sleeplessness at night	38%
Irritability and moodiness	23%
Emotionalism	10%
Fatigability	9%
General weakness	21%
Convulsion	1%
Palpitation	1%
Stuttering and stammering	3%
Nausea	12%
Vomiting	6%

Delayed traumatic apoplexy

Dementia pugilistica

Dementia traumatica

Encephalopathia traumatica

Litigation neurosis

Postconcussion neurosis

Postconcussion syndrome

Posttraumatic concussion state

Posttraumatic head syndrome

Posttraumatic psychoneurosis

Punch drunk, punch-drunk state[138]

Terror neurosis

Traumatic constitution

Traumatic encephalitis

Traumatic encephalopathy

Traumatic encephalopathy of boxers

Traumatic hysterias

Traumatic insanity

Traumatic neurosis

Traumatic psychosis

POSTTRAUMATIC ENCEPHALOPATHY VERSUS CHRONIC TRAUMATIC ENCEPHALOPATHY

Posttraumatic encephalopathy (PTE) and CTE are two distinct sequelae of traumatic brain injury. However, they can occur together in the same individual.[99] Posttraumatic encephalopathy is not a neurodegenerative disease and is not progressive; CTE is a neurodegenerative disease and is progressive. Posttraumatic encephalopathy is a clinicopathologic syndrome that temporally follows brain trauma and is induced by focal or diffuse (or both), gross or microscopic (or both) destruction of brain tissue caused by primary or secondary brain trauma.[99, 121] Geddes and colleagues[46] reported a case of CTE in a 23-year-old boxer in 1996 using recently emerged tissue immunohistochemical technology. Their findings were confirmed by Omalu's reports in football players in 2005 and 2006,[102, 103] further confirming the distinction between PTE and CTE. In their report, Geddes and colleagues noted that the only abnormality detected in the brain in their case was taupathy, without any of the abnormalities previously reported and pathognomonic for DP in boxers.[46] Omalu's first case (Mike Webster) exhibited similar features, but with diffuse amyloid plaques.[103] Both cases showed a topographic distribution of taupathy that was distinct from that of Alzheimer's disease (AD), relatively sparing the hippocampus.[46, 103]

In isolated CTE, without PTE, the brain shows evidence of progressive neurodegeneration with proteinopathies (primary taupathy with or without amyloidopathy, TDP-43 proteinopathy, or other secondary proteinopathies), with no evidence of structural destruction of the brain or loss or necrosis of brain tissue (figure 10.1). In isolated PTE, without CTE, the brain shows evidence of structural destruction of the brain with loss or necrosis of brain tissue and no evidence of neurodegeneration or progressive proteinopathy. There is no clear relationship between PTE brain changes or symptoms (hippocampal sclerosis, seizure type, seizure frequency, age of onset or duration of epilepsy) and CTE brain changes

(Braak staging of taupathy) and symptoms, further confirming that PTE and CTE are distinct diseases.[152]

Posttraumatic encephalopathy includes persistent sequelae of primary and secondary brain trauma including, but not limited to, contusions of the brain, lacerations of the brain, secondary ischemic–hypoxic injury of the brain following brain trauma, intracranial hemorrhages and compression of the brain, traumatic cerebral herniations, and surgical tissue excisions and lobectomies to control secondary consequences of brain trauma. Posttraumatic encephalopathy injuries typically induce necrosis of brain tissue; cavitation and loss of brain tissue; topographic death and loss of neurons as in hippocampal sclerosis; anisomorphic astrogliosis; activation of microglia; and infiltration by histiocytes with many foamy and possibly pigment-laden histiocytes, resulting in scarring of the brain.[4, 18, 24, 112, 165] Posttraumatic epilepsy is a widely recognized subtype of PTE[4, 36, 37, 63, 116, 120] that originates from a variety of pathogenetic mechanisms, including epileptogenic astroglial scars of the brain and mesial temporal lobe sclerosis.[143, 149] When posttraumatic changes similar to those of PTE occur in the spinal cord, a similar syndrome applies, which is posttraumatic myelopathy (PTM). Distribution of PTE changes in the brain or in the spinal cord are more likely to be topographically focal and lobar,[51] or focal and segmental in the spinal cord, with attendant Wallerian degeneration of nerve fibers, and are more likely to present with focal lateralizing neurological symptoms and signs.[118]

In the majority of CTE cases reported by Omalu and colleagues[99-105] and Geddes and colleagues[46] there were no PTE changes. However, CTE can occur with PTE, whereby changes of PTE are present, accompanied by the neurodegenerative proteinopathies of CTE.[99] One of Dr. Omalu's reported CTE cases[99] is a good example of the co-occurrence or comorbidity of CTE and PTE. This 50-year-old professional boxer had suffered a remote severe traumatic brain injury that included a large right acute subdural hemorrhage with cerebral hemispheric compression and cerebral herniation. At autopsy, his brain revealed CTE changes in addition to diffuse right cerebral hemispheric multicystic necrosis and xanthochromia (PTE).

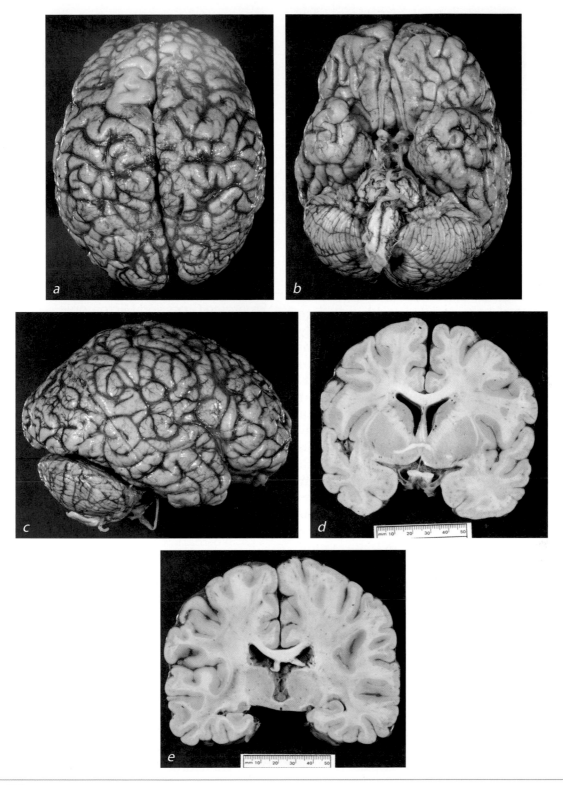

Figure 10.1 (a) Gross photograph of the brain of a deceased NFL football player who was diagnosed with CTE, showing the dorsal surfaces of the cerebral hemispheres without any significant gross pathologic changes. (b) Gross photograph of the brain of a deceased NFL football player who was diagnosed with CTE, showing the basal surfaces of the brain without any significant gross pathologic changes. (c) Gross photograph of the brain of a deceased NFL football player who was diagnosed with CTE, showing the right lateral surfaces of the brain without any significant gross pathologic changes. (d) Gross photograph of the brain of a deceased NFL football player who was diagnosed with CTE, showing a coronal section of the cerebral hemispheres at the level of the anterior commissure with no significant pathologic changes, especially the absence of cortical or subcortical atrophy that would be seen in a brain with AD. (e) Gross photograph of the brain of a deceased NFL football player who was diagnosed with CTE, showing a coronal section of the cerebral hemispheres at the level of the cornu ammonis with no significant pathologic changes, especially the absence of hippocampal atrophy that would be seen in a brain with AD.

GROSS MORPHOLOGY AND HISTOMORPHOLOGY OF CHRONIC TRAUMATIC ENCEPHALOPATHY

Chronic traumatic encephalopathy is not AD. It is not Parkinson's disease (PD). While CTE exhibits an AD-like neuropathology, it does not exhibit PD neuropathology. In younger CTE patients, that is, those less than 50 years old, CTE neuropathology is clearly distinct from that of AD. However, as the patients get older, the neuropathology of CTE progresses, with increasing simulation of AD neuropathology. In older CTE patients, that is, those older than 65 years, advanced or end-stage CTE shows a neuropathology that progressively resembles AD neuropathology and may be difficult to distinguish from AD neuropathology. In such older CTE patients, the compounding effects of AD pathology, mild cognitive impairment (MCI) pathology, and normal aging changes in the brain, not related to CTE, may not be reasonably delineated. In these older patients who may be suspected to be suffering from CTE and whose brains show AD neuropathology without any reasonable distinction from CTE, a diagnosis of AD should be made with a comment that end-stage CTE may resemble AD and cannot be ruled out. One should therefore exercise caution when diagnosing CTE in elderly patients in cases in which AD cannot be ruled out.[99]

Chronic traumatic encephalopathy and PTE can also occur in the same patient, whose brain would show both CTE and PTE pathology. In these patients, both CTE and PTE should be reported as comorbidities. Chronic traumatic encephalopathy pathology frequently co-occurs with PTE pathology in the brains of boxers, who may show evidence of tissue destruction of the brain including, but not limited to, fenestrations of the septum pellucidum, lobar contusional necrosis, topographic lobar infarcts, and chronic intracranial hemorrhages, especially subdural hemorrhages.[28, 82, 99, 125]

The following list enumerates the gross and microscopic changes that may be seen in the brains of CTE sufferers. Table 10.2 enumerates the four Omalu-Bailes histomorphologic subtypes of CTE, which were introduced by Omalu and colleagues[99] to facilitate easier identification and diagnosis of CTE. These histomorpho-

logic subtypes of CTE are based on topographic and quantitative distribution of neurofibrillary tangles (figure 10.2), neuropil threads, and amyloid plaques (figure 10.3) in the brain. Chronic traumatic encephalopathy patients who suffer also from PTE show additional PTE neuropathology superimposed on CTE neuropathology. These CTE pathologic changes will progressively resemble AD pathology as the patient ages and CTE progresses to end-stage CTE.[64, 71-73, 90, 91, 99] Similarly, more or different pathologic changes may be seen in atypical CTE cases, which may deviate slightly from the changes enumerated in table 10.2.

Emerging Gross and Microscopic Neuropathologic Features of CTE

1. Brain may appear unremarkable or within normal limits for age on conventional computerized tomography (CT) scanning and magnetic resonance imaging (MRI) without cortical atrophy or ventriculomegaly

2. No xanthochromia of the dura mater or arachnoid mater, and no epidural or subdural membranes

3. No lobar cortical cavitatory contusional necrosis

4. No marked cortical lobar or subcortical ganglionic atrophy (figure 10.1)
   a. Minimal to mild cortical atrophy of the frontal, parietal, and temporal lobes may be present
   b. No hippocampal atrophy
   c. No cerebellar folial atrophy
   d. No brain stem atrophy

5. Normal pigmentation or minimal to mild hypopigmentation of the substantia nigra, locus ceruleus, dorsal raphe nucleus, or more than one of these

6. No hydrocephalus ex vacuo

7. Negligible, minimal to mild neocortical neuronal dropout
   a. No hippocampal sclerosis

8. Possible presence of sparse to many subpial, subventricular, and neuropil corpora amylaceae

9. No to sparse multifocal perivascular infiltration of Virchow-Robin spaces by few

Table 10.2   Omalu–Bailes Histomorphology Subtypes of CTE

CTE subtype	Histologic features and criteria
0	Negative for CTE: NFTs and NTs absent in the cerebral cortex, subcortical nuclei or basal ganglia, brain stem, and cerebellum No diffuse amyloid plaques in the cerebral cortex, subcortical nuclei or basal ganglia, brain stem, or cerebellum
1	Sparse to frequent NFTs and NTs present in the cerebral cortex and brain stem, may be present in subcortical nuclei or basal ganglia No diffuse amyloid plaques in the cerebral cortex No NFTs and NTs in the cerebellum
2	Sparse to frequent NFTs and NTs present in the cerebral cortex and brain stem, may be present in subcortical nuclei or basal ganglia Sparse to frequent diffuse amyloid plaques present in the cerebral cortex No NFTs and NTs in the cerebellum
3	Moderate to frequent NFTs and NTs present in brain stem nuclei (brain stem predominant) No to sparse NFTs and NTs in cerebral cortex and subcortical nuclei or basal ganglia No NFTs and NTs in the cerebellum No diffuse amyloid plaques in the cerebral cortex
4	No to sparse (several) NFTs and NTs present in cerebral cortex, brain stem, and subcortical nuclei or basal ganglia (incipient) No NFTs and NTs in the cerebellum No diffuse amyloid plaques in the cerebral cortex
A	Moderate to frequent NFTs and NTs present in the hippocampus; diffuse amyloid plaques may or may not be present in the hippocampus
B	No to sparse NFTs and NTs in the hippocampus; diffuse amyloid plaques may or may not be present in the hippocampus
C	Sections of hippocampus unavailable for histologic analysis

NFT, neurofibrillary tangle; NT, neuropil thread.

hemosiderin-laden histiocytes and lymphocytes, without vascular wall necrosis

10. Low-grade, minimal to mild diffuse isomorphic fibrillary astrogliosis, subcortical white matter, and centrum semiovale

11. Low-grade, minimal to mild diffuse microglial activation and neuropil histiocytes, subcortical white matter, and centrum semiovale

12. Low-grade, minimal to mild rarefaction of the subcortical white matter and centrum semiovale

13. Sparse to frequent tau-immunopositive neurofibrillary tangles and neuritic–neuropil threads, neocortex, subcortical ganglia, and brain stem ganglia (figure 10.2)

    a. Neurofibrillary tangles and neuropil threads in the cerebellar cortex, medial occipital cortex, and calcarine cortex are extremely rare

    b. There may be neurofibrillary tangles in the neocortex while the hippocampus is relatively spared

    c. Neurofibrillary tangles may assume different configurations: flame shaped, band shaped, small globose, and large globose

    d. Ghost tangles may be present as well as tau-immunopositive neuritic neuropil plaques

    e. Glial tau inclusions, astrocytic plaques, and tufted and thorn astrocytes may be present and are frequently absent

    f. Neurofibrillary tangles and neuropil threads show random unpredictable differential topographic involvement

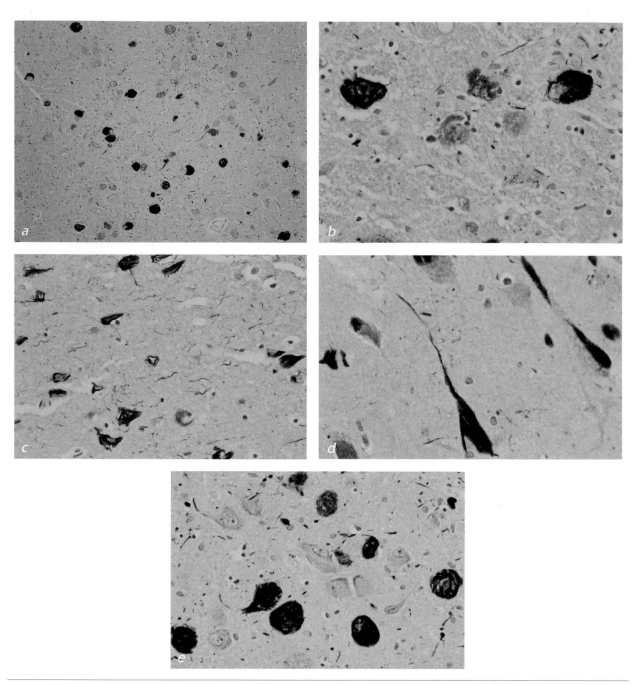

Figure 10.2 (a) Photomicrograph of a tau-immunostained section of the pons (locus ceruleus) from the brain of a deceased NFL player with CTE showing frequent neurofibrillary tangles and neuritic threads (x100 magnification). (b) Photomicrograph of tau-immunostained section of a brain stem nucleus from the brain of a deceased NFL player with CTE showing globose neurofibrillary tangles and neuropil threads, accompanied by scattered ghost tangles and dying or dead neurons (x400 magnification) (c) Photomicrograph of tau-immunostained section of the neocortex from the brain of a deceased World Wrestling Entertainment (WWE) professional wrestler with CTE showing frequent flame-shaped neurofibrillary tangles and large numbers of neuropil threads (x200 magnification). (d) Photomicrograph of tau-immunostained section of the subiculum of the hippocampus from the brain of a retired NFL player with CTE showing flame-shaped neurofibrillary tangles and neuropil threads (x600 magnification). (e) Photomicrograph of tau-immunostained section of a brain stem nucleus from the brain of a retired NFL player with CTE showing neurofibrillary tangles and neuropil threads (x600 magnification).

of the neocortex displaying a "skip phenomenon," whereby different neocortical regions show no tangles or threads whatsoever, while other adjacent neocortical regions show sparse to frequent densities of tangles and threads in the same lobe

g. There may be larger numbers and densities of tangles and threads in the depths of the sulci and around blood vessels

h. Sparse to frequent neurofibrillary tangles and neuropil threads with or without ghost tangles may be found in the subcortical ganglia and brain stem ganglia, including the corpus striatum, thalamus, subthalamus, amygdala, nucleus accumbens, basal nucleus of Meynert, dorsal raphe nucleus, substantia nigra, and locus ceruleus

i. Involved subcortical and brain stem ganglia may show neuronal dropout

j. Ubiquitin immunostains may highlight the neurofibrillary tangles and neuropil threads

14. Sparse to frequent diffuse amyloid plaques may be present in the neocortex, hippocampus, subcortical ganglia, and brain stem nuclei (figure 10.3)

    a. No to sparse neuritic amyloid plaques may be present

    b. Frequent neuritic amyloid plaques, as in AD, are more likely to be present in advanced or end-stage CTE, especially in older patients

    c. Cerebral amyloid angiopathy may or may not be present, and is frequently absent

15. There are no alpha-synuclein neuronal or glial inclusions; no Lewy bodies or Lewy neurites in the neocortex, subcortical ganglia, and brain stem nuclei

    a. The substantia nigra does not show Lewy bodies or Lewy neurites

16. Secondary ubiquitin and TDP-43 proteinopathy may be present

This classification system is a two-tier system based on the presence or absence of neurofibril-

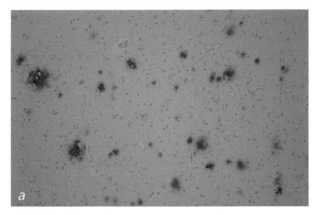

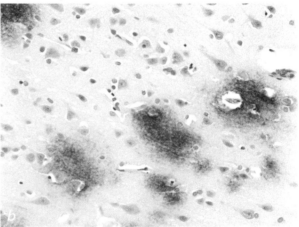

Figure 10.3 (a) Photomicrograph of betaA4 amyloid-immunostained section of the neocortex of a deceased NFL player with CTE showing diffuse amyloid plaques (x100 magnification). (b) Photomicrograph of diffuse amyloid plaques in betaA4-immunostained section of the neocortex of a deceased NFL player with CTE (x400 magnification).

lary tangles (NFTs), neutropil threads (NTs), and diffuse amyloid plaques in the cerebral cortex, subcortical nuclei or basal ganglia, hippocampus, and cerebellum, as well as the quantitative topographic distribution of NFTs and NTs in the cerebral cortex, subcortical nuclei or basal ganglia, hippocampus, and cerebellum. The first-tier classification has five subtypes represented by five Arabic numerals, 0, 1, 2, 3, and 4. The second-tier classification has three subtypes represented by the first three letters of the English alphabet, capitalized: A, B, and C. This second-tier classification applies to the presence or absence of NFTs and NTs and to the quantitative distribution of NFTs and NTs in the hippocampus. Applying this classification scheme, each CTE case should be designated as 0, 1, 2, 3, or 4 and A, B, or C, connected by a hyphen. A negative CTE case is represented as 0.

Historically, DP has been regarded as a primary parkinsonian syndrome with predominant sensorimotor impairment.[82, 125] With advancing tissue technology, it is becoming increasingly evident that CTE is not a primary parkinsonian syndrome and does not exhibit the pathognomonic neuropathology of PD.[99] Parkinson's disease is a primary alpha-synucleinopathy, with Lewy bodies and Lewy neurites destroying the substantia nigra and other brain stem nuclei. Chronic traumatic encephalopathy is not a primary alpha-synucleinopathy, but rather a primary taupathy with neurofibrillary tangles and neuropil threads destroying the substantia nigra and other brain stem nuclei (figure 10.2). If and when motor symptoms occur in CTE patients, they may be driven, in part, by a taupathy or other secondary proteinopathy,[83] and not an alpha-synucleinopathy as in PD.[6, 7, 56, 57, 170]

Historically as well, CTE has been regarded as a primary amyloidopathy.[4, 32, 46, 52, 128, 129] Still, with advancing tissue technology and immunohistochemistry, it is increasingly evident that CTE is a primary taupathy accompanied by other possible secondary proteinopathies including amyloidopathy (figure 10.3), TDP-43 proteinopathy, and ubiquinopathy.[45, 82, 99] Some researchers concluded that the presence of TDP-43 proteinopathy in CTE cases meant that motor neuron disease (primary TDP-43 proteinopathy) was part of the spectrum of CTE, or caused by repetitive traumatic brain and spinal injury.[83] This conclusion may be precipitate or premature,[10, 15] since TDP-43 proteinopathy may occur as a secondary proteinopathy in a variety of neurodegenerative diseases including AD.[11, 25, 47, 95, 164] Chronic traumatic encephalopathy changes may also be seen in the spinal medulla and anterior horn neurons as part of the long-term consequences of repetitive blunt force traumas, as well as acceleration–deceleration injuries of the head, neck, and trunk. In such instances, the involvement of the spinal medulla does not create a novel disease that is distinct from CTE. The term chronic traumatic encephalomyelopathy (CTEM) may be used for such instances. Chronic traumatic encephalomyelopathy is the same disease entity as CTE,[83, 144] with the involvement of both the brain and spinal cord.

Published reports have suggested that posttraumatic stress disorder (PTSD) in military veterans may belong to the CTE spectrum.[100] Omalu identified CTE changes in the brain of a 61-year-old deceased Vietnam war veteran who was diagnosed with PTSD. He identified similar CTE changes in the brain of a 27-year-old deceased Iraq war veteran who was diagnosed with PTSD and committed suicide by hanging.[100, 124] The emerging pathoetiology would be similar to that of sport-related repetitive acceleration–deceleration injuries of the brain, but due to combat and noncombat military activities, especially blast exposures including mortar shells, rocket-propelled grenades, and improvised explosive devices (IEDs).[49, 100, 131, 132] Goldstein and colleagues[49] have confirmed and validated Omalu's findings of CTE-related neuropathology in war veterans diagnosed with PTSD. The link between CTE and PTSD in war veterans remains to be further investigated and may result in the eventual reclassification and subclassification of PTSD in war veterans as a subtype of CTE caused by traumatic brain damage and not simply a neuropsychiatric disease without microstructural or cellular traumatic brain damage.[100] In the near future, we believe that PTSD in war veterans will be delineated from PTSD in patients who were exposed to strictly emotional and psychological traumatic experiences without any physical traumatic brain injury involving transfer of forces to the brain.[49, 100]

The clinical symptoms of CTE as a progressive disease may initially involve qualitative impairment of neuronal and axonodendritic functioning by hyperphosphorylated tau and other possible secondary proteinopathies, accompanied by neuropil inflammatory changes, myelinopathy, and astrogliosis.[99, 100] This impaired functioning may result, in part, from an impairment of the delicate homeostatic neurotransmitter milieu of the brain. As CTE advances in severity as the patient becomes older, there is an accompanying loss of axons and loss of cortical, subcortical, and brain stem neurons, progressing further to additional quantitative impairment of the delicate homeostatic neurotransmitter milieu, with progressive global deficiency of neurotransmitters in the brain. Multidomain destruction and loss of neurons in subcortical and brain stem nuclei result in quantitative deficiency of a variety of neurotransmitters and neurochemicals synthesized by these damaged nuclei.[150] For example, damage by hyperphosphorylated tau and death of neurons in the substantia nigra, locus ceruleus, dorsal raphe nucleus, and basal nucleus of Meynert eventually result in quantitative deficiencies of dopamine, noradrenaline, serotonin, and acetyl choline, respectively, further impairing the homeostatic balance of neurotransmitters in the brain.

Neurometabolic and neuromolecular cellular cascades, which are induced by and which follow a concussion injury of the brain, may include, but are not limited to, nonspecific depolarization and initiation of action potentials; release of excitatory neurotransmitters; massive efflux of potassium; increased activity of membrane ionic pumps; hyperglycolysis to generate more adenosine triphosphate (ATP); lactate accumulation; axolemmal disruption; calcium influx and sequestration in mitochondria; impaired oxidative metabolism; decreased ATP production; calpain activation; initiation of apoptosis; beta-amyloid precursor protein (βAPP) overexpression and accumulation[32, 65]; neurofilament compaction via phosphorylation or sidearm cleavage; destabilization of microtubules; and axonal swelling and eventual axotomy.[13, 48]

While the specific pathophysiological cascades linking traumatic brain injury to CTE have not been clearly elucidated, it is believed that single and repetitive traumatic brain injuries induce upregulation, accumulation, and abnormal enzymatic cellular processing of transmembrane and cytoskeletal neuroaxonal proteins including amyloid precursor protein and microtubule-associated proteins, accompanied by cytokine inflammatory and excitotoxic cellular cascades. [4, 45, 51, 52, 65, 133] Other possible pathophysiological cascades are possible seeding, aggregation, and self-perpetuating transcellular propagation (prionopathy) of abnormal pathogenic proteins like hyperphosphorylated tau protein.[55, 93, 96, 117]

Young children and adolescents may possess a higher risk of developing CTE following single and repetitive traumatic brain injury than adults. [12, 40, 41, 59, 122] This increased vulnerability to CTE in children is in part underlain by their developing and myelinating brain, which responds differently to trauma than the developed adult brain.[14, 69, 84] The CTE risk may even be higher the younger the child is.[8]

The neuropathology of CTE has evolved with improvements and advances in tissue processing and staining technology, as well as immunohistochemistry. Historically, the autopsy and postmortem examination of brains have played a pivotal role in this evolution. In 1954, Brandenburg and Hallervorden[21] were the first to report frequent "senile" plaques in the atrophic cortex of a 51-year-old deceased punch-drunk boxer who had boxed as an amateur for 11 years and become a German middleweight champion. Ten years after his retirement, at the age of 38 years, he became forgetful, excitable, and his speech became unclear. In the year before his death he developed obvious signs of a parkinsonian syndrome with dementia. He died from intracerebral hemorrhage at the age of 51 years without arteriosclerosis or hypertension. The brain showed cortical atrophy with many neurofibrillary tangles and AD-like amyloid–senile plaques,[28, 29] accompanied by amyloid vascular degeneration. The brain also showed scattered loss of Purkinje neurons and mild loss of nigral neurons, with many of the residual nigral neurons displaying neurofibrillary tangles.

In 1957, Graham and Ule[53] reported cortical cerebral atrophy with ventriculomegaly in the brain of a deceased 48-year-old retired boxer who had developed progressive parkinsonian symptoms and dementia approximately 10 years after his retirement, at the age of 25 years, following a 10-year career. He was noted to have developed by the age of 46 years what was described as dull-euphoric dementia, with poorly defined focal symptoms, extrapyramidal disturbances, and progressive external and internal hydrocephalus. He died as a result of hemorrhagic infarction of the right frontal and parietal lobes due to thrombosis of the dural sinuses and meningeal veins. Brain histology confirmed neuronal loss with neurofibrillary tangles in the neocortex, subcortical ganglia, and brain stem nuclei. There were no amyloid senile plaques in any region of the brain. Old contusions were absent.[53]

In 1956 and 1961, Strich[147, 148] reported brain degeneration and posttraumatic dementia following uncomplicated head injury in 20 patients who died from 2 days to 24 months after sustaining head injury. A majority of these patients had no fractures of the skull, no intracranial hemorrhages, and no large lacerations of the brain. Their brains showed diffuse white matter degeneration and demyelination admixed with axonal retraction bulbs, histiocytes, and activated astrocytes. The cortex showed slight generalized neuronal loss accompanied by other gross findings of focal cortical contusions and scattered remote white matter microhemorrhages. Ventriculomegaly or necrotic foci or both were present in some cases.

In 1968, Oppenheimer[109] demonstrated four diffuse microscopic neuropathologic changes following survival for more than 12 hours in the brains of 59 deceased individuals who suffered all types of brain trauma, from mild concussion to virtual decerebration. These diffuse changes comprised (1) anoxic cell injury; (2) multiple capillary hemorrhages, which were indistinguishable from gross vascular markings of cerebral parenchymal congestion; (3) microscopic disruption of nervous tissue and white matter tract degeneration by silver impregnation, which was not identified grossly; and (4) microglial reaction. Oppenheimer attributed these diffuse changes to acceleration injuries of the brain and concluded that they are seen in both trivial concussions and severe brain trauma. Oppenheimer[109] identified microglial activation beginning at about 15 hours posttrauma, which became more pronounced at 24 to 48 hours posttrauma. Axonal retraction balls accompanying clusters of activated microglia were observed at about 48 hours posttrauma, as well as microscopic foci of pallor demonstrated by myelin stains. Activated microglia and histiocytes remained pronounced even at 2 weeks following trauma, and at about 3 weeks, reactive astrocytes were seen. Pronounced microglial activation, histiocytes, and activated astrocytes remained present at 6 weeks posttrauma; and in patients who survived for months and years, microglial and astrocytic activation remained present, constituting the major residual features of the trauma at this time. These changes were also noted in five cases of clinically trivial brain injuries involving concussions.[109]

Also in 1968, Payne[113] enumerated the neuropathological findings in six deceased retired professional boxers who suffered from chronic alcoholism, manic-depressive psychosis, depression, compulsive gambling, violent behavior, emotional lability, paranoia, insomnia, marital disharmony, inability to remain employed for long durations, headaches, memory impairment, impaired concentration, confusion, intel-

lectual deterioration, dysarthria, and ataxia. The prevalent neuropathological findings in all cases included, but were not limited to, leptomeningeal thickening, slight to moderate cerebral atrophy, some enlargement of the ventricular system, fenestrations of the septum pellucidum and presence of cavum septi pellucidi, multifocal cortical scarring and gliosis with minimal to mild cortical neuronal dropout, multifocal cortical white matter and myelin degeneration, chronic inflammation with perivascular lymphocytes and pigment-laden and foamy histiocytes, and neuropil histiocytes, as well as a small number of cortical and hippocampal senile amyloid plaques in only one case and early neurofibrillary changes in only two cases.[113]

Cassasa (1924),[23] Osnato and Giliberti (1927),[110] and Martland and Beling (1927)[77] reported the findings for a total of 414 autopsied brains in individuals who died after sustaining concussions. Martland and Beling described "multiple miliary hemorrhages" or "multiple concussion hemorrhages," which were not immediately related to the traumatic focus. Over a 2-year period, Martland,[77] as chief medical examiner of Essex County, New Jersey, performed 309 autopsies on persons who had died of cerebral injuries exclusive of gunshot and penetrating force wounds of the head. In this cohort, Martland and Beling[77] reported only nine cases (2.9%) of multiple, small, discrete, punctuate, and sometimes confluent parenchymal hemorrhages of the cerebral white matter and gray matter of the basal nuclei. These hemorrhages were the only gross evidence of brain injury without cortical cerebral contusion, cortical cerebral laceration, or fracture of the skull (except in one case, which showed negligible fracture of the supraorbital plate of the frontal bone). There were no hemorrhages in the cerebellum or brain stem except in one case, which showed small hemorrhages in the rostral cervical spinal medulla. Microscopically, these "concussion hemorrhages" comprised marked vascular congestion of the penetrating parenchymal blood vessels with perivascular microextravasates. These "concussion hemorrhages" may occur in concussions of the brain without causing symptoms.[77]

Cassasa[23] reported similar "concussion hemorrhages" in his cases and noted that these hemorrhages almost never occurred when the calvarium of the skull was fractured. He reported multiple and punctate cerebral parenchymal hemorrhages in five autopsied decedents from the New York medical examiner's office who died following head trauma without any laceration of the scalp, fractures of the skull, cortical lacerations, or contusions, except occasional pial hemorrhages. He found only five of these types of cases over a 10-year period of work with the chief medical examiner of New York County and thought them to be relatively rare. The hemorrhages were perivascular and limited either to the Virchow-Robin spaces or to the perivascular neuropil.

Combined, Osnato and Giliberti[110] and Neubuerger and colleagues[94] reported their findings on a total of 102 cases of brain trauma and concussions. Neubuerger and coworkers[94] reported the following neuropathological findings in a middle-aged boxer who suffered from DP: cortical brain atrophy, ventriculomegaly, mild to moderate cortical neuronal loss with astrogliosis, cortical white matter astrogliosis accentuated around the blood vessels, cortical white matter fiber loss and demyelination, neuronal loss in the presubiculum of the hippocampus, and mild loss of the cerebellar internal granule neurons. They concluded that concussion injuries of the brain may not undergo complete resolution and can result in secondary degenerative changes and dementia.[110]

In 1973, Corsellis and coauthors[28] published characteristic patterns of brain changes observed over a period of 16 years in the brains of 15 retired boxers who suffered from symptoms of DP or punch-drunk syndrome. Their ages at death ranged from 57 to 91 years with a mean of 69 years. Based on their review and findings in the individual cases, Corsellis and colleagues[28] surmised that the following changes may be characteristic findings in brains of DP sufferers: fenestrations of the septum pellucidum; prominent or enlarged cavum septi pellucidi and cavum vergae; inferior cerebellar cortical astrogliosis and atrophy; neuronal loss and demyelination of the subcortical folial white matter, accentuated in the tonsillar regions; hypopigmentation of the substantia nigra and locus ceruleus with neuronal loss and neurofibrillary tangles in many residual neurons without Lewy bodies; and non-AD topographic pattern of neurofibrillary tangles, diffusely spread in the neocortex and brain stem, accentuated in the mesial tem-poral lobe and amygdala, temporal, frontal and insular cortex, relatively sparing the parietal and occipital lobes, and accompanied by no to sparse senile amyloid plaques. Other frequent findings were brain atrophy and loss of volume of cerebral hemispheres; atrophy of the corpus callosum; ventriculomegaly of the lateral and third ventricles; varying degrees of mild to severe topographic neuronal loss; and varying degrees of cerebral white matter pallor, demyelination, and astrogliosis. These authors[28] noted the following symptoms that were common to their cohort: alcohol abuse, rage reactions, memory impairment, memory loss, and dementia.

With the advent and evolution of immunohistochemical tissue technology in the 1980s and 1990s, many case reports, case series, and animal studies reported the neuropathology of DP with the immunohistochemical identification and confirmation of abnormal protein accumulations. In 1996, Geddes and coauthors[46] reported a unique immunophenotype of isolated taupathy in a 23-year-old professional boxer who had begun boxing at the age of 11 years. Computerized tomography scans of his brain had been normal, but he was described as somewhat forgetful. He had died days after sustaining a subdural hemorrhage from a fight. At autopsy his brain appeared grossly within normal limits except for congestive brain swelling and cerebral edema with mass effect and transtentorial and transforaminal cerebral herniation, accompanied by brain stem herniation (Duret) hemorrhages. His brain did not show brain atrophy or any other gross evidence of brain damage.[46] Histologically there was evidence of his terminal acute brain trauma, with excitotoxic neuronal injury and focal axonal injury in the splenium of the corpus callosum. No neocortical neuronal loss was detected, and no obvious cell loss of the cerebellar cortex, locus ceruleus, and substantia nigra was present. No cerebral or cerebellar cortical scarring was seen. The principal histomorphologic and immunophenotypic findings were tau-immunopositive neocortical neurofibrillary tangles and neuritic threads, which were accentuated in the inferolateral surfaces of the brain, fusiform gyrus, and inferior temporal, middle frontal, and orbital gyri, with focal collections in the supramarginal gyrus of the parietal cortex and the frontal cortex. Very rare tangles were found in the occipital cortex and cingulum. The tangles were distributed in all layers of the neocortex in a patchy fashion, and appeared to be closely associated and grouped around penetrating parenchymal blood vessels. Uniquely, there were no tangles or neuritic threads in the mesial temporal cortex, including the amygdala and hippocampal complex (dentate fascia, cornu ammonis, subiculum, transentorhinal and entorhinal cortex), other subcortical nuclei, and brain stem nuclei. Just one tangle was found in the nucleus basalis of Meynert. There was no astrogliosis associated with the tangles. Geddes and colleagues[46] revolutionized CTE with this case report, nearly completely changing the way this disease had been envisioned and characterized.

With the advent and proliferation of tissue immunohistochemistry, many other valuable animal model-, autopsy-, and tissue-based reports on CTE have been published over the years, leading us to our current neuropathologic definition and characterization of CTE.[5, 30, 32, 42, 45, 52, 65, 82, 92, 126-130, 135, 139, 140, 153, 163, 166, 174] However, the House of Lords of the United Kingdom, the Royal College of Physicians of London, and Dr. A. H. Roberts must be given credit for reaffirming in 1969 that CTE was a valid disease entity that was caused by traumatic brain injury, especially repeated concussions and subconcussions.[125, 134]

CONCLUDING THOUGHTS

Chronic traumatic encephalopathy is an emerging public health concern. The long-term risks of chronic repetitive mild traumatic brain injury are far greater than once appreciated. Chronic traumatic encephalopathy represents a devastating deterioration of neurological function and resides at the severe end of the spectrum of consequences of repetitive mild traumatic brain injury. There is a clear need for improved diagnostic and prognostic tests. In addition, we need to more clearly elucidate disease pathophysiology, imaging, and biomarker-based tests. Long-term prospective studies will allow us to learn more about the true incidence and prevalence of posttraumatic neurodegenerative disease. Animal models of disease will hopefully allow us to understand the factors that contribute to developing CTE—sex, genetics, environmental factors, and so on—and create avenues for prevention and treatment.

REFERENCES

1. Editorial: Brain damage in sport. Lancet 1976;1(7956):401-402.

2. Letter: Brain damage in sport. Lancet 1976;1(7959):585.

3. Adams FS. The genuine works of Hippocrates. Translated . . . with a preliminary discourse and annotations by F. Adams: London; 1849.

4. Adams JH, Graham DI, Jennett B. The structural basis of moderate disability after traumatic brain damage. J Neurol Neurosurg Psychiatry 2001;71(4):521-524.

5. Allsop D, Haga S, Bruton C, Ishii T, Roberts GW. Neurofibrillary tangles in some cases of dementia pugilistica share antigens with amyloid beta-protein of Alzheimer's disease. Am J Pathol 1990;136(2):255-260.

6. Amen DG, Newberg A, Thatcher R, Jin Y, Wu J, Keator D, et al. Impact of playing American professional football on long-term brain function. J Neuropsychiatry Clin Neurosci 23(1):98-106.

7. Amen DG, Wu JC, Taylor D, Willeumier K. Reversing brain damage in former NFL players: implications for traumatic brain injury and substance abuse rehabilitation. J Psychoactive Drugs 2011;43(1):1-5.

8. Anderson V, Moore C. Age at injury as a predictor of outcome following pediatric head injury: a longitudinal perspective. Child Neuropsychol 1995;1(3):187-202.

9. Aotsuka A, Kojima S, Furumoto H, Hattori T, Hirayama K. [Punch drunk syndrome due to repeated karate kicks and punches]. Rinsho Shinkeigaku 1990;30(11):1243-1246.

10. Armon C, Miller RG. Correspondence regarding: TDP-43 proteinopathy and motor neuron disease in chronic traumatic encephalopathy. J Neuropathol Exp Neurol 2010;69:918-929. J Neuropathol Exp Neurol 2011;70(1):97-98; author reply 98-100.

11. Armstrong RA, Ellis W, Hamilton RL, Mackenzie IR, Hedreen J, Gearing M, et al. Neuropathological heterogeneity in frontotemporal lobar degeneration with TDP-43 proteinopathy: a quantitative study of 94 cases using principal components analysis. J Neural Transm 2010;117(2):227-239.

12. Baillargeon A, Lassonde M, Leclerc S, Ellemberg D. Neuropsychological and neurophysiological assessment of sport concussion in children, adolescents and adults. Brain Inj 2012;26(3):211-220.

13. Barkhoudarian G, Hovda DA, Giza CC. The molecular pathophysiology of concussive brain injury. Clin Sports Med 2011;30(1):33-48, vii-viii.

14. Bauer R, Fritz H. Pathophysiology of traumatic injury in the developing brain: an introduction and short update. Exp Toxicol Pathol 2004;56(1-2):65-73.

15. Bedlack RS, Genge A, Amato AA, Shaibani A, Jackson CE, Kissel JT, et al. Correspondence regarding: TDP-43 proteinopathy and motor neuron disease in chronic traumatic encephalopathy. J Neuropathol Exp Neurol 2010;69:918-929. J Neuropathol Exp Neurol 2011;70(1):96-97; author reply 98-100.

16. Bell B. A System of Surgery. Edinburgh: C. Elliott; 1787.

17. Bennet W. Some milder forms of concussion of the brain. In: Allbutt TC, Rolleston HD, eds. A System of Medicine by Many Writers. London: Macmillan; 1910:231.

18. Bigler ED. Neuropathology of acquired cerebral trauma. J Learn Disabil 1987;20(8):458-473.

19. Boden BP, Kirkendall DT, Garrett WE Jr. Concussion incidence in elite college soccer players. Am J Sports Med 1998;26(2):238-241.

20. Boyer A. Traité des maladies chirurgicales, et des opérations qui leur conviennent. 3rd ed. Paris: Migneret; 1882.

21. Brandenburg W, Hallervorden J. [Dementia pugilistica with anatomical findings]. Virchows Arch 1954;325(6):680-709.

22. Breasted JH. The Edwin Smith Surgical Papyrus. Chicago: University of Chicago Press; 1930.

23. Cassasa CB. Multiple traumatic cerebral hemorrhages. Proc New York Path Soc 1924;24:101.

24. Cervos-Navarro J, Lafuente JV. Traumatic brain injuries: structural changes. J Neurol Sci 1991;103 Suppl:S3-14.

25. Chen-Plotkin AS, Lee VM, Trojanowski JQ. TAR DNA-binding protein 43 in neurodegenerative disease. Nat Rev Neurol 2010;6(4):211-220.

26. Collins MW, Grindel SH, Lovell MR, Dede DE, Moser DJ, Phalin BR, et al. Relationship between concussion and neuropsychological performance in college football players. JAMA 1999;282(10):964-970.

27. Cooper AP. Lectures on the Principles and Practice of Surgery, with additional notes and cases by Frederick Tyrrel. Philadelphia: Haswell, Barrington & Haswell; 1839.

28. Corsellis JA, Bruton CJ, Freeman-Browne D. The aftermath of boxing. Psychol Med 1973;3(3):270-303.

29. Critchley M. Medical aspects of boxing, particularly from a neurological standpoint. Br Med J 1957;1(5015):357-362.

30. Critchley M. Punch drunk syndromes: the chronic traumatic encephalopathy of boxers. Hommage à Clovis Vincent. Paris: Maloine; 1949:131.

31. Daneshvar DH, Riley DO, Nowinski CJ, McKee AC, Stern RA, Cantu RC. Long-term consequences: effects on normal development profile after concussion. Phys Med Rehabil Clin N Am 2011;22(4):683-700, ix.

32. DeKosky ST, Abrahamson EE, Ciallella JR, Paljug WR, Wisniewski SR, Clark RS, et al. Association of increased cortical soluble abeta42 levels with diffuse plaques after severe brain injury in humans. Arch Neurol 2007;64(4):541-544.

33. Denny-Brown D, Russell WR. Experimental cerebral concussion. Brain 1941;64:93-164.

34. Denny-Brown D, Russell WR. Experimental cerebral concussion. J Physiol 1940;99(1):153.

35. Denny-Brown DE, Russell WR. Experimental concussion: (Section of Neurology). Proc R Soc Med 1941;34(11):691-692.

36. Diaz-Arrastia R, Agostini MA, Madden CJ, Van Ness PC. Posttraumatic epilepsy: the endophenotypes of a human model of epileptogenesis. Epilepsia 2009;50 Suppl 2:14-20.

37. Dichter MA. Posttraumatic epilepsy: the challenge of translating discoveries in the laboratory to pathways to a cure. Epilepsia 2009;50 Suppl 2:41-45.

38. Dupuytren G. Leçons orales de clinique chirurgicale faites â l'Hôtel-dieu de Paris. 2nd ed. Paris: Germer-Baillière; 1839.

39. Erichsen JE. On Concussion of the Spine, Nervous Shock and Other Obscure Injuries to the Nervous System. New ed. Baltimore: William Wood; 1886.

40. Field M, Collins MW, Lovell MR, Maroon J. Does age play a role in recovery from sports-related concussion? A comparison of high school and collegiate athletes. J Pediatr 2003;142(5):546-553.

41. Franklin CC, Weiss JM. Stopping sports injuries in kids: an overview of the last year in publications. Curr Opin Pediatr 2012;24(1):64-67.

42. Gabbita SP, Scheff SW, Menard RM, Roberts K, Fugaccia I, Zemlan FP. Cleaved-tau: a biomarker of neuronal damage after traumatic brain injury. J Neurotrauma 2005;22(1):83-94.

43. Gavett BE, Cantu RC, Shenton M, Lin AP, Nowinski CJ, McKee AC, et al. Clinical appraisal of chronic traumatic encephalopathy: current perspectives and future directions. Curr Opin Neurol 2011;24(6):525-531.

44. Gavett BE, Stern RA, McKee AC. Chronic traumatic encephalopathy: a potential late effect of sport-related concussive and subconcussive head trauma. Clin Sports Med 2011;30(1):179-188, xi.

45. Geddes JF, Vowles GH, Nicoll JA, Revesz T. Neuronal cytoskeletal changes are an early consequence of repetitive head injury. Acta Neuropathol 1999;98(2):171-178.

46. Geddes JF, Vowles GH, Robinson SF, Sutcliffe JC. Neurofibrillary tangles, but not Alzheimer-type pathology, in a young boxer. Neuropathol Appl Neurobiol 1996;22(1):12-16.

47. Geser F, Lee VM, Trojanowski JQ. Amyotrophic lateral sclerosis and frontotemporal lobar degeneration: a spectrum of TDP-43 proteinopathies. Neuropathology 2010;30(2):103-112.

48. Giza CC, Hovda DA. The neurometabolic cascade of concussion. J Athl Train 2001;36(3):228-235.

49. Goldstein LE, Fisher AM, Tagge CA, Zhang XL, Velisek L, Sullivan JA, et al. Chronic traumatic encephalopathy in blast-exposed military veterans and a blast neurotrauma mouse model. Sci Transl Med 2012;4(134):134ra160.

50. Gonzales TA. Fatal injuries in competitive sports. JAMA 1951;146(16):1506-1511.

51. Graham DI, Adams JH, Nicoll JA, Maxwell WL, Gennarelli TA. The nature, distribution and causes of traumatic brain injury. Brain Pathol 1995;5(4):397-406.

52. Graham DI, Gentleman SM, Lynch A, Roberts GW. Distribution of beta-amyloid protein in the brain following severe head injury. Neuropathol Appl Neurobiol 1995;21(1):27-34.

53. Graham H, Ule G. Beitrag zur kenntnis der chronischen cerebralen krankheitsbilder bei boxern. Psychiatria et Neurologia 1957;134:261-283.

54. Gronwall D, Wrightson P. Cumulative effect of concussion. Lancet 1975;2(7943):995-997.

55. Guo JL, Lee VM. Seeding of normal Tau by pathological Tau conformers drives pathogenesis of Alzheimer-like tangles. J Biol Chem 2011;286(17):15317-15331.

56. Guskiewicz KM, Marshall SW, Bailes J, McCrea M, Cantu RC, Randolph C, et al. Association between recurrent concussion and late-life cognitive impairment in retired professional football players. Neurosurgery 2005;57(4):719-726; discussion 719-726.

57. Guskiewicz KM, Marshall SW, Bailes J, McCrea M, Harding HP Jr, Matthews A, et al. Recurrent concussion and risk of depression in retired professional football players. Med Sci Sports Exerc 2007;39(6):903-909.

58. Haase E. Bemerkenswerte pathologisch-anatomische befunde nach gehirnerschütterung. Zentralbl f d ges Neurol u Psychiatrie 1929-1930;54:637.

59. Halstead ME, Walter KD. American Academy of Pediatrics. Clinical report—sport-related concussion in children and adolescents. Pediatrics 2010;126(3):597-615.

60. Harvey PK, Davis JN. Traumatic encephalopathy in a young boxer. Lancet 1974;2(7886):928-929.

61. Honey CR. Brain injury in ice hockey. Clin J Sport Med 1998;8(1):43-46.

62. Horn P. Ueber Symptomatologie und Prognose der cerebralen Kommotionsneurosen unter vergleichender Berücksichtigung der Kopfkontusionen der Schädeldach-und Basisbrüche. Ztschr f d ges Neurol u Psychiatrie 1916;34:206.

63. Hunt RF, Scheff SW, Smith BN. Posttraumatic epilepsy after controlled cortical impact injury in mice. Exp Neurol 2009;215(2):243-252.

64. Hyman BT, Phelps CH, Beach TG, Bigio EH, Cairns NJ, Carrillo MC, et al. National Institute on Aging-Alzheimer's Association guidelines for the neuropathologic assessment of Alzheimer's disease. Alzheimers Dement 2012;8(1):1-13.

65. Ikonomovic MD, Uryu K, Abrahamson EE, Ciallella JR, Trojanowski JQ, Lee VM, et al. Alzheimer's pathology in human temporal cortex surgically excised after severe brain injury. Exp Neurol 2004;190(1):192-203.

66. Jordan BD. Medical Aspects of Boxing. Boca Raton, FL: CRC Press; 1993.

67. Jordan BD, Bailes JE. Concussion history and current neurological symptoms among retired professional football players. Neurology 2000;54(Suppl 3):A410-A411.

68. Kaplan HA, Browder J. Observations on the clinical and brain wave patterns of professional boxers. JAMA 1954;156(12):1138-1144.

69. Karlin AM. Concussion in the pediatric and adolescent population: "different population, different concerns." PM R 2011;3(10 Suppl 2):S369-379.

70. Kelly JP, Rosenberg JH. The development of guidelines for the management of concussion in sports. J Head Trauma Rehabil 1998;13(2):53-65.

71. Khachaturian ZS. Diagnosis of Alzheimer's disease. Arch Neurol 1985;42(11):1097-1105.

72. Khachaturian ZS. Diagnosis of Alzheimer's disease: two decades of progress. Alzheimers Dement 2005;1(2):93-98.

73. Khachaturian ZS. Diagnosis of Alzheimer's disease: two decades of progress. J Alzheimers Dis 2006;9(3 Suppl):409-415.

74. Kutner KC, Erlanger DM, Tsai J, Jordan B, Relkin NR. Lower cognitive performance of older football players possessing apolipoprotein E epsilon4. Neurosurgery 2000;47(3):651-657; discussion 657-658.

75. Littré A. Diverses observations anatomiques. Hist Acad Sci 1705:54-55.

76. Martland HS. Punch drunk. JAMA 1928;91(15):1103-1107.

77. Martland HS, Beling CC. Traumatic cerebral hemorrhage. Arch Neurol Psychiatry 1929;22(5):1001-1023.

78. Matser EJ, Kessels AG, Lezak MD, Jordan BD, Troost J. Neuropsychological impairment in amateur soccer players. JAMA 1999;282(10):971-973.

79. Matser JT, Kessels AG, Jordan BD, Lezak MD, Troost J. Chronic traumatic brain injury in professional soccer players. Neurology 1998;51(3):791-796.

80. McCown IA. Boxing injuries. Am J Surg 1959;98:509-516.

81. McCown IA. Protecting the boxer. JAMA 1959;169(13):1409-1413.

82. McKee AC, Cantu RC, Nowinski CJ, Hedley-Whyte ET, Gavett BE, Budson AE, et al. Chronic traumatic encephalopathy in athletes: progressive tauopathy after repetitive head injury. J Neuropathol Exp Neurol 2009;68(7):709-735.

83. McKee AC, Gavett BE, Stern RA, Nowinski CJ, Cantu RC, Kowall NW, et al. TDP-43 proteinopathy and motor neuron disease in chronic traumatic encephalopathy. J Neuropathol Exp Neurol 2010;69(9):918-929.

84. Meehan WP III, Taylor AM, Proctor M. The pediatric athlete: younger athletes with sport-related concussion. Clin Sports Med 2011;30(1):133-144, x.

85. Meyer A. The anatomical facts and clinical varieties of traumatic insanity, 1904. J Neuropsychiatry Clin Neurosci 2000;12(3):407-410.

86. Meyer A. The anatomical facts and clinical varieties of traumatic insanity. Am J Insan 1904;6:374, 377, 382, 388.

87. Miles A. On the mechanism of brain injuries: preliminary considerations, various theories of concussion. Brain 1892;15(2):153-189.

88. Miller GG. Cerebral concussion. Arch Surg 1927;14(4):891-916.

89. Millspaugh JA. Dementia pugilistica. US Naval Medicine Bulletin 1937;35:297-303.

90. Mirra SS, Hart MN, Terry RD. Making the diagnosis of Alzheimer's disease. A primer for practicing pathologists. Arch Pathol Lab Med 1993;117(2):132-144.

91. Mirra SS, Heyman A, McKeel D, Sumi SM, Crain BJ, Brownlee LM, et al. The Consortium to Establish a Registry for Alzheimer's Disease (CERAD). Part II. Standardization of the neuropathologic assessment of Alzheimer's disease. Neurology 1991;41(4):479-486.

92. Mortimer JA, van Duijn CM, Chandra V, Fratiglioni L, Graves AB, Heyman A, et al. Head trauma as a risk factor for Alzheimer's disease: a collaborative re-analysis of case-control studies. EURODEM Risk Factors Research Group. Int J Epidemiol 1991;20 Suppl 2:S28-35.

93. Murayama S. [Seed, aggregation and propagation of abnormal proteins could explain neurodegeneration?]. Rinsho Shinkeigaku 2011;51(11):1097-1099.

94. Neubuerger KT, Sinton DW, Denst J. Cerebral atrophy associated with boxing. AMA Arch Neurol Psychiatry 1959;81(4):403-408.

95. Neumann M, Sampathu DM, Kwong LK, Truax AC, Micsenyi MC, Chou TT, et al. Ubiquitinated TDP-43 in frontotemporal lobar degeneration and amyotrophic lateral sclerosis. Science 2006;314(5796):130-133.

96. Nussbaum JM, Schilling S, Cynis H, Silva A, Swanson E, Wangsanut T, et al. Prion-like behaviour and tau-dependent cytotoxicity of pyroglutamylated amyloid-beta. Nature 2012;485(7400):651-655.

97. Obersteiner H. Ueber Erschütterung des Rückenmarkes. Med Jahrb 1879:531.

98. Omalu B. Play Hard, Die Young: Football Depression, Dementia, and Death. 1st ed. Lodi, CA: NeoForenxis Books; 2008.

99. Omalu B, Bailes J, Hamilton RL, Kamboh MI, Hammers J, Case M, et al. Emerging histomorphologic phenotypes of chronic traumatic encephalopathy in American athletes. Neurosurgery 2011;69(1):173-183; discussion 183.

100. Omalu B, Hammers JL, Bailes J, Hamilton RL, Kamboh MI, Webster G, et al. Chronic traumatic encephalopathy in an Iraqi war veteran with posttraumatic stress disorder who committed suicide. Neurosurg Focus 2011;31(5):E3.

101. Omalu BI, Bailes J, Hammers JL, Fitzsimmons RP. Chronic traumatic encephalopathy, suicides and parasuicides in professional American athletes: the role of the forensic pathologist. Am J Forensic Med Pathol 2009;31(2):130-132.

102. Omalu BI, DeKosky ST, Hamilton RL, Minster RL, Kamboh MI, Shakir AM, et al. Chronic traumatic encephalopathy in a national football league player: part II. Neurosurgery 2006;59(5):1086-1092; discussion 1092-1083.

103. Omalu BI, DeKosky ST, Minster RL, Kamboh MI, Hamilton RL, Wecht CH. Chronic traumatic encephalopathy in a National Football League player. Neurosurgery 2005;57(1):128-134; discussion 128-134.

104. Omalu BI, Fitzsimmons RP, Hammers J, Bailes J. Chronic traumatic encephalopathy in a professional American wrestler. J Forens Nurs 2010;6(3):130-136.

105. Omalu BI, Hamilton RL, Kamboh MI, DeKosky ST, Bailes J. Chronic traumatic encephalopathy in a national football league player: case report and emerging medico-legal practice questions. J Forensic Nurs 2010;6(1):40-46.

106. Ommaya AK, Gennarelli TA. Cerebral concussion and traumatic unconsciousness. Correlation of experimental and clinical observations of blunt head injuries. Brain 1974;97(4):633-654.

107. Oppenheim H. Die traumatischen Neurosen. Berlin: A. Hirschwald; 1889.

108. Oppenheim H. Die traumatischen Neurosen nach den in der Nervenklinik der Charité in den 8 Jahren 1883-1891. 2nd ed. Berlin: A. Hirschwald; 1892.

109. Oppenheimer DR. Microscopic lesions in the brain following head injury. J Neurol Neurosurg Psychiatry 1968;31(4):299-306.

110. Osnato M, Giliberti V. Postconcussion neurosis-traumatic encephalitis. Arch Neurol Psychiatry 1927;18:181-211.

111. Parker HL. Traumatic encephalopathy ("punch drunk") of professional pugilists. J Neurol Psychopathol 1934;15(57):20-28.

112. Patt S, Brodhun M. Neuropathological sequelae of traumatic injury in the brain. An overview. Exp Toxicol Pathol 1999;51(2):119-123.

113. Payne EE. Brains of boxers. Neurochirurgia (Stuttg) 1968;11(5):173-188.

114. Peterson F, Haines WS, Webster RW. Legal Medicine and Toxicology: Saunders; 1923.

115. Petit JL. Traité des maladies chirurgicales, et des opérations qui leur conviennent. Paris: Méquignon l'Aineé; 1790.

116. Pitkanen A, Immonen RJ, Grohn OH, Kharatishvili I. From traumatic brain injury to posttraumatic epilepsy: what animal models tell us about the process and treatment options. Epilepsia 2009;50 Suppl 2:21-29.

117. Polymenidou M, Cleveland DW. Prion-like spread of protein aggregates in neurodegeneration. J Exp Med 2012;209(5):889-893.

118. Povlishock JT, Katz DI. Update of neuropathology and neurological recovery after traumatic brain injury. J Head Trauma Rehabil 2005;20(1):76-94.

119. Powell JW, Barber-Foss KD. Traumatic brain injury in high school athletes. JAMA 1999;282(10):958-963.

120. Prince DA, Parada I, Scalise K, Graber K, Jin X, Shen F. Epilepsy following cortical injury: cellular and molecular mechanisms as targets for potential prophylaxis. Epilepsia 2009;50 Suppl 2:30-40.

121. Proceedings of the Congress of Neurological Surgeons in 1964. Report of the Ad Hoc Committee to Study Head Injury Nomenclature. Clin Neurosurg 1966;12:386-394.

122. Purcell L, LeBlanc CM. Policy statement—boxing participation by children and adolescents. Pediatrics 2011;128(3):617-623.

123. Rabadi MH, Jordan BD. The cumulative effect of repetitive concussion in sports. Clin J Sport Med 2001;11(3):194-198.

124. Robbins S. Doctors study link between combat and brain disease. Stars and Stripes, January 23, 2010.

125. Roberts AH. Brain Damage in Boxers. A Study of the Prevalence of Traumatic Encephalopathy Among Ex-Professional Boxers. London: Pitman Medical and Scientific; 1969.

126. Roberts GW. Immunocytochemistry of neurofibrillary tangles in dementia pugilistica and Alzheimer's disease: evidence for common genesis. Lancet 1988;2(8626-8627):1456-1458.

127. Roberts GW, Allsop D, Bruton C. The occult aftermath of boxing. J Neurol Neurosurg Psychiatry 1990;53(5):373-378.

128. Roberts GW, Gentleman SM, Lynch A, Graham DI. Beta A4 amyloid protein deposition in brain after head trauma. Lancet 1991;338(8780):1422-1423.

129. Roberts GW, Gentleman SM, Lynch A, Murray L, Landon M, Graham DI. Beta amyloid protein deposition in the brain after severe head injury: implications for the pathogenesis of Alzheimer's disease. J Neurol Neurosurg Psychiatry 1994;57(4):419-425.

130. Roberts GW, Whitwell HL, Acland PR, Bruton CJ. Dementia in a punch-drunk wife. Lancet 1990;335(8694):918-919.

131. Ropper A. Brain injuries from blasts. N Engl J Med 2011;364(22):2156-2157.

132. Rosenfeld JV, Ford NL. Bomb blast, mild traumatic brain injury and psychiatric morbidity: a review. Injury 2010;41(5):437-443.

133. Rovegno M, Soto PA, Saez JC, von Bernhardi R. [Biological mechanisms involved in the spread of traumatic brain damage]. Med Intensiva 2012;36(1):37-44.

134. Royal College of Physicians of London. Committee on Boxing. Report on the Medical Aspects of Boxing. London: Royal College of Physicians of London; 1969.

135. Rudelli R, Strom JO, Welch PT, Ambler MW. Posttraumatic premature Alzheimer's disease. Neuropathologic findings and pathogenetic considerations. Arch Neurol 1982;39(9):570-575.

136. Russell WR. Cerebral involvement in head injury: a study based on the examination of 200 cases. Brain 1932;55(4):549-603.

137. Saulle M, Greenwald BD. Chronic traumatic encephalopathy: a review. Rehabil Res Pract 2012;2012:816069.

138. Schaller WF. After-effects of head injury: the post-traumatic concussion state (concussion, traumatic encephalopathy) and the post-traumatic psychoneurotic state (psychoneurosis, hysteria): a study in differential diagnosis. JAMA 1939;113(20):1779-1785.

139. Smith DH, Chen XH, Nonaka M, Trojanowski JQ, Lee VM, Saatman KE, et al. Accumulation of amyloid beta and tau and the formation of neurofilament inclusions following diffuse brain injury in the pig. J Neuropathol Exp Neurol 1999;58(9):982-992.

140. Smith DH, Chen XH, Pierce JE, Wolf JA, Trojanowski JQ, Graham DI, et al. Progressive atrophy and neuron death for one year following brain trauma in the rat. J Neurotrauma 1997;14(10):715-727.

141. Smodlaka VN. Medical aspects of heading the ball in soccer. Phys Sportsmed 1984;12:127-131.

142. Sortland O, Tysvaer AT. Brain damage in former association football players. An evaluation by cerebral computed tomography. Neuroradiology 1989;31(1):44-48.

143. Statler KD. Pediatric posttraumatic seizures: epidemiology, putative mechanisms of epileptogen-

esis and promising investigational progress. Dev Neurosci 2006;28(4-5):354-363.

144. Stern RA, Riley DO, Daneshvar DH, Nowinski CJ, Cantu RC, McKee AC. Long-term consequences of repetitive brain trauma: chronic traumatic encephalopathy. PM R 2011;3(10 Suppl 2):S460-467.

145. Stevenson LD. Head injuries: effects and their appraisal: II. The role of the microglia. Arch Neurol Psychiatry 1932;27(784):784-789.

146. Strauss I, Savitsky N. Head injury, neurologic and psychiatric aspects. Arch Neurol Psychiatry 1934;31(5):893-955.

147. Strich SJ. Diffuse degeneration of the cerebral white matter in severe dementia following head injury. J Neurol Neurosurg Psychiatry 1956;19(3):163-185.

148. Strich SJ. Shearing of the nerve fibers as a cause of brain damage due to head injury: a pathological study of twenty cases. Lancet 1961;278(7200):443-498.

149. Swartz BE, Houser CR, Tomiyasu U, Walsh GO, DeSalles A, Rich JR, et al. Hippocampal cell loss in posttraumatic human epilepsy. Epilepsia 2006;47(8):1373-1382.

150. Symonds C. Concussion and its sequelae. Lancet 1962;1;7219(7219):1-5.

151. Tanzi E, Lugaro E. Malattie Mentali. 2nd ed. Milan; 1914.

152. Thom M, Liu JY, Thompson P, Phadke R, Narkie-wicz M, Martinian L, et al. Neurofibrillary tangle pathology and Braak staging in chronic epilepsy in relation to traumatic brain injury and hippocampal sclerosis: a post-mortem study. Brain 2011;134(Pt 10):2969-2981.

153. Tokuda T, Ikeda S, Yanagisawa N, Ihara Y, Glenner GG. Re-examination of ex-boxers' brains using immunohistochemistry with antibodies to amyloid beta-protein and tau protein. Acta Neuropathol 1991;82(4):280-285.

154. Tromner E. Erinnerungen an die traumatische Hirnschwäche (Encephalopathia traumatica). Deutsche Ztschr f Nervenh 1921;68-69:491.

155. Trotter W. Certain minor injuries of the brain. Lancet 1924;1:935.

156. Trotter W. On Certain Minor Injuries of the Brain: Being the Annual Oration, Medical Society of London. Br Med J 1924;1(3306):816-819.

157. Tucker AM. Common soccer injuries. Diagnosis, treatment and rehabilitation. Sports Med 1997;23(1):21-32.

158. Tysvaer AT. Head and neck injuries in soccer. Impact of minor trauma. Sports Med 1992;14(3):200-213.

159. Tysvaer AT, Lochen EA. Soccer injuries to the brain. A neuropsychologic study of former soccer players. Am J Sports Med 1991;19(1):56-60.

160. Tysvaer AT, Sortland O, Storli OV, Lochen EA. [Head and neck injuries among Norwegian soccer players. A neurological, electroencephalographic, radiologic and neuropsychological evaluation]. Tidsskr Nor Laegeforen 1992;112(10):1268-1271.

161. Tysvaer AT, Storli OV. Soccer injuries to the brain. A neurologic and electroencephalographic study of active football players. Am J Sports Med 1989;17(4):573-578.

162. Tysvaer AT, Storli OV, Bachen NI. Soccer injuries to the brain. A neurologic and electroencephalographic study of former players. Acta Neurol Scand 1989;80(2):151-156.

163. Uryu K, Laurer H, McIntosh T, Pratico D, Martinez D, Leight S, et al. Repetitive mild brain trauma accelerates Abeta deposition, lipid peroxidation, and cognitive impairment in a transgenic mouse model of Alzheimer amyloidosis. J Neurosci 2002;22(2):446-454.

164. Uryu K, Nakashima-Yasuda H, Forman MS, Kwong LK, Clark CM, Grossman M, et al. Concomitant TAR-DNA-binding protein 43 pathology is present in Alzheimer disease and corticobasal degeneration but not in other tauopathies. J Neuropathol Exp Neurol 2008;67(6):555-564.

165. Valsamis MP. Pathology of trauma. Neurosurg Clin N Am 1994;5(1):175-183.

166. Van Duijn CM, Clayton DG, Chandra V, Fratiglioni L, Graves AB, Heyman A, et al. Interaction between genetic and environmental risk factors for Alzheimer's disease: a reanalysis of case-control studies. EURODEM Risk Factors Research Group. Genet Epidemiol 1994;11(6):539-551.

167. Von Sarbó A. Granatenfernwirkungsfolgen und Kriegshysterie. Neurol Centralbl 1917;36:360.

168. Ward AA Jr. The physiology of concussion. Clin Neurosurg 1964;12:95-111.

169. Wilkins RH. Neurosurgical classic. XVII. J Neurosurg 1964;21:240-244.

170. Willeumier K, Taylor DV, Amen DG. Elevated body mass in National Football League players linked to cognitive impairment and decreased prefrontal cortex and temporal pole activity. Transl Psychiatry 2012;2:e68.

171. Winterstein CE. Head injuries attributable to boxing. Lancet 1937;2:719-720.

172. Yarnell PR, Lynch S. The "ding": amnestic states in football trauma. Neurology 1973;23(2):196-197.

173. Yarnell PR, Lynch S. Retrograde memory immediately after concussion. Lancet 1970;1(7652):863-864.

174. Yoshiyama Y, Uryu K, Higuchi M, Longhi L, Hoover R, Fujimoto S, et al. Enhanced neurofibrillary tangle formation, cerebral atrophy, and cognitive deficits induced by repetitive mild brain injury in a transgenic tauopathy mouse model. J Neurotrauma 2005;22(10):1134-1141.

The Emerging Role of Subconcussion

Clinical care of the athlete with concussion has traditionally centered on the recognition of signs and symptoms associated with a concussive event. As discussed previously, grading scales have been largely replaced by the recognition and characterization of concussion symptoms and their duration for determination of severity. Additionally, appropriate management centers on a symptom-free waiting period of physical and cognitive rest to allow the athlete to, usually, subsequently return to play. However, emerging research now suggests that head impacts may commonly occur during contact or collision sports in which symptoms may not develop and there are no outward or visible signs of neurological dysfunction—a phenomenon termed subconcussion. While these impacts are often not recognized or identified as a concussion at the clinical level, their importance cannot be overstated. The concept of minimal or "subconcussive" injuries thus requires examination and consideration regarding the role they may play in accruing sufficient anatomical or physiological damage or both. Emerging evidence is drawn from laboratory data in animal models of mild traumatic brain injury, biophysics data, advanced neuroimaging studies, and forensic analyses of brains of former athletes who did not have a diagnosis of concussion during their playing career. Thus, subconcussion is a previously underrecognized phenomenon that needs to be further explored and also contemporaneously appreciated for its ability to cause important current and future detrimental neurological effects, such that the effects of these injuries are potentially expressed later in life.[3]

A WORKING DEFINITION

Subconcussion is a cranial impact that does not result in known or diagnosed concussion on clinical grounds. It may also occur with rapid acceleration-deceleration to the body or torso, particularly when the brain is free to move within the cranium, creating a "slosh" phenomenon. Subconcussion has its greatest effect through repetitive occurrences whereby cumulative exposure becomes deleterious. It should be stressed that not all head impacts should be considered potentially harmful. The athlete's risk of experiencing longstanding effects of repetitive subconcussive blows is likely measured as a cumulative dose over a lifetime, and could include factors such as age at exposure, type and magnitude of exposure, recovery periods, differential rates of recovery, genotype, and individual vulnerability. The role of protective equipment and variability in equipment also are factors that may come into play, but their contribution is unknown.

LABORATORY EVIDENCE OF SUBCONCUSSIVE EFFECTS

As discussed earlier in the book, traumatic brain injury (TBI) is traditionally thought of as involving both primary and secondary injury phases. [18] In addition to primary and secondary injury, a tertiary phase of TBI may now be thought of as involving ongoing abnormalities in glucose utilization and cellular metabolism, as well as membrane fluidity, synaptic function, and structural integrity. [4, 26, 34-36, 51, 52, 56, 60] This phase of TBI potentially could become chronic and also compounded if the individual is subjected to repetitive minor head impacts.

Little attention was paid to repetitive mild head injury before the year 2000, with only a few repetitive injury studies having been published. [27, 43, 64] Since that time there has been an increased interest in laboratory research focused on repetitive mild TBI. [1, 7, 11, 13, 19, 21, 28, 31, 33, 54, 58, 62, 65] Most of these studies were performed in rodents; a few were performed in pig models of TBI. In one study, DeFord and colleagues showed that as compared to a single episode of mild TBI, repeat injury was associated with impairments of complex spatial learning and cognitive impairment. [19] Interestingly, this was despite no overt cell death in the cortex or hippocampus or blood–brain barrier compromise.

Researchers have demonstrated that repetitive mild TBI (mTBI) causes changes in cortical and hippocampal cytoskeletal proteins and increases the brain's vulnerability to subsequent head injury compared to single TBI. [27, 31] Some studies have reported evidence of central nervous system injury despite no overt behavioral deficits, consistent with subconcussive injury. One study used microtubule-associated protein-2 (MAP-2) staining techniques to demonstrate that local and remote injury was significantly greater if it occurred in a shorter time window following the initial injury in mice that exhibited minimal behavioral response following experimental head injury. [33]

Some researchers have demonstrated evidence of deleterious effects following a single subconcussive experimental head injury. Some have modified the Marmarou weight drop method concussion model to diminish impact forces to effect a non–response-altering reaction, thus simulating less than concussive injury. [2, 40-42] In these mice, staining for amyloid precursor protein (APP) has shown that these subconcussive impacts reliably produce tearing of axons and the formation of axonal retraction bulbs in the brain stem–level descending motor pathways. These animals exhibited no alteration of consciousness or responsiveness, but significant numbers of APP-positive axons were found compared to observations in control animals. In another rodent vertical impact mTBI model, Lado and Persinger found that there was minimal change in the animals' behavioral response following injury, yet at sacrifice the animals showed dark, swollen neuronal soma. [30]

Lifshitz and Lisembee, in a rodent fluid percussion brain injury model, found at 28 days that thalamic ventral basal neurons exhibited atrophic changes without neuronal death. [32] It has been noted that persistence in a chronic atrophic state after ipsilateral hippocampal injury deprives the deafferented basal cholinergic neurons of trophic support, a finding consistent with detailed autopsy studies on chronic traumatic encephalopathy (CTE) athletes. [45-49] Creed and coauthors showed that, compared to sham-injured mice, concussive brain-injured mice had abnormal spatial acquisition and working memory as measured by Morris water maze over the first 3 days (p < 0.001) but not later than the fourth day postinjury. [12] At 1 and 3 days postinjury, intra-axonal accumulation of APP in the corpus callosum and cingulum was associated with neurofilament dephosphorylation, abnormal transport of Fluoro-Gold and synaptophysin, and deficits in axonal conductance, which continued until 14 days when axonal degeneration was apparent. What this showed was that although there may be recovery from acute cognitive deficits, even subconcussive brain trauma leads to axonal degeneration and abnormal axonal function. [12]

Shultz and colleagues investigated the effects of a mild lateral fluid percussion injury (0.50-0.99 atmosphere (atm) on rat behavior and neuropathological changes in an attempt to better understand subconcussive brain injury. [59] In their study, male Long-Evans rats received either a single mild lateral fluid percussion injury or a sham injury, followed by either a short (24 hours) or long (4 weeks) recovery period. No significant group differences were found on behavioral and axonal injury measures; however, rats given one subconcussive mild fluid percussion injury displayed a significant increase in microglial activation and reactive astrogliosis at 4 days postinjury.[59] These findings are thought to be consistent with observations in humans experiencing a subconcussive impact.[8, 59]

As noted in these studies, such animal models of mTBI have resulted in a significant number of damaged corticospinal tract axons, created permeability in the blood–brain barrier, caused remote effects away from the cortical impact site, and altered neuronal soma. All of these alterations can occur in the absence of behavioral changes. Thus, there is laboratory evidence that subconcussive-level impacts can lead to anatomical and physiological alterations and that these occur particularly if the blows are repetitive.

CLINICAL EVIDENCE OF SUBCONCUSSION

Much of the current clinical work in subconcussion was born out of advanced neuroimaging studies. Recent biophysics and autopsy studies have also been suggestive of the phenomenon of subconcussion. Here we review these clinical data.

Biophysics Data

Concussion and subconcussion can occur in any sport; however, American football has a high incidence of concussion, largely due to the style of play, the high rate of impacts, and the expanse of participation.[25] The mandatory use of helmets in American football has allowed for the systematic analysis of injury biomechanics and real-time measurements of forces, velocities, accelerations, and frequencies of head impacts via implanted telemetry devices (figure 11.1). Our understanding of the issue of subconcussion is clouded by the marked variability between the thresholds for clinically diagnosed concussion in terms of linear acceleration, rotational acceleration, and location and number of impacts.[6, 9, 10, 14, 23, 24, 39, 50, 55, 57, 61]

Broglio and colleagues studied 95 high school football players across four seasons using a helmet telemetry system to record total number of head impacts and the associated acceleration forces.[10] The number of impacts varied with the athletes' playing position and starting status. The average player sustained 652 impacts during a 14-week season. Linemen had the greatest number of impacts per season (868); the group with the next highest number of impacts consisted of tight ends, running backs, and linebackers (619), followed by quarterbacks (467), receivers, cornerbacks,

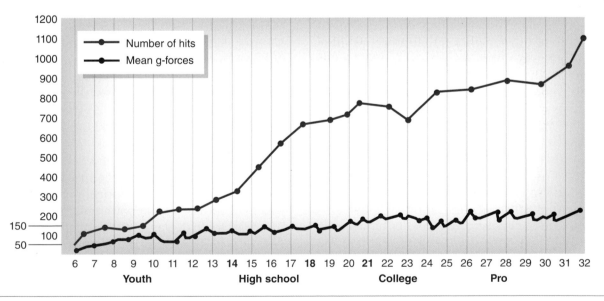

Figure 11.1 Subconcussion curve of head impacts and forces over age change and playing level.

and safeties (372). The seasonal linear acceleration burden averaged 16,746.1 g, while the rotational acceleration burden was 1,090,697.7 rad/s^2. These findings indicate that high school football players sustain a high number of head impacts each season, with associated cumulative impact burdens that are equally impressive.[10] Talavage and colleagues, using similar technology, found comparable numbers and rates of hit accumulations.[61]

Eckner and coauthors explored the characteristics of 20 concussion-invoking impacts in 19 high school football players, analyzing the total number of head impacts, the severity profile values, and cumulative linear and rotational acceleration values during the same game or practice session as well as the 30-minute and 1-week periods preceding these impacts.[20] Concussions occurred over a wide range of impact magnitudes. Interestingly, cumulative impact burden before a concussion was not different from nonconcussive impacts of greater magnitudes in the same athletes. Therefore, the authors concluded that an athlete's concussion threshold may be a dynamic feature over time and that there is a lack of cumulative effects of nonconcussive impacts on concussion threshold. Thus, the types of impacts that occur in players who sustain a concussion may be no different from those that occur in asymptomatic players, further pointing to the role and potential importance of subconcussive impacts.

Crisco and colleagues have investigated impact characteristics in collegiate football players.[14-16] The authors found that player position and impact location were the largest factors accounting for differences in head impacts. The total number of head impacts was a median of 420 and a maximum of 2,492. Studies have shown variance in the total number of head impacts in collegiate players, from 950 head impacts per season[22, 23] to 1,353 per season.[57] Schnebel and colleagues used accelerometers embedded in the crown of the helmets in both high school and collegiate football players.[57] They found the expected number of high-speed, open-field collisions occurring in skill position athletes with forces in the range of 90 to 120 g and a duration of about 15 ms. One of the most intriguing and unexpected findings of this study was that linemen experienced impacts of 20 to 30 g on nearly every play. Due to the football tradition of linemen starting every play in the three-point stance and lunging forward to immediately encounter the opposing player, head contact occurs on a constant and ubiquitous basis.

Youth football players constitute about 70% of all American football players and a total of 3.5 million participants. A recent study monitored seven youth football participants, aged 7 and 8 years, during a football season and noted an average of 107 impacts per player for the season.[17] Linear accelerations ranged from 10 to 100 g, and rotational accelerations ranged from 52 to 7,694 rad/s^2. This study was the first to document that very high velocity impacts are possible at the youth level of football play. Thus, while youth football players may have fewer helmet impacts and lower-force hits than their older counterparts, high-magnitude impacts may occur nonetheless, and their long-term implications in an exposure paradigm are uncertain.[18]

Neuropsychological Evaluation

In a recent study, Gysland and colleagues sought to investigate the relationship between subconcussive impacts and concussion history on clinical measures of neurological function.[24] Forty-six collegiate football players completed five clinical measures of neurological function commonly employed in the evaluation of concussion before and after a single season. These tests included the Automated Neuropsychological Assessment Metrics, Sensory Organization Test, Standardized Assessment of Concussion, Balance Error Scoring System, and Graded Symptom Checklist; impact data were recorded with the Head Impact Telemetry System (HITS). Even though players averaged 1,177.3 ± 772.9 head impacts over the course of a season, the authors found that they did not demonstrate any clinically meaningful changes from preseason to postseason on the measures of neurological function employed.[24] Similar findings were reported in another study of college football players.[39] There may be a dose response with regard to impacts that must be considered over the course of a player's career. Additionally, it is possible that the measures of neurological function employed were not sensitive enough to detect subclinical neurological dysfunction in athletes sustaining many repetitive subconcussive impacts.

Other research, though, now suggests that these nonconcussive impacts may not be benign. Killam and coauthors found that nonconcussed collegiate athletes in contact sports actually scored lower than control subjects in two memory domains and had lower total scores on the Repeatable Battery for the Assessment of Neuropsychological Status (RBANS).[29] Their data suggest that participation in contact sports may produce subclinical cognitive impairments in the absence of a diagnosable concussion, presumably resulting from the cumulative consequences of multiple mild head injuries. This investigation showed, and other studies have continued to demonstrate, that measures of peak acceleration may not be sufficient to predict cognitive deficit, and that greater impact forces do not necessarily correlate with a greater likelihood of neurological impairment.

McAllister and colleagues studied 214 collegiate Division I football and ice hockey players, analyzing their accelerometer data and neuropsychological outcomes compared to those for a control group of noncontact sport athletes. They found that the athletes in contact sports had worse performance on tests for new learning, and postseason cognitive testing correlated with greater head impact exposure. This was despite the fact that none of the subjects had a documented sport concussion during the period of study.[37] Other studies, though, have failed to detect differences between preseason baseline, midseason, and postseason assessments in players who did not sustain concussions.[39] Thus, there may be specific neuropsychological metrics that are better suited to or more sensitive for detecting the effects of repetitive subconcussion forces. It may also be that the symptoms or sequelae of repetitive subconcussion could require a greater length of time to develop than a single season.

Neuroradiological Findings

The role of advanced neuroimaging in concussion has been a progressive one. The use of these new techniques is especially relevant in the case of subconcussion because even in cases of concussion, conventional computed tomography and magnetic resonance imaging (MRI) sequences are unable to detect macroscopic structural abnormalities.[53] To test the hypothesis that subconcussive blows cause an accumulation of neurophysiological changes, it is necessary to measure changes in neurological function over time.

Talavage and colleagues studied a group of high school football players by performing MRI, functional MRI (fMRI), and neurocognitive assessments at three distinct times: (1) before the start of contact practices, (2) during the season, and (3) 2 to 5 months after the season concluded.[61] In addition to these assessments, the HIT system was used to record head collisions during all contact practices and games. The authors demonstrated quantifiable neurophysiological changes, in both fMRI and ImPACT testing, in the absence of outwardly observable symptoms of concussion. This finding of neuropsychological disturbance in the absence of classical symptoms of concussion is consistent with prior observations in seven former National Football League (NFL) offensive linemen and a wide receiver as reported by Omalu and colleagues.[46, 47, 49] A follow-up study by Breedlove and colleagues demonstrated that the fMRI changes in many regions of the brain were statistically correlated to the number and (spatial) distribution of hits received subsequent to the beginning of contact practices.[9] This study went on to suggest that the clinical diagnosis of neurological system deficits may be dependent on which systems have been compromised, and that the entire (recent) history of blows to the head plays a causal role in overall neurological changes.

A new study using diffusion tensor imaging (DTI) highlights the emerging clinical evidence for subconcussive brain injury.[6] Bazarian and colleagues investigated the ability to detect subject-specific changes in brain white matter (WM) before and after sport-related concussion. This prospective cohort study was performed in nine high school athletes engaged in hockey or football and six controls. Subjects underwent DTI pre- and postseason within a 3-month interval. Only one athlete was diagnosed with a concussion (scanned within 72 hours), and eight suffered between 26 and 399 subconcussive head blows.[6] While analysis detected significantly changed WM in a single concussed athlete as expected, the most striking findings were in those athletes who did not sustain a concussion. Asymptomatic athletes with multiple subconcussive head blows had abnormalities in a percentage of their WM that was over three times higher than in controls. The significance of these WM changes and their relationship to head impact forces are currently unknown.

Necropsy Tissue Analysis

It is now appreciated that the syndrome of CTE, initially described by Omalu and colleagues in 2005,[47] occurs not only in football players but also in boxers, wrestlers, hockey players, and even military personnel.[38, 44, 45] It is believed to be a lesser form of injury than dementia pugilistica (DP), initially described by Martland in 1928. In a series of eight former professional football players, autopsy analysis using detailed and specialized staining techniques for the presence of tau protein was performed (table 11.1). In all cases, similar neurobehavioral, neuropsychiatric, and neuropathological abnormalities were found, consistent with CTE. Interestingly, none of these athletes had a history of concussion noted as a part of the medical and athletic history. It is unknown whether the methodology at the time was insufficient to detect the presence of a concussion or whether underreporting occurred due to player ignorance, motivation, or sport cultural issues. Seven of the athletes were football linemen, a position associated with constant, mandatory, and often gratuitous head-to-head impacts. Autopsy data from McKee and coauthors[5, 38]

demonstrate that a subset of athletes in contact sports, particularly former football players, do not have a prominent history of known or identified concussions but nonetheless have typical tauopathy seen in autopsy examination.[38, 45-49] Taken together, these necropsy tissue findings point to subconcussion as a pathophysiological mechanism for unsuspected brain injury in those exposed to contact and collision sports.

CONCLUDING THOUGHTS

In recent years there have been major advances in our understanding of the incidence of mTBI and the biomechanical forces and cellular responses. The amount of laboratory research, both animal-based experiments and investigations of the cellular responses underlying concussion, as well as clinical studies to determine the effects of concussion, has exponentially increased.[63] In fact, it is now often stated that the information from mTBI research produced during the past decade supersedes the volume and knowledge of all previous information. An emerging concept is the phenomenon of subconcussive impacts, as new evidence highlights their ubiquity in sports, as well as their potential to contribute to the development of subacute and chronic sequelae.

As noted previously, Talavage and colleagues discovered a new category of injured athletes: those who had no readily observable symptoms but who instead exhibited functional impairment as measured by neuropsychological testing

Table 11.1 Autopsy Analysis of Former NFL players

Case	Age	Duration of professional career	Symptoms	Cause of death
1	50 years	17 years	Dep, FB, FM, SA	Cardiac
2	45 years	7 years	Dep, FB, FM, SA	Suicide
3	45 years	10 years	Dep, FB, FM	OD
4	35 years	10 years	Dep, FB, FM	Suicide
5	45 years	12 years	Dep, drugs, FM	OD
6	39 years	7 years	Dep, drugs, FM	OD
7	50 years	10 years	Dep, drugs, FM	OD
8	26 years	5 years	Dep, personality changes	Fall from vehicle

Dep, depression; FB, failed business; FM, failed marriage; NFL, National Football League; OD, overdose; SA, substance abuse.
Adapted, by permission, from J.E. Bailes et al., 2013, "Role of subconcussion in repetitive mild traumatic brain injury," *Journal of neurosurgery* 119(5): 1235-45.

and fMRI studies.[61] This group of individuals, who demonstrated abnormal neurological performance despite a lack of symptoms typically associated with a clinically diagnosed concussion, may shed light on the issue of subconcussive impacts and their relationship to chronic neurological syndromes. The research reviewed in this chapter suggests that the sequence of blows experienced by a player can mediate the severity of the observed symptoms that lead to the clinical diagnosis of concussion, or the absence thereof (e.g., in the case of functionally observed impairment).

Biophysics data gathered through football helmet accelerometer studies have shown that youth, high school, and college players may experience a wide range of head impacts, from 100 to over 1,000 during the course of a season (table 11.2). Compared to location and magnitude of forces, it may likely be that the cumulative number of head impacts best correlates with the potential for concussion occurrence or chronic effects. It is uncertain whether head impacts have a threshold for magnitude or number (or both) that could result in a cumulative risk for detrimental effects on brain structures or physiological function.[18]

Our understanding of subconcussion is still early and evolving but will likely in the future determine the ultimate risk for those who are exposed to repetitive mTBI in athletic endeavors. For now, there is a lack of evidence to permit a recommendation regarding the number of subconcussive impacts that should be allowed prior to ending an athlete's season or career. As our knowledge about this emerging concept continues to evolve, refined and advanced adjunct measures of assessment may someday be able to help guide such decisions with the aim of decreasing the incidence of delayed chronic neurological deficits associated with repetitive subconcussion. Strategies should be developed to minimize exposure to recurring cranial impacts during practice sessions, as Pop Warner Football has recently done at the youth level. Another possibility is to change styles of play. Just one example would be to have linemen in football start in a squatting "two-point" position or stance, rather than in a down stance, to remove them from head contact on every play. It is clear that further research is needed, but for the time being, limiting the overall head impact burden as best as possible is the most prudent recommendation for today's athlete.

Table 11.2   Comparison of Head Impacts in Football by Level of Competition

Citations	Level of competition	Age range	Average head impacts per season	Range of head impacts per season
Daniel et al. 2012	Youth	5-14 years	107	n/a
Breedlove et al. 2012 Broglio et al. 2011 Eckner et al. 2011 Schnebel et al. 2007 Talavage et al. 2010	High school	14-18 years	625§	5-2,235
Crisco et al. 2010 Crisco et al. 2011 Guskiewicz et al. 2007 Gysland et al. 2012 Rowson et al. 2012 Schnebel et al. 2007	Collegiate	18-22 years	1,125§	125-2,492
Extrapolation	Professional	>22 years	>1200*	n/a

n/a, not available. *Note:* The number of impacts accrued each season varies by position.
*Estimate based on practice patterns and style of play
§Head impacts averaged from mean data available from accelerometer studies at each level of competition.
Adapted from: J.E. Bailes et al., 2013, "Role of subconcussion in repetitive mild traumatic brain injury," *Journal of Neurosurgery* 119(5): 1235-1245.

REFERENCES

1. Allen GV, Gerami D, Esser MJ. Conditioning effects of repetitive mild neurotrauma on motor function in an animal model of focal brain injury. Neuroscience 2000;99(1):93-105.

2. Bailes JE, Mills JD. Docosahexaenoic acid reduces traumatic axonal injury in a rodent head injury model. J Neurotrauma 2010;27(9):1617-1624.

3. Bailes JE, Petraglia AL, Omalu BI, Nauman E, Talavage T. Role of subconcussion in repetitive mild traumatic brain injury. J Neurosurg 2013; 119(5):1235-45.

4. Barkhoudarian G, Hovda DA, Giza CC. The molecular pathophysiology of concussive brain injury. Clin Sports Med 2011;30(1):33-48, vii-iii.

5. Baugh CM, Stamm JM, Riley DO, Gavett BE, Shenton ME, Lin A, et al. Chronic traumatic encephalopathy: neurodegeneration following repetitive concussive and subconcussive brain trauma. Brain Imaging Behav 2012; 6(2):244-254.

6. Bazarian JJ, Zhu T, Blyth B, Borrino A, Zhong J. Subject-specific changes in brain white matter on diffusion tensor imaging after sports-related concussion. Magn Reson Imaging 2012;30(2):171-180.

7. Bennett RE, Mac Donald CL, Brody DL. Diffusion tensor imaging detects axonal injury in a mouse model of repetitive closed-skull traumatic brain injury. Neurosci Lett 2012;513(2):160-165.

8. Blaylock RL, Maroon J. Immunoexcitotoxicity as a central mechanism in chronic traumatic encephalopathy—a unifying hypothesis. Surg Neurol Int 2011;2:107.

9. Breedlove EL, Robinson M, Talavage TM, Morigaki KE, Yoruk U, O'Keefe K, et al. Biomechanical correlates of symptomatic and asymptomatic neurophysiological impairment in high school football. J Biomech 2012;45(7):1265-1272.

10. Broglio SP, Eckner JT, Martini D, Sosnoff JJ, Kutcher JS, Randolph C. Cumulative head impact burden in high school football. J Neurotrauma 2011;28(10):2069-2078.

11. Conte V, Uryu K, Fujimoto S, Yao Y, Rokach J, Longhi L, et al. Vitamin E reduces amyloidosis and improves cognitive function in Tg2576 mice following repetitive concussive brain injury. J Neurochem 2004;90(3):758-764.

12. Creed JA, DiLeonardi AM, Fox DP, Tessler AR, Raghupathi R. Concussive brain trauma in the mouse results in acute cognitive deficits and sustained impairment of axonal function. J Neurotrauma 2011;28(4):547-563.

13. Creeley CE, Wozniak DF, Bayly PV, Olney JW, Lewis LM. Multiple episodes of mild traumatic brain injury result in impaired cognitive performance in mice. Acad Emerg Med 2004;11(8):809-819.

14. Crisco JJ, Fiore R, Beckwith JG, Chu JJ, Brolinson PG, Duma S, et al. Frequency and location of head impact exposures in individual collegiate football players. J Athl Train 2010;45(6):549-559.

15. Crisco JJ, Wilcox BJ, Beckwith JG, Chu JJ, Duhaime AC, Rowson S, et al. Head impact exposure in collegiate football players. J Biomech 2011;44(15):2673-2678.

16. Crisco JJ, Wilcox BJ, Machan JT, McAllister TW, Duhaime AC, Duma SM, et al. Magnitude of head impact exposures in individual collegiate football players. J Appl Biomech 2011; 28(2):174-183.

17. Daniel RW, Rowson S, Duma SM. Head impact exposure in youth football. Ann Biomed Eng 2012;40(4):976-981.

18. Dashnaw ML, Petraglia AL, Bailes JE. An overview of the basic science of concussion and subconcussion: where we are and where we are going. Neurosurg Focus 2012;33(6):E5.

19. DeFord SM, Wilson MS, Rice AC, Clausen T, Rice LK, Barabnova A, et al. Repeated mild brain injuries result in cognitive impairment in B6C3F1 mice. J Neurotrauma 2002;19(4):427-438.

20. Eckner JT, Sabin M, Kutcher JS, Broglio SP. No evidence for a cumulative impact effect on concussion injury threshold. J Neurotrauma 2011;28(10):2079-2090.

21. Friess SH, Ichord RN, Ralston J, Ryall K, Helfaer MA, Smith C, et al. Repeated traumatic brain injury affects composite cognitive function in piglets. J Neurotrauma 2009;26(7):1111-1121.

22. Guskiewicz KM, Mihalik JP. Biomechanics of sport concussion: quest for the elusive injury threshold. Exerc Sport Sci Rev 2011;39(1):4-11.

23. Guskiewicz KM, Mihalik JP, Shankar V, Marshall SW, Crowell DH, Oliaro SM, et al. Measurement of head impacts in collegiate football players: relationship between head impact biomechanics and acute clinical outcome after concussion. Neurosurgery 2007;61(6):1244-1252; discussion 1252-1253.

24. Gysland SM, Mihalik JP, Register-Mihalik JK, Trulock SC, Shields EW, Guskiewicz KM. The relationship between subconcussive impacts and concussion history on clinical measures of neurologic function in collegiate football players. Ann Biomed Eng 2012;40(1):14-22.

25. Hootman JM, Dick R, Agel J. Epidemiology of collegiate injuries for 15 sports: summary and recommendations for injury prevention initiatives. J Athl Train 2007;42:311-319.

26. Johnson GV, Greenwood JA, Costello AC, Troncoso JC. The regulatory role of calmodulin in the proteolysis of individual neurofilament proteins by calpain. Neurochem Res 1991;16(8):869-873.

27. Kanayama G, Takeda M, Niigawa H, Ikura Y, Tamii H, Taniguchi N, et al. The effects of repetitive mild brain injury on cytoskeletal protein and behavior. Methods Find Exp Clin Pharmacol 1996;18(2):105-115.

28. Kane MJ, Angoa-Perez M, Briggs DI, Viano DC, Kreipke CW, Kuhn DM. A mouse model of human repetitive mild traumatic brain injury. J Neurosci Methods 2012;203(1):41-49.

29. Killam C, Cautin RL, Santucci AC. Assessing the enduring residual neuropsychological effects of head trauma in college athletes who participate in contact sports. Arch Clin Neuropsychol 2005;20(5):599-611.

30. Lado WE, Persinger MA. Mechanical impacts to the skulls of rats produce specific deficits in maze performance and weight loss: evidence for apoptosis of cortical neurons and implications for clinical neuropsychology. Percept Mot Skills 2003;97(3 Pt 2):1115-1127.

31. Laurer HL, Bareyre FM, Lee VM, Trojanowski JQ, Longhi L, Hoover R, et al. Mild head injury increasing the brain's vulnerability to a second concussive impact. J Neurosurg 2001;95(5):859-870.

32. Lifshitz J, Lisembee AM. Neurodegeneration in the somatosensory cortex after experimental diffuse brain injury. Brain Struct Funct 2012;217(1):49-61.

33. Longhi L, Saatman KE, Fujimoto S, Raghupathi R, Meaney DF, Davis J, et al. Temporal window of vulnerability to repetitive experimental concussive brain injury. Neurosurgery 2005;56(2):364-374; discussion 364-374.

34. Mata M, Staple J, Fink DJ. Changes in intra-axonal calcium distribution following nerve crush. J Neurobiol 1986;17(5):449-467.

35. Maxwell WL, McCreath BJ, Graham DI, Gennarelli TA. Cytochemical evidence for redistribution of membrane pump calcium-ATPase and ecto-Ca-ATPase activity, and calcium influx in myelinated nerve fibres of the optic nerve after stretch injury. J Neurocytol 1995;24(12):925-942.

36. Maxwell WL, Povlishock JT, Graham DL. A mechanistic analysis of nondisruptive axonal injury: a review. J Neurotrauma 1997;14(7):419-440.

37. McAllister TW, Flashman LA, Maerlender A, Greenwald RM, Beckwith JG, Tosteson TD, et al. Cognitive effects of one season of head impacts in a cohort of collegiate contact sport athletes. Neurology 2012;78(22):1777-1784.

38. McKee AC, Cantu RC, Nowinski CJ, Hedley-Whyte ET, Gavett BE, Budson AE, et al. Chronic traumatic encephalopathy in athletes: progressive tauopathy after repetitive head injury. J Neuropathol Exp Neurol 2009;68(7):709-735.

39. Miller JR, Adamson GJ, Pink MM, Sweet JC. Comparison of preseason, midseason, and postseason neurocognitive scores in uninjured collegiate football players. Am J Sports Med 2007;35(8):1284-1288.

40. Mills JD, Bailes JE, Sedney CL, Hutchins H, Sears B. Omega-3 fatty acid supplementation and reduction of traumatic axonal injury in a rodent head injury model. J Neurosurg 2011;114(1):77-84.

41. Mills JD, Bailes JE, Turner RC, Dodson SC, Sakai J, Maroon JC. Anabolic steroids and head injury. Neurosurgery 2012;70(1):205-209; discussion 209-210.

42. Mills JD, Hadley K, Bailes JE. Dietary supplementation with the omega-3 fatty acid docosahexaenoic acid in traumatic brain injury. Neurosurgery 2011;68(2):474-481; discussion 481.

43. Olsson Y, Rinder L, Lindgren S, Stalhammar D. Studies on vascular permeability changes in experimental brain concussion. A comparison between the effects of single and repeated sudden mechanical loading of the brain. Acta Neuropathologica 1971;19(3):225-233.

44. Omalu B, Bailes J, Hamilton RL, Kamboh MI, Hammers J, Case M, et al. Emerging histomorphologic phenotypes of chronic traumatic encephalopathy in American athletes. Neurosurgery 2011;69(1):173-183; discussion 183.

45. Omalu BI, Bailes J, Hammers JL, Fitzsimmons RP. Chronic traumatic encephalopathy, suicides and parasuicides in professional American athletes: the role of the forensic pathologist. Am J Forens Med Pathol 2010;31(2):130-132.

46. Omalu BI, DeKosky ST, Hamilton RL, Minster RL, Kamboh MI, Shakir AM, et al. Chronic traumatic encephalopathy in a national football league player: part II. Neurosurgery 2006;59(5):1086-1092; discussion 1092-1093.

47. Omalu BI, DeKosky ST, Minster RL, Kamboh MI, Hamilton RL, Wecht CH. Chronic traumatic encephalopathy in a National Football League player. Neurosurgery 2005;57(1):128-134; discussion 128-134.

48. Omalu BI, Fitzsimmons RP, Hammers J, Bailes J. Chronic traumatic encephalopathy in a professional American wrestler. J Forens Nurs 2010;6(3):130-136.

49. Omalu BI, Hamilton RL, Kamboh MI, DeKosky ST, Bailes J. Chronic traumatic encephalopathy (CTE) in a National Football League player: case report and emerging medicolegal practice questions. J Forens Nurs 2010;6(1):40-46.

50. Pellman EJ, Viano DC, Tucker AM, Casson IR, Waeckerle JF. Concussion in professional football: reconstruction of game impacts and injuries. Neurosurgery 2003;53:799-812.

51. Pettus EH, Povlishock JT. Characterization of a distinct set of intra-axonal ultrastructural changes associated with traumatically induced alteration in

axolemmal permeability. Brain Res 1996;722(1-2):1-11.

52. Povlishock JT, Pettus EH. Traumatically induced axonal damage: evidence for enduring changes in axolemmal permeability with associated cytoskeletal change. Acta Neurochir Suppl 1996;66:81-86.

53. Prabhu SP. The role of neuroimaging in sport-related concussion. Clin Sports Med 2011;30(1):103-114, ix.

54. Raghupathi R, Mehr MF, Helfaer MA, Margulies SS. Traumatic axonal injury is exacerbated following repetitive closed head injury in the neonatal pig. J Neurotrauma 2004;21(3):307-316.

55. Rowson S, Duma SM, Beckwith JG, Chu JJ, Greenwald RM, Crisco JJ, et al. Rotational head kinematics in football impacts: an injury risk function for concussion. Ann Biomed Eng 2012;40(1):1-13.

56. Saatman KE, Abai B, Grosvenor A, Vorwerk CK, Smith DH, Meaney DF. Traumatic axonal injury results in biphasic calpain activation and retrograde transport impairment in mice. J Cereb Blood Flow Metab 2003;23(1):34-42.

57. Schnebel B, Gwin JT, Anderson S, Gatlin R. In vivo study of head impacts in football: a comparison of National Collegiate Athletic Association Division I versus high school impacts. Neurosurgery 2007;60(3):490-495; discussion 495-496.

58. Shitaka Y, Tran HT, Bennett RE, Sanchez L, Levy MA, Dikranian K, et al. Repetitive closed-skull traumatic brain injury in mice causes persistent multifocal axonal injury and microglial reactivity. J Neuropathol Exp Neurol 2011;70(7):551-567.

59. Shultz SR, MacFabe DF, Foley KA, Taylor R, Cain DP. Sub-concussive brain injury in the Long-Evans rat induces acute neuroinflammation in the absence of behavioral impairments. Behav Brain Res 2012;229(1):145-152.

60. Spain A, Daumas S, Lifshitz J, Rhodes J, Andrews PJ, Horsburgh K, et al. Mild fluid percussion injury in mice produces evolving selective axonal pathology and cognitive deficits relevant to human brain injury. J Neurotrauma 2010;27(8):1429-1438.

61. Talavage TM, Nauman E, Breedlove EL, Yoruk U, Dye AE, Morigaki K, et al. Functionally-detected cognitive impairment in high school football players without clinically-diagnosed concussion. J Neurotrauma 2010; 31(4):327-338.

62. Uryu K, Laurer H, McIntosh T, Pratico D, Martinez D, Leight S, et al. Repetitive mild brain trauma accelerates Abeta deposition, lipid peroxidation, and cognitive impairment in a transgenic mouse model of Alzheimer amyloidosis. J Neurosci 2002;22(2):446-454.

63. Weber JT. Experimental models of repetitive brain injuries. Prog Brain Res 2007;161:253-261.

64. Weitbrecht WU, Noetzel H. [Autoradiographic investigations in repeated experimental brain concussion (author's transl)]. Arch Psychiatr Nervenk 1976;223(1):59-68.

65. Yoshiyama Y, Uryu K, Higuchi M, Longhi L, Hoover R, Fujimoto S, et al. Enhanced neurofibrillary tangle formation, cerebral atrophy, and cognitive deficits induced by repetitive mild brain injury in a transgenic tauopathy mouse model. J Neurotrauma 2005;22(10):1134-1141.

Severe Head Injury and Second Impact Syndrome

The last 30 to 40 years have seen a dramatic decrease in the incidence of severe head injury in athletics. Rule changes, better equipment standards and design, increased awareness, and improved medical care have all accounted for fewer injuries. While severe closed head injuries are relatively rare in organized sporting events, the injuries can have devastating consequences. Understanding the fundamentals of severe and catastrophic injuries allows the sports medicine practitioner to be prepared in the event of these occurrences.

CEREBRAL CONTUSIONS AND INTRAPARENCHYMAL HEMORRHAGE

Hemorrhagic brain contusions and intraparenchymal hemorrhages (also known as traumatic intracerebral hemorrhage) represent regions of primary neuronal and vascular injury. Contusions are frequent sequelae of head injury and most commonly occur following acceleration–deceleration mechanisms. A contusion represents a heterogeneous area of brain injury that consists of hemorrhage, cerebral infarction, and necrosis. These regions of the brain are usually edematous with areas of punctuate hemorrhages that can extend deep into the white matter or even the subdural and subarachnoid spaces. Contusions commonly occur in coup or contrecoup fashion. In coup injuries, the brain is injured directly under the area of impact. The degree of injury to the underlying brain depends on the energy transmitted, the area of contact, and the region of the brain involved, as well as other factors. Contrecoup injuries occur on the side opposite the impact as the brain glides and strikes the skull surface. This results in a hemorrhagic lesion diametrically opposed to the impact site. After impact, the brain may also become contused if it collides with bony protuberances on the inside surface of the skull. The frontal and temporal lobes are particularly susceptible to this type of injury; however, contusions can be observed in the midbrain and cerebellum, as well.

Contusions vary in size from small, localized areas to larger areas of injury (figure 12.1). The important aspect to remember about these types of brain injuries is that they can demonstrate progression over time with respect to size and number of contusions. This progression typically occurs over the first 24 to 48 hours, with a proportion of cases demonstrating delayed hemorrhage occurring in areas that were previously free of blood on imaging. Multiple smaller areas of contusion can coalesce into a larger-appearing lesion, more commonly referred to as an intraparenchymal hemorrhage. Contusions can be associated with other intra- or extra-axial hemorrhages, and skull fractures can be present quite frequently.

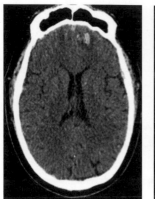
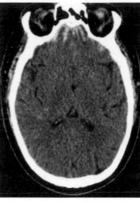

Figure 12.1 Representative axial computed tomography images demonstrating bifrontal hemorrhagic contusions.

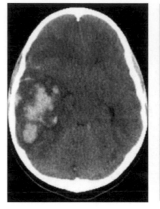
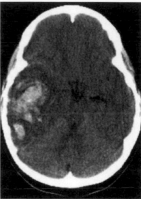

Figure 12.2 Representative axial CT images demonstrating an intraparenchymal hemorrhage in the right frontal, parietal, and temporal lobes.

The clinical course of these patients varies greatly depending on the location of the hemorrhagic lesion, as well as the number and extent of the hemorrhagic contusions. A patient can present with a neurological exam ranging from essentially normal to focal neurological deficits or even a coma. Involvement of the frontal and temporal lobes often results in behavioral or mental status changes. Some athletes have never suffered initial unconsciousness or focal neurological deficit but may have a headache or period of confusion after their head injury. The apparent failure to rapidly clear their mental status is usually what leads to the diagnosis. Diagnosis is usually made with a computed tomography (CT) scan, which is also frequently used for radiographic surveillance when following patients through their clinical course. Management is typically conservative with close observation, but depends on many factors including the size of the contusion, location, and the patient's clinical exam.

A traumatic intracerebral hemorrhage is a parenchymal lesion. It is very similar in radiographic appearance and pathophysiology to a contusion. It represents a localized collection of blood within the brain and is recognized as a confluent area of homogenous hemorrhage, which is what distinguishes it from a contusion (figure 12.2). As with cerebral contusions, diagnosis is readily established by CT scan. Patients usually present with focal neurological deficits but may progress to further neurological deterioration. Intraparenchymal hemorrhages are among the most common causes of lethal sport-related brain injuries.

Some patients present with a delayed intracerebral hemorrhage. This entity is typically seen in older patient populations but should be kept in mind during evaluation of any patient who has sustained a significant head impact and has delayed symptoms. The reported incidence varies with the resolution of the CT scanner, timing of the scan, and definition.[103] In those patients with a Glasgow Coma Scale (GCS) less than or equal to 8, the reported incidence is approximately 10%.[27, 32, 42, 48, 77, 96] The hemorrhage forms in the hours to days after the initial trauma, although most occur within 72 hours after the trauma.[26, 42] The athlete is generally at risk because these hematomas are seen more commonly when rotational head trauma has occurred. Factors believed to contribute to delayed traumatic intracerebral hemorrhage include local or systemic coagulopathy, hemorrhage into an already contused region of the brain or an area of necrotic brain softening, vascular injury, or coalescence of extravasated microhematomas.[26] The outcome reported in the literature has generally been poor for these patients.

TRAUMATIC SUBARACHNOID HEMORRHAGE

Another acute neurological injury observed in athletics is traumatic subarachnoid hemorrhage (SAH). As its name implies, traumatic SAH is bleeding into the fluid-filled space around the

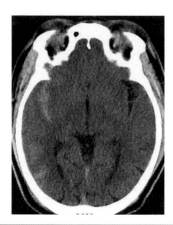

Figure 12.3 Representative axial CT image demonstrating traumatic subarachnoid hemorrhage along the right sylvian fissure.

brain called the subarachnoid space (figure 12.3). A large percentage of serious traumatic brain injuries involve some component of this type of bleeding. While the hemorrhage can cause meningeal irritation, the condition is usually not life threatening, and no immediate treatment is required for a good outcome. Larger amounts of SAH may lead to vasospasm, although this is more typically observed with spontaneous aneurysmal SAH. Communicating hydrocephalus can occur in a delayed fashion as a result of SAH and may clinically present with late clinical deterioration.

SUBDURAL HEMATOMA

Subdural hematomas (SDHs) are the most common form of serious and lethal brain injuries in athletics. A SDH is a collection of blood that occurs beneath the dura (which is the membrane overlying the brain). Subdural hematomas in younger athletes do not behave in the same manner as those usually seen in the elderly population. The younger athlete does not possess a large potential subdural space as elderly people do. As a result, mass effect, increases in intracranial pressure, and clinical deterioration occur much more rapidly. These hematomas can occur both acutely and chronically.

Acute SDHs usually present within 48 to 72 hours after a head injury. According to reports from the National Center for Catastrophic Sports Injury Research, an acute SDH is the most common cause of death due to head injury in sport.[73] With their research on American football players, Boden and colleagues demonstrated that 38% of athletes receiving such an injury were playing while still symptomatic from a prior head injury that season.[6] Acute SDHs can occur at any location in the brain and generally occur by two main mechanisms. These hemorrhages can result from a tearing of surface or bridging veins secondary to rotational acceleration-deceleration during violent head motion. With this etiology, primary brain damage may be less severe. The other common cause is a parenchymal laceration leading to a surrounding subdural accumulation of blood. In this case there is usually severe primary brain injury. Frequently, the athlete with a SDH has a small blood collection with underlying brain contusion and hemispheric swelling. In either case, significant associated underlying contusions or edema can further compound brain injury.

Chronic SDHs occur in a later time frame with more variable clinical manifestations. A chronic SDH is defined as a hematoma present at 3 weeks or more after a traumatic injury. The initial hemorrhage that occurs into the subdural space may be a small amount that fails to generate any significant brain compression and thus may not be identified early on. The bleeding or oozing of blood may continue, and by 4 to 7 days, a chronic SDH begins to involve the infiltration of fibroblasts to organize an outer membrane around the clot.[74] Subsequently, an inner membrane can form and turn the hematoma into an encapsulated osmotic membrane that interacts with the production and absorption of cerebrospinal fluid (CSF), creating an active dynamic process within the membrane layers.

Subdural hematomas can result in a wide variety of sequelae, ranging from mild symptoms such as headaches to focal neurological deficits and even death. Athletes may become unconscious or experience focal neurological deficits (or both) immediately, or symptoms may develop more insidiously over time. Typically athletes with any sizable acute SDH have a significant neurological deficit. Chronic SDHs have more protean clinical manifestations and may become symptomatic in a more insidious manner. Although not common in athletes, a chronic SDH must always be in the differential diagnosis, especially in those presenting with a remote history of head impact. Emergent CT diagnosis is mandatory for the expeditious and successful treatment of these patients. Acute SDHs appear as a crescent-shaped mass of increased attenuation (hyperdense), usually overlying the convexity of the brain, adjacent to the inner table of the skull[39, 40] (figure 12.4). However, acute SDHs can also be interhemispheric, along the tentorium, or in the posterior fossa. Chronic SDHs have a similar appearance, although they appear hypodense (approaching the appearance of CSF) on the CT scan (figure 12.5). Subdural hematomas in general differ from epidural hematomas in that they are more diffuse, less uniform in appearance, and usually concave over the surface of the brain.

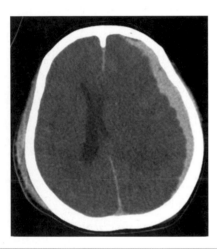

Figure 12.4 Representative axial CT image demonstrating a left frontoparietal, hyperdense, concave collection that is consistent with an acute subdural hematoma. Also note the midline shift to the right.

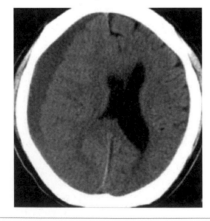

Figure 12.5 Representative axial CT image demonstrating a right frontoparietal, hypodense, concave collection that is consistent with a chronic subdural hematoma. Also note the midline shift to the left.

Patients with a suspected SDH should be immediately transported to a facility with neurosurgical services, where an emergent CT can be obtained and appropriate treatment carried out. Rapid surgical evacuation of the hematoma should be considered for symptomatic acute SDHs that are greater than about 1 cm at the thickest point (or greater than 5 mm in pediatric patients).[39, 40] In patients with an underlying brain contusion, surgical decompression and evacuation of the hematoma may not improve the symptoms due to the primary parenchymal injury.[3]

SKULL FRACTURES

Head injury resulting in the fracture of the skull is a common occurrence in sports, especially those in which helmets are not regularly employed. Additionally, any recreational or sporting activity in which inadvertent head impacts occur can predispose to skull fracture. Baseball, for example, is a sport in which an athlete on the field is unhelmeted and if hit in the head by a line drive could sustain a skull fracture. Not uncommonly, spectators are also at risk if struck in the head with a ball or puck. Diagnosis can be made with either plain skull radiographs or a CT scan; the latter can identify any underlying associated injuries.

Fractures can be linear or comminuted, and they can also be depressed or nondepressed. Linear skull fractures are common and can involve the frontal, parietal, temporal, or occipital bones (figure 12.6). They usually are the result of a direct blow to the skull. Linear skull fractures are not typically depressed, although they can be. They may occur with a concomitant overlying scalp laceration, in which case they are considered a compound fracture. More often than not, there is no misalignment of the bone edges, and the fractures are not generally considered serious. They are more important as markers of potential underlying cerebral injury given the large magnitude of blunt force necessary to create the fracture. Injury to blood vessels in close proximity can also occur. Most linear, nondepressed skull fractures do not require specific treatment other than conservative observation for any neurological dysfunction or deterioration. These fractures can heal within several months to years and, in the absence of any other issues, often do not prevent the athlete from resuming participation, even in contact sports.

Fractures can also be comminuted and depressed. Depressed, comminuted skull fractures, like linear fractures, can occur to any of the surface bones of the skull (figure 12.7). They usually occur when a relatively small object makes impact with the skull, resulting in the depression of the underlying bone. Impacts with large objects (stationary or moving) can also result in these complex fractures. Bone fragments can separate and be driven deep, potentially lacerating the underlying dura or even invading the brain surface itself. Many patients with depressed skull fractures do not have significant brain injury; however, hematomas, CSF leak, or infection may occur. In contrast to linear skull fractures, comminuted or depressed skull frac-

tures often require treatment based on the location, contamination, potential regarding cosmetic appearance, and degree of skull depression.

EPIDURAL HEMATOMA

Skull fractures that cross the bony grooves harboring blood vessels may cause bony fragments to lacerate the meningeal vessels, resulting in an epidural hematoma (EDH). Epidural hematomas are not an uncommon occurrence secondary to traumatic brain injury in athletes, especially in sports in which the participants are not helmeted such as baseball or golf, although they occur less commonly than acute SDH. The overall incidence of EDH is 1% of head trauma admissions, which is approximately 50% of the incidence of acute SDH.[39, 40]

An EDH is a collection of blood that occurs between the dura and the skull (figure 12.8). Blood accumulates between the skull and outside the dura, with the dura dissecting until the point of dural attachment to the overlying cranium. The bleeding is frequently arterial and fails to tamponade quickly because of the high arterial pressure. Approximately 85% of EDHs are due to arterial bleeding; the middle meningeal artery is the most common source of middle fossa EDHs.[39, 40] The remainder of cases are mainly due to bleeding from the middle meningeal vein or dural sinuses. It is important to note that fractured bone

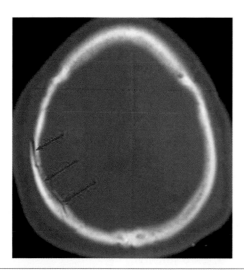

Figure 12.6 Representative axial CT image demonstrating a right-sided linear skull fracture (arrows).

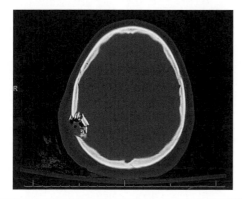

Figure 12.7 Representative axial CT image demonstrating a depressed occipital skull fracture (arrows).
Courtesy of University of Rochester Medical Center.

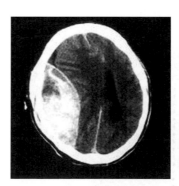
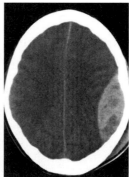

Figure 12.8 Representative axial CT images demonstrating (on the left) a large right frontotemporal, hyperdense, biconvex collection that is consistent with an acute epidural hematoma. The darker (hypodense) areas within the hematoma represent hyperacute hemorrhage. Also note the significant midline shift to the left. On the right is a left frontal epidural hematoma with a typical "lentiform" appearance.

edges or bleeding from a diploic space can also result in significant epidural hemorrhage, especially in the pediatric population. A skull fracture is present in approximately 75% of patients with an EDH.[53, 76] The majority (70%) of cases occur laterally over the hemisphere with their epicenter at the pterion.[39, 40] Epidural hematomas can also occur in the frontal, occipital, and posterior fossa.

The classic clinical picture of a patient with an EDH involves a brief posttraumatic loss of consciousness (LOC), secondary to the force of impact. This is usually followed by arousal to an essentially normal level of consciousness. This is often referred to as a "lucid interval," which can last a variable period of time. A short time thereafter, the athlete may experience a sudden, excruciating headache followed by a progressive neurological deterioration. The patient will progress to obtundation, contralateral hemiparesis, and ipsilateral (same side as clot) pupillary dilation. If this remains untreated, the patient can go on to exhibit decerebrate posturing-rigidity, hypertension, respiratory distress, and death (secondary to brain herniation).[39, 40] While classically clinically characterized this way, a true "lucid interval" and "textbook" presentation occurs in less than 10% to 27% of patients with an EDH,[3, 39, 40] although it has been characterized in some studies as occurring in as many as 47% of patients.[1] The clinical manifestations of EDH depend on the type of head injury, forces imparted, and time course of the hematoma formation.

Any patient or athlete who has sustained a significant head impact such that a significant LOC or neurological deficit is present should undergo a more immediate and thorough medical evaluation including a CT scan. Epidural hematomas generally (85% of the time) have a classic appearance of a hyperdense, biconvex (lenticular) shape adjacent to the skull on head CT scans[39] (figure 12.8). Mass effect is also frequently associated with EDH. Management can vary from observation to surgical evacuation of the EDH and depends on the presence of symptoms, size of the EDH, and age of the patient. It is essential to recognize this injury early on in order to commence appropriate management. If it is treated early, complete neurological recovery can typically be expected, as EDHs are usually not associated with other underlying brain injuries.

DIFFUSE AXONAL INJURY

Diffuse axonal injury (DAI) is a less localized but more severe type of acute neurological injury that can occur in sport. It is a type of injury seen most commonly in victims of motor vehicle accidents due to significant acceleration–deceleration forces but is occasionally seen in severe athletic-related head trauma as well. Diffuse axonal injury occurs in half of patients with severe TBI and is responsible for one-third of all head injury-related deaths.[34] It is the most common cause of persistent vegetative state and significant disability following traumatic brain injury.

Diffuse axonal injury is the result of shearing of multiple axons secondary to rotational forces (acceleration) on the brain. Parts of the brain such as the cortex (gray matter) and white matter have various densities and different physical properties that accelerate at different speeds upon impact, resulting in shearing. There is usually a lack of a mass lesion with severe DAI. Additionally, the rotational acceleration of the head results in a swirling motion of the brain around pedicles of blood vessels. A consequence of such an injury is punctuate hemorrhages from small vessel tears, in addition to the diffuse tearing of white matter fiber tracts (figure 12.9). Management varies based on the clinical manifestations and the severity of the pathophysiology, which can occur along a spectrum from mild to severe.

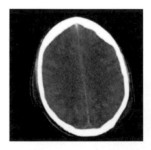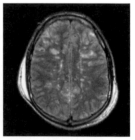

Figure 12.9 Diffuse axonal injury in a comatose patient 2 days after a motor vehicle accident. Computed tomography scan displays minimal shear and often can appear quite normal (left). The corresponding T2-weighted MRI image (right) reveals extensive bilateral foci of microhemorrhage.

Reprinted from Seminars in Pediatric Surgery, 19(4), S.E. Morrow and M. Pearson, "Management strategies for severe closed head injuries in children," pgs. 279-285, copyright 2010, with permission from Elsevier.

ARTERIAL DISSECTION AND STROKE

Athletic trainers, team physicians, pediatricians, or emergency room physicians are the first providers to see athletes with sport-related stroke. Thus, it is particularly important that these professionals be aware of the possibility of ischemic stroke occurring after any form of head or neck athletic injury. Any athlete with recent head or neck trauma who presents with acute stroke-like symptoms should be immediately evaluated for possible acute ischemic stroke.[29, 82]

Craniocervical arterial dissection is a condition in which the layers of blood vessel separate from each other, either spontaneously or secondary to trauma. Most often this separation occurs between the intima and media, and it is often associated with a tear in the luminal lining of the intima. Craniocervical arterial dissection and stroke has been reported in a wide spectrum of athletic activities; among these are soccer, boxing, wakeboarding, mixed martial arts, scuba diving, treadmill running, triathlon, springboard diving, taekwondo, rugby, winter activities, baseball, golf, volleyball, and softball.[4, 24, 31, 36, 37, 43, 51, 56, 62, 70, 72, 75, 78, 80, 84-86, 88, 90, 92, 94, 100]

Injuries to the head that cause sudden flexion or extremely rapid rotation of the neck can tear the intima of the carotid or vertebral arteries. Injuries to these vessels must not be overlooked as potential acute neurological injuries. Such tears or dissections can extend near the skull base, resulting in vessel occlusion and possible cerebral ischemia or infarction. Stroke is the most significant complication of craniocervical arterial dissection. Dissection occurs more commonly in the extracranial carotid and vertebral arteries as compared to the intracranial portions of these vessels. Cervical internal carotid artery dissections occur typically 2 cm distal to the bifurcation and may extend distally for a variable distance (figure 12.10). Extracranial vertebral artery dissection commonly involves the V3 segment at the C1-C2 levels, where it is most susceptible to mechanical trauma (figure 12.11).

Athletes with craniocervical arterial dissections can present with nonspecific complaints and in all settings. Maintaining a high index of suspicion for carotid or vertebral artery dissection is critical whenever a patient presents with

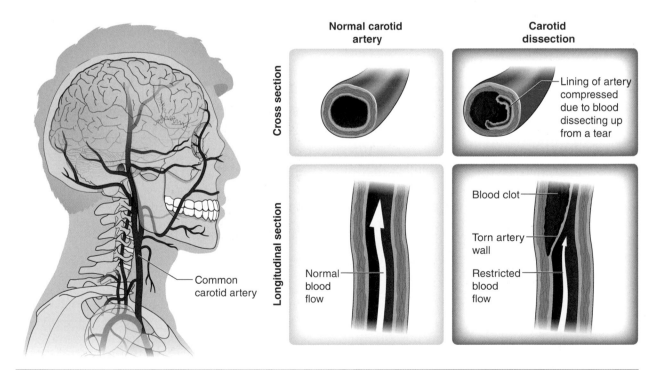

Figure 12.10 Illustration of a carotid dissection.

Vertebral Artery Dissection with Development of Emboli Resulting in Cerebral Infarction

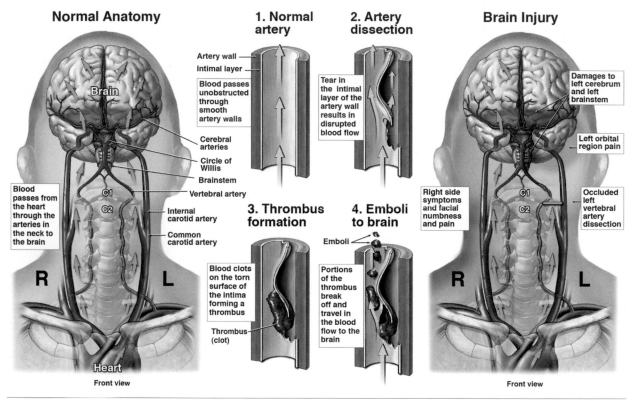

Figure 12.11 Vertebral artery dissection.

unusual focal neurological complaints, particularly if the cranial nerves are involved and if the patient has a suspicious mechanism of trauma. A history of cervical hyperextension, flexion, or rotation should alert the physician to the possibility of dissection. That being said, a direct impact on the neck can also result in a dissection or arterial injury. One example is that of a lacrosse player who was struck in the back of the neck with a ball and sustained a vertebral artery dissection with diffuse subarachnoid hemorrhage and subsequently progressed to death (figure 12.12). Injury to the craniocervical vessels can occur in sports typically felt to be benign, such as golf. "Golfer's stroke" has been described by Maroon and colleagues,[62] as well as others,[24, 46, 93] and can result in injury or dissection to either the vertebral or carotid arteries with the minor repetitive neck motion used in golf.

The diagnosis of an arterial dissection or a significant hemodynamic process or injury may require multiple imaging modalities. While catheter angiography is still considered the gold standard, recent evidence in the literature suggests that magnetic resonance imaging (MRI), computed tomography angiogram (CTa), or both provide highly sensitive and specific diagnostic information.[23] Thus, catheter angiography may be needed only in cases in which noninvasive imaging is negative or inconclusive.[98] It should be noted that vertebral artery dissections represent a greater diagnostic challenge than carotid dissections for both MRI (e.g., flow artifacts and periarterial venous enhancement simulating a mural hematoma) and CTa (bone artifact, particularly at the skull base).[82]

Expeditious identification and management are essential for good outcome. There are no clear recommendations to guide return to participation. Most agree that patients can be encouraged to participate in noncontact and low-contact sports. Some have suggested waiting at least 6

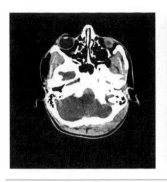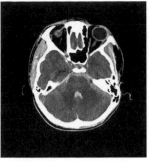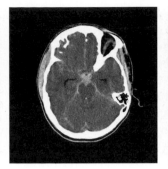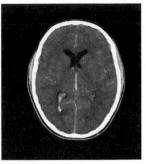

Figure 12.12   Representative axial CT images in an athlete who was struck in the back of the neck with a ball and who presented to the hospital emergently for rapid neurological deterioration. The patient was found to have significant subarachnoid and intraventricular hemorrhage throughout the basal cisterns and ventricular system, secondary to a traumatic vertebral artery dissection.

months before resumption of contact sports, while others have reported that they would never recommend participation in high-contact sports after arterial dissection and acute ischemic stroke. [5] There seems to be more hesitation about letting a patient with an arterial dissection return to athletics in comparison to a patient with idiopathic stroke.[5] Though most studies find that the recurrence risk for arterial dissection is approximately 1% per year,[23] the recurrence risk in athletes (particularly children) with sport-related stroke may be higher, with rates of up to 30% having been cited.[5, 55, 82]

Other less common mechanisms of injury to the craniocervical arteries have been described. Bow hunter's stroke is a symptomatic vertebra-basilar insufficiency caused by stenosis or occlusion of the vertebral artery with physiologic head rotation.[87] In 1978, Sorensen coined the term bow hunter's stroke to refer to the sudden onset of right-sided hemiparesis, contralateral hemisensory changes, and a dilated right pupil in a 39-year-old man after he turned his head during archery practice.[87] Since that time, additional series have described patients with bow hunter's stroke who presented with either a completed stroke or transient ischemic attack (TIA) referable to changes in head position.[35, 38, 44, 57, 64, 83, 101] It is important to note that although the term stroke is used throughout the literature to refer to the condition, the condition encompasses a wide spectrum of rotational hemodynamic insufficiency ranging from a TIA to an acute ischemic stroke.[54] Various other pathologic conditions have been reported as causes of bow hunter's stroke, including far lateral cervical disc herniation reported by Vates and coauthors[97] and

C1-C2 facet hypertrophy reported by Chough and colleagues.[25] Bow hunter's stroke most commonly occurs at the junction of C1 and C2 and less commonly as the vertebral artery enters the C6 transverse foramen.[69] The predominance of this site for occlusion is accounted for by the immobilization of the vertebral artery at the transverse foramina of C1 and C2 and along the sulcus arteriosus to where it inserts into the dura. [54] Management has varied from conservative treatment with anticoagulation to surgical fixation and fusion at C1-C2. An alternative treatment is surgical decompression of the vertebral artery at the site of compression. The long-term outcome of patients with this disease is not clearly understood given the overall rarity of the condition; however, any intervention that alleviates the compression and restores blood flow should significantly improve outcomes.[54]

FATALITIES

While participation in sport is usually regarded as healthy and safe, athletes are nevertheless subject to an unpredictable risk of sudden death during participation.[58, 95] Although most data regarding these tragic events have had to do with cardiovascular causes,[59-61] neurological injury can also lead to fatalities.[21, 22]

An excellent recent study by Thomas and colleagues sought to define the clinical profile, epidemiology, and frequency of trauma-related deaths in young U.S. athletes by analyzing the 30-year U.S. National Registry of Sudden Death in Young Athletes (1980-2009) using systematic identification and tracking strategies.[95] Of the

1,827 deaths of athletes aged 21 years or younger, 261 (14%) were caused by trauma-related injuries, usually involving the head or neck.[95] This was noted in 22 different sports. The majority (90%) of deaths occurred in male athletes. The highest number of events in a single year was 16, with an average of 9 athletic trauma-related deaths per year throughout 30 years.[95] The mortality rate in this retrospective study was 0.11 per 100,000 participations. Sports in which trauma-related deaths occurred included track and field (predominantly pole vaulting), baseball, soccer, horseback riding, skiing, gymnastics, softball, basketball, cheerleading, hockey, wrestling, cycling, lacrosse, triathlon or cross country running, rugby, surfing, weightlifting, American football, and boxing. The largest number of deaths was in American football, accounting for 148 fatalities (57%), including 17 deaths in which there were documented concussions shortly before a fatal head injury ("second impact syndrome").[95] Trauma-related deaths, in this review, occurred either in competitive events (62%) or during practice (38%).[95] The majority of the trauma-related deaths were due to injury of the head, neck, or both (89% of trauma-related deaths), with other deaths resulting from abdominal, thoracic, or multiple organ damage. These data corroborate findings from other similar studies. [6-14, 21, 22]

Boxing is another sport that has received substantial attention in the media for sport-related fatalities in recent years. Unfortunately, there is a paucity of validated epidemiological data on which to accurately base boxing fatality rates. [66-68] Instead, many of the reported fatality data have been obtained from a combination of media sources, industry reports, and individual case reports. From what can be ascertained based on the available reviews of boxing deaths, it appears that the rate of boxing fatalities has declined over the last few decades and that this can in part be attributed to rule changes, as well as medical advances that have improved both the diagnosis and treatment of the acutely injured fighter. The majority of boxing fatalities result from SDHs, and typically these are associated with an immediate LOC during the fight. While death as a result of participation in boxing and other combat sports has received plenty of media attention, the fatality rate in boxing actually compares favorably to that in many other sports receiving less attention with respect to participant safety, such as horse racing, sky diving, hang gliding, and mountaineering.

Miele and Bailes analyzed the number and types of punches landed in a typical professional match, in bouts considered to be competitive and in those that ended in fatalities, to determine whether or not this would be a practical method of differentiating between these groups. [66] Several statistically significant differences were discovered between matches that resulted in fatalities and the control group; these included the number of punches landed per round, the number of power punches landed per round, and the number of power punches thrown per round by losing boxers.[66] When the fatal bouts were compared with the most competitive bouts, though, these differences were no longer evident. Thus, based on their findings, the authors concluded that a computerized method of counting landed blows at ringside could provide sufficient data to stop matches that might result in fatalities; however, such a process would become less effective as matches became more competitive.[66]

OTHER POSTTRAUMATIC SEQUELAE

Posttraumatic seizures are thought to occur in approximately 5% of all patients with cranial cerebral trauma and approximately 15% of those with severe head injuries, although these may be underestimates. Certain factors in TBI predispose the athlete to developing posttraumatic epilepsy. Patients with lesions such as a contusion or hematoma (particularly in the temporal lobe), those with a depressed skull fracture impinging on the cortical surface, and those experiencing delayed seizures (later than 1 week following trauma) are believed to have a higher incidence of posttraumatic epilepsy.

In the setting of TBI, seizures can occur at a variety of time points. "Impact seizures" occur immediately at the time of trauma and are believed to occur secondary to altered electromechanical conductance due to the impact. "Immediate seizures" occur within the first 24 hours after trauma, while "early seizures" occur within the first week after TBI. "Later seizures" occur at a time remote from the initial injury and are most typically considered to be congruent with posttraumatic epilepsy. While the use of prophylactic anticonvulsants (such as phenytoin) in patients believed to be at greater risk for developing posttraumatic seizures has helped reduce the incidence of seizures within the first week, there is no effect on the development of seizures in a delayed fashion. The management of patients with posttraumatic epilepsy follows the guidelines for the treatment of patients with epilepsy of nontraumatic origin.

Another sequela of TBI includes posttraumatic hydrocephalus. Hydrocephalus is the enlargement of the ventricular system (figure 12.13). This typically occurs only with more severe forms of TBI. The incidence of posttraumatic ventriculomegaly has been reported to range from 30% to 86%.[49] The enlargement can represent ventriculomegaly alone or symptomatic hydrocephalus.[41] Particularly following severe TBI, it is not uncommon to see loss of cerebral tissue. Imaging with CT or MRI demonstrates areas of porencephaly, venous–arterial infarction, or atrophy.[41] The loss of tissue allows for passive dilation of the ventricular system as the ventricles expand to fill a void. Diagnosis is typically made clinically with the aid of imaging. Sometimes the presentation is as subtle as a leveling off of neurological improvement in the rehabilitation of TBI. Some of these patients can improve with procedures such as a ventriculoperitoneal shunt, which is commonly used to divert cerebrospinal fluid away from the point of obstruction.

Another rare complication of traumatic brain injury is cerebral venous sinus thrombosis (CVST). Cerebral venous sinus thrombosis is rare,

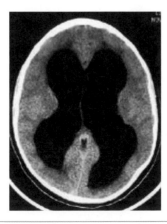

Figure 12.13 Representative axial CT image demonstrating significantly enlarged lateral ventricles.

with an incidence of around three or four cases per million people.[30] Overall, in adults, 75% of CVST cases occur in females.[89] Clinically, CVST can present with a variety of symptoms. More commonly patients present with a headache that develops over several days; much less commonly, with an acute decrease in consciousness. In some cases, CVST can result in death. While most cases of CVST are idiopathic or associated with thrombophilia, pregnancy, or chronic inflammatory conditions, a rare cause that is often overlooked is traumatic closed head injury. There have been several reports of CVST associated with TBI.[2, 15, 45, 52, 63, 102] Cases are sometimes associated with an overlying skull fracture, and many may even be small and go unrecognized.[102] The actual occurrence in traumatic injuries may be higher than realized if overlooked in the acute TBI setting. One retrospective review study of 195 patients with acute traumatic head injuries identified 15.8% of patients as having an occlusive CVST on imaging.[28] Imaging studies should be carried out to enable prompt and exacting management. Treatment with thrombolytics or other potential interventional procedures may be required to prevent serious neurological consequences or even death.

SECOND IMPACT SYNDROME

The term second impact syndrome (SIS) was coined in 1984 by Saunders and Harbaugh[79]; however, the phenomenon was actually first described in 1973 by renowned neurosurgeon Richard C. Schneider.[20, 81] Second impact syndrome is defined as a fatal, malignant, and uncontrollable increase in intracranial pressure caused by diffuse cerebral edema that occurs after a head impact has been sustained before complete recovery from a previous head trauma. The syndrome occurs when an athlete experiences a head injury, possibly a concussion or even worse, and then sustains a second injury before the symptoms associated with the first injury have cleared.[17-20] The second blow may be remarkably minor and involve only a blow to the chest or torso that may impart forces to the brain.[20] The affected athlete does not necessarily lose consciousness and in most cases even remains on the playing field or walks off under his own power. Then the stunned but conscious athlete, in a matter of seconds to minutes, may precipitously collapse to the ground, with rapidly dilating pupils, loss of eye movement, and evidence of respiratory failure.[17-20]

Significant controversy exists about the validity of this condition, and its precise frequency in sport is unknown; however, numerous cases have been reported in the literature, and most involve adolescent males or young adults.[18, 20, 33, 50, 65, 71, 99] The precise incidence per 100,000 participants is not known because the population at risk has not been clearly defined. Second impact syndrome is associated with a high mortality rate (approaching 50%) and a nearly 100% morbidity rate.[19] It is an important acute neurological injury to keep in mind when one is making return-to-play decisions about an athlete who has suffered a TBI, as clearly prevention is of utmost importance.

The pathophysiological mechanism is thought to involve a dysfunction or loss of autoregulation of the cerebral vasculature, leading to vascular engorgement and diffuse cerebral edema.[20, 47, 91] This hyperemic brain swelling markedly increases intracranial pressure and can lead to brain herniation syndromes. The increased pressure can cause subsequent inferomedial herniation of the temporal lobes (transtentorial herniation),

subfalcine herniation, or herniation of the cerebellar tonsils through the foramen magnum with resultant brain stem compression (figure 12.14). The deterioration is extremely rapid and often faster than that seen with EDHs. While MRI can more precisely delineate and characterize the injury, CT scanning is the initial imaging modality of choice because it can rapidly identify a potential lesion or brain shift that may require neurosurgical intervention.[99] On imaging, the brain appears edematous with a hemispheric asymmetry; and there is often a small SDH that can be associated with the injury (figure 12.15). The notable finding is that the shift is out of proportion to the amount of SDH present. The basal cisterns may be effaced due to temporal lobe or diencephalic herniation.[20] If the patient survives the initial episode of intracranial hypertension, multifocal bilateral nonhemorrhagic infarction ensues. This highlights the importance of early recognition because there is usually little primary brain injury, and serious or fatal neurological outcomes are due to secondary brain injury from raised intracranial pressure and resultant brain herniation. Prompt treatment with intubation, hyperventilation, osmotic agents, and surgical intervention (if ultimately needed) has helped to reduce the mortality associated with SIS.[16, 19]

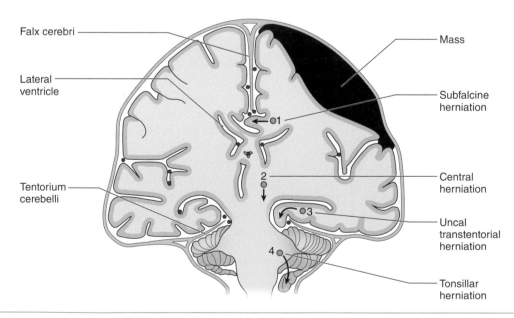

Figure 12.14 A mass lesion (like a large hematoma) or significant cerebral edema can cause the brain to herniate in many different ways, as illustrated, with resultant brain compression.

Reprinted, by permission, from B. Blumenfeld, 2002, Neuroanatomy through clinical cases (Sunderland, MA: Sinauer Associates, Inc.).

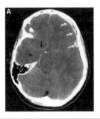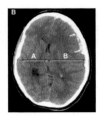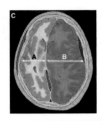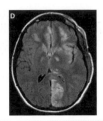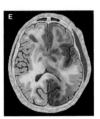

Figure 12.15 Typical imaging findings of dysautoregulation/second impact syndrome (DSIS). (a, b) Admission non-contrast axial CT images and (c) artist's rendition demonstrate a small heterogeneous left frontal subdural hematoma (SDH; white arrows) that causes complete effacement of the basal cisterns and brain stem distortion. Note the subtle linear increased density in the region of the circle of Willis (black arrow), consistent with "pseudosubarachnoid hemorrhage," resulting from the marked elevation in intracranial pressure. Although preservation of the gray–white matter differentiation is seen, there is asymmetric enlargement of the left hemisphere, consistent with hyperemic cerebral swelling (dysautoregulation). Note that (a) is smaller than (b) even though the left hemisphere is mildly compressed by the overlying SDH. The extent of mass effect and midline shift is disproportional to the volume of the SDH (compare with figures 12.3 and 12.4). This 3-day-postoperative Fluid attenuated inversion recovery (FLAIR) magnetic resonance image (d) and artist's rendition (e) demonstrate bilateral multifocal ischemic lesions involving several vascular territories, including the left posterior cerebral artery, thalamus, insular cortex, basal ganglia, and orbitofrontal cortex.

Reprinted, by permission, from R. Cantu and A.D. Gean, 2010, "Second-impact syndrome and a small subdural hematoma: An uncommon catastrophic result of repetitive head injury with a characteristic imaging appearance," Journal of Neurotrauma 27(9): 1557-1564. The publisher for this copyrighted material is Mary Ann Liebert, Inc. publishers.

CONCLUDING THOUGHTS

While the incidence of severe head injury has decreased, it is important for caregivers at athletic contests to be cognizant of the spectrum of injuries that occur in response to brain trauma. Two important goals in evaluating the potentially head-injured athlete include recognizing that a head injury may have occurred and that athletes requiring transport to a medical facility for further workup and treatment must be accurately identified. While mild traumatic brain injury or concussion occurs more frequently and has received a lot of attention lately, other injuries include intracranial hemorrhage, subdural hematomas, epidural hematomas, skull fractures, neurovascular injury, and diffuse axonal injury and can even result in death. Although extremely rare, second impact syndrome is deadly, and concern regarding its occurrence has shaped the conservative, modern-day management of mild traumatic brain injury.

REFERENCES

1. Araujo JL, Aguiar Udo P, Todeschini AB, Saade N, Veiga JC. Epidemiological analysis of 210 cases of surgically treated traumatic extradural hematoma. Rev Col Bras Cir 2012;39(4):268-271.

2. Barbati G, Dalla Monta G, Coletta R, Blasetti AG. Post-traumatic superior sagittal sinus thrombosis. Case report and analysis of the international literature. Minerva Anestesiol 2003;69(12):919-925.

3. Begso JJ, Lehman RC. Field evaluation and management of head and neck injuries. Clin Sports Med 1987;6:1.

4. Benedict WJ, Prabhu V, Viola M, Biller J. Carotid artery pseudoaneurysm resulting from an injury to the neck by a fouled baseball. J Neurol Sci 2007;256(1-2):94-99.

5. Bernard TJ, deVeber GA, Benke TA. Athletic participation after acute ischemic childhood stroke: a survey of pediatric stroke experts. J Child Neurol 2007;22(8):1050-1053.

6. Boden B, Tacchetti R, Cantu R, Knowles S, Mueller F. Catastrophic head injuries in high school and college football players. Am J Sports Med 2000;35:1-7.

7. Boden BP. Direct catastrophic injury in sports. J Am Acad Orthop Surg 2005;13(7):445-454.

8. Boden BP, Boden MG, Peter RG, Mueller FO, Johnson JE. Catastrophic injuries in pole vaulters: a prospective 9-year follow-up study. Am J Sports Med 2012;40(7):1488-1494.

9. Boden BP, Lin W, Young M, Mueller FO. Catastrophic injuries in wrestlers. Am J Sports Med 2002;30(6):791-795.

10. Boden BP, Pasquina P, Johnson J, Mueller FO. Catastrophic injuries in pole-vaulters. Am J Sports Med 2001;29(1):50-54.

11. Boden BP, Tacchetti R, Mueller FO. Catastrophic cheerleading injuries. Am J Sports Med 2003;31(6):881-888.

12. Boden BP, Tacchetti R, Mueller FO. Catastrophic injuries in high school and college baseball players. Am J Sports Med 2004;32(5):1189-1196.

13. Boden BP, Tacchetti RL, Cantu RC, Knowles SB, Mueller FO. Catastrophic cervical spine injuries in high school and college football players. Am J Sports Med 2006;34(8):1223-1232.

14. Boden BP, Tacchetti RL, Cantu RC, Knowles SB, Mueller FO. Catastrophic head injuries in high school and college football players. Am J Sports Med 2007;35(7):1075-1081.

15. Brors D, Schafers M, Schick B, Dazert S, Draf W, Kahle G. Sigmoid and transverse sinus thrombosis after closed head injury presenting with unilateral hearing loss. Neuroradiology 2001;43(2):144-146.

16. Bruce DA, Alavi A, Bilaniuk L, Dolinskas C, Obrist W, Uzzell B. Diffuse cerebral swelling following head injuries in children: the syndrome of "malignant brain edema." J Neurosurg 1981;54(2):170-178.

17. Cantu RC. Second impact syndrome a risk in any contact sport. Phys Sportsmed 1995;23:27-34.

18. Cantu RC. Second impact syndrome: immediate management. Phys Sportsmed 1992;20:55-58.

19. Cantu RC. Second-impact syndrome. Clin Sports Med 1998;17(1):37-44.

20. Cantu RC, Gean AD. Second-impact syndrome and a small subdural hematoma: an uncommon catastrophic result of repetitive head injury with a characteristic imaging appearance. J Neurotrauma 2010;27(9):1557-1564.

21. Cantu RC, Mueller FO. Brain injury-related fatalities in American football, 1945-1999. Neurosurgery 2003;52(4):846-852; discussion 852-843.

22. Cantu RC, Mueller FO. Catastrophic football injuries: 1977-1998. Neurosurgery 2000;47(3):673-675; discussion 675-677.

23. Caplan LR. Dissections of brain-supplying arteries. Nat Clin Pract Neurol 2008;4(1):34-42.

24. Choi KD, Oh SJ, Yang TI, Lee TH. Golfer's stroke from internal carotid artery dissection. Arch Neurol 2008;65(8):1122-1123.

25. Chough CK, Cheng BC, Welch WC, Park CK. Bow hunter's stroke caused by a severe facet hypertrophy of C1-2. J Korean Neurosurg Soc 2010;47(2):134-136.

26. Cooper PR. Delayed traumatic intracerebral hemorrhage. Neurosurg Clin N Am 1992;3(3):659-665.

27. Cooper PR, Maravilla K, Moody S, Clark WK. Serial computerized tomographic scanning and the prognosis of severe head injury. Neurosurgery 1979;5(5):566-569.

28. Delgado Almandoz JE, Kelly HR, Schaefer PW, Lev MH, Gonzalez RG, Romero JM. Prevalence of traumatic dural venous sinus thrombosis in high-risk acute blunt head trauma patients evaluated with multidetector CT venography. Radiology 2010;255(2):570-577.

29. Dharmasaroja P, Dharmasaroja P. Sports-related internal carotid artery dissection: pathogenesis and therapeutic point of view. Neurologist 2008;14(5):307-311.

30. Dobbs TD, Barber ZE, Squier WL, Green AL. Cerebral venous sinus thrombosis complicating traumatic head injury. J Clin Neurosci 2012;19(7):1058-1059.

31. Echaniz-Laguna A, Fleury MC, Petrow P, Arnould G, Beaujeux R, Warter JM. Internal carotid artery dissection caused by a kick during French boxing. Presse Med 2001;30(14):683.

32. Erol FS, Kaplan M, Topsakal C, Ozveren MF, Tiftikci MT. Coexistence of rapidly resolving acute subdural hematoma and delayed traumatic intracerebral hemorrhage. Pediatr Neurosurg 2004;40(5):238-240.

33. Fekete JF. Severe brain injury and death following minor hockey accidents: the effectiveness of the "safety helmets" of amateur hockey players. Can Med Assoc J 1968;99(25):1234-1239.

34. Fick DS. Management of concussion in collision sports. Guidelines for the sidelines. Postgrad Med 1995;97(2):53-56, 59-60.

35. Fox MW, Piepgras DG, Bartleson JD. Anterolateral decompression of the atlantoaxial vertebral artery for symptomatic positional occlusion of the vertebral artery. Case report. J Neurosurg 1995;83(4):737-740.

36. Fridley J, Mackey J, Hampton C, Duckworth E, Bershad E. Internal carotid artery dissection and stroke associated with wakeboarding. J Clin Neurosci 2011;18(9):1258-1260.

37. Furtner M, Werner P, Felber S, Schmidauer C. Bilateral carotid artery dissection caused by springboard diving. Clin J Sport Med 2006;16(1):76-78.

38. George B, Laurian C. Impairment of vertebral artery flow caused by extrinsic lesions. Neurosurgery 1989;24(2):206-214.

39. Greenberg MS, Arredondo N. Handbook of Neurosurgery. 6th ed. Lakeland, FL/New York: Greenberg Graphics/Thieme Medical; 2006.

40. Greenberg MS. Handbook of Neurosurgery. 7th ed. Tampa, FL: Greenberg Graphics; 2010.

41. Gudeman SK, Kishore PR, Becker DP, Lipper MH, Girevendulis AK, Jeffries BF, et al. Computed tomography in the evaluation of incidence and significance of post-traumatic hydrocephalus. Radiology 1981;141(2):397-402.

42. Gudeman SK, Kishore PR, Miller JD, Girevendulis AK, Lipper MH, Becker DP. The genesis and significance of delayed traumatic intracerebral hematoma. Neurosurgery 1979;5(3):309-313.

43. Hafner F, Gary T, Harald F, Pilger E, Groell R, Brodmann M. Dissection of the internal carotid artery after SCUBA-diving: a case report and review of the literature. Neurologist 2011;17(2):79-82.

44. Hanakita J, Miyake H, Nagayasu S, Nishi S, Suzuki T. Angiographic examination and surgical treatment of bow hunter's stroke. Neurosurgery 1988;23(2):228-232.

45. Hesselbrock R, Sawaya R, Tomsick T, Wadhwa S. Superior sagittal sinus thrombosis after closed head injury. Neurosurgery 1985;16(6):825-828.

46. Hong JM, Kim TJ, Lee JS, Lee JS. Neurological picture. Repetitive internal carotid artery compression of the hyoid: a new mechanism of golfer's stroke? J Neurology Neurosurg Psychiatry 2011;82(2):233-234.

47. Junger EC, Newell DW, Grant GA, Avellino AM, Ghatan S, Douville CM, et al. Cerebral autoregulation following minor head injury. J Neurosurg 1997;86(3):425-432.

48. Kaplan M, Ozveren MF, Topsakal C, Erol FS, Akdemir I. Asymptomatic interval in delayed traumatic intracerebral hemorrhage: report of two cases. Clin Neurol Neurosurg 2003;105(3):153-155.

49. Katz RT, Brander V, Sahgal V. Updates on the diagnosis and management of posttraumatic hydrocephalus. Am J Phys Med Rehabil 1989;68(2):91-96.

50. Kelly JP, Nichols JS, Filley CM, Lillehei KO, Rubinstein D, Kleinschmidt-DeMasters BK. Concussion in sports. Guidelines for the prevention of catastrophic outcome. JAMA 1991;266(20):2867-2869.

51. Kocyigit A, Cinar C, Kitis O, Calli C, Oran I. Isolated PICA dissection: an unusual complication of scuba diving: case report and review of the literature. Clin Neuroradiol 2010;20(3):171-173.

52. Kuether TA, O'Neill O, Nesbit GM, Barnwell SL. Endovascular treatment of traumatic dural sinus thrombosis: case report. Neurosurgery 1998;42(5):1163-1166; discussion 1166-1167.

53. Kvarnes TL, Trumpy JH. Extradural haematoma. Report of 132 cases. Acta Neurochir 1978;41(1-3):223-231.

54. Lemole GM Jr, Henn JS, Spetzler RF, Zabramski JM. Bow hunter's stroke. BNI Q2001;17:4-10..

55. Lynch JK, Pavlakis S, Deveber G. Treatment and prevention of cerebrovascular disorders in children. Curr Treat Options Neurol 2005;7(6):469-480.

56. Macdonald DJ, McKillop EC. Carotid artery dissection after treadmill running. Br J Sports Med 2006;40(4):e10; discussion e10.

57. Mapstone T, Spetzler RF. Vertebrobasilar insufficiency secondary to vertebral artery occlusion froma fibrous band. Case report. J Neurosurg 1982;56(4):581-583.

58. Maron BJ. Sudden death in young athletes. New Engl J Med 2003;349(11):1064-1075.

59. Maron BJ, Doerer JJ, Haas TS, Tierney DM, Mueller FO. Sudden deaths in young competitive athletes: analysis of 1866 deaths in the United States, 1980-2006. Circulation 2009;119(8):1085-1092.

60. Maron BJ, Haas TS, Doerer JJ, Thompson PD, Hodges JS. Comparison of U.S. and Italian experiences with sudden cardiac deaths in young competitive athletes and implications for preparticipation screening strategies. Am J Cardiol 2009;104(2):276-280.

61. Maron BJ, Shirani J, Poliac LC, Mathenge R, Roberts WC, Mueller FO. Sudden death in young competitive athletes. Clinical, demographic, and pathological profiles. JAMA 1996;276(3):199-204.

62. Maroon JC, Gardner P, Abla AA, El-Kadi H, Bost J. "Golfer's stroke": golf-induced stroke from vertebral artery dissection. Surg Neurol 2007;67(2):163-168; discussion 168.

63. Matsushige T, Nakaoka M, Kiya K, Takeda T, Kurisu K. Cerebral sinovenous thrombosis after closed head injury. J Trauma 2009;66(6):1599-1604.

64. Matsuyama T, Morimoto T, Sakaki T. Comparison of C1-2 posterior fusion and decompression of the vertebral artery in the treatment of bow hunter's stroke. J Neurosurg 1997;86(4):619-623.

65. McQuillen JB, McQuillen EN, Morrow P. Trauma, sport, and malignant cerebral edema. Am J Forens Med Pathol 1988;9(1):12-15.

66. Miele VJ, Bailes JE. Objectifying when to halt a boxing match: a video analysis of fatalities. Neurosurgery 2007;60(2):307-315; discussion 315-316.

67. Miele VJ, Bailes JE, Cantu RC, Rabb CH. Subdural hematomas in boxing: the spectrum of consequences. Neurosurg Focus 2006;21(4):E10.

68. Miele VJ, Bailes JE, Voelker JL. Boxing and the neurosurgeon. Clin Neurosurg 2002;49:396-406.

69. Miele VJ, France JC, Rosen CL. Subaxial positional vertebral artery occlusion corrected by decompression and fusion. Spine 2008;33(11):E366-370.

70. Miyata M, Yamasaki S, Hirayama A, Tamaki N. Traumatic middle cerebral artery occlusion. No Shinkei Geka 1994;22(3):253-257.

71. Mori T, Katayama Y, Kawamata T. Acute hemispheric swelling associated with thin subdural hematomas: pathophysiology of repetitive head injury in sports. Acta Neurochir Suppl 2006;96:40-43.

72. Motohashi O, Kameyama M, Kon H, Fujimura M, Onuma T. A case of vertebral artery occlusion following heading play in soccer. No Shinkei Geka 2003;31(4):431-434.

73. Mueller FO, Cantu RC. National Center for Catastrophic Sports Injury Research 27th annual report. Fall 1982 to spring 2009. Chapel Hill, NC National Center for Catastrophic Sport Injury Research: 2009.

74. Munro D, Merritt HH. Surgical pathology of subdural hematoma: based on a study of one hundred and five cases. Arch Neurol Psychiatry 1936;35:64-78.

75. Pary LF, Rodnitzky RL. Traumatic internal carotid artery dissection associated with taekwondo. Neurology 2003;60(8):1392-1393.

76. Phonprasert C, Suwanwela C, Hongsaprabhas C, Prichayudh P, O'Charoen S. Extradural hematoma: analysis of 138 cases. J Trauma 1980;20(8):679-683.

77. Ramina R, Kruger J, Marcu H. [Delayed traumatic intracerebral hemorrhage. Report of 5 cases]. Arquivos de Neuro-Psiquiatria 1980;38(3):252-260.

78. Reess J, Pfandl S, Pfeifer T, Kornhuber HH. Traumatic occlusion of the internal carotid artery as an injury sequela of soccer. Sportverletz Sportschaden 1993;7(2):88-89.

79. Saunders RL, Harbaugh RE. The second impact in catastrophic contact-sports head trauma. JAMA 1984;252(4):538-539.

80. Schievink WI, Atkinson JL, Bartleson JD, Whisnant JP. Traumatic internal carotid artery dissections caused by blunt softball injuries. Am J Emerg Med 1998;16(2):179-182.

81. Schneider RL. Head and Neck Injuries in Football. Baltimore: Williams & Wilkins; 1973.

82. Sepelyak K, Gailloud P, Jordan LC. Athletics, minor trauma, and pediatric arterial ischemic stroke. Eur J Pediatr 2010;169(5):557-562.

83. Shimizu T, Waga S, Kojima T, Niwa S. Decompression of the vertebral artery for bow-hunter's stroke. Case report. J Neurosurg 1988;69(1):127-131.

84. Skurnik YD, Sthoeger Z. Carotid artery dissection after scuba diving. Isr Med Assoc J 2005;7(6):406-407.

85. Slankamenac P, Jesic A, Avramov P, Zivanovic Z, Covic S, Till V. Multiple cervical artery dissection in a volleyball player. Arch Neurol 2010;67(8):1024.

86. Slowey M, Maw G, Furyk J. Case report on vertebral artery dissection in mixed martial arts. Emerg Med Australas 2012;24(2):203-206.

87. Sorensen BF. Bow hunter's stroke. Neurosurgery 1978;2(3):259-261.

88. Sparing R, Hesse MD, Schiefer J. Traumatic internal carotid artery dissection associated with triathlon: a rare differential diagnosis. Sportverletz Sportschaden 2005;19(4):211-213.

89. Stam J. Thrombosis of the cerebral veins and sinuses. New Engl J Med 2005;352(17):1791-1798.

90. Stampfel G. Winter sport injuries to the carotid artery. Radiologe 1983;23(9):426-430.

91. Strebel S, Lam AM, Matta BF, Newell DW. Impaired cerebral autoregulation after mild brain injury. Surg Neurol 1997;47(2):128-131.

92. Suzuki R, Osaki M, Endo K, Amano T, Minematsu K, Toyoda K. Common carotid artery dissection caused by a frontal thrust in Kendo (Japanese swordsmanship). Circulation 2012;125(17):e617-619.

93. Taniguchi A, Wako K, Naito Y, Kuzuhara S. Wallenberg syndrome and vertebral artery dissection probably due to trivial trauma during golf exercise. Rinsho Shinkeigaku 1993;33(3):338-340.

94. Tascilar N, Ozen B, Acikgoz M, Ekem S, Aciman E, Gul S. Traumatic internal carotid artery dissection associated with playing soccer: a case report. Turk J Trauma Emerg Surg 2011;17(4):371-373.

95. Thomas M, Haas TS, Doerer JJ, Hodges JS, Aicher BO, Garberich RF, et al. Epidemiology of sudden death in young, competitive athletes due to blunt trauma. Pediatrics 2011;128(1):e1-8.

96. Tseng SH. Delayed traumatic intracerebral hemorrhage: a study of prognostic factors. J Formos Med Assoc 1992;91(6):585-589.

97. Vates GE, Wang KC, Bonovich D, Dowd CF, Lawton MT. Bow hunter stroke caused by cervical disc herniation. Case report. J Neurosurg 2002;96(1 Suppl):90-93.

98. Vertinsky AT, Schwartz NE, Fischbein NJ, Rosenberg J, Albers GW, Zaharchuk G. Comparison of multidetector CT angiography and MR imaging of cervical artery dissection. AJNR 2008;29(9):1753-1760.

99. Weinstein E, Turner M, Kuzma BB, Feuer H. Second impact syndrome in football: new imaging and insights into a rare and devastating condition. J Neurosurg Pediatr 2013;11(3):331-334.

100. Weinstein SM, Cantu RC. Cerebral stroke in a semi-pro football player: a case report. Med Sci Sports Exerc 1991;23(10):1119-1121.

101. Yang PJ, Latack JT, Gabrielsen TO, Knake JE, Gebarski SS, Chandler WF. Rotational vertebral artery occlusion at C1-C2. AJNR 1985;6(1):96-100.

102. Yokota H, Eguchi T, Nobayashi M, Nishioka T, Nishimura F, Nikaido Y. Persistent intracranial hypertension caused by superior sagittal sinus stenosis following depressed skull fracture. Case report and review of the literature. J Neurosurg 2006;104(5):849-852.

103. Young HA, Gleave JR, Schmidek HH, Gregory S. Delayed traumatic intracerebral hematoma: report of 15 cases operatively treated. Neurosurgery 1984;14(1):22-25.

Neurological Considerations in Return to Sport Participation

In the last few years, it has become apparent that allowing a brain-injured athlete to reappear within the same game or practice is not beneficial for the athlete in the present and may be deleterious for the future. The last decade has seen many advances in our knowledge of the pathophysiology of concussion, how concussions occur on a cellular and ultrastructural basis, and the potential for ongoing metabolic disturbances. Generally speaking, symptom onset, severity, type, and duration have been the identifying factors through which concussion is managed. In addition, several important concussion tools, such as the Sideline Assessment of Concussion (SAC) and the Sports Concussion Assessment Tool (SCAT3), have come to be routinely employed to improve player management.

It is imperative that those in attendance of athletes in training, practice, and game settings have a considered, robust, and qualified concussion management strategy. It is generally now accepted, at all levels of play from professional to youth sports, that athletes do not resume sport participation on the same day a concussion injury is suspected or diagnosed. The focused neurological assessment, initial action plan, and determination of disposition are important and should be in place for all those involved in the care of athletes. In addition, it is invaluable for those in attendance to determine the mechanism of injury, which will often come into play later when decisions are made about the athlete's future. This chapter focuses on the assessment of the extent of injury, its potential for continuous brain dysfunction, and judgment processes regarding resumption of athletic activities.

HISTORY OF RETURN TO PLAY

Return-to-play (RTP) decisions in sport are most often difficult and involve many and complex factors. The practice of neurological sports medicine is fraught with innumerable potential facts and circumstances, which means that each decision is individualized. The circumstances involved in the various sports, those that entail regular contact as well as those that have the potential for frequent collisions, are all considered before a final course of action is formulated.

In sports that involve regular, often purposeful blows to the head (such as boxing, mixed martial arts, and American gridiron football) and others that have the potential for such collisions (including soccer, ice hockey, basketball, and lacrosse), never before has the issue of RTP been so important. Due to our ever-increasing fund of knowledge of the pathophysiology of concussion and a better appreciation of the long-term implications of repetitive concussions, we have greater concern regarding the outcomes. In addition, caretakers are under greater scrutiny than ever before, and having knowledge of the many features and nuances of concussion is helpful.

Historically, the acute clinical symptoms of concussion are believed to primarily reflect a functional disturbance; we know that the mechanical trauma of a concussion may result in neuropathological changes at the ultrastructural level (particularly in patients with subacute or chronic symptoms), which ultimately initiates a complex cascade of neurochemical and neurometabolic events.[12, 16, 25, 34, 35] At the cellular level, it is appreciated that neuronal membrane disruption, or mechanoporation, leads to ionic shifts and an increase in intracellular glutamate and calcium.[12, 16, 34] Additionally, mitochondrial dysfunction leads to a failure in adenosine triphosphate and an increase in reactive oxygen species (see chapter 4). Concussion may also compromise or alter the control of cerebral blood flow, cerebrovascular reactivity, and cerebral oxygenation. There is also the possibility after concussion for repetitive subconcussive injury.

The spectrum of postconcussive disease includes acute symptoms, postconcussion syndrome (PCS), persistent or prolonged PCS (PPCS), mild cognitive impairment, chronic traumatic encephalopathy (CTE), and dementia pugilistica (figure 13.1). We also know that prior brain injury is the leading environmental cause of Parkinson's disease (PD) later in life. The role of ongoing neuroinflammation and immunoexcitotoxicity mechanisms in the genesis of these

postconcussive processes has been appreciated recently. The acute and chronic timing of some of these cascades may have important implications in the treatment of concussed individuals[5, 12, 15, 20, 34] (table 13.1).

Traditionally, most patients who sustain a concussion have a spontaneous, sequential resolution of their symptoms within a period of 7 to 10 days. Some patients have a prolonged recovery and display signs and symptoms of concussion past the usual period. As noted in the earlier chapter on PCS, different time points have been suggested in the literature as to when a patient can be considered to be exhibiting a PCS. For some, a diagnosis of PCS may be made when symptoms resulting from concussion last

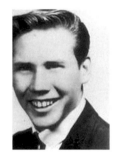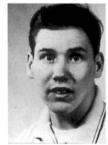

Figure 13.1 The impact of repetitive mild traumatic brain injury.

Reprinted, by permission, from R.C. Schnieder, 1973, *Head and neck injuries in football* (Philadelphia, PA: Lippincott, Williams, and Wilkins), 192.

Table 13.1 Stages of Concussive Injury

Stage	Symptoms
Acute concussion	Physical symptoms Headaches, dizziness, hearing loss, balance difficulty, nausea and vomiting, sensitivity to light or noise, diminished athletic performance Cognitive deficits Loss of short-term memory, difficulty with focus or concentration, decreased attention, diminished work or school performance Emotional disturbances Irritability, anger, fear, mood swings, decreased libido
Postconcussion syndrome	Persistent concussion symptoms, usually lasting 6 weeks to 3 months after mild traumatic brain injury; self-limiting
Prolonged postconcussion syndrome	Symptoms lasting over 3 months Lowered concussion threshold, diminished athletic performance, diminished work or school performance
Chronic traumatic encephalopathy	Latency period (usually 6-10 years), personality disturbances, emotional disturbances, emotional lability, marriage and personal problems, relationship failures, depression, alcohol or substance abuse, suicide attempt or completion

for months after the injury. Postconsussion syndrome has also been characterized in the literature as symptoms lasting 10 days. A small minority of patients have symptoms lasting for several months or longer; this is referred to as PPCS.[29, 34]

Still, discrepancy exists in the literature regarding the timing of the phenomenon because PPCS has been defined by other standards as symptoms lasting 3 months. It is now considered that the persistence of symptoms between 6 weeks and 3 months is consistent with PCS and that any symptoms lasting longer than 3 months constitute a PPCS.[34] When deciding who should be treated pharmacologically, one should first consider whether the patient's symptoms have exceeded the typical recovery period, and secondly whether the symptoms are sufficient that the possible benefit of treatment outweighs the potential adverse effects of the given medication.

The clinical care of the athlete with mild TBI has always centered on recognition of the concussion symptoms and the diagnosis of a concussive event. During the past two decades, concussion manifestations and their cataloging into a tiered grading scale enabled the identification and ultimately the management of those injured to allow for their proper recovery and ultimate safe return to participation in their sport. Among the guiding principles in sport concussion have been that loss of consciousness occurs in the vast minority, about 10%, and that other symptoms including confusion, amnesia, postural abnormalities, visual disturbances, and headache are characteristic. In addition, a symptom-free waiting period of physical and mental rest is appropriate before the athlete is allowed to return to play. A period of time off from school or classroom participation and other academic accommodations, such as allowing a longer time to complete school assignments, are often necessary and beneficial.

Recent findings indicate that impacts during contact sports may occur that are not identified at the clinical level because no outward or visible sign of neurological dysfunction or symptomatology develops. As discussed in the earlier chapter on subconcussion, this emerging evidence includes extensive tauopathy changes seen through autopsy analysis of brains of former professional football players who did not have a diagnosis of concussion during their playing career; accelerometer data gathered in football players not known to have had a concussion or

concussion-like symptoms during play; and data on laboratory animals subjected to mild TBI forces and later proven to have injury. Subconcussion is cranial impact that does not result in known or diagnosed concussion on clinical grounds. It may also occur with rapid acceleration-deceleration to the body or torso, particularly when the brain is free to move within the cranium, creating a "slosh" phenomenon.

Subconcussion has its greatest effect via repetitive occurrences whereby cumulative exposure becomes deleterious. The concept of minimal or "subconcussive" injury requires further exploration for its potential role in accruing sufficient anatomical damage so as to have a clinical expression later in life.[12] Subconcussion may need to be considered in RTP or retirement decisions due to the extent of exposure to repetitive head blows.

The care of the athlete involved in contact or collision sports has traditionally been based on clinical factors meshed with concussion grading scales. In recent years, the grading of concussions has fallen into disfavor for several reasons. First, there is an inherent assumption that all ages, level of competition, sex, sport, concussion and medical history, and other important factors can all be lumped into the same category. We understand now, more than ever, that the heterogeneity of sport concussion requires taking these numerous factors into account. In addition, the full spectrum of postconcussion symptomatology should be considered in every case in order to arrive at an optimal plan for continuation in the given sport or for retirement in some instances. In the past, it was customary that for each grade of concussion one could take a predetermined and standardized approach regarding the length of time off and the safe return strategy. However, with further clinical experience, we now know that RTP must be approached within a flexible, graded, and individualized system of care.

Current Recommendations for Return to Play

1. No activity—complete physical and cognitive rest until asymptomatic; objective is rest and recovery

2. Light aerobic exercise—walking, stationary bike at >70% intensity

3. Sport-specific exercise—skating drills, running, soccer drills, and so on

4. Noncontact training drills—more advanced drills, for example, movement drills, coordination, passing drills; may add resistance training

5. Full contact practice—participation in normal training activities

6. Return to game play

The concepts of RTP have now been codified at many levels in sport and in our society. Following the lead of the State of Washington, more than 40 states have passed laws that govern allowing an athlete with a brain injury to return to play and the providers who are able to participate in the decision-making process. In a pioneering effort, Washington passed the Lystedt Law in 2009. This law states that athletes under the age of 18 who are suspected of having sustained a concussion are to be removed from the practice or game and are not allowed to return until cleared; they must obtain a written RTP authorization from a medical professional trained in the diagnosis and management of concussions. The law also requires that athletes, parents, and coaches be educated annually about concussions and their dangers and implications, and that they read and sign a head injury information sheet annually. School districts are required to work with their various state interscholastic governing bodies to develop guidelines for safe play, and private nonprofit youth leagues must comply as well.

In addition, various sport and sports medicine organizations have stressed that under no circumstances may an athlete with a suspected concussion return to a practice or game until the head injury issues have been addressed and resolved. This implies that even if the symptoms that day seem to resolve, the athlete is disqualified pending further evaluation and clearance. Athletes will no longer be under inflexible guidelines, timelines, or the demands of a particular sport for RTP decisions.

The National Federation of State High School Associations (NFHS), the governing body for high school sports in the United States, has enacted several initiatives aimed at improved concussion management. Effective starting from the 2010 high school football season, any player showing signs, symptoms, or behavior associated with a concussion must be removed from the game or practice and shall not return to play until cleared by an appropriate health care professional. While the earlier rule directed officials to remove an athlete from play if he was "unconscious or apparently unconscious," officials are now mandated to remove any player who shows features of concussion such as loss of consciousness, headache, dizziness, confusion, or balance problems.

That same year, the National Collegiate Athletic Association (NCAA) enacted similar rules to govern the management of college athletes at all three divisions of play. The rule requires that those in attendance at athletic events, including games and practices, focus first on the identification of any player who possibly exhibits concussion signs and symptoms. Once identified, athletes are to be pulled from the game or practice; and if diagnosed with or suspected of concussion, they are not allowed to return that day. Once concussion has been confirmed, they must be cleared by an appropriate health care provider. The successful RTP must follow a written, codified plan that involves a graded exercise and sport-specific regimen without a relapse into concussion symptoms.

At the youth level, several organizations, including Pop Warner Football (PWF) and USA Football, have continued the concussion education and management policy that applies at higher levels of play. Pop Warner Football follows the rules promulgated by the NFHS concerning concussion and its management, and has also passed rule changes effective as of the 2012 football season to eliminate head contact in practice sessions, including reducing all contact drills to only one-third of practice time.

Numerous (more than 20) concussion grading and management scales have been developed in the past two decades (see chapter 4). These were not, however, developed as a result of prospective, randomized, clinical studies. They also were not sport, age, or concussion history specific. Previous studies have demonstrated that migraine headache, cognitive symptoms, visual memory, and processing speed are neuropsychological parameters that predict a prolonged recovery from concussion in high school athletes. It has been noted that these findings of prior concussion history do not necessarily discriminate between simple and complex concussion classifications. Therefore, we now rely heavily on adjunctive measures, including neuropsychological testing, in athletes who do not recover as expected.

SYMPTOM COMPLEX AND IDENTIFICATION

Our primary marker for the resolution of concussion at both the cellular and ultrastructural levels has been the symptom checklist. The most common symptoms of concussion are well known; these include headache, dizziness, visual or balance difficulties, sleep disturbance, and diminished school or job performance.[37] However, ancillary testing, most commonly neuropsychological assessment, can show ongoing abnormalities. Makdissi and colleagues found cognitive deficits on neuropsychological evaluation, even after concussion symptoms had resolved.[25] Among other factors, age, as well as concussion history, should weigh prominently in the evaluation for RTP, as it is believed that concussion resolution takes longer in high school players than in their older counterparts.[10, 14, 33]

The role of neuroimaging in concussion had been a progressive one. Magnetic resonance imaging (MRI) is becoming more widely used in determining ongoing brain dysfunction. Most standard MRI sequences have been designed to evaluate for structural damage at the macroscopic level; however, advanced sequences have recently been developed that have the potential to increase the sensitivity of MRI to detect both structural and functional abnormalities associated with concussion, in the acute setting as well as later in the subacute and chronic phases of recovery. The use of these new techniques, such as diffusion tensor imaging (DTI), is especially relevant in cases in which conventional CT and MRI sequences are unable to detect macroscopic structural abnormalities.

Talavage and colleagues, in a group of high school football players, performed MRI, functional MRI (fMRI), and neurocognitive assessments at three distinct times: (1) before the start of contact practices, (2) during the season, and (3) 2 to 5 months after the season ended. Also, helmet-mounted accelerometers were used to record head collisions during all contact practices and games. The authors demonstrated quantifiable neurophysiological changes in both fMRI and ImPACT testing in the absence of outwardly observable symptoms of concussion. Players with functionally observed impairments (FOI+) showed differences in fMRI activation for a working memory task that were at least as large as those in players in whom a diagnosis of concussion (i.e., a clinically observed impairment, COI+) had been made by the team physician. Of particular interest, the FOI+ group comprised primarily linemen, individuals who experience helmet-to-helmet contact on nearly every play from scrimmage.[41] This finding of diminished neurological performance in the absence of classical symptoms of concussion is similar to previous observations of tauopathy in eight former National Football League (NFL) players, seven of whom were offensive linemen.[31]

Breedlove and colleagues corroborated this finding by showing that fMRI changes in many regions of the brain were statistically correlated to the number and spatial distribution of head hits received after the beginning of contact practices. Regression models constructed to relate the hits experienced to observed fMRI changes were found to explain an even greater proportion of the variance for a concussed group (COI+) than for an asymptomatic group (COI−). The COI− group exhibited substantial impact-correlated involvement of the visual processing systems in the upper parietal and occipital lobes. In contrast, the COI+ group demonstrated significant relationships between the number and locations of hits and those regions involved in verbal working memory.[7] This last observation implies that clinical diagnosis of neurological system deficits may be dependent on which brain functional units have been compromised, and that the entire sport history of blows to the head plays a causal role in overall neurological changes.

As noted in the chapters on subconcussion and neuroimaging, DTI highlights the emerging clinical evidence we are finding for subconcussive brain injury. A prospective study by Bazarian and coauthors was performed in high school athletes engaged in hockey or football compared with controls.[3] The authors investigated the ability to detect subject-specific changes in brain white matter (WM) before and after sport-related concussion. Subjects underwent DTI pre- and postseason within a 3-month interval. Only one athlete was diagnosed with a concussion (scanned within 72 hours), and eight suffered between 26 and 399 subconcussive head blows. Fractional anisotropy (FA) and mean diffusivity (MD) were measured, and the percentage of WM voxels with significant ($p < .05$) pre–post FA and MD changes was highest for the concussion subject, intermediary for those with subconcussive head blows, and lowest for controls. While analysis detected significantly changed WM in a single concussed athlete as expected, the most striking findings were in those athletes who had not sustained a concussion. Asymptomatic athletes with multiple subconcussive head blows had significant changes in a percentage of their WM, over three times higher than in controls. The significance of these WM changes and their relationship to head impact forces are currently uncertain and require further study. Overall, findings in these fMRI and DTI studies point to the potential future role of functional neuroimaging in making RTP decisions.

The athlete's risk of experiencing longstanding effects of repetitive blows is likely to be measured as a cumulative dose over the lifetime, and could include factors such as age at exposure, type and magnitude of exposure, recovery periods, differential rates of recovery, and genotype.[12] There are likely other important factors, such as the number of cranial hits within the same game or practice, the interval between the hits, the severity and effects of each impact, and the weekly cranial impact burden. The ultimate consequence likely is mediated through the effect on brain cells' metabolic disturbance and recovery therefrom. The role of protective equipment and variability in equipment also are factors that may come into play, but their contribution is unknown. The athlete's concussion history is of utmost importance with respect to considering RTP. Although a few studies have questioned the contribution of previous concussions to the issue of recurrence and length of symptoms, most have confirmed that prior events increase subsequent risk. On the horizon is the potential for emerging biomarkers to elucidate concussion diagnosis.[3]

At the high school, collegiate, and professional levels, there appears to be greater risk of concussion, prolonged symptomatology, and ongoing or chronic effects in athletes who have experienced prior events. In general, it seems that having sustained three or more concussions at any level of play increases one's risk of having either season- or career-ending symptoms. Excellent studies at both the high school and NCAA levels have shown that prior concussions increase both the susceptibility to and severity of subsequent concussions. Studies at the Center for Study of Retired Athletes, at the University of North Carolina, Chapel Hill, have shown that having had three or more concussions necessitating loss of playing time in professional football markedly increased the chances of being diagnosed with and treated for mild cognitive impairment and depression during the retirement years.[18, 19] A 2009 study at the University of Michigan School of Social Research found that former NFL players, who were not yet 50 years of age, were at a 19 times greater risk of being diagnosed with dementia or Alzheimer's disease compared to other men their age.[38]

RETURN TO PLAY AND BRAIN ABNORMALITIES

The participation of athletes with prior diagnosed brain lesions or abnormalities is a complex issue and has long been a source of confusion for the athletes and their caretakers, as well as physicians. Several relatively common diagnoses occur in those who have already played their specific sport or desire to become involved at either a recreational or organized sporting level.[28]

Returning to participation in contact sports following the diagnosis of a structural brain lesion has been one of the most complicated decisions the sports medicine practitioner must make. The advisability of allowing athletes with a previous craniotomy to reinstitute participation in contact and collision sports, including American football, ice hockey, soccer, boxing, and several other high-velocity sports, remains unclear.[28] The published literature concerning safety in these situations is minimal and there are no randomized, controlled studies, so our current state of knowledge is primarily anecdotal.

In several instances following craniotomy, athletes have successfully returned to contact sports, including American football, ice hockey, and boxing. In these sports, an advantage is that the use of helmets may provide some protection. The criterion that has generally been used to allow return to contact sports is a radiographically demonstrated healing or healed craniotomy bone flap. In general, this occurs satisfactorily within 1 year in nonsmokers. Often a frontal sinus anterior or posterior wall fracture has occurred, most commonly in soccer or ice hockey players. Many athletes, after definitive repair, have returned to play without adverse effects.

Contraindications to Returning to Sport*

Persistent postconcussion symptoms

Increasing symptoms in the setting of decreased number or severity of impacts

Space-occupying brain mass

Craniotomy

Permanent central nervous system sequelae

Hydrocephalus (untreated)

Intracranial hemorrhage from any cause

Second impact syndrome

*General recommendations, decision individualized.

Chiari Malformation

The Chiari I malformation (CM-I) is a congenital disorder of unknown incidence, characterized by the caudal herniation of cerebellar tonsils through the foramen magnum (figure 13.2). This is an increasingly recognized finding on MRI, with a mean age at onset of symptoms and diagnosis of 15 years, which overlaps with the most common years of participation in contact or collision sports.[4] The variable clinical symptoms result from brain stem compression by the herniating tonsils and from disorders of cerebrospinal fluid (CSF) circulation. Classic symptoms are severe throbbing headache and neck pain starting shortly after coughing, sneezing, straining, changing posture, or physical exertion. Because symptoms may be brought out or aggravated

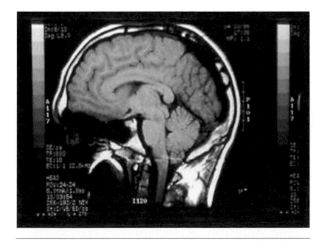

Figure 13.2　A sagittal T1-weighted MRI demonstrating cerebellar tonsillar ectopia consistent with a diagnosis of Chiari I malformation.

by increased intracranial pressure, some have questioned whether the presence of a CM-I can alter the normal CSF capacity for buffering of the brain in instances of high-velocity impacts. Although of no apparent consequence during normal activities, this abnormality may prevent the normal buoyancy of the CSF from protecting the brain from the strong forces that can be generated during impact in contact sports.

Numerous football players at the high school and college levels who sustained concussions were later found to have CM-I as their only abnormality on radiographic evaluations. Whether these findings were incidental or whether the CM-I was a contributing factor to their injury is a matter of debate. Also of concern is the rare fatality associated with the condition; several cases of sudden cardiorespiratory arrest in children with no prior neurological abnormalities have been reported. Cardiac arrest has also been described following a brisk head movement in an adult with a CM-I, as have deaths following minor head trauma in two adults (it is likely that these fatalities were the result of respiratory arrest). This could be the result of medullary compression from the cerebellar tonsillar herniation, which may have depressed the function of the respiratory center, producing hypoxia.[2, 4]

There are several football players at the high school and college levels who sustained concussions and whose radiographic evaluations showed CM-I as their only abnormality. A CM-I malformation is currently not considered an absolute, only a relative, contraindication to further participation in contact sports in asymptomatic patients. When this abnormality is discovered during a diagnostic evaluation for concussion, the authors of this book have generally reacted conservatively and recommended against returning to contact sports, especially for players with repetitive symptoms.

Arachnoid Cysts

Arachnoid cysts may occur in 1% of the general population (figure 13.3). They are frequently associated with symptoms that result from focal compression, mass effect, or hydrocephalus. The decision to surgically treat cysts usually involves a strategy to reduce the mass effect. Athletes who are asymptomatic have typically been allowed to continue to participate in their sport, and no significant associated trends or adverse events have

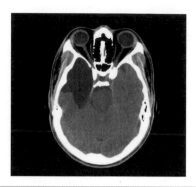

Figure 13.3 Computed tomography scan of the head of a patient with a right-sided (temporal) arachnoid cyst.

been reported.[28] The potential for an arachnoid cyst to hemorrhage is another consideration. Hemorrhage occurs from fragile vessels within the cyst wall or leptomeninges or from bridging veins.[44] This can result in intracystic, subdural, or epidural hemorrhage. With regards to the risk of hemorrhage, there is no direct correlation with cyst location, size, or symptomatic state. Despite the relative frequency of arachnoid cysts in the general population, sparse information exists in the medical literature concerning the likelihood of hemorrhage into the cyst in the setting of athletic participation. A rare but well-known propensity exists for arachnoid cysts to present with hemorrhage (either spontaneous or traumatic), thought to occur in approximately 0.1% of people with these cysts.[23, 28, 44] Bleeding into the subdural space from an arachnoid cyst has been reported in soccer and football players.[2] An arachnoid cyst may present increased risk for a traumatically induced hemorrhage, and although it is not an absolute contraindication to participation in contact sports, patients and their family members should be carefully counseled that the risk is present but uncertain.[32]

We reported a case of a 16-year-old female soccer player who presented with subdural hemorrhage 4 weeks after heading a soccer ball without loss of consciousness.[36] Her symptoms of hemisensory loss and seizures heralded the large hematoma, which required craniotomy for evacuation. Although she made a complete recovery, she chose not to participate any further in the sport. This case points out that merely striking the soccer ball with the head, without losing consciousness, is sufficient to lead to intracranial hemorrhage, especially if there is an underlying structural lesion. Since that publication, other cases of similar hemorrhage in soccer and basketball have been reported.

It is felt that disturbances in the CSF pathways and normal CSF circulation by anatomic abnormalities are perhaps the major implication for CM-I malformations as well as arachnoid cysts. Some have questioned whether the presence of a CM-I malformation can alter the normal CSF capacity for buffering the brain in instances of high-velocity impacts.[2] While this is of no apparent consequence during normal activities, the high-gravity forces that can be generated during impact in contact sports may prevent the normal buoyancy of the CSF from protecting the brain.

Ventriculoperitoneal Shunts

The outlook for children in whom shunts have been placed to treat hydrocephalus has become positive during the past decade, and a large percentage of these children attain high levels of neurological functioning. They are often able to participate in organized sports. The estimated prevalence of ventriculoperitoneal (VP) shunts is about 125,000 in the United States alone. The medical literature contains few articles that specifically address the issue of sport-related shunt complications.[6] Additionally, a recent review of the legal literature failed to locate any cases of sport-related shunt complications. For several reasons, this population is thought to be at a higher risk for neurological sequelae during participation in sport. Some of these patients have persistent ventriculomegaly despite shunt placement.

These athletes may be at risk for cortical collapse over their enlarged ventricles, with secondary tearing of bridging veins and development of subdural hematomas. Patients who have had longstanding hydrocephalus sometimes have a thinner cranium. This could increase the risk for brain injury from impacts to the head. The physiological reserve of the central nervous system to respond to injury may be significantly reduced in this population due to the original insult that caused the hydrocephalus. The CSF acts in part as a shock absorber for the brain. Patients who have undergone shunt placement for hydrocephalus have a change in the dynamics of the CSF flow that could have a negative impact on this buffering effect.[6]

The Joint Section on Pediatric Neurosurgery of the American Association of Neurological Surgeons and the Congress of Neurological Surgeons conducted a study on VP shunts and sports. [6] The study revealed a very low incidence of sport-related complications with VP shunts; the incidence was significantly less than 1%. There was no reported instance of a neurological morbidity or a fatality. The most commonly discussed issues were shunt fractures and shunt dysfunction occurring close in time to participation in an active sport. The catheters of the currently used systems can become calcified along their tracks over time and may become adherent to adjacent tissue, which can increase the risk of fracture or disconnection of the catheter during participation in sport. Dysfunction of the shunt caused by a sport-related fall directly onto the shunt valve has also been reported. The sporting events most frequently implicated by providers were wrestling and soccer. Three providers specifically indicated that the observed adverse event could be attributed to supervised wrestling. All such events involved catheter disconnections or fractures. Accumulation of a clot or other subdural fluid collection was reported by four providers. Three of these involved subacute subdural fluid accumulations in patients with enlarged ventricles, and one acute clot was reported that occurred in an athlete with normal-sized ventricles who directly headed a fast-traveling soccer ball. Football, turning cartwheels, rapid somersaulting, and sledding or tobogganing were also linked to adverse effects. Overall, this report established that the incidence of observed problems attributable to sport participation in shunt-treated children seems very low.

There are no specific guidelines for suggested activities or contact sport restrictions in this population.[28] The majority (89%) of surveyed neurosurgeons do not restrict participation in noncontact sports, and one-third of responding neurosurgeons do not restrict participation in contact sports.[6] Another third prohibit or strongly advise against participation in all contact sports.[6] Football was the most commonly prohibited sport, yet data from this survey did not implicate football-related problems in children treated with shunts. This could be the result of a low incidence of football participation in these children or of improved protective equipment. Boxing and wrestling were also specifically prohibited.[6]

Prior Craniotomy

In general, most experts have not allowed patients who have had a craniotomy for any parenchymal lesion to return to contact sports. It has been felt that obliteration by scar tissue of the normal CSF pathways and buoyancy may alter the brain's ability to withstand repetitive concussive effects. However, recently, rigid cranial fixation in a patient with a normal neurological examination has not been considered an absolute contraindication to later return to contact sport participation. The newer cranial reconstruction plates are thought to confer a major advantage in terms of rigid fixation and promotion of bridging of the kerf line in the craniotomy flap by osteoblastic activity[28] (figure 13.4).

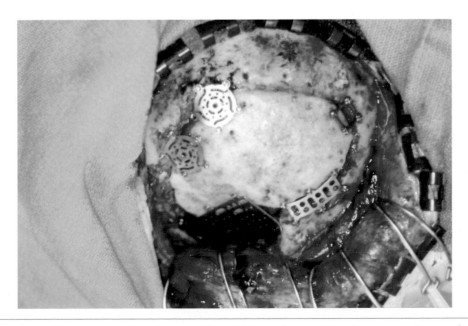

Figure 13.4   Newer cranial reconstruction plates are thought to confer a major advantage in terms of rigid fixation.

Epilepsy

Epilepsy is seen in about 2% of the general population and has led to mixed emotions but a generally conservative attitude on the part of patients, parents, and physicians regarding participation in contact or collision sports. Thus, the question of participation in athletic activities by individuals with epilepsy has been controversial. However, no convincing evidence indicates that epilepsy is an absolute contraindication to participation in most contact sports.[1, 11] The American Medical Association's Committee on Medical Aspects of Sports stated in 1974, "There is ample evidence to show that patients with epilepsy will not be adversely affected by indulging in any sport, including football, provided the normal safeguards for sports participation are followed, including adequate head protection."[11] In 1983, the American Academy of Pediatrics agreed that epilepsy should not exclude a child from participation in contact sports.[1] In addition, it seems that repetitive minor impacts in contact sports do not cause athletes with epilepsy to experience any deterioration in their condition.[2, 28, 43] According to most experts, the psychological, emotional, social, and physical benefits of exercise seem to generally outweigh concerns regarding sport activities in people with seizure disorders.[30] The authors of this book recommend an individualized approach because many factors must be considered, such as the inherent danger in a sport (e.g., parachuting and hang gliding), the degree of seizure control, and seizure precipitants during exercise (e.g., excessive fatigue, electrolyte disturbances, and hyperthermia).[9, 26] For some, boxing and full-contact karate have been absolutely contraindicated.

ADDRESSING AND RESOLVING RETURN-TO-PLAY ISSUES

The basis for retirement from contact sports is complex, and athletes may need to consider many factors at any stage of their career, from high school to professional levels. Retirement after concussion generally reflects the underlying brain injury and falls into one of the four categories (discussed previously) depending on the timing of concussion.

Factors for Consideration in Retirement[a]

Season Ending

- Prolonged postconcussion syndrome
- Three or more concussions in single season
- Two or more major concussions[b] in single season
- Diminished academic performance
- Diminished athletic performance
- CT or MRI brain scan abnormality

Career Ending

- Chiari malformation
- Intracranial hemorrhage
- Diminished academic performance or cognitive abilities
- Persistent prolonged postconcussion syndrome
- Lowering of threshold for concussion (as judged by physicians, athletes, coaches, certified athletic trainers)
- Three or more major career concussions
- CT or MRI brain scan documentation of structural brain injury
- Nonresolving functional MRI scan deficits
- CTE syndrome

[a]All return-to-play and retirement decisions are individualized; some features are relative contraindications for return to play.
[b]Major concussion: symptomatic for more than 1 week.

Some athletes choose to retire due to intractable acute symptoms after concussion. Others may choose to retire due to PCS, which usually consists of self-limited sequelae of concussion such as dizziness, headaches, and declining academic or athletic performance. Thirdly, more prolonged postconcussive effects may result in a decision to retire due to changes in performance, motivation, or personality, which again may manifest in declining athletic or academic abilities.[8] Finally, in unique subsets of patients, displaying signs or symptoms of CTE may prompt a decision to retire.

Concussion and Traumatic Brain Injury History

Exposure to mild TBI is the primary historical information used in a decision to retire an athlete. As stated earlier, recent research has shed light on the issue of subconcussive impacts and the potential for their cumulative number to be significant. Now more than ever, the collective burden of these impacts—either the quantity of hits, or more likely, playing years as a surrogate—can greatly influence the estimation of potential for brain injury. The number, symptoms, and time to recovery after concussion are all important factors, as is a history of returning to play while still symptomatic (table 13.2). Although they are rare, a history of postconcussive seizures should be sought. The mechanism of concussion, if known, and the type of protective equipment worn are also considered. Information regarding current postconcussive symptomatology should be sought; this is best gleaned from the patient, family, and athletic trainers, among others.[21]

The frequency and severity of headaches should be recorded. Mood swings, irritability, insomnia, lack of concentration, or impaired memory are pertinent. Personality changes may occur. Any persistent postconcussive symptoms or permanent neurological symptoms from a concussion, such as organic dementia, hemiplegia, and homonymous hemianopsia, should prompt investigation into the possibility of retiring an athlete. A history of declining school or athletic performance may be a sensitive indicator of both early and chronic changes after concussion, and this is particularly important to elicit if present.

For a subset of patients with a long history of exposure, symptoms suggestive of CTE should be sought, such as explosive behavior, alcohol or substance abuse, excessive jealousy, mood disorders, and paranoia. These symptoms often demonstrate latency from initial exposure and are progressive. Omalu and colleagues performed an extensive postmortem psychological history in their series of patients and unearthed a variety of common historical clues pointing to chronic cognitive and neuropsychological decline. These included drug and alcohol abuse, increasing religiosity, suicidal ideations or attempts, insomnia, hyperactivity, breakdown of intimate or family relationships, exaggerated responses to stressors, poor business or financial management, bankruptcy, and others.[31] Although the latency period of symptoms in CTE is not known, these should be investigated when an athlete and family are interviewed for possible retirement after concussion.[27, 31]

Past Traumatic Brain Injury

Specific potentially catastrophic events after concussion, such as second impact syndrome and surgically treated brain injuries (e.g., subdural hematoma), would ordinarily disqualify an athlete from further participation in contact sports. Any athlete surviving a second impact syndrome should retire from contact sports. In addition, any athlete requiring surgery for evacuation of an intracranial hemorrhage should be considered for retirement due to multiple factors, including changes in CSF dynamics and the decrease in structural integrity of the skull, although some

Table 13.2 Risk Factors That May Extend or Complicate Recovery From Concussion

Factors	Modifiers
Concussion history	Total number, proximity, severity (duration)
Symptoms	Total number, severity (intensity and especially duration)
Signs	Prolonged loss of consciousness (>1 min)
Susceptibility	Concussions occurring with lower impact magnitude, requiring longer recovery, or both
Age	Youth and adolescent athletes may recover more slowly; older athletes may have cumulative effects
Preexisting conditions	Migraine, depression, anxiety or panic attacks, attention deficit hyperactivity disorder, learning disabilities, other medical illnesses

investigators have reported that, rarely, an athlete may be considered for RTP after craniotomy following healing of bony defect (discussed earlier in this chapter). Concussions that occur earlier during the athlete's life and are not sport related, including childhood injuries, may also contribute to the magnitude of injury burden and should be documented and considered in RTP decisions. These principles assist in making a decision to retire an athlete.

The physical examination should center on any abnormal neurological findings. A complete and detailed neurological examination should be performed to search for any focal abnormalities. Visual field testing should be completed. Tests of balance and coordination should be performed to assess for ataxia. Examination of reflexes for hyperreflexia, as well as other long tract findings, should be documented. Patients should be observed for signs of parkinsonism. Mental status examination is an important clinical prelude to further neuropsychological testing. Even with an extensive neurological examination, findings may be normal in a large percentage of patients with recurrent concussion.

Neuropsychological testing has undergone an evolution in its sport applications, and the neurocognitive and neuropsychological features may be measured with current methods.[10, 14, 31, 33, 37] Neuropsychological impairment has been related to concussive and subconcussive injury in boxers and football and soccer players, and neuropsychological testing is crucial in determining the consequences of concussive injury. The number of concussive events has been shown to be significantly related to lifetime risk of depression as well as late-life cognitive impairment, with a suggestion that increasing number of concussions leads to higher prevalence.

Several recent studies show the subtle cognitive effects of concussive injury and suggest that specialized testing of attention and information processing be used for assessment of postconcussive effects. These discoveries led to a consensus statement from the participants in the 3rd International Conference on Concussion in Sport held in Zurich, which emphasized the importance of neuropsychological testing. It has been recommended by Echemendia and colleagues that clinical neuropsychologists, rather than athletic trainers or others, administer the complex psychometric tests to evaluate for these subtle abnormalities.[13] Furthermore, it has been suggested that computer-based tests be used, such as ImPACT, CogSport, and Automated Neuropsychological Assessment Metrics (ANAM).

The advent of these computerized platforms, with access to the Internet and qualified neuropsychological opinion, make neuropsychological testing all the more practical and available for a larger population.[43] For accurate assessment of the effects of concussive injury on athletes before a decision is made to end a career, it is imperative that these tests be administered. Many sources have shown that simple tests of intellectual and mental function do not reveal the true extent of cognitive decline. Furthermore, baseline neuropsychological examinations are important and preferred for comparison and more sensitive detection of decline. Although many nuances are involved in correctly applying neuropsychological testing and interpreting the results, both traditional and computer-based instruments have proven invaluable in athletic concussion management. Therefore, neuropsychological testing, either computer-based or in consultation with a neuropsychologist, provides objective data that greatly aid sports medicine clinicians when deciding if retirement from sport should be pursued.

Imaging studies are integral to a full evaluation and should be performed. Although a CT scan may be performed to rule out any obvious abnormalities (e.g., intracranial hemorrhage), the standard imaging method is MRI, including DTI sequencing of the brain for further anatomic signs of trauma. Diffuse cerebral atrophy or ventriculomegaly may be encountered as well as other signs of chronic injury. Imaging studies may reveal further, nontraumatic anatomic abnormalities; and although these aspects may not be directly related to concussion, they too may prompt a decision to retire an athlete. Discovery of any symptomatic abnormalities of the foramen magnum, such as a Chiari I malformation, should prompt consideration of retirement, especially when combined with syringomyelia, obliteration of subarachnoid space, or indentation of the anterior medulla. This has also been suggested for discovery of hydrocephalus or the incidence of spontaneous subarachnoid hemorrhage from any cause, although no guidelines are currently in place. More recently, MRI diffusion tensor imaging has demonstrated a correlation of increased fractional anisotropy and decreased radial diffusivity with increasing severity of post-concussive symptoms in adolescents after concussion.[3] This is currently increasing the ability to visualize and characterize postconcussive effects.

Potential for Future Genetic Testing

Early research in CTE and other neurodegenerative diseases has shown a trend toward developing these diseases among people with certain genetic traits. Specifically, the ApoE4 and the ApoE3 alleles, in both homozygous and heterozygous forms, have been implicated in the development of Alzheimer's disease and CTE after brain trauma. This was first discovered in a population of 30 career boxers and has since been confirmed in other populations with neurotrauma. These proteins are various alleles of the apolipoprotein E, which is important for lipid transport and is widely produced in the brain. Although this clinical science is still in its infancy, it may be possible someday to predict who will develop long-term problems from repeated head trauma in sport. Genetic testing, although raising ethical questions, may be a valuable tool for athletes who wish to know their risk for sustaining repeated concussive injury and may play a role in the decision to retire athletes in the future. Furthermore, although the presence of hetero- or homozygous ApoE4 or ApoE3 confers a three- to nine-fold increased risk of developing various forms of dementia after traumatic brain injury, its implications with regard to modern sport are uncertain.[22, 24]

The pathophysiological mechanism for this association may be that beta-amyloid is deposited in the brain to a greater extent after head trauma in individuals with the ApoE4 allele. The allele may also affect the efficiency of neuronal repair, which is suggested by the poorer outgrowth of neurites observed in cell cultures containing ApoE4 after traumatic injury; this could lead to the accumulation of residual tissue damage after repeated episodes of trauma. ApoE4-related alterations in the neuronal cytoskeleton, increased susceptibility to reactive oxygen species in association with ApoE4, and altered intracerebral cholesterol trafficking are other mechanisms proposed to be the cause of increased susceptibility to chronic TBI in athletes with the ApoE4 gene.[22]

However, the link between ApoE4 and chronic TBI is not universally accepted. Most studies relating to mild TBI in sport have included a relatively small population of patients, and this has been a major criticism. Also, investigators have relied on brief cognitive assessments or coarse measures of global functioning, thereby limiting their conclusions. In other research on the role of the ApoE4 allele in mild to moderate brain injury in which a more detailed evaluation of neuropsychiatric outcome was performed, no link was found between the presence of the ApoE4 allele and poor outcome across all measures.

Many, if not most, questions remain unanswered. The extent of the risk is not known, nor is the relationship between this gene and an increased risk of chronic TBI; but the implications are major. Should all athletes in contact or collision sports be tested for ApoE4 as a part of the preparticipation physical, and should those with positive results be banned from participation? Issues such as the genetic profile of an athlete could be useful in determining if the participant is predisposed to a particular injury. If this information is known before participation, the athlete can be properly counseled concerning risks, given special techniques and equipment to minimize risk, and offered alternative sporting activities. In addition, several societal concerns exist with regard to DNA-based testing. When testing is performed, who should be allowed access to the acquired information? Other questions arise, for example whether sport regulatory agencies should have access to information about an individual's ApoE4 status before granting a boxing license or taking other actions.

Social and Legal Implications in the Decision to Retire

Concerning retirement based on concussive injury, it should be recognized that athletes generally desire to continue play and thus continue their exposure to potential concussions. While the decision to retire an athlete is difficult in view of the factors already discussed, it is made even more challenging because of the many social factors involved. In addition to the athlete, the coach, team members, agents, and athlete's family have considerable input and stake in the decision to retire. Athletes may be under significant financial stress to continue in their sport. This can extend to all levels of competition, from high school athletes desiring a college scholarship to professional athletes who may have limited alternative vocational skills and are supporting a family or have other responsibilities. Athletes are often reluctant to describe their full symptomatology after concussive injury. This may have less of an impact on the decision to retire an athlete than on a RTP decision because these debates often take place only after evidence of postconcussive injury has become apparent to everyone.[39]

Despite the many complexities of the retirement decision-making process, the athlete must be involved in this milestone event. The decision should be made with the athlete and family in discourse and engagement. At times, however, the very cognitive and neuropsychological decline that may prompt a decision to retire interferes with the executive functioning and judgment of the athlete. Neuropsychological testing should be performed and integrated into decision making regarding the extent of a patient's ability to participate in the retirement decision.

The decision to retire an athlete after concussion may be complicated by other factors. According to Goldberg, team-employed physicians have frequently been cited as downplaying injury and encouraging RTP. Goldberg makes the case that sport-related health decisions should be made by independent physicians as in workers' compensation claims.[17] To avoid this complicating factor, some have advised that retirement assessments be performed by an independent physician or that a second opinion by an independent physician be encouraged. The NFL and other organizations are implementing this suggestion to provide local neurosurgeons and neurologists for second-opinion consultations on concussion.

The decision to allow or disallow RTP when a question of retirement arises has several legal implications for treating physicians. The decision to retire is usually symptom driven. Until biomarkers become reliable and are implemented, their value is uncertain.[42] Furthermore, much is still to be learned about the potential for chronic brain injury and CTE. A recent preliminary study suggests that positron emission tomography scanning may be useful for determining the distribution and extent of tau protein deposition[40] (figure 13.5).

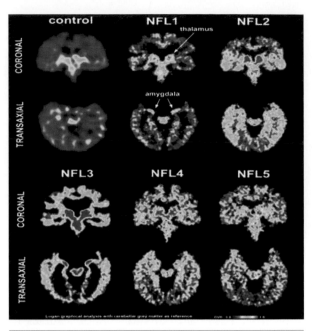

Figure 13.5 Figure legend: FDDNP-PET scan results for NFL players and a control. Coronal and transaxial FDDNP-PET scans of the retired NFL players include: NFL1: 59-year-old linebacker with MCI, who experienced momentary loss of consciousness after each of two concussions; NFL2: 64-year-old quarterback with age-consistent memory impairment, who experienced momentary loss of consciousness and 24-hour amnesia following one concussion; NFL3: 73-year-old guard with dementia and depression, who suffered brief loss of consciousness after 20 concussions, and a 12-hour coma following 1 concussion; NFL4: 50-year-old defensive lineman with MCI and depression, who suffered two concussions and loss consciousness for 10 minutes following one of them; NFL5: 45-year-old center with MCI, who suffered 10 concussions and complained of light sensitivity, irritability, and decreased concentration after the last two. The players' scans show consistently high signals in the amygdala and subcortical regions and a range of cortical binding from extensive to limited, whereas the control subject shows limited binding in these regions. Red and yellow areas indicate high FDDNP binding signals.

Reprinted from **American Journal of Geriatric Psychiatry** Vol. 21(2), G.W. Small et al., "PET scanning of brain tau in retired National Football League players: Preliminary findings," pgs. 138-44, copyright 2013, with permission from Elsevier.

In spite of the uncertainty about the impact of concussive injury on long-term functioning, however, physicians must carefully weigh the benefits and risks of RTP and counsel athletes accordingly; some have advocated a conservative approach. Physicians also have a responsibility to provide athletes with full information about their medical condition and the possible consequences of return to play so that their decision is informed. Throughout this process, the obligation of a physician is to protect the health, safety, and future welfare of the athlete to the extent possible, regardless of whether the individual wants to return to play.

CONCLUDING THOUGHTS

Among the main concerns of the injured athlete is always "How soon can I return to sports?" The answer to this question is not always easy because each athlete and each injury is unique. Return-to-play decisions are fundamental to the practice of sports medicine but vary greatly for a given medical condition and circumstance, and often from one provider to another. Returning too soon can increase one's risk of reinjury or of developing a chronic problem that will lead to a longer recovery. On the other hand, keeping the athlete out too long can lead to unnecessary deconditioning.

Attempts have been made to develop consensus regarding such decisions. Grading systems for concussion are a thing of the past; and appropriately, a conservative approach has been taken regarding RTP for these athletes. The available evidence and literature on RTP in contact sports following the diagnosis of a structural brain lesion are sparse, and these decisions are among most complicated the sports medicine practitioner needs to make. We do have some literature to help guide the decisions for patients with a prior craniotomy, epilepsy, Chiari malformation, and ventriculoperitoneal shunts. Adding case series to the literature will provide increased support for the decisions that sports medicine practitioners need to make regarding return to play.

REFERENCES

1. Sports and the child with epilepsy. Pediatrics 1983;72(6):884-885.

2. Bailes JE, Cantu RC. Head injury in athletes. Neurosurgery 2001;48(1):26-45; discussion 45-46.

3. Bazarian JJ, Zhu T, Blyth B, Borrino A, Zhong J. Subject-specific changes in brain white matter on diffusion tensor imaging after sports-related concussion. Magn Reson Imaging 2012;30(2):171-180.

4. Beuls EA, Vandersteen MA, Vanormelingen LM, Adriaensens PJ, Freling G, Herpers MJ, et al. Deformation of the cervicomedullary junction and spinal cord in a surgically treated adult Chiari I hindbrain hernia associated with syringomyelia: a magnetic resonance microscopic and neuropathological study. Case report. J Neurosurg 1996;85(4):701-708.

5. Blaylock RL, Maroon J. Immunoexcitotoxicity as a central mechanism in chronic traumatic encephalopathy—a unifying hypothesis. Surg Neurol Int 2011;2:107.

6. Blount JP, Severson M, Atkins V, Tubbs RS, Smyth MD, Wellons JC, et al. Sports and pediatric cerebrospinal fluid shunts: who can play? Neurosurgery 2004;54(5):1190-1196; discussion 1196-1198.

7. Breedlove EL, Robinson M, Talavage TM, Morigaki KE, Yoruk U, O'Keefe K, et al. Biomechanical correlates of symptomatic and asymptomatic neurophysiological impairment in high school football. J Biomech 2012;45(7):1265-1272.

8. Cantu RC. Return to play guidelines after a head injury. Clin Sports Med 1998;17(1):45-60.

9. Cantu RC. Epilepsy and athletics. Clin Sports Med 1998;17(1):61-69.

10. Collins MW, Lovell MR, Iverson GL, Cantu RC, Maroon JC, Field M. Cumulative effects of concussion in high school athletes. Neurosurgery 2002;51(5):1175-1179; discussion 1180-1171.

11. Corbitt RW, Cooper DL, Erickson DJ, Kriss FC, Thornton ML, Craig TT. Editorial: Epileptics and contact sports. JAMA 1974;229(7):820-821.

12. Dashnaw ML, Petraglia AL, Bailes JE. An overview of the basic science of concussion and subconcussion: where we are and where we are going. Neurosurg Focus 2012;33(6):E5:1-9.

13. Echemendia RJ, Herring S, Bailes J. Who should conduct and interpret the neuropsychological assessment in sports-related concussion? Br J Sports Med 2009;43 Suppl 1:i32-35.

14. Field M, Collins MW, Lovell MR, Maroon J. Does age play a role in recovery from sports-related concussion? A comparison of high school and collegiate athletes. J Pediatr 2003;142(5):546-553.

15. Gagnon I, Galli C, Friedman D, Grilli L, Iverson GL. Active rehabilitation for children who are slow to recover following sport-related concussion. Brain Inj 2009;23(12):956-964.

16. Giza CC, Hovda DA. The neurometabolic cascade of concussion. J Athl Train 2001;36(3):228-235.

17. Goldberg DS. Concussions, professional sports, and conflicts of interest: why the national football league's current policies are bad for its (players') health. HEC Forum 2008;20(4):337-355.

18. Guskiewicz KM, Marshall SW, Bailes J, McCrea M, Cantu RC, Randolph C, et al. Association

between recurrent concussion and late-life cognitive impairment in retired professional football players. Neurosurgery 2005;57(4):719-726; discussion 719-726.

19. Guskiewicz KM, Marshall SW, Bailes J, McCrea M, Harding HP Jr, Matthews A, et al. Recurrent concussion and risk of depression in retired professional football players. Med Sci Sports Exerc 2007;39(6):903-909.

20. Iverson G. Predicting slow recovery from sport-related concussion: the new simple-complex distinction. Clin J Sport Med 2007;17(1):31-37.

21. Johnson LS. Return to play guidelines cannot solve the football-related concussion problem. J School Health 2012;82(4):180-185.

22. Katzman R, Galasko DR, Saitoh T, Chen X, Pay MM, Booth A, et al. Apolipoprotein-epsilon4 and head trauma: synergistic or additive risks? Neurology 1996;46(3):889-891.

23. Kawanishi A, Nakayama M, Kadota K. Heading injury precipitating subdural hematoma associated with arachnoid cysts—two case reports. Neurol Med Chir (Tokyo) 1999;39(3):231-233.

24. Kutner KC, Erlanger DM, Tsai J, Jordan B, Relkin NR. Lower cognitive performance of older football players possessing apolipoprotein E epsilon4. Neurosurgery 2000;47(3):651-657; discussion 657-658.

25. Makdissi M, Darby D, Maruff P, Ugoni A, Brukner P, McCrory PR. Natural history of concussion in sport: markers of severity and implications for management. Am J Sports Med 2010;38(3):464-471.

26. McCrory PR, Bladin PF, Berkovic SF. Retrospective study of concussive convulsions in elite Australian rules and rugby league footballers: phenomenology, aetiology, and outcome. Br Med J 1997;314(7075):171-174.

27. McKee AC, Cantu RC, Nowinski CJ, Hedley-Whyte ET, Gavett BE, Budson AE, et al. Chronic traumatic encephalopathy in athletes: progressive tauopathy after repetitive head injury. J Neuropathol Exp Neurol 2009;68(7):709-735.

28. Miele VJ, Bailes JE, Martin NA. Participation in contact or collision sports in athletes with epilepsy, genetic risk factors, structural brain lesions, or history of craniotomy. Neurosurg Focus 2006;21(4):E9.

29. Moser RS, Schatz P, Jordan BD. Prolonged effects of concussion in high school athletes. Neurosurgery 2005;57(2):300-306; discussion 300-306.

30. Nakken KO, Bjorholt PG, Johannessen SI, Loyning T, Lind E. Effect of physical training on aerobic capacity, seizure occurrence, and serum level of antiepileptic drugs in adults with epilepsy. Epilepsia 1990;31(1):88-94.

31. Omalu B, Bailes J, Hamilton RL, Kamboh MI, Hammers J, Case M, et al. Emerging histomorphologic phenotypes of chronic traumatic encephalopathy in American athletes. Neurosurgery 2011;69(1):173-183; discussion 183.

32. Parsch CS, Krauss J, Hofmann E, Meixensberger J, Roosen K. Arachnoid cysts associated with subdural hematomas and hygromas: analysis of 16 cases, long-term follow-up, and review of the literature. Neurosurgery 1997;40(3):483-490.

33. Pellman EJ, Lovell MR, Viano DC, Casson IR. Concussion in professional football: recovery of NFL and high school athletes assessed by computerized neuropsychological testing—part 12. Neurosurgery 2006;58(2):263-274; discussion 263-274.

34. Petraglia AL, Maroon JC, Bailes JE. From the field of play to the field of combat: a review of the pharmacological management of concussion. Neurosurgery 2012;70(6):1520-1533; discussion 1533.

35. Petraglia AL, Winkler EA, Bailes JE. Stuck at the bench: potential natural neuroprotective compounds for concussion. Surg Neurol Int 2011;2:146.

36. Prabhu VC, Bailes JE. Chronic subdural hematoma complicating arachnoid cyst secondary to soccer-related head injury: case report. Neurosurgery 2002;50(1):195-197; discussion 197-198.

37. Sabini RC, Nutini DN. Return-to-play guidelines in concussion: a closer look at the literature. Phys Sportsmed 2011;39(3):23-30.

38. Schwarz A. Dementia risk seen in NFL players. New York Times. September 29, 2009.

39. Sedney CL, Orphanos J, Bailes JE. When to consider retiring an athlete after sports-related concussion. Clin Sports Med 2011;30(1):189-200, xi.

40. Small GW, Kepe V, Siddarth P, Ercoli LM, Merrill DA, Donoghue N, et al. PET scanning of brain tau in retired National Football League players: preliminary findings. Am J Geriatr Psychiatry 2013;21(2):138-144.

41. Talavage TM, Nauman E, Breedlove EL, Yoruk U, Dye AE, Morigaki K, et al. Functionally-detected cognitive impairment in high school football players without clinically-diagnosed concussion. J Neurotrauma 2010;31(4):327-338.

42. Turner RC, Lucke-Wold BP, Robson MJ, Omalu BI, Petraglia AL, Bailes JE. Repetitive traumatic brain injury and development of chronic traumatic encephalopathy: a potential role for biomarkers in diagnosis, prognosis, and treatment? Front Neurol 2012;3:186.

43. van Linschoten R, Backx FJ, Mulder OG, Meinardi H. Epilepsy and sports. Sports Med 1990;10(1):9-19.

44. Vigil DV, DiFiori JP, Puffer JC, Peacock WJ. Arachnoid cyst and subdural hygroma in a high school football player. Clin J Sport Med 1998;8(3):234-237.

The Role of Pharmacologic Therapy and Rehabilitation in Concussion

Traditionally, the medical management of concussion has involved close observation as well as physical and cognitive rest. As we have learned more about concussion over the years, it has become clear that the use of a multifaceted assessment and serial testing can provide a better framework for determining effective individualized patient management strategies. Treatment for patients with concussion centers on symptom management and education of the patient, family, and other significant contacts (athletic trainers, teachers, coaches, employers, and so on). While the role of education in the management of these patients has been investigated at length,[20, 41, 71, 76, 84, 85, 90, 91, 105, 126, 127] there have been no randomized, controlled trials regarding the pharmacologic treatment of concussion symptoms. As has been demonstrated in several reviews, the evidence is equivocal for many of the medications used to manage the postconcussive patient.[14, 20, 73, 86] In most cases, the studies involve patients with moderate and severe traumatic brain injury (TBI) and fail to look at the efficacy of these medications in a concussion cohort alone. The symptomatic treatment of concussion can be challenging, in part due to patient heterogeneity. While no standardized approach exists, there are a number of effective adjunctive medical therapies for symptoms that when used appropriately, in an individualized manner, can improve outcomes. Additionally, rehabilitation strategies may be effective for some patients with persistent postconcussive symptoms.

THE DECISION TO TREAT PHARMACOLOGICALLY

As mentioned in previous chapters, most patients who sustain a concussion have a spontaneous, sequential resolution of their symptoms within a period of 7 to 10 days.[30, 36, 45, 72, 135] That being said, it must be emphasized that some patients do have a prolonged recovery and display signs and symptoms of concussion past the "usual period." Different time points have been suggested in the literature as to when a patient can be considered to exhibit a postconcussion syndrome (PCS) or prolonged postconcussion syndrome (PPCS). The persistence of symptoms between 6 weeks and 3 months is consistent with PCS, and any symptoms lasting longer than 3 months can be considered PPCS.[86, 110] When deciding who should be treated pharmacologically, one should consider first whether or not the patient's symptoms have exceeded the typical recovery period and second, whether or not the symptoms are negatively affecting the patient's life to such a degree that the possible benefit of treatment outweighs the potential adverse effects of the medication under consideration.[73, 86]

An appreciation of the basic pathophysiology of concussion provides a basis for understanding the potential treatments. Following a concussion is a complex cascade of neurochemical and neurometabolic events.[8, 21, 47, 67-69, 86, 88, 93, 104, 116] Concussion may also compromise or alter mitochondrial function, the control of cerebral blood flow (CBF), cerebrovascular reactivity, and cerebral oxygenation.[21, 59, 86] There is also accumulating evidence that neuroinflammatory cascades and excitotoxicity play a significant role in the pathogenesis of disease following concussion and possibly repetitive subconcussive injury.[10, 21, 86] Overall, the acute and chronic timing of some of these cascades may have important implications in the treatment of concussed individuals.

The use of naturally occurring supplements and compounds as an initial therapeutic approach to concussion patients has been described.[86, 87] An alternative approach with natural neuroprotective compounds such as eicosapentaenoic acid (EPA)–docosahexaenoic acid (DHA) or fish oil, curcumin, resveratrol, and various vitamins is discussed further in the next chapter. In the authors' opinion, such compounds address the underlying pathophysiological processes (particularly neuroinflammation) and thus aid in patient and disease management. When patients have persistent symptoms despite conservative efforts and a natural therapeutic approach, then pharmacologic symptom treatment options can be considered.[86] While no clinically validated pharmacologic treatment has been shown to speed recovery or ameliorate the deficits attributed to TBI,[9] patients with PCS or PPCS may benefit from symptomatic medical treatment while they are healing.[9, 75, 76, 98]

One should note several general points when considering using medication for the treatment of postconcussion symptoms. It is best to avoid medications that lower the seizure threshold, cause confusion, or contribute to cognitive slowing, fatigue, or daytime drowsiness—all of which could potentially confound the clinical exam. In general, therapies should be initiated at the lowest effective dose and be titrated slowly based on tolerability, side effects, and clinical response. All patient medications and over-the-counter supplements should be reviewed to try to prevent unwanted interactions. These basic principles have been echoed in most reviews on concussion management.[20, 72, 73, 86] Treatment of concussion should be symptom specific, and these symptoms are generally grouped into four categories[72, 73, 98]: somatic complaints, sleep disturbance, and emotional and cognitive symptoms. It is important to keep in mind that a complex relationship exists between the various concussion symptoms and also that alleviating one symptom may improve others.

SOMATIC SYMPTOMS

The initial treatment of somatic complaints in a concussion patient starts with a thorough clinical evaluation and is based on individual symptom presentation. Posttraumatic headaches are the most common symptom reported after a concussion; these occur acutely in upward of 90% of patients[6, 26, 37, 83] (table 14.1). There may be an increased risk of hemorrhage within the first 24 to 48 hours following concussion.[35] In general, aspirin and other nonsteroidal anti-inflammatory drugs (NSAIDs) are avoided in the acute period so as not to induce or exacerbate intracranial hemorrhage. No controlled trials have demonstrated this theoretical small risk, though.[135] Rebound headaches are also common with prolonged NSAID and narcotic use and can potentially complicate the recovery process, particularly in athletes.[53, 60, 80] For this reason, acetaminophen is a logical choice for the treatment of postconcussion headache in the acute period. Most patients have a spontaneous resolution of their headache; however, those patients that go on to develop persistent headaches as a part of a PCS may require further treatment.

Management of headache in brain injury is difficult and complex because there are many possible underlying factors. Medication selection is guided by the character of the headaches. Most of the evidence is weak (level III), in part due to poor study design, heterogeneous patient populations, and a lack of adequate controls.[20, 73, 86] Additionally, the variation in medication regimens (i.e., dose, duration, start of treatment) across studies makes it difficult to synthesize the data. Most patients who develop persistent headaches after concussion have tension-type or migraine-like headaches.[38, 60, 63, 80] Patients

Table 14.1   Pharmacotherapy for Somatic Symptoms—Headache[a]

Class	Medication	Brand names	Dosing	Side effects
Analgesics	Acetamin-ophen	Tylenol	500-1,000 mg TID-QID (max daily dose 4,000 mg)	Usually rare; at high doses or over-doses, vomiting, liver and kidney failure
	Aspirin	Bayer, Bufferin, Ecotrin	81 or 325 mg daily	GI upset, ulcers, bleeding, nausea, headache
NSAIDs	Ibuprofen	Advil, Motrin	600-800 mg TID	GI upset, GI ulcers, GI bleeding, dizziness, nausea, vomiting, loss of appetite, arrhythmia, confusion; *prolonged use in concussion patients can lead to rebound headaches*
	Naproxen	Aleve, Naprosyn	550-850 mg BID	
	Diclofenac	Voltaren, Cataflam	50-100 mg daily (divided doses)	
Anti-depressants	Ami-triptyline	Elavil, Endep, Vanatrip	10-25 mg QHS; titrate up for effect (usually doses of 150 mg or less employed)	Nausea, GI upset, weakness, blurred vision, changes in appetite, drowsiness, dizziness, arrhythmia, motor tics, seizures, hallucination, unusual bleeding
	Nor-triptyline	Aventyl, Pamelor	10-25 mg QHS; titrate as above	
Anti-convulsants	Valproic acid	Depakene, Depakote	250 mg BID; can titrate up in increments of 250 mg for effect (max daily dose 1,500 mg)	Drowsiness, dizziness, headache, diarrhea, constipation, heartburn, appetite changes, weight changes, back pain, agitation, mood swings
	Topiramate	Topamax, Topiragen	15-25 mg QHS and slowly raised to as high as 100 mg BID	Lack of coordination, impaired memory and concentration, irritability, headache, weakness, motor tics, GI upset, hair loss, appetite changes
	Gaba-pentin	Neurontin, Gabarone, Fanatrex, Horizant	300 mg TID and may be slowly raised as high as 1,200 mg TID	Dizziness, headache, blurred vision, anxiety, memory problems, motor tics, increased appetite
Beta-adrenergic antagonists	Propran-olol	Inderal, Inno-Pran	40-320 mg daily (divided doses)	Abdominal cramps, fatigue, insomnia, nausea, depression, impotence, light-headedness, slow heart rate, low blood pressure, cold extremities, shortness of breath or wheezing; *not to be used in patients with asthma*
	Metoprolol	Lopressor, Toprol	25 mg BID; can increase dose up to 100 mg BID if needed	
Ergot preparations (abortive)	Dihydro-ergotamine (DHE)	DHE45, Migranal	Intranasal versus IM/SQ versus IV (0.5-1 mg, max 2 mg/day)	Abnormal skin sensations, anxiety, diarrhea, dizziness, flushing, sweating, nausea, vomiting
Triptans (abortive)	Suma-triptan	Imitrex, Alsuma	Oral: 25-100 mg prn Intranasal: 10-20 mg BID prn SQ: 6 mg	Unusual taste (nasal formulation), paresthesias, hyperesthesia, dizziness, chest tightness, vertigo, tingling, hypertension, injection site reactions, flushing, chest pressure, heaviness, jaw or neck pain
	Zolmi-triptan	Zomig	Oral: 5-10 mg Intranasal: 5 mg	
	Rizatriptan	Maxalt	5-10 mg; can repeat dose 2 h from first dose (max 30 mg/day)	

[a]mg, milligrams; TID, three times a day; QID, four times a day; max, maximum; GI, gastrointestinal; NSAIDs, nonsteroidal anti-inflammatory drugs; BID, twice a day; QHS, at bedtime; IM, intramuscular; SQ, subcutaneous; IV, intravenous; prn, as needed.

with cervicogenic pain, myofascial injury, temporomandibular joint injury, or muscle spasms in the superior trapezius and semispinalis capitis muscles in the suboccipital region can also present with headaches.[115, 135] These patients may benefit from treatment with a muscle relaxant. Headaches frequently noted in the athletic population are covered further in a later chapter.

Antidepressants are commonly used to treat postconcussion headaches despite the equivocal evidence in the literature.[20, 76, 86] The antidepressant amitriptyline has shown efficacy in the treatment of postconcussion headaches in some studies.[20, 123, 130] In one retrospective review that looked at 23 mild TBI patients treated with amitriptyline for posttraumatic headaches, 56% and 34% of patients had an "excellent" and "good" recovery, respectively.[123] This study also seemed to show more favorable outcomes for patients who were younger, female, and started on medication shortly after injury.[123] It is important to recognize that such a study is limited by its design and very small sample size, making it difficult to draw any definitive conclusions from the findings. Another study looked at amitriptyline treatment in 12 depressed control patients with headaches and compared them to 10 depressed concussion patients with headaches.[107] The authors concluded that postconcussive headaches were not successfully managed with amitriptyline. Interestingly, all of the patients in the depressed control group exhibited headache improvement following 4 weeks of amitriptyline. None of the patients in the depressed mild TBI group exhibited improvement with their headaches.[107] Amitriptyline is used in the treatment of tension-type and migraine-like headache not associated with trauma and thus still remains a good option for postconcussive headaches.[38, 60, 63, 73, 86] Amitriptyline can also be sedating, which may provide relief for those also suffering from sleep disturbances following a concussion.[53, 60, 63, 73]

McBeath and Nanda reviewed repetitive administration of intravenous dihydroergotamine (DHE) and metoclopramide for postconcussion headache.[70] Patients varied in the period of time they had headaches following trauma, ranging from 1 day to more than 3 years. All patients displayed at least three other PCS symptoms including memory problems, impaired concentration, sleep problems, dizziness, and

anxiety. A "good to excellent" overall headache response to DHE therapy was achieved in 28 (85%) of the patients.[70] Patients also obtained "good to excellent" relief of memory problems (91% of patients), sleep problems (94%), and dizziness (88%). Dihydroergotamine seemed to be well tolerated, and no serious or unexpected adverse reactions were reported.[70]

Valproic acid is a medication believed to enhance the neurotransmission of gamma-aminobutyric acid (GABA), via inhibition of GABA transaminase; however, several other mechanisms of action have been proposed in recent years.[102] Valproic acid also blocks voltage-gated sodium channels and T-type calcium channels. While valproic acid has been traditionally used as a broad-spectrum anticonvulsant drug, it also has been found useful for the treatment of migraine and chronic daily headaches. Packard sought to determine the effectiveness of divalproex sodium in the treatment of chronic daily posttraumatic headaches.[81] They performed a retrospective review of 100 patients treated with divalproex sodium for posttraumatic headaches of 2 months or longer duration. All headaches in the study resulted from mild head injuries, defined in the study as having a period of unconsciousness less than 20 minutes, a Glasgow Coma Scale of 13 or more, and posttraumatic amnesia lasting less than 48 hours. For inclusion in the study, charts had to show patients with at least 1 month (or more) of treatment with divalproex. Dosing had been individualized for optimum therapeutic effect. Starting dose was generally 250 mg daily (sometimes as 125 mg taken twice a day). This was increased by 250 mg per week depending on patient response. Maximum doses were 500 mg three times a day. No other prophylactic medications were used. Sixty percent of patients in the study had mild to moderate improvement in their headaches after at least 1 month of treatment; 26% showed no response, and another 14% discontinued treatment because of side effects that included nausea, weight gain, hair loss, and tremor. Fifty-eight percent of the patients who did show improvement had a change in their headache pattern from daily to episodic. The authors concluded that divalproex sodium appears to be safe and effective for the treatment of persistent postconcussive headaches.[81]

Although the subjects were not a cohort of athletes, Erickson and colleagues performed a retrospective study in 100 U.S. Army soldiers with chronic posttraumatic headaches after mild head trauma.[23] Response rates to various headache abortive medications were measured, with the goal of determining outcomes with acute and prophylactic medical therapies. Treatment outcomes were also compared between subjects with blast-induced injury and non-blast posttraumatic headache. Headache frequency decreased by 41% among nonblast patients compared to the 9% decrease seen among blast injury patients. A significant decline in headache frequency occurred in the 29 patients treated with topiramate (100 mg divided, daily) but not in the 48 patients treated with a low-dose tricyclic antidepressant. Additionally, a significantly greater proportion of patients (70%) who used a triptan-class medication experienced reliable headache relief within 2 hours compared to the 42% of subjects using other headache abortive medications. The authors concluded that triptan-class medications appeared to be effective for aborting posttraumatic headaches attributed to a concussion from a blast injury or nonblast injury in military troops, and that topiramate appeared to be an effective headache prophylactic therapy in those same patients.[23]

Other options exist for persistent headaches following a concussion; however, as with the previously mentioned treatments, there is scant literature on which to base treatment selection.[86] Other pharmacologic treatments discussed in the literature include the use of beta-blockers, calcium channel blockers, triptans, and gabapentin as potential medical therapies for persistent postconcussive headaches, mostly based on their use in other headache disorders.[53, 60, 63, 73] Some small reports and studies have addressed the use of some of these other treatments in patients with posttraumatic headaches.[3, 17, 23, 29, 111, 130] For example, triptans are a family of tryptamine-based drugs traditionally used as abortive medication in the treatment of migraines and cluster headaches.[86] Their action is attributed to their binding to serotonin 5-HT$_{1B}$ and 5-HT$_{1D}$ receptors in cranial blood vessels, causing their constriction and subsequent inhibition of proinflammatory neuropeptide release. These drugs may be effective because they act on serotonin receptors in nerve endings as well as the blood vessels.[95, 120, 121] One case series reported on four patients with posttraumatic headaches after mild TBI who

were treated with subcutaneous sumatriptan.[111] Adequate headache relief occurred in 95% of 32 treated attacks, with an average time to relief of 51 minutes. Another small case series discussed the treatment of seven patients with posttraumatic headaches following mild TBI with subcutaneous sumatriptan and reported headache relief by 20 minutes.[29]

Another example is the use of beta-blockers for the treatment of migraine-like headaches. Beta-blockers may work by decreasing prostaglandin production, though they may also prevent headaches through their effect on serotonin or a direct effect on arteries. One study reported the use of propranolol alone or in combination with amitriptyline in 30 patients with headache following minor head trauma.[130] Seventy percent of patients reported a dramatic reduction in the frequency and severity of their headaches. Thus, in certain circumstances in which trials with other medications have proven ineffective, such medications may be reasonable choices, albeit anecdotally.[86]

Dizziness and disequilibrium are also common somatic symptoms experienced by the postconcussive patient and may occur in upward of 30% of people sustaining a concussion[16] (table 14.2). The differential diagnosis for these symptoms is broad; thus the patient interview, medication review, and clinical exam often guide the clinician in determining the plan of care. Although vestibular suppressants have been shown to be effective acutely for vestibular disorders, the same cannot be said for chronic dizziness after a concussion.[137] No studies have investigated the role of pharmacotherapy for vestibular symptoms in concussion; however, if chronic postconcussive dizziness is severe enough to significantly limit functional activities of daily living, then a brief trial of a vestibular suppressant may be warranted. Careful consideration should be given to the use of these medications in PCS patients in view of the effects on arousal and memory, as well as their addictive qualities.[6] Potential medical therapies for persistent postconcussive dizziness include meclizine, scopolamine, and dimenhydrinate.[86] In general, treatment with benzodiazepines (although possibly effective) should be avoided if possible given their sedating and addictive qualities.

Fatigue is another common symptom reported in postconcussion patients (table 14.2).

Table 14.2   Pharmacotherapy for Somatic Symptoms—Dizziness, Fatigue, Nausea[a]

Class	Medication	Brand names	Dosing	Side effects
DIZZINESS				
Vestibular suppressants	Meclizine	Antivert, Bonine, Medivert	12.5-50 mg every 4-6 h prn	Hallucinations, blurred vision, dry mouth, constipation, dizziness, drowsiness
	Scopolamine	Scopace, Transderm-Scop, Maldemar	0.5 mg patch every 3 days prn	Dry mouth, topical allergy, tachyarrythmia, drowsiness, dizziness, restlessness, blurred vision, dry or itchy eyes, flushing, nausea, vomiting, headache
	Dime-hydrinate	Dramamine, Driminate	50 mg every 4-6 h prn	Dizziness, drowsiness, dry mouth or throat
Benzo-diazepines	Lorazepam	Ativan	0.5 mg BID	Sedation, dizziness, weakness, unsteadiness, depression, loss of orientation, headache, respiratory depression; *caution should be used as these medications can cause physical dependence*
	Clonazepam	Ceberclon, Klonopin, Valpax	0.25-0.5 mg BID	
	Diazepam	Valium, Valrelease	2-10 mg daily	
FATIGUE				
Neuro-stimulants	Methyl-phenidate	Ritalin, Concerta, Metadate	5 mg BID; can titrate up total daily dose by 5 mg every 2 weeks to a max of 20 mg BID	Insomnia, decreased appetite, GI upset, headaches, dizziness, motor tics, irritability, anxiousness, tearfulness
	Dextro-amphetamine	Adderall, Dexedrine, ProCentra	5 mg daily; can titrate up for effect (max daily dose 40 mg)	Anxiety, GI upset, insomnia, irritability, euphoria, staring episodes
	Modafanil	Provigil	100 mg every morning; can increase by 100 mg amounts, using divided doses (max daily dose 400 mg)	Headache, dizziness, feeling nervous or agitated, nausea, diarrhea, insomnia, dry mouth, hallucinations, depression
	Amantadine	Symadine, Symmetrel	100-400 mg daily	Dizziness, blurred vision, anxiety, insomnia
	Atomoxetine	Strattera	40 mg daily (single or divided doses); can titrate up for effect (max daily dose 100 mg)	Dry mouth, irritability, nausea, decreased appetite, constipation, dizziness, sweating, dysuria, sexual problems, weight changes, palpitations, tachycardia, hypertension
NAUSEA				
Antiemetics	Ondansetron	Zofran	4 mg every QID prn	Dizziness, drowsiness, anxiety, diarrhea, blurred vision, dry mouth, stuffy nose, tinnitus, weight gain, swelling, impotence, constipation, light-headedness
	Phenergan	Phenergan, Pentazine, Promethagan	12.5-25 mg QID prn	

[a]mg, milligrams; prn, as needed; BID, twice a day; max, maximum; QID, four times a day.

Medications, substance use, and lifestyle can also contribute to fatigue; thus all medical and psychological issues and modifiable factors should be addressed first.[86] All conservative measures should be taken before pharmacotherapy for fatigue is started. Although neurostimulants are widely used in TBI (particularly severe TBI),[28, 46, 48, 73, 131] there is no research evidence to support the use of these medications for fatigue in concussion. The pharmacologic agents that have been trialed in mild to severe TBI, with variable success, include methylphenidate, modafinil, and amantadine.[46, 48, 73]

In general, posttraumatic nausea occurs frequently in the acute period after concussion and less commonly as part of PCS (table 14.2). Persistent nausea in postconcussion patients most commonly occurs in association with persistent dizziness or secondary to medication effects.[2] Before treating patients with antiemetics such as ondansetron, the clinician should be sure to thoroughly review the patient's history and attempt to define any triggers or patterns.[86] Other somatic symptoms that typically follow a concussion acutely, such as vision difficulties (i.e., diplopia, blurred vision, photophobia), hearing difficulties (i.e., altered acuity, phonophobia), and changes in appetite, tend to resolve spontaneously with conservative measures and rarely require further treatment.[2]

SLEEP DISTURBANCE SYMPTOMS

Difficulties with sleep often occur acutely following a concussion and are a common source of significant morbidity, especially for student-athletes, as they tend to markedly affect school performance.[73, 83] Patients may have difficulty falling asleep or staying asleep, or may have insomnia. Sleep hygiene is one of the first issues that should be addressed and discussed with patients.[6, 73, 94] Patients should be advised to eliminate distractions from the bedroom (i.e., television, stereo, video games, phones, computers). Bedtime should be spent sleeping. Reducing sources of stimulation can help the patient fall asleep and stay asleep. Having patients return to and engage in daytime physical and mental activities, within each individual's functional limits, will help to establish a regular, normalized sleep–wake pattern.[86] Additionally, people

with sleep disturbances should avoid caffeine, nicotine, and alcohol use, and minimize daytime naps.[73] If conservative measures do not suffice, sleep agents may assist patients with PCS (table 14.3).

Trazodone is an antidepressant with 5-HT$_{2A}$ receptor antagonist and some serotonin reuptake inhibitor properties.[27, 73] It has anxiolytic and hypnotic effects, with less anticholinergic and sexual side effects than other antidepressants, and thus is a commonly used agent to treat sleep disturbances following concussion.[27, 73] Some clinicians prefer other commonly used agents such as zolpidem or tricyclic antidepressants.[94] Prazosin is a selective alpha-1 receptor antagonist, best known for its use in the treatment of hypertension, anxiety, and posttraumatic stress disorder. Ruff and colleagues examined whether treatment with sleep hygiene counseling and oral prazosin would improve sleep, headaches, and cognitive performance.[103] The cohort of patients included 126 veteran soldiers with blast-induced mild TBI during deployment in Operation Iraqi Freedom or Operation Enduring Freedom (OIF/OEF). Seventy-four of the 126 veterans had comorbidities including frequent severe headaches and residual deficits on neurological examination, neuropsychological testing, or both. Of these veterans, only five had restful sleep. After 9 weeks of treatment, 65 veterans reported restful sleep; a significant number of patients had improved headaches and cognitive assessment scores.

Other clinicians prefer to use melatonin as a sleep agent. Melatonin is an endogenous hormone produced primarily by the pineal gland and converted from serotonin. Melatonin's high efficacy, high safety profile, and virtual lack of toxicity make it of interest in clinical medicine.[99] Studies have shown it to be effective and safe for use in TBI patients, with most studies using 5 mg dosing.[13, 27, 50, 64, 79, 106] Melatonin is an over-the-counter supplement, and the recommended dosage is 0.3 mg to 5 mg.[1, 12] This is considered a safe and effective dosage.[1, 12] Generally, it is a good idea to start at lower melatonin doses and then gradually increase the dosage until the most effective one is found. The basic mechanism by which melatonin produces sleepiness in humans is unclear, although three main hypotheses have been proposed. Melatonin's mechanism of action may involve a phase shift of the endogenous

Table 14.3 Pharmacotherapy for Sleep Disturbances[a]

Class	Medication	Brand names	Dosing	Side effects
Sedative hypnotics	Zolpidem	Ambien, Edluar, Zolpimist	5 mg QHS; can increase to 10 mg QHS if poor results	Drowsiness, headache, dizziness, light-headedness, unsteady walking, difficulty with coordination, constipation, diarrhea, heartburn, stomach pain, changes in appetite, paresthesias, unusual dreams
Serotonin modulators	Trazodone	Desyrel, Oleptro	25-50 mg QHS	Headache or heaviness in head, nausea, vomiting, bad taste in mouth, stomach pain, diarrhea, constipation, changes in appetite or weight, weakness, nervousness, decreased concentration, confusion, nightmares, tinnitus
Alpha-adrenergic antagonists	Prazosin	Minipress	1 mg QHS; may slowly increase/titrate dose for effect (max daily dose is 10 mg QHS)	Dizziness, drowsiness, dry mouth, frequent urination, headache, lack of energy, nausea, light-headedness, nasal congestion, weakness
Supplement	Melatonin	Health Aid Melatonin, Ves-Pro Melatonin, Melaxen	0.3 mg to 5 mg QHS	Daytime sleepiness, sleepwalking, confusion, headache, dizziness, abdominal discomfort

[a]mg, milligrams; QHS, at bedtime; max, maximum.

circadian pacemaker, a reduction in core body temperature, a direct action on somnogenic structures of the brain, or more than one of these.[100]

EMOTIONAL SYMPTOMS

Emotional symptoms are common in postconcussive patients.[72, 83] Patients may report irritability, depression, apathy, anxiety, posttraumatic stress disorder, personality changes, disinhibited behavior, or emotional lability. Restrictions on activity, in addition to the removal of athletes from their teammates, can also lead to depression. Many of the acute emotional symptoms are short-lived and can be managed conservatively with coping strategies, professional counseling, and support of family and friends.[73, 86] However, patients with persistent postconcussive emotional or behavioral symptoms may benefit from pharmacologic treatment in addition to nonpharmacologic therapeutic measures (table 14.4).

In general, antidepressants have been globally used for most emotional symptoms.[73, 86] Tricyclic antidepressants and selective serotonin reuptake inhibitors (SSRIs) have both been investigated as therapeutic options in the treatment of TBI-related depression.[114, 129] Some studies suggest that while amitriptyline has been useful in treating primary depression, it may not be as effective for treating post-TBI depression.[20, 22, 108, 129] As with the medical treatments for other concussion symptoms, most of the evidence for SSRI use in concussion comes from small, uncontrolled or open studies and case reports rather than large randomized trials. That being said, SSRIs have become the primary treatment for TBI-associated depression because of their perceived clinical efficacy and relatively few side effects. Once a response or remission is achieved, it is uncertain as to how long therapy should be continued in this patient population.[97]

Fann and coauthors performed an 8-week nonrandomized, single-blind, placebo run-in trial of sertraline in 15 patients diagnosed with

Table 14.4   Pharmacotherapy for Emotional Symptoms[a]

Class	Medication	Brand names	Dosing	Side effects
DEPRESSION				
Tricyclic anti-depressants	Amitriptyline	Elavil, Endep, Vanatrip	10-25 mg QHS; titrate up for effect (usually doses of 150 mg or less employed)	Nausea, GI upset, weakness, blurred vision, changes in appetite, drowsiness, dizziness, arrhythmia, motor tics, seizures, hallucination, unusual bleeding
	Nortriptyline	Aventyl, Pamelor	10-25 mg QHS; titrate as above	
Selective serotonin reuptake inhibitors	Sertraline	Zoloft	25 mg daily; can increase weekly in 25 mg increments (max daily dose 200 mg)	Aggressiveness, strange changes in behavior, suicidal thoughts/behavior, extreme changes in mood, insomnia, nausea, dry mouth, decreased libido, dizziness, diarrhea
	Citalopram	Celexa	10 mg daily; can titrate dose up for effect (max daily dose 80 mg)	Constipation, decreased sexual desire or ability, diarrhea, dizziness, drowsiness, dry mouth, increased sweating, light-headedness
	Escitalo-pram	Lexapro	10-20 mg daily	Nausea, dizziness, GI upset, increased appetite, hallucination, arrhythmia
	Paroxetine	Paxil	20 mg daily; can titrate dose up for effect (max daily dose 50 mg)	Anxiety, blurred vision, constipation, decreased sexual desire or ability, diarrhea, dizziness, drowsiness, dry mouth, loss of appetite, nausea, nervousness, stomach upset
	Fluoxetine	Prozac	20 mg daily; can increase to maintenance dose up to 80 mg daily	Anxiety, nausea, motor tics, decreased appetite, weakness
Other anti-depressants	Bupropion	Wellbutrin, Zyban	Dose depends on if immediate versus sustained versus extended release (max daily dose 450 mg)	Seizures, delirium, hallucinations
ANXIETY				
Benzo-diazepines	Lorazepam	Ativan	0.5 mg BID	Sedation, dizziness, weakness, unsteadiness, depression, loss of orientation, headache, respiratory depression; *caution should be used as these medications can cause physical dependence*
	Clonazepam	Ceberclon, Klonopin, Valpax	0.25-0.5 mg BID	
	Diazepam	Valium, Valrelease	2-10 mg daily	

[a]mg, milligrams; QHS, at bedtime; GI, gastrointestinal; max, maximum; BID, twice a day.

major depression between 3 and 24 months after a mild TBI.[25] On the Hamilton Depression Rating Scale (HAMD), at least 13 patients (87%) had a decrease in their score greater than or equal to 50% ("response"), and 10 patients (67%) achieved "remission" of their depression by week 8 of sertraline treatment.[25] There was also a statistically significant improvement in other postconcussive symptoms, including psychological distress, anger, aggression, and cognitive variables of psychomotor speed and recent verbal/visual memory. Thus, as previously mentioned, treating depression following a concussion may also improve other cognitive symptoms or deficits in patients.[24]

Rapoport and colleagues examined the rates of response and remission associated with citalopram treatment for major depression following TBI.[96] Patients with major depression following mild to moderate TBI were treated with citalopram for either 6 weeks (n = 54) or 10 weeks (n = 26). The HAMD was used to assess depression severity and treatment effect. After 6 weeks of treatment, 54 subjects were assessed; 27.7% responded, with 24.1% in remission. Following 10 weeks of treatment, 26 subjects were assessed; 46.2% responded, with 26.9% in remission. Other SSRIs have also been investigated for post-TBI depression.[14, 44, 77] Paroxetine was found to be just as effective as citalopram in improving emotional symptoms in one study,[77] and another study found significant improvement in mood with fluoxetine treatment in post-TBI patients,[44] although the TBI populations were heterogeneous in these studies.

COGNITIVE SYMPTOMS

Cognitive complaints and symptoms are extremely common in the first hours and days following a concussion.[18, 19, 72, 73, 83] Patients frequently report difficulty with memory and concentration. Advances in computerized neuropsychological testing have revealed qualitative deficits in memory, complex attention or working memory, and speed of mental and motor performance.[18, 19, 45, 72, 124] A subgroup of individuals continue to have both subjective symptoms and persistent deficits on formal neuropsychological testing, and these patients may benefit from a trial of medications if symptoms are interfering with activities of daily living (table 14.5).

Though methylphenidate has been studied more than most other cognitive agents in TBI, no studies have investigated the role of methylphenidate strictly in the setting of concussion.[89, 118, 133, 134, 136] There is evidence to support the use of methylphenidate in treating deficits in attention, processing speed, and general cognitive functioning following brain injury.[73, 129] Whyte and colleagues investigated 34 adults with moderate to severe TBI and attention complaints in the postacute phase of recovery in a 6-week randomized, double-blind, placebo-controlled, repeated crossover study of methylphenidate administration.[134] They found that methylphenidate had a clinically significant effect on processing speed, attention, and some aspects of on-task behavior in naturalistic tasks. The effect of subacute administration of methylphenidate on recovery from moderate to moderately severe closed head injury was also explored in a double-blind, placebo-controlled trial.[89] The study included 23 patients ranging in age from 16 to 64 years. Head injury severity ranged from moderately severe to "complicated mild" (defined as Glasgow Coma Scale from 13 to 15 with evidence of cerebral contusion on computed tomography scan). Thirty-day follow-up was based on 12 patients, whereas 90-day evaluation was based on 9 patients; complicated mild head injuries were excluded from the analyses. This study was clearly limited by a small and very heterogeneous patient group; however, subacute administration of methylphenidate after moderately severe head injury appeared to enhance the rate but not the ultimate degree of recovery.[89] Not all studies have shown such a benefit from methylphenidate, though, and caution is in order when one is prescribing methylphenidate due to its potential to lower seizure thresholds.[14, 73, 136]

Amantadine is another potential medication used to manage postconcussive neurocognitive recovery.[61, 109] Amantadine appears to act through several pharmacologic mechanisms, but no dominant mechanism of action has been identified.[86] It is a dopaminergic and noradrenergic agent and may also be a weak N-methyl-D-aspartate (NMDA) receptor antagonist. The role of amantadine in TBI has been investigated, with equivocal evidence in the literature regarding its efficacy.[86] Several studies have suggested that amantadine is safe and may improve cognitive functioning.[52, 74] In one study of 22 patients with

Table 14.5 Pharmacotherapy for Cognitive Symptoms[a]

Class	Medication	Brand names	Dosing	Side effects
Neuro-stimulants	Methylphe-nidate	Ritalin, Concerta, Metadate	5 mg BID; can titrate up total daily dose by 5 mg every 2 weeks to a max of 20 mg BID	Insomnia, decreased appetite, GI upset, headaches, dizziness, motor tics, irritability, anxiousness, tearfulness
	Dextroam-phetamine	Adderall, Dexadrine, ProCentra	5 mg daily; can titrate up for effect (max daily dose 40 mg)	Anxiety, GI upset, insomnia, irritability, euphoria, staring episodes
	Modafanil	Provigil	100 mg every morning; can increase by 100 mg amounts, using divided doses (max daily dose 400 mg)	Headache, dizziness, feeling nervous or agitated, nausea, diarrhea, insomnia, dry mouth, hallucinations, depression
	Amantadine	Symadine, Symmetrel	100-400 mg daily	Dizziness, blurred vision, anxiety, insomnia
	Atomoxetine	Strattera	40 mg daily (single or divided dose); can titrate up for effect (max daily dose 100 mg)	Dry mouth, irritability, nausea, decreased appetite, constipation, dizziness, sweating, dysuria, sexual problems, weight changes, palpitations, tachycardia
Selective serotonin reuptake inhibitors	Sertraline	Zoloft	25 mg daily; can increase weekly in 25 mg increments (max daily dose 200 mg)	Aggressiveness, strange changes in behavior, extreme changes in mood, insomnia, nausea, dry mouth, decreased libido, dizziness, diarrhea
	Fluoxetine	Prozac	20 mg daily; can increase to maintenance dose up to 80 mg daily	Anxiety, nausea, motor tics, decreased appetite, weakness
Acetylcho-linesterase inhibitors	Donepezil	Aricept	5-10 mg daily	Severe diarrhea, severe nausea or vomiting, weight loss, stomach pain, fainting spells, bradycardia, difficulty passing urine, worsening of asthma, stomach ulcers
	Rivastig-mine	Exelon	1.5 mg BID; can be titrated for effect (max daily dose 200 mg)	Diarrhea, dizziness, drowsiness, headache, loss of appetite, nausea, stomach upset, vomiting
	Galan-tamine	Razadyne	4 mg BID initially, then increased to goal 8-12 mg BID (also available in extended release form)	Diarrhea, dizziness, headache, loss of appetite, nausea, stomach upset, drowsiness, weight loss
Others	Cytidine diphos-phate-cho-line (CDP-choline)	Citicoline	250-500 mg daily	Increased body temperature, sweating, nausea, loss of appetite

[a]mg, milligrams; BID, twice a day; max, maximum; GI, gastrointestinal.

mild, moderate, and severe TBI, amantadine significantly improved executive function testing.[52] Additionally, positron emission tomography scans demonstrated a significant increase in left prefrontal cortex glucose metabolism that correlated with improved cognitive testing.

Cholinergic dysfunction is thought to underlie the memory impairment in patients with Alzheimer's disease (AD), and postconcussive patients with cognitive symptoms share some similarity with AD patients in relation to memory and attention deficits.[135] Donepezil is a long-acting acetyl-cholinesterase inhibitor that has been shown to improve cognition in AD patients. There is accumulating evidence that donepezil administration can improve overall function, as well as short- and long-term memory.[49, 66, 128, 132] Donepezil also reduced anxiety, depression, and apathy in some patients.[66] Newer-generation acetylcholinesterase inhibitors, such as rivastigmine and galantamine, have also been investigated, with similar promising results.[78, 112, 113, 117, 119, 138]

Cytidine diphosphate-choline (CDP-choline), an intermediate precursor in the synthesis of phosphatidylcholine, is thought to lead to increased brain acetylcholine levels. Levin and colleagues explored CDP-choline treatment of postconcussional symptoms for 1 month after mild to moderate TBI.[62] This small, double-blinded, placebo-controlled study of 14 patients found that CDP-choline produced a significantly greater reduction of postconcussion symptoms than placebo. The patients also had a significant improvement in recognition memory for designs.[62] There is still a need for further studies to determine the efficacy of cholinergic agents in treating the neurocognitive symptoms in postconcussion patients. Several other pharmacologic agents, such as fluoxetine, sertraline, atomoxetine, bromocriptine, and pramiracetam, have been investigated as treatment for postconcussive cognitive symptoms; however, the evidence is limited.[14, 44, 73, 86, 129]

THE ROLE OF REHABILITATION IN CONCUSSION MANAGEMENT

Each athlete must be assessed on an individualized basis. Athletes with persistent symptoms may not respond or may find only little relief from pharmacologic treatments. Certainly more conservative measures such as reassurance, discussions of expected recovery time, and compensatory strategies can improve symptoms of PCS.[20, 51, 76, 125, 127] Other studies have found that an information booklet can reduce PCS symptoms at 3 to 6 months after injury in adults.[91] One reported that particularly in children, an information booklet on strategies for dealing with posttraumatic symptoms resulted in fewer symptoms and less behavioral changes at 3 months after injury.[90] That being said, Al Sayegh and colleagues identified six randomized controlled trials that concluded no benefit versus three that demonstrated an improvement in symptoms.[4] According to these authors, one can argue that elements of this intervention may be justified as cost-effective in preventing the development of PCS, perhaps in selected patients such as those whose head injury warranted admission, although they felt that support for its usefulness has been perhaps overstated.[4]

As with the pharmacologic interventions, a recent systematic review of psychological interventions for PCS revealed equivocal evidence in the literature.[4] Cognitive behavioral therapy (CBT) is a form of psychological intervention that focuses on identifying and changing patterns of maladaptive thinking and behavior that can exacerbate (or in some cases even cause) affective symptoms often associated with persistent effects of direct brain injury, including depression and anxiety.[58] Studies using either single-case designs or trials with limited controls have demonstrated that psychosocial treatment with cognitive–behavioral components may be effective in addressing particular persistent symptoms after mixed-severity TBI.[92] Such studies have shown improvement in symptoms such as dizziness,[34] headache,[33, 65] and depression.[11] There is also some evidence for broader improvements in activities of daily living in uncontrolled studies of CBT for mild TBI.[42] In their systematic review on investigations of the potential efficacy of CBT for PCS, Al Sayegh and colleagues found 10 studies, three of which used a randomized controlled design, and all 10 concluded a benefit.[4] Robust conclusions about the efficacy of CBT were difficult to make due to relatively small numbers and short durations of follow-up. There is also limited evidence that multifaceted rehabilitation programs that include a psychotherapeutic element are of benefit in the management of persisting symptoms.

Neurocognitive rehabilitation uses cognitive tasks to improve cognitive processes, or it may involve developing compensatory strategies to address difficulties with aspects of cognition such as attention, memory, and executive functioning.[58] Studies have demonstrated that neurocognitive rehabilitation improves performance on selected neuropsychological test scores and cognitive function in patients with mild or mild-to-moderate TBI.[15, 39, 40] The evidence supporting the efficacy of neurocognitive rehabilitation following TBI varies for different cognitive processes. Several studies have demonstrated evidence supporting neurocognitive rehabilitation of attention processes in head-injured patients. [15, 39, 82, 101] One randomized controlled trial of an 11-week program of combined neurocognitive rehabilitation and cognitive behavioral therapy, in symptomatic mild-to-moderate TBI patients, showed improved divided auditory attention, anxiety, and depression.[122]

While there have been no studies demonstrating the effectiveness of vestibular suppressants following a concussion, investigations using objective balance assessments have shown that nonpharmacologic interventions, such as vestibular rehabilitation, may be a useful alternative for treating postconcussive dizziness and disequilibrium.[5, 31, 32, 43] Vestibular rehabilitation may reduce dizziness and improve gait and balance in children and adults.[5, 31] Customized exercise programs of gaze stabilization, dynamic visual acuity, static postural stability, dynamic postural stability, desensitization of head motion, and aerobic conditioning yield the best results in symptom resolution.[31] Rehabilitation options and length of treatment will differ depending on the symptoms and other associated variables in these patients. Most mild TBI patients respond to vestibular physical therapy intervention over 8 weeks, although some may continue to improve with an additional 4 to 8 weeks of gaze stabilization and dynamic gait training.[31, 32] Using vestibular therapy in coordination with a structured multidisciplinary program can dramatically improve symptom control and realization of functional self-goals.[31]

Recent developments have supported the use of standardized exercise testing and controlled aerobic exercise treatment as an approach to treating PCS.[7, 54-56, 58] Drs. John Leddy, Barry Willer, and colleagues at the University of Buffalo in New York have pioneered much of this work. This rehabilitative treatment approach proposes that one fundamental cause of refractory PCS is persistent physiologic dysfunction, which may include altered autonomic function and impaired autoregulation as well as distribution of CBF.[55, 57] Previous studies by Leddy and coauthors have demonstrated the efficacy, safety, and reliability of a progressive subsymptom threshold exercise rehabilitation program in ameliorating PCS.[54, 56] The authors of these studies postulate that exercise assessment and aerobic exercise training could possibly reduce concussion-related physiological dysfunction by restoring autonomic balance and by improving autoregulation of CBF. A similar rehabilitation program has been established for children with PCS after sport-related concussion that combines gradual, closely monitored physical conditioning, general coordination exercises, visualization, education, and motivation activities.

A recent pilot study by Leddy and colleagues compared functional magnetic resonance imaging (fMRI) activation patterns during a cognitive task, exercise capacity, and symptoms in PCS patients who received exercise treatment with (a) a PCS placebo stretching group and (b) a healthy control group.[55] The number of study participants was limited, with only four patients per group. Patients completed a math processing task during fMRI and an exercise treadmill test before (time 1) and after approximately 12 weeks (time 2) of the exercise treatment.[55] Those in the exercise treatment group performed aerobic exercise at 80% of the heart rate (HR) attained on the treadmill test for 20 minutes per day with an HR monitor at home, 6 days per week.[55] At time 1, there was no difference in fMRI activation between the two PCS groups; however, the healthy controls had significantly greater activation in the posterior cingulate gyrus, lingual gyrus, and cerebellum versus all PCS subjects. At time 2, the PCS patients in the exercise group did not differ from healthy controls, whereas PCS patients in the placebo stretching group had significantly less activity in the cerebellum, anterior cingulate gyrus, and thalamus than healthy controls.[55] After 12 weeks of the exercise program, PCS patients achieved a significantly greater exercise HR and had fewer symptoms than the placebo stretching group. Interestingly, cognitive performance did not differ by group or time. The authors concluded that controlled aerobic exercise rehabilitation might help restore normal CBF regulation, as indicated by fMRI activation, in PCS patients.[55] These studies need to be further explored with a larger group of patients; however, these preliminary results are extremely encouraging.

CONCLUDING THOUGHTS

Treating patients with postconcussive symptoms is not an easy task. It is paramount to have a consistent and cohesive multidisciplinary approach when treating concussion patients with somatic, sleep, cognitive, or behavioral impairments.[86] Fortunately, most postconcussive symptoms resolve spontaneously and require only conservative treatment. Subgroups of patients do have prolonged recoveries, however, and may benefit from treatment with medications. While we have a variety of medications at our disposal, at this time there exists a clear inability to precisely treat concussion symptoms pharmacologically in this difficult population. The choice of which medication to use for a patient depends on the characteristic nature of the symptoms, and each decision should be made on an individual case basis.[86] Additionally, paradigms such as vestibular therapy, CBT, or controlled aerobic exercise rehabilitation should be considered as adjunct treatment measures for postconcussive patients with persistent symptoms. Future research should be geared toward developing well-designed studies to explore the effectiveness of these various treatment modalities.

REFERENCES

1. Medline Plus: Melatonin. 2010. Available from: www.nlm.nih.gov/medlineplus/druginfo/natural/940.html.

2. VA/DoD clinical practice guideline for management of concussion/mild traumatic brain injury. J Rehabil Res Dev 2009;46(6):CP1-68.

3. Abend NS, Nance ML, Bonnemann C. Subcutaneous sumatriptan in an adolescent with acute posttraumatic headache. J Child Neurol 2008;23(4):438-440.

4. Al Sayegh A, Sandford D, Carson AJ. Psychological approaches to treatment of postconcussion syndrome: a systematic review. J Neurol Neurosurg Psychiatry 2010;81(10):1128-1134.

5. Alsalaheen BA, Mucha A, Morris LO, Whitney SL, Furman JM, Camiolo-Reddy CE, et al. Vestibular rehabilitation for dizziness and balance disorders after concussion. J Neurol Phys Ther 2010;34(2):87-93.

6. Arciniegas DB, Anderson CA, Topkoff J, McAllister TW. Mild traumatic brain injury: a neuropsychiatric approach to diagnosis, evaluation, and treatment. Neuropsychiatr Dis Treat 2005;1(4):311-327.

7. Baker JG, Freitas MS, Leddy JJ, Kozlowski KF, Willer BS. Return to full functioning after graded exercise assessment and progressive exercise treatment of postconcussion syndrome. Rehabil Res Pract 2012;2012:705309.

8. Barkhoudarian G, Hovda DA, Giza CC. The molecular pathophysiology of concussive brain injury. Clin Sports Med 2011;30(1):33-48, vii-viii.

9. Beauchamp K, Mutlak H, Smith WR, Shohami E, Stahel PF. Pharmacology of traumatic brain injury: where is the "golden bullet"? Mol Med 2008;14(11-12):731-740.

10. Blaylock RL, Maroon J. Immunoexcitotoxicity as a central mechanism in chronic traumatic encephalopathy—a unifying hypothesis. Surg Neurol Int 2011;2:107.

11. Bradbury CL, Christensen BK, Lau MA, Ruttan LA, Arundine AL, Green RE. The efficacy of cognitive behavior therapy in the treatment of emotional distress after acquired brain injury. Arch Phys Med Rehabil 2008;89(12 Suppl):S61-68.

12. Buscemi N, Vandermeer B, Hooton N, Pandya R, Tjosvold L, Hartling L, et al. The efficacy and safety of exogenous melatonin for primary sleep disorders. A meta-analysis. J Gen Intern Med 2005;20(12):1151-1158.

13. Buscemi N, Vandermeer B, Pandya R, Hooton N, Tjosvold L, Hartling L, et al. Melatonin for treatment of sleep disorders. Evid Rep Technol Assess (Summ) 2004(108):1-7.

14. Chew E, Zafonte RD. Pharmacological management of neurobehavioral disorders following traumatic brain injury—a state-of-the-art review. J Rehabil Res Dev 2009;46(6):851-879.

15. Cicerone KD. Remediation of "working attention" in mild traumatic brain injury. Brain Inj 2002;16(3):185-195.

16. Cicerone KD, Kalmar K. Persistent post concussive syndrome: the structure of subjective complaints after mild traumatic brain injury. J Head Trauma Rehabil 1995;10(3):1-17.

17. Cohen SP, Plunkett AR, Wilkinson I, Nguyen C, Kurihara C, Flagg A II, et al. Headaches during war: analysis of presentation, treatment, and

factors associated with outcome. Cephalalgia 2012;32(2):94-108.

18. Collins MW, Grindel SH, Lovell MR, Dede DE, Moser DJ, Phalin BR, et al. Relationship between concussion and neuropsychological performance in college football players. JAMA 1999;282(10):964-970.

19. Collins MW, Lovell MR, McKeag DB. Current issues in managing sports-related concussion. JAMA 1999;282(24):2283-2285.

20. Comper P, Bisschop SM, Carnide N, Tricco A. A systematic review of treatments for mild traumatic brain injury. Brain Inj 2005;19(11):863-880.

21. Dashnaw ML, Petraglia AL, Bailes JE. An overview of the basic science of concussion and subconcussion: where we are and where we are going. Neurosurg Focus 2012;33(6):E5:1-9.

22. Dinan TG, Mobayed M. Treatment resistance of depression after head injury: a preliminary study of amitriptyline response. Acta Psychiatr Scand 1992;85(4):292-294.

23. Erickson JC. Treatment outcomes of chronic post-traumatic headaches after mild head trauma in US soldiers: an observational study. Headache 2011;51(6):932-944.

24. Fann JR, Uomoto JM, Katon WJ. Cognitive improvement with treatment of depression following mild traumatic brain injury. Psychosomatics 2001;42(1):48-54.

25. Fann JR, Uomoto JM, Katon WJ. Sertraline in the treatment of major depression following mild traumatic brain injury. J Neuropsychiatry Clin Neurosci 2000;12(2):226-232.

26. Faux S, Sheedy J. A prospective controlled study in the prevalence of posttraumatic headache following mild traumatic brain injury. Pain Med 2008;9(8):1001-1011.

27. Flanagan SR, Greenwald B, Wieber S. Pharmacological treatment of insomnia for individuals with brain injury. J Head Trauma Rehabil 2007;22(1):67-70.

28. Frenette AJ, Kanji S, Rees L, Williamson DR, Perreault MM, Turgeon AF, et al. Efficacy and safety of dopamine agonists in traumatic brain injury: a systematic review of randomized controlled trials. J Neurotrauma 2012;29(1):1-18.

29. Gawel MJ, Rothbart P, Jacobs H. Subcutaneous sumatriptan in the treatment of acute episodes of posttraumatic headache. Headache 1993;33(2):96-97.

30. Giza CC, Hovda DA. The neurometabolic cascade of concussion. J Athl Train 2001;36(3):228-235.

31. Gottshall K. Vestibular rehabilitation after mild traumatic brain injury with vestibular pathology. NeuroRehabilitation 2011;29(2):167-171.

32. Gottshall KR, Hoffer ME. Tracking recovery of vestibular function in individuals with blast-induced head trauma using vestibular-visual-cognitive interaction tests. J Neurol Phys Ther 2010;34(2):94-97.

33. Gurr B, Coetzer BR. The effectiveness of cognitive-behavioural therapy for post-traumatic headaches. Brain Inj 2005;19(7):481-491.

34. Gurr B, Moffat N. Psychological consequences of vertigo and the effectiveness of vestibular rehabilitation for brain injury patients. Brain Inj 2001;15(5):387-400.

35. Guskiewicz KM, Bruce SL, Cantu RC, Ferrara MS, Kelly JP, McCrea M, et al. Recommendations on management of sport-related concussion: summary of the National Athletic Trainers' Association position statement. Neurosurgery 2004;55(4):891-895; discussion 896.

36. Guskiewicz KM, McCrea M, Marshall SW, Cantu RC, Randolph C, Barr W, et al. Cumulative effects associated with recurrent concussion in collegiate football players: the NCAA Concussion Study. JAMA 2003;290(19):2549-2555.

37. Guskiewicz KM, Weaver NL, Padua DA, Garrett WE Jr. Epidemiology of concussion in collegiate and high school football players. Am J Sports Med 2000;28(5):643-650.

38. Haas DC. Chronic post-traumatic headaches classified and compared with natural headaches. Cephalalgia 1996;16(7):486-493.

39. Helmick K. Cognitive rehabilitation for military personnel with mild traumatic brain injury and chronic post-concussional disorder: results of April 2009 consensus conference. NeuroRehabilitation 2010;26(3):239-255.

40. Hicks RR, Smith DH, Lowenstein DH, Saint Marie R, McIntosh TK. Mild experimental brain injury in the rat induces cognitive deficits associated with regional neuronal loss in the hippocampus. J Neurotrauma 1993;10(4):405-414.

41. Hinkle JL, Alves WM, Rimell RW, Jane JA. Restoring social competence in minor head injury patients. J Neurosci Nurs 1986;18(5):268-271.

42. Ho MR, Bennett TL. Efficacy of neuropsychological rehabilitation for mild-moderate traumatic brain injury. Arch Clin Neuropsychol 1997;12(1):1-11.

43. Hoffer ME, Gottshall KR, Moore R, Balough BJ, Wester D. Characterizing and treating dizziness after mild head trauma. Otol Neurotol 2004;25(2):135-138.

44. Horsfield SA, Rosse RB, Tomasino V, Schwartz BL, Mastropaolo J, Deutsch SI. Fluoxetine's effects on cognitive performance in patients with traumatic brain injury. Int J Psychiatry Med 2002;32(4):337-344.

45. Iverson GL, Brooks BL, Collins MW, Lovell MR. Tracking neuropsychological recovery following concussion in sport. Brain Inj 2006;20(3):245-252.

46. Jha A, Weintraub A, Allshouse A, Morey C, Cusick C, Kittelson J, et al. A randomized trial of modafinil for the treatment of fatigue and excessive daytime sleepiness in individuals with chronic traumatic brain injury. J Head Trauma Rehabil 2008;23(1):52-63.

47. Johnson GV, Greenwood JA, Costello AC, Troncoso JC. The regulatory role of calmodulin in the proteolysis of individual neurofilament proteins by calpain. Neurochem Res 1991;16(8):869-873.

48. Kaiser PR, Valko PO, Werth E, Thomann J, Meier J, Stocker R, et al. Modafinil ameliorates excessive daytime sleepiness after traumatic brain injury. Neurology 2010;75(20):1780-1785.

49. Kaye NS, Townsend JB III, Ivins R. An open-label trial of donepezil (aricept) in the treatment of persons with mild traumatic brain injury. J Neuropsychiatry Clin Neurosci 2003;15(3):383-384; author reply 384-385.

50. Kemp S, Biswas R, Neumann V, Coughlan A. The value of melatonin for sleep disorders occurring post-head injury: a pilot RCT. Brain Inj 2004;18(9):911-919.

51. King NS. Post-concussion syndrome: clarity amid the controversy? Br J Psychiatry 2003;183:276-278.

52. Kraus MF, Smith GS, Butters M, Donnell AJ, Dixon E, Yilong C, et al. Effects of the dopaminergic agent and NMDA receptor antagonist amantadine on cognitive function, cerebral glucose metabolism and D2 receptor availability in chronic traumatic brain injury: a study using positron emission tomography (PET). Brain Inj 2005;19(7):471-479.

53. Lane JC, Arciniegas DB. Post-traumatic headache. Curr Treat Options Neurol 2002;4(1):89-104.

54. Leddy JJ, Baker JG, Kozlowski K, Bisson L, Willer B. Reliability of a graded exercise test for assessing recovery from concussion. Clin J Sport Med 2011;21(2):89-94.

55. Leddy JJ, Cox JL, Baker JG, Wack DS, Pendergast DR, Zivadinov R, et al. Exercise treatment for postconcussion syndrome: a pilot study of changes in functional magnetic resonance imaging activation, physiology, and symptoms. J Head Trauma Rehabil 2013;28(4):241-249.

56. Leddy JJ, Kozlowski K, Donnelly JP, Pendergast DR, Epstein LH, Willer B. A preliminary study of subsymptom threshold exercise training for refractory post-concussion syndrome. Clin J Sport Med 2010;20(1):21-27.

57. Leddy JJ, Kozlowski K, Fung M, Pendergast DR, Willer B. Regulatory and autoregulatory physiological dysfunction as a primary characteristic of post concussion syndrome: implications for treatment. NeuroRehabilitation 2007;22(3):199-205.

58. Leddy JJ, Sandhu H, Sodhi V, Baker JG, Willer B. Rehabilitation of concussion and post-concussion syndrome. Sports Health 2012;4(2):147-154.

59. Len TK, Neary JP. Cerebrovascular pathophysiology following mild traumatic brain injury. Clin Physiol Funct Imaging 2011;31(2):85-93.

60. Lenaerts ME, Couch JR. Posttraumatic headache. Curr Treat Options Neurol 2004;6(6):507-517.

61. Leone H, Polsonetti BW. Amantadine for traumatic brain injury: does it improve cognition and reduce agitation? J Clin Pharm Ther 2005;30(2):101-104.

62. Levin HS. Treatment of postconcussional symptoms with CDP-choline. J Neurol Sci 1991;103 Suppl:S39-42.

63. Lew HL, Lin PH, Fuh JL, Wang SJ, Clark DJ, Walker WC. Characteristics and treatment of headache after traumatic brain injury: a focused review. Am J Phys Med Rehabil 2006;85(7):619-627.

64. Maldonado MD, Murillo-Cabezas F, Terron MP, Flores LJ, Tan DX, Manchester LC, et al. The potential of melatonin in reducing morbidity-mortality after craniocerebral trauma. J Pineal Res 2007;42(1):1-11.

65. Martelli MF, Grayson RL, Zasler ND. Posttraumatic headache: neuropsychological and psychological effects and treatment implications. J Head Trauma Rehabil 1999;14(1):49-69.

66. Masanic CA, Bayley MT, VanReekum R, Simard M. Open-label study of donepezil in traumatic brain injury. Arch Phys Med Rehabil 2001;82(7):896-901.

67. Mata M, Staple J, Fink DJ. Changes in intra-axonal calcium distribution following nerve crush. J Neurobiol 1986;17(5):449-467.

68. Maxwell WL, McCreath BJ, Graham DI, Gennarelli TA. Cytochemical evidence for redistribution of membrane pump calcium-ATPase and ecto-Ca-ATPase activity, and calcium influx in myelinated nerve fibres of the optic nerve after stretch injury. J Neurocytol 1995;24(12):925-942.

69. Maxwell WL, Povlishock JT, Graham DL. A mechanistic analysis of nondisruptive axonal injury: a review. J Neurotrauma 1997;14(7):419-440.

70. McBeath JG, Nanda A. Use of dihydroergotamine in patients with postconcussion syndrome. Headache 1994;34(3):148-151.

71. McCrea M, Hammeke T, Olsen G, Leo P, Guskiewicz K. Unreported concussion in high school football players: implications for prevention. Clin J Sport Med 2004;14(1):13-17.

72. McCrory P, Meeuwisse W, Johnston K, Dvorak J, Aubry M, Molloy M, et al. Consensus statement on concussion in sport: the 3rd International Conference on Concussion in Sport held in Zurich, November 2008. Br J Sports Med 2009;43 Suppl 1:i76-90.

73. Meehan WP III. Medical therapies for concussion. Clin Sports Med 2011;30(1):115-124, ix.

74. Meythaler JM, Brunner RC, Johnson A, Novack TA. Amantadine to improve neurorecovery in traumatic brain injury-associated diffuse axonal injury: a pilot double-blind randomized trial. J Head Trauma Rehabil 2002;17(4):300-313.

75. Mittenberg W, Burton DB. A survey of treatments for post-concussion syndrome. Brain Inj 1994;8(5):429-437.

76. Mittenberg W, Canyock EM, Condit D, Patton C. Treatment of post-concussion syndrome following mild head injury. J Clin Exp Neuropsychol 2001;23(6):829-836.

77. Muller U, Murai T, Bauer-Wittmund T, von Cramon DY. Paroxetine versus citalopram treatment of pathological crying after brain injury. Brain Inj 1999;13(10):805-811.

78. Noble JM, Hauser WA. Effects of rivastigmine on cognitive function in patients with traumatic brain injury. Neurology 2007;68(20):1749; author reply 1750.

79. Orff HJ, Ayalon L, Drummond SP. Traumatic brain injury and sleep disturbance: a review of current research. J Head Trauma Rehabil 2009;24(3):155-165.

80. Packard RC. Epidemiology and pathogenesis of posttraumatic headache. J Head Trauma Rehabil 1999;14(1):9-21.

81. Packard RC. Treatment of chronic daily post-traumatic headache with divalproex sodium. Headache 2000;40(9):736-739.

82. Palmese CA, Raskin SA. The rehabilitation of attention in individuals with mild traumatic brain injury, using the APT-II programme. Brain Inj 2000;14(6):535-548.

83. Paniak C, Reynolds S, Phillips K, Toller-Lobe G, Melnyk A, Nagy J. Patient complaints within 1 month of mild traumatic brain injury: a controlled study. Arch Clin Neuropsychol 2002;17(4):319-334.

84. Paniak C, Toller-Lobe G, Durand A, Nagy J. A randomized trial of two treatments for mild traumatic brain injury. Brain Inj 1998;12(12):1011-1023.

85. Paniak C, Toller-Lobe G, Reynolds S, Melnyk A, Nagy J. A randomized trial of two treatments for mild traumatic brain injury: 1 year follow-up. Brain Inj 2000;14(3):219-226.

86. Petraglia AL, Maroon JC, Bailes JE. From the field of play to the field of combat: a review of the pharmacological management of concussion. Neurosurgery 2012;70(6):1520-1533; discussion 1533.

87. Petraglia AL, Winkler EA, Bailes JE. Stuck at the bench: potential natural neuroprotective compounds for concussion. Surg Neurol Int 2011;2:146.

88. Pettus EH, Povlishock JT. Characterization of a distinct set of intra-axonal ultrastructural changes associated with traumatically induced alteration in axolemmal permeability. Brain Res 1996;722(1-2):1-11.

89. Plenger PM, Dixon CE, Castillo RM, Frankowski RF, Yablon SA, Levin HS. Subacute methylphenidate treatment for moderate to moderately severe traumatic brain injury: a preliminary double-blind placebo-controlled study. Arch Phys Med Rehabil 1996;77(6):536-540.

90. Ponsford J, Willmott C, Rothwell A, Cameron P, Ayton G, Nelms R, et al. Impact of early intervention on outcome after mild traumatic brain injury in children. Pediatrics 2001;108(6):1297-1303.

91. Ponsford J, Willmott C, Rothwell A, Cameron P, Kelly AM, Nelms R, et al. Impact of early intervention on outcome following mild head injury in adults. J Neurol Neurosurg Psychiatry 2002;73(3):330-332.

92. Potter S, Brown RG. Cognitive behavioural therapy and persistent post-concussional symptoms: integrating conceptual issues and practical aspects in treatment. Neuropsychol Rehabil 2012;22(1):1-25.

93. Povlishock JT, Pettus EH. Traumatically induced axonal damage: evidence for enduring changes in axolemmal permeability with associated cytoskeletal change. Acta Neurochir Suppl 1996;66:81-86.

94. Rao V, Rollings P. Sleep disturbances following traumatic brain injury. Curr Treat Options Neurol 2002;4(1):77-87.

95. Rapoport AM, Tepper SJ. Triptans are all different. Arch Neurol 2001;58(9):1479-1480.

96. Rapoport MJ, Chan F, Lanctot K, Herrmann N, McCullagh S, Feinstein A. An open-label study of citalopram for major depression following traumatic brain injury. J Psychopharmacol 2008;22(8):860-864.

97. Rapoport MJ, Mitchell RA, McCullagh S, Herrmann N, Chan F, Kiss A, et al. A randomized controlled trial of antidepressant continuation for major depression following traumatic brain injury. J Clin Psychiatry 2010;71(9):1125-1130.

98. Reddy C. A treatment paradigm for sports concussion. Brain Injury Professional 2004;4:24-25.

99. Reiter RJ, Korkmaz A. Clinical aspects of melatonin. Saudi Med J 2008;29(11):1537-1547.

100. Rogers NL, Dinges DF, Kennaway DJ, Dawson D. Potential action of melatonin in insomnia. Sleep 2003;26(8):1058-1059.

101. Rohling ML, Faust ME, Beverly B, Demakis G. Effectiveness of cognitive rehabilitation following acquired brain injury: a meta-analytic re-examination of Cicerone et al's (2000, 2005) systematic reviews. Neuropsychology 2009;23(1):20-39.

102. Rosenberg G. The mechanisms of action of valproate in neuropsychiatric disorders: can we

see the forest for the trees? Cell Mol Life Sci 2007;64(16):2090-2103.

103. Ruff RL, Ruff SS, Wang XF. Improving sleep: initial headache treatment in OIF/OEF veterans with blast-induced mild traumatic brain injury. J Rehabil Res Dev 2009;46(9):1071-1084.

104. Saatman KE, Abai B, Grosvenor A, Vorwerk CK, Smith DH, Meaney DF. Traumatic axonal injury results in biphasic calpain activation and retrograde transport impairment in mice. J Cereb Blood Flow Metab 2003;23(1):34-42.

105. Salazar AM. Impact of early intervention on outcome following mild head injury in adults. J Neurol Neurosurg Psychiatry 2002;73(3):239.

106. Samantaray S, Das A, Thakore NP, Matzelle DD, Reiter RJ, Ray SK, et al. Therapeutic potential of melatonin in traumatic central nervous system injury. J Pineal Res 2009;47(2):134-142.

107. Saran A. Antidepressants not effective in headache associated with minor closed head injury. Int J Psychiatry Med 1988;18(1):75-83.

108. Saran AS. Depression after minor closed head injury: role of dexamethasone suppression test and antidepressants. J Clin Psychiatry 1985;46(8):335-338.

109. Sawyer E, Mauro LS, Ohlinger MJ. Amantadine enhancement of arousal and cognition after traumatic brain injury. Ann Pharmacother 2008;42(2):247-252.

110. Sedney CL, Orphanos J, Bailes JE. When to consider retiring an athlete after sports-related concussion. Clin Sports Med 2011;30(1):189-200, xi.

111. Sheftell FD, Weeks RE, Rapoport AM, Siegel S, Baskin S, Arrowsmith F. Subcutaneous sumatriptan in a clinical setting: the first 100 consecutive patients with acute migraine in a tertiary care center. Headache 1994;34(2):67-72.

112. Silver JM, Koumaras B, Chen M, Mirski D, Potkin SG, Reyes P, et al. Effects of rivastigmine on cognitive function in patients with traumatic brain injury. Neurology 2006;67(5):748-755.

113. Silver JM, Koumaras B, Meng X, Potkin SG, Reyes PF, Harvey PD, et al. Long-term effects of rivastigmine capsules in patients with traumatic brain injury. Brain Inj 2009;23(2):123-132.

114. Silver JM, McAllister TW, Arciniegas DB. Depression and cognitive complaints following mild traumatic brain injury. Am J Psychiatry 2009;166(6):653-661.

115. Solomon S. Posttraumatic headache. Med Clin North Am 2001;85(4):987-996, vii-viii.

116. Spain A, Daumas S, Lifshitz J, Rhodes J, Andrews PJ, Horsburgh K, et al. Mild fluid percussion injury in mice produces evolving selective axonal pathology and cognitive deficits relevant to human brain injury. J Neurotrauma 2010;27(8):1429-1438.

117. Tenovuo O. Central acetylcholinesterase inhibitors in the treatment of chronic traumatic brain injury-clinical experience in 111 patients. Prog Neuropsychopharmacol Biol Psychiatry 2005;29(1):61-67.

118. Tenovuo O. Pharmacological enhancement of cognitive and behavioral deficits after traumatic brain injury. Curr Opin Neurol 2006;19(6):528-533.

119. Tenovuo O, Alin J, Helenius H. A randomized controlled trial of rivastigmine for chronic sequels of traumatic brain injury-what it showed and taught? Brain Inj 2009;23(6):548-558.

120. Tepper SJ. Safety and rational use of the triptans. Med Clin North Am 2001;85(4):959-970.

121. Tepper SJ, Millson D. Safety profile of the triptans. Expert Opin Drug Saf 2003;2(2):123-132.

122. Tiersky LA, Anselmi V, Johnston MV, Kurtyka J, Roosen E, Schwartz T, et al. A trial of neuropsychologic rehabilitation in mild-spectrum traumatic brain injury. Arch Phys Med Rehabil 2005;86(8):1565-1574.

123. Tyler GS, McNeely HE, Dick ML. Treatment of post-traumatic headache with amitriptyline. Headache 1980;20(4):213-216.

124. Van Kampen DA, Lovell MR, Pardini JE, Collins MW, Fu FH. The "value added" of neurocognitive testing after sports-related concussion. Am J Sports Med 2006;34(10):1630-1635.

125. Vidal PG, Goodman AM, Colin A, Leddy JJ, Grady MF. Rehabilitation strategies for prolonged recovery in pediatric and adolescent concussion. Pediatric Ann 2012;41(9):1-7.

126. Wade DT, Crawford S, Wenden FJ, King NS, Moss NE. Does routine follow up after head injury help? A randomised controlled trial. J Neurol Neurosurg Psychiatry 1997;62(5):478-484.

127. Wade DT, King NS, Wenden FJ, Crawford S, Caldwell FE. Routine follow up after head injury: a second randomised controlled trial. J Neurol Neurosurg Psychiatry 1998;65(2):177-183.

128. Walker W, Seel R, Gibellato M, Lew H, Cornis-Pop M, Jena T, et al. The effects of Donepezil on traumatic brain injury acute rehabilitation outcomes. Brain Inj 2004;18(8):739-750.

129. Warden DL, Gordon B, McAllister TW, Silver JM, Barth JT, Bruns J, et al. Guidelines for the pharmacologic treatment of neurobehavioral sequelae of traumatic brain injury. J Neurotrauma 2006;23(10):1468-1501.

130. Weiss HD, Stern BJ, Goldberg J. Post-traumatic migraine: chronic migraine precipitated by minor head or neck trauma. Headache 1991;31(7):451-456.

131. Wheaton P, Mathias JL, Vink R. Impact of pharmacological treatments on cognitive and behavioral outcome in the postacute stages of adult traumatic brain injury: a meta-analysis. J Clin Psychopharmacol 2011;31(6):745-757.

132. Whelan FJ, Walker MS, Schultz SK. Donepezil in the treatment of cognitive dysfunction associated with traumatic brain injury. Ann Clin Psychiatry 2000;12(3):131-135.

133. Whyte J, Hart T, Schuster K, Fleming M, Polansky M, Coslett HB. Effects of methylphenidate on attentional function after traumatic brain injury. A randomized, placebo-controlled trial. Am J Phys Med Rehabil 1997;76(6):440-450.

134. Whyte J, Hart T, Vaccaro M, Grieb-Neff P, Risser A, Polansky M, et al. Effects of methylphenidate on attention deficits after traumatic brain injury: a multidimensional, randomized, controlled trial. Am J Phys Med Rehabil 2004;83(6):401-420.

135. Willer B, Leddy JJ. Management of concussion and post-concussion syndrome. Curr Treat Options Neurol 2006;8(5):415-426.

136. Williams SE, Ris MD, Ayyangar R, Schefft BK, Berch D. Recovery in pediatric brain injury: is psychostimulant medication beneficial? J Head Trauma Rehabil 1998;13(3):73-81.

137. Zee DS. Perspectives on the pharmacotherapy of vertigo. Arch Otolaryngol 1985;111(9):609-612.

138. Zhang L, Plotkin RC, Wang G, Sandel ME, Lee S. Cholinergic augmentation with donepezil enhances recovery in short-term memory and sustained attention after traumatic brain injury. Arch Phys Med Rehabil 2004;85(7):1050-1055.

The Research Behind Natural Neuroprotective Approaches to Concussion

In collaboration with
Ethan A. Winkler, MD, PhD

Significant efforts have been made in recent years to discover substances that can provide neuroprotection against diseases of the central nervous system (CNS). Regarding traumatic brain injury (TBI), no therapies generated in the laboratory have successfully translated from the bench to the bedside. Concussion is a unique form of TBI in that the current mainstay of treatment focuses on both physical and cognitive rest. There has been immense interest in natural compounds, nutraceuticals (i.e., food derivatives or dietary supplements and herbal remedies that provide health benefits), and other natural alternative treatment measures such as hyperbaric oxygen. [164] Some of these preparations and compounds have been used for centuries to treat illness and have become more popular in society lately, particularly because of their relatively few side effects.[164] With so many ineffective treatments, it is important to continue to explore potential neuroprotective translational therapies for TBI. Encouraging results from laboratory studies demonstrate the multimechanistic neuroprotective properties of many naturally occurring compounds and treatments. Similarly, some intriguing clinical observational studies potentially suggest both acute and chronic

neuroprotective effects. Here we review some of the research behind a few of these natural treatment approaches.

EICOSAPENTAENOIC ACID AND DOCOSAHEXAENOIC ACID

Omega-3 polyunsaturated fatty acids are important structural components of all cell membranes modulating membrane fluidity, thickness, cell signaling, and mitochondrial function.[63, 185] Long-chain polyunsaturated fatty acids, including eicosapentaenoic acid (EPA) and docosahexaenoic acid (DHA), are highly enriched in neuronal synaptosomal plasma membranes and vesicles. [63] The predominant CNS polyunsaturated fatty acid is DHA, which is readily retained in neuronal plasma membranes.[139] Neuronal DHA, in turn, influences the phospholipid content of the plasma membrane, increasing phosphatidylserine and phosphatidylethanolamine production and promoting neurite outgrowth during both development and adulthood.[34, 176] Despite DHA's importance for CNS function, the predominant dietary polyunsaturated fatty is linolenic acid obtained through ingestion of certain nuts and vegetable oils, which is inefficiently converted to

EPA or DHA.[96] Therefore, effective supplementation or increased ingestion of dietary sources rich in EPA and DHA, such as cold-water fish species and fish oil, may help improve a multitude of neuronal functions, including long-term potentiation and cognition[114, 141, 146].

With respect to neuroprotection in the context of improving outcomes following TBI, multiple preclinical studies have suggested that supplementation with DHA, EPA, or both may have potential benefit through a multitude of diverse but complementary mechanisms.[13, 145, 232, 233] Studies using rodent models of experimental injury have shown that preinjury dietary supplementation with fish oil effectively reduces posttraumatic elevations in protein oxidation, resulting in stabilization of multiple molecular mediators of learning, memory, cellular energy homeostasis, and mitochondrial calcium homeostasis, as well as improving cognitive performance[232, 233] (table 15.1). Not only have the benefits of pretraumatic DHA supplementation been independently confirmed,[145] but DHA supplementation has been shown to significantly reduce the number of swollen, disconnected, and injured axons when administered following TBI. [13, 145] Of note, DHA has provided neuroprotection in experimental models of both focal and diffuse TBI.[13, 145, 232, 233] Studies in other models of neurological injury have revealed a variety of potential mechanisms of neuroprotection in addition to DHA's and EPA's well-established antioxidant and anti-inflammatory properties[32, 34, 35, 66, 87, 131, 132, 140, 144, 166, 176, 188, 203, 223, 232, 233] (table 15.1).

Despite abundant laboratory evidence supporting its neuroprotective effects in experimental models, the role of dietary DHA or EPA supplementation in human neurological diseases remains uncertain. To date, no clinical trials have investigated the effects of DHA or EPA dietary supplementation on the treatment or prevention of TBI. Several population-based observational studies have suggested that increased consumption of dietary fish, omega-3 polyunsaturated fatty acid, or both may reduce risk for ischemic stroke in several populations[83, 93, 148]; however, such benefit has not been observed in all populations studied.[31] Randomized controlled trials have also demonstrated significant reductions in ischemic stroke recurrence,[212] relative risk for ischemic stroke,[2] and reduced incidence of both symptomatic vasospasm and mortality

following subarachnoid hemorrhage.[248] Multiple studies, on the other hand, have found no statistically significant reduction in neurological impairment following ischemic stroke[73, 168] or reductions in epileptic seizure frequency.[28, 58, 169, 250] Clinical trials in Alzheimer's disease have also been largely ineffective.[170] The clinical evidence thus far appears equivocal; however, the overall difficulty in controlling for basal dietary intake of polyunsaturated fatty acids between experimental groups, lack of good study design, and the significant heterogeneity of the studied patient populations make these studies difficult to interpret collectively. Nonetheless, the multimechanistic neuroprotective properties and the positive preclinical findings associated with omega-3 polyunsaturated fatty acid supplementation warrant well-designed clinical trials in the future to determine whether supplementation may improve outcomes following mild TBI.

CURCUMIN

Curcumin is a flavonoid compound that is the principal curcuminoid of the Indian spice turmeric. It is also a member of the ginger family. While this natural phenol is most commonly known for providing the yellow pigment seen in many curries, curcumin has long been a staple of traditional remedies offered by practitioners of Oriental and Aryurvedic medicine.[74] More recently, curcumin has gained much attention from Western researchers for its potential therapeutic benefits in large part due to its potent antioxidant[127, 189, 231] and anti-inflammatory properties.[3, 115, 138] Curcumin is highly lipophilic and crosses the blood–brain barrier, enabling it to exert a multitude of established neuroprotective effects (table 15.2). Multiple experimental animal models have suggested that curcumin supplementation may offer benefit in the treatment of chronic neurodegenerative processes such as Alzheimer's disease,[127, 242] as well as of acute neurological insults including ischemic stroke[62, 95, 198, 216, 241, 254] and subarachnoid hemorrhage.[222]

Specifically in the context of TBI, a series of preclinical studies suggested that pretraumatic and posttraumatic curcumin supplementation may bolster the brain's resilience to injury and serve as a valuable therapeutic option.[115, 196, 197, 231, 234] Curcumin may confer significant neuro-

Table 15.1 Eicosapentaenoic Acid– and Docosahexaenoic Acid–Mediated Multimechanstic Neuroprotection

Mechanism	Model	Agent	Summary	References
Antioxidant	Cell culture	Docosa-hexaenoic acid (DHA)	Increased activity of glutathione peroxidase and glutathione reductase	223
	Rat corpus callosum	Fish oil	Increased activity of superoxide dismutase Reduced activity of xanthine oxidase activity and nitric oxide levels	188
	Rat hypo-thalamus	Fish oil	Reduced activity of superoxide dismutase Decreased nitric oxide and tissue malondialde-hyde (lipid peroxidation) levels	203
	Gerbil isch-emia	DHA	Increased activity of glutathione peroxidase and catalase levels	35
	Rat TBI	Fish oil	Reduced protein oxidation	232, 233
Anti-inflammatory	Isolated monocytes Isolated monocytes	Fish oil	Decreased synthesis of interleukin-1β (IL-1β) and tumor necrosis factor-α (TNF-α) Decreased synthesis of TNF-α, IL-1, IL-6, and IL-8 Reduced monocyte–endothelium adhesion and transendothelial migration	66 140
	Cell culture	Eicosa-pentaenoic acid (EPA)	Inhibition of downstream mediators of c-Jun N-terminal kinases (JNK) pathway	131
	Cell culture	DHA	Reduced expression of TNF-α, IL-6, nitric oxide synthase, and Cyclooxygenase-2 (COX-2) in microglia	132
Reduction in excitoxicity	Cell culture	DHA	Inhibition of glutamate-induced neuronal toxic-ity	223
	Rat nucleus basalis	Fish oil	Increased neuronal survival following N-Methyl-D-aspartate (NMDA) receptor activation	87
	Organotypic hippocampal slices	DHA	Reduced neuronal toxicity following α-Amino-3-hydroxy-5-methyl-4-isoxazolepropionic acid (AMPA) receptor activation	144
Mitochondrial protection	Rat traumatic brain injury (TBI)	Fish oil	Counteracted posttraumatic reductions in ubiq-uitous mitochondrial creatinine kinase (uMtCK)	233
Protection of brain me-tabolism	Cell culture	EPA/DHA	Increased blood–brain barrier glucose transport	166
	Rat TBI	Fish oil	Counteracted posttraumatic reductions in the silent information regulator 2 (Sir2) and uMtCK	233
Neurite growth and neurogenesis	Cell culture	DHA	Increased neuron population and increased length of neurites	32
	Cell culture	DHA	Increased neuronal viability and increased length of neurites	34
	Cell culture	EPA/DHA	Increased neurite outgrowth	176
Protection of synaptic plasticity	Rat TBI	Fish oil	Counteracted posttraumatic reductions in brain-derived neurotrophic factor (BDNF), synapsin I, and cyclic adenosine monophosphate (cAMP) responsive element binding protein (CREB)	232

Table 15.2 Mechanisms of Curcumin–Mediated Neuroprotection

Mechanism	Model	Agent	Summary	References
Antioxidant	Alzheimer's mice	Curcumin	Reduced protein oxidation	131
	Rat TBI	Curcumin	Reduced protein oxidation	231
	Rat TBI	CNB-001	Reduced lipid peroxidation	196
	Rat TBI	CNB-001	Normalized posttraumatic superoxide dismutase levels	234
	Rat ischemia	Curcumin	Counteracted reductions in glutathione peroxidase Decreased levels of reactive oxygen species, peroxynitrite, and nitric oxide	62, 95, 216
	Rat ischemia	Curcumin	Increased activity of superoxide dismutase and reduced lipid peroxidation	198
Anti-inflammatory	Alzheimer's mice	Curcumin	Reduced levels of IL-1β and perineuronal microgliosis	127
	Mouse TBI	Curcumin	Reduced expression of IL-1β and inhibited nuclear factor kappa B (NFκB) Reduced reactive astrogliosis	115
	Rat ischemia	Curcumin	Counteracted post-ischemic neutrophil infiltration	62
Anti-apoptotic	Rat ischemia	Curcumin	Decreased levels of cytochrome c and cleaved caspase 3 expression Increased B-cell lymphoma-2 (Bcl-2) expression	254
Protects blood–brain barrier	Rat ischemia	Curcumin	Reduced blood–brain barrier disruption	95
Decreases edema	Mouse TBI	Curcumin	Counteracted posttraumatic upregulation of astrocyte aquaporin-4	115
	Rat ischemia	Curcumin	Reduced edema following ischemic injury	62, 95
Mitochondrial protection	Rat TBI	Curcumin	Counteracted posttraumatic reductions in uMtCK, uncoupling protein 2 (UCP-2), and Cyclooxygenase-2 (COX-2)	197
	Rat ischemia	Curcumin	Decreased levels of cytochrome c and increased Bcl-2 expression	254
Protection of brain metabolism	Rat TBI	Curcumin	Counteracted posttraumatic reductions in the Sir2, adenosine monophosphate (AMP)-activated protein kinase (AMPK), uMtCK, UCP-2	231
	Rat TBI	CNB-001	Counteracted posttraumatic reductions in Sir2	234
Plasma membrane turnover	Rat TBI	CNB-001	Counteracted posttraumatic reductions in phospholipase A2 protein levels	196
Protects synaptic plasticity	Rat TBI	Curcumin	Counteracted posttraumatic reductions in BDNF, synapsin I, and CREB	231
	Rat TBI	CNB-001	Counteracted posttraumatic reductions in NMDA receptor NR2B subunit and syntaxin 3	196
	Rat TBI	CNB-001	Counteracted posttraumatic reductions in BDNF, synapsin I, CREB, and calcium/calmodulin-dependent protein kinase (CaMKII)	234

protection because of its ability to act on multiple deleterious posttraumatic molecular cascades. For example, pretraumatic curcumin supplementation improved posttraumatic cognitive deficits and stabilized levels of certain proteins implicated in the molecular mechanisms underlying learning, memory, and cellular energy homeostasis[115, 197, 231] (table 15.2). Additionally, these studies demonstrated that both pre- and posttraumatic curcumin administration resulted in a significant reduction of neuroinflammation via inhibition of the proinflammatory molecules interleukin-1β (IL-1β) and nuclear factor kappa B (NFκB). More importantly, the reduced neuroinflammatory response mitigated posttraumatic reactive astrogliosis and prevented upregulation of the water channel aquaporin 4, thus reducing the magnitude of cellular edema. It was determined, though, that prophylactic administration of curcumin exerted greater neuroprotective effects than posttraumatic treatment and that the therapeutic window for significant neuroprotection in these studies was less than 1 hour post-TBI.[115]

Other studies have further evaluated the benefits of posttraumatic administration of a curcumin derivative, CNB-001, with enhanced neuroprotective properties.[130, 196, 234] These studies demonstrate that this compound is capable of significantly reducing posttraumatic elevations in lipid peroxidation and protein oxidation, as well as disturbances in plasma membrane turnover and phospholipid metabolism. Additionally, this curcumin derivative prevented reductions in proteins important for learning, memory, and synaptic transmission and promoted cellular energy homeostasis (table 15.2). Posttraumatic administration of CNB-001 also improved injury-associated behavioral impairment,[196, 234] thereby suggesting that curcumin-induced normalization of multiple molecular systems may help preserve neuronal structure and function during the postinjury period.

Therapeutic administration of curcumin in human patients has been shown to be well tolerated.[15, 60] However, despite a tremendous amount of laboratory evidence demonstrating the neuroprotective effects of curcumin, to date no human studies have been conducted with respect to the effects of curcumin administration on the treatment of TBI, subarachnoid or intracranial hemorrhage, epilepsy, or stroke. Preliminary clinical evidence in support of curcumin's neuroprotective properties has come from several epidemiologic studies. One study suggested that curcumin, a spice highly consumed in the Indian culture, may be partially responsible for the significant reductions in Alzheimer's disease prevalence observed in India when compared to the United States.[39] Another study suggested that increased curry consumption in an elderly population is associated with higher Mini Mental Status Examination scores.[154] In spite of these initial favorable findings, the results of more recent clinical trials in several Alzheimer's disease populations remain equivocal.[80] Whether curcumin intake or administration can afford significant neuroprotection in human TBI remains largely unknown and underexplored.

RESVERATROL

Resveratrol is a naturally occurring phytoalexin and stilbenoid compound found in multiple dietary sources including red wine, grapes, and peanuts[17]. Since its discovery in 1940, resveratrol has gained media attention as the cardioprotective agent in red wine[26] and for its capability to extend vertebrate life span.[16] Resveratrol has been demonstrated to effectively cross the blood–brain barrier and improve outcomes in animal models following multiple acute neurologic insults including stroke,[71, 90, 122, 171, 201] global cerebral ischemia,[59] spinal cord injury,[100, 111, 243] and TBI.[11, 200, 204] Resveratrol has also been demonstrated to slow the development of chronic neurodegenerative disease in animal models.[102, 174] Although many of resveratrol's therapeutic benefits are classically attributed to its potent antioxidant effects,[11, 17] numerous studies have identified additional mechanisms of neuroprotection (table 15.3).

Preclinical studies have also explored resveratrol's therapeutic effect on experimental TBI. Studies have demonstrated that the posttraumatic administration of resveratrol reduces neuropathologic and behavioral sequelae in both immature and adult rodents.[11, 200, 204] Resveratrol treatment in immature rodents reduced posttraumatic neuronal loss and improved behavioral measures of locomotion, anxiety, and novel object recognition memory.[204] In adult rodents, administration of resveratrol resulted in reduced levels of oxidative stress and lipid peroxidation

Table 15.3   Mechanisms of Resveratrol Neuroprotection

Mechanism	Model	Agent	Summary	References
Antioxidant	Rat ischemia	Resveratrol	Counteracted post-ischemia elevations in tissue malondialdehyde (lipid peroxidation) and reductions in brain glutathione	201
	Rabbit spinal cord ischemia	Resveratrol	Reduced spinal cord malondialdehyde (lipid peroxidation) levels	100
	Rabbit spinal cord ischemia	Resveratrol	Reduced spinal cord malondialdehyde (lipid peroxidation) and nitric oxide levels	111
	Rat TBI	Resveratrol	Counteracted posttraumatic elevations in malondialdehyde, xanthine oxidase, and nitric oxide levels. Increased posttraumatic glutathione levels	11
Anti-inflammatory	Rabbit spinal cord ischemia	Resveratrol	Reduced spinal cord neutrophil infiltration	100
	Cell culture	Resveratrol	Inhibited NFκB	101
Reduces excitoxicity	Rat ischemia	Resveratrol	Reduced glutamate release and lessened excitotoxic index	122
Alters intraneuronal mediators	Organotypic hippocampal slices	Resveratrol	Activated nicotinamide adenine dinucleotide-dependent deacetylase sirtuin 1 (SIRT1)	171
	Rat ischemia	Resveratrol	Activated nicotinamide adenine dinucleotide-dependent deacetylase SIRT1	59
Maintains extracellular matrix	Mouse ischemia	Resveratrol	Counteracted post-ischemic upregulation of matrix metalloproteinase-9 (MMP-9)	71
Decreases edema	Rat spinal cord injury	Resveratrol	Reduced posttraumatic edema and improved Na+/K+-adenosine triphosphatase (ATPase) activity	243
	Rat TBI	Resveratrol	Reduced posttraumatic edema	11, 200

and stabilized endogenous antioxidants following TBI.[11] Furthermore, studies have demonstrated that resveratrol treatment reduces brain edema and lesion volume, as well as improving neurobehavioral functional performance following TBI.[11, 200] The molecular mechanisms underlying the neuroprotection remain largely unknown.

To date, no human trials have investigated the effects of resveratrol on the prevention or treatment of TBI. Administration of resveratrol in some clinical studies has shown that it is capable of increasing cerebral blood flow[105] and reducing inflammation via inhibition of the proinflammatory molecule NFκB.[101] Epidemiological studies have also suggested that increased red wine consumption is associated with reductions in stroke risk.[150] However, it remains to be

determined whether such protection is a result of improvements in other vascular and neuronal parameters or if it is even dependent on the presence of resveratrol. Therefore, further studies are needed to fully elucidate resveratrol's potential neuroprotective benefit, particularly in TBI.

CREATINE

Creatine is an amino acid-like compound favored as a dietary supplement by many athletes for its promotion of muscle mass production. It also plays an integral role in the endogenous maintenance of cellular energy reserves in tissues with high and fluctuating energy demands, such as the brain and skeletal muscle. Central nervous system creatine is derived both from its local biosynthesis from the essential amino acids methionine, glycine, and arginine and through the transport of circulating peripherally derived or dietary creatine across the blood–brain barrier.[18, 156] Dietary creatine is predominantly found in protein-rich foods such as meat, fish, and poultry. Biochemically, creatine is readily phosphorylated by creatine kinase to yield the high-energy analogue phosphocreatine. Phosphocreatine may then transfer its N-phosphoryl group to adenosine diphosphate (ADP), creating one molecule of adenosine triphosphate (ATP) and thereby replenishing cellular energy stores.[18] In the CNS, maintenance of cellular ATP levels is necessary for proper development and provides the cellular energy required to maintain the various cellular processes necessary for proper neuronal structure and function; these include the maintenance of neuronal membrane potential, ion gradients underlying signal propagation, intracellular calcium homeostasis, neurotransmission, intracellular and intercellular signal transduction, and neuritic transport.[18, 236] More recent evidence also suggests that creatine may serve as a neuronal cotransmitter augmenting postsynaptic gamma-aminobutyric acid (GABA) signal transduction.[5, 54, 153, 163] Studies of patients with CNS creatine deficiency and murine models with genetic ablation of creatine kinase have consistently demonstrated significant neurologic impairment in the absence of proper creatine, phosphocreatine, or creatine kinase function, thus highlighting its functional importance.[18, 152]

Preclinical studies in a variety of experimental models have suggested that dietary creatine may provide neuroprotection in animal models of chronic neurodegenerative disease, including Alzheimer's disease, Parkinson's disease, Huntington's disease, and amyotrophic lateral sclerosis.[18, 78] The neuroprotective effects may also be conferred in acute neurologic injuries, such as TBI.[190, 209] It is important to note that mild TBI reduces brain creatine and phosphocreatine levels in rodent models, suggesting that resulting impairments in the maintenance of cellular energy may play a role in the evolution of secondary brain injury.[199] In rodents, pretraumatic dietary supplementation with creatine monohydrate significantly reduced the magnitude of cortical tissue damage and the concentration of two biomarkers of cellular injury, free fatty acids and lactic acid, following experimental injury.[190,

209] It was further elucidated that creatine-mediated neuroprotection is in part mediated by the maintenance of cellular ATP levels and improvements in mitochondrial bioenergetics, including increased mitochondrial membrane potential and reductions in mitochondrial permeability, reactive oxygen species, and calcium levels.[209] Additional mechanisms of neuroprotection in the context of TBI remain to be determined.

In humans, studies using nuclear magnetic spectroscopy have demonstrated that creatine supplementation indeed increases cerebral creatine and phosphocreatine stores. Additionally, chronic dosing may partially reverse neurologic impairments in human CNS creatine deficiency syndromes.[78, 152] Acute supplementation of creatine may also improve cognition in elderly patients and in adults following sleep deprivation.[142, 143] Several studies have suggested that creatine supplementation may also reduce oxidative DNA damage and brain glutamate levels in Huntington's disease patients.[20, 86] Another study highlighted that creatine supplementation marginally improved indices of mood and reduced the need for increased dopaminergic therapy in patients with Parkinson's disease.[21] Together, these data suggest that dietary creatine supplementation may effectively increase CNS creatine–phosphocreatine stores and may modulate human neurologic disease.

No human studies have addressed the effects of prophylactic creatine supplementation on increasing brain resilience to TBI. However, preliminary results in a pediatric population have suggested that posttraumatic oral creatine administration (0.4 g/kg), given within 4 hours of TBI and then daily thereafter, may improve both acute and long-term outcomes.[183, 184] Acutely, posttraumatic creatine administration seemed to reduce duration of posttraumatic amnesia, length of time spent in the intensive care unit, and duration of intubation.[183] At 3 and 6 months postinjury, subjects in the creatine treatment group demonstrated improvement on indices of self-care, communication abilities, locomotion, sociability, personality or behavior, and cognitive function when compared to untreated controls. [183] Further analysis of the same population revealed that patients in the creatine treatment group were less likely to experience headaches, dizziness, and fatigue over 6 months of follow-up.[184] Most importantly, creatine treatment appeared to be well tolerated and no significant side effects were reported,[183, 184] which was consistent with other human studies using higher dosages.[10, 21, 86] While initial studies have also provided encouraging preliminary evidence supporting the use of creatine supplementation in the treatment of primary depression,[178] whether creatine may serve as an effective treatment for posttraumatic or postconcussive depression remains to be determined.

GREEN TEA

Although enjoyed by many for simply its taste and ability to bolster alertness during a time of fatigue, green tea is composed of a trio of protective compounds that have independently drawn the attention of researchers from diverse disciplines, including cardiology, oncology, rheumatology, and neurology. At the core of green tea's neuroprotective properties are the flavonoid epigallocatechin-3-gallate (EGCG), the amino acid theanine, and the methylxanthine caffeine (discussed later). All three of these compounds have been shown to exert multiple in vitro and in vivo neuroprotective effects[14, 79, 98, 106, 108, 137, 173] (table 15.4).

One of the most abundant compounds in green tea extract is the potent antioxidant EGCG, which is capable of crossing the blood–nerve and blood–brain barrier[151, 207] and exerting neuroprotective benefits in animal models of peripheral nerve injury,[228] spinal cord trauma,[106] and ischemic stroke.[49, 120, 159] Epigallocatechin-3-gallate also displays neuroprotective properties in animal models of chronic neurodegenerative diseases including amyotrophic lateral sclerosis,[113, 249] Parkinson's disease,[48, 121, 136] and Alzheimer's disease.[108, 173] Epigallocatechin-3-gallate's neuroprotection has largely been attributed to its potent antioxidant[14, 108, 173, 228] and anti-inflammatory properties[106, 137]; however, a number of studies have identified additional neuroprotective mechanisms (table 15.4).

Other animal studies have also demonstrated that theanine, another important component of green tea extract, exerts a multitude of neuroprotective benefits in experimental models of ischemic stroke,[64, 98] Alzheimer's disease[109] and Parkinson's disease.[43] Theanine, like EGCG, contains multiple mechanisms of neuroprotec-

tive action, including protection from excitotoxic injury[98] and inhibition of inflammation (table 15.4).[109]

As with most other natural compounds, no human trials have been conducted to investigate the effects of EGCG or theanine on reducing or treating brain injury following TBI; however, preliminary evidence has suggested that green tea–derived compounds may indeed modulate neuronal function in human subjects. For example, a randomized, placebo-controlled trial demonstrated that administration of green tea extract and L-theanine, over 16 weeks of treatment, improved indices of memory and brain theta wave activity on electroencephalography, suggesting greater cognitive alertness.[161] Additional studies have suggested that green tea extract may decrease cognitive decline in the elderly[155] and that L-theanine- and theogallin-enriched green tea or caffeine may increase brain theta wave activity and performance on tasks requiring attention, respectively.[61, 103] Collectively, these studies suggest that green tea consumption or supplementation with its derivatives may bolster cognitive function acutely and may slow cognitive decline. However, sound evidence demonstrating green tea's neuroprotection in chronic neurodegenerative disease is lacking. At least one population-based study, though, did demonstrate that increased green tea consumption was associated with a reduced risk for Parkinson's disease independent of total caffeine intake.[40] Future clinical and preclinical studies are needed to definitively address whether green tea may provide significant neuroprotection in TBI.

CAFFEINE

Caffeine has assumed a unique position in Western popular culture as a readily available psychoactive agent in tea, carbonated soft drinks, and coffee to combat periods of fatigue and increase mental alertness. Much less appreciated are the potential neuroprotective benefits from chronic caffeine consumption. Caffeine is a nonselective adenosine receptor antagonist that may also influence CNS adenosine receptor levels following chronic, but not acute, treatment.[124] Caffeine-mediated neuroprotection arises through adenosine-dependent effects such as modulation of glutaminergic synaptic

Table 15.4 Mechanisms of Neuroprotection Mediated by the Green Tea Ingredients Epigallocatechin–3–Gallate (EGCG) and Theanine

Mechanism	Model	Agent	Summary	References
Antioxidant	Diabetic rats	EGCG	Reduced levels of malondialdehyde (lipid peroxidation) and nitrites	14
	Rat spinal cord injury	EGCG	Reduced inducible nitric oxide synthase and nitrotyrosine levels	106
	Rat peripheral nerve injury		Reduced neuronal nicotinamide adenine dinucleotide phosphate-diaphorase (NADPH-d) and neuronal nitric oxide synthase (nNOS)	228
	Rat ischemia	EGCG	Reduced malondialdehyde (lipid peroxidation) and the level of oxidized:total glutathione ratio	49
	Parkinson's mouse	EGCG	Reduced neuronal nitric oxide synthase	48
	Parkinson's mouse	EGCG	Prevented 1-methyl-4-phenyl-1,2,3,6-tetrahydropyridine (MPTP)-induced elevations in superoxide dismutase and catalase	121
	Mouse brain	Theanine	Increased brain glutathione levels and decreased protein oxidation and lipid damage	109
Anti-inflammatory	Rat spinal cord injury	EGCG	Reduced myeloperoxidase activity Attenuated postinjury elevations in TNF-α, IL-1β, COX-2	106
	Mouse ischemia	Theanine	Reduced post-ischemic microgliosis	64
	Mouse brain	Theanine	Inhibited activation of NFκB	109
Reduction in excitotoxicity	Organotypic spinal cord slices	EGCG	Reduced glutamate level	249
Extracellular matrix	Mouse ischemia	EGCG	Counteracted post-ischemic upregulation of MMP-9	159
Neurite growth and neurogenesis	Cell culture	EGCG	Potentiated nerve growth factor-induced neurite outgrowth	79
	Cell culture	Theanine	Prevented downregulation of BDNF and glial-derived neurotrophic factor	43
Synaptic transmission	Mouse ischemia	Theanine	Modulated postsynaptic gamma-aminobutyric acid (GABA)$_A$ receptors	64
Tau and beta-amyloid	Alzheimer's mice	EGCG	Reduced tau phosphorylation and beta-amyloid deposition	173

transmission, cell survival signal transduction, and inhibition of neuroinflammation, as well as through adenosine-independent effects such as protection of the blood–brain barrier.[41] Significant caffeine-mediated neuroprotection has been demonstrated in animal models of chronic neu-rodegenerative disease like Alzheimer's disease[7, 8, 33, 55] and Parkinson's disease.[99, 192, 239]

The preclinical evidence regarding the neuroprotective effects of caffeine administration in TBI is equivocal.[4, 24, 41, 124, 227] It seems that chronic but not acute caffeine treatment leads to significant reductions in neurological deficits, cerebral edema, cellular apoptosis, and inflammatory cell infiltrate following experimental injury. These improvements were attributed to upregulation of adenosine A$_1$ receptors, which in turn suppressed synthesis of proinflammatory cytokines and reduced glutamate release and subsequent excitotoxic injury.[124] Consistent with this report, studies have also suggested that chronic caffeine treatment is associated with diminished hippocampal neuronal cell death following TBI.[227] Other studies have demonstrated that selective adenosine A$_1$ agonists improve neuropathology following experimental injury,[220] whereas adenosine A$_1$ receptor genetic ablation worsens posttraumatic neuroinflammation and seizure activity.[82, 112] Together, these studies suggest that chronic caffeine consumption may exert neuroprotective effects by modulating adenosine signaling in the brain. Yet another study demonstrated that posttraumatic caffeine treatment was associated with reductions in intracranial pressure.[24] Furthermore, the protective effects of posttraumatic caffeine administration were shown to be potentiated by its coadministration with alcohol.[56] In stark contrast, an independent study has reported that acute administration of high concentrations of caffeine just before traumatic injury worsened mortality, inflammatory cell infiltrate, edema, and blood–brain barrier disruption.[4] The reasons underlying these apparent contradictions remain unclear but would necessitate careful consideration and caution regarding dosing, timing, and duration of treatment if caffeine administration were to be translated into the clinical arena.

Population-based studies have also yielded conflicting results regarding the utility of dietary caffeine intake in the prevention of human neurologic disease. Several studies have identified that ingestion of coffee, tea, or both is associated with reduced risk for cognitive decline,[187] Alzheimer's disease,[67, 135, 186] and Parkinson's disease,[9, 53, 179, 181] suggesting that caffeine intake may provide protection from chronic neurodegenerative processes. One large population-based observational study found that consumption of three cups of coffee or tea per day for 10 years led to a 22% and a 28% reduction in risk for the development of Parkinson's disease.[211] The benefits are less clear for acute neurologic

diseases such as stroke. In certain populations, such as women, chronic coffee consumption was associated with a lower risk of ischemic stroke and subarachnoid hemorrhage.[117] However, in other populations, chronic coffee intake did not change stroke risk[77] and in one study even transiently increased stroke risk immediately following ingestion.[147] Caffeine use has also been identified as a risk factor for subarachnoid hemorrhage[27] and intracerebral hemorrhage[70] in young patients.

To date no formal clinical trials have been conducted to establish the effects of caffeine on reducing or treating TBI. Adenosine levels have been shown to be elevated in brain interstitial and cerebrospinal fluid (CSF) following TBI,[19, 50, 175] although the significance of these changes is unclear. Elevated CSF caffeine levels were associated with more favorable outcomes 6 months following TBI in one study.[182] While this was only a preliminary finding, it suggests that pretraumatic caffeine ingestion may afford some degree of neuroprotection and improve outcomes following TBI.[182] It is still uncertain whether this benefit is associated with acute or chronic caffeine consumption and if so, what amount.

VITAMINS E AND C

Vitamins generally have a positive connotation with respect to perceived health benefits. Preclinical and more recently clinical studies have begun to support the use of vitamins E and C in reducing neuropathology and cognitive deficits following brain trauma.[51, 89, 172, 235] Of the numerous vitamins commercially available, vitamin E has been at the forefront of many studies investigating the potential neuroprotective benefits of vitamin supplementation. Vitamin E is a collective term for eight naturally occurring compounds, four tocopherols (alpha-, beta-, gamma-, and delta-) and four tocotrienols (alpha-, beta-, gamma-, and delta-).[219] Vitamin E is a potent, lipid-soluble antioxidant that is present in high concentrations in the mammalian brain.[205] In several animal models of brain injury such as ischemic stroke,[107, 158] subarachnoid hemorrhage,[104, 218] and Alzheimer's disease,[210] administration of alpha-tocopherol or its potent derivative alpha-tocotrienol has been shown to lessen oxidative stress and neuropathology. Other laboratory studies have demonstrated that pretraumatic alpha-tocopherol supplementation reduces TBI-induced increases in lipid peroxidation and oxidative injury and impairments in spatial memory.[89, 235] Other studies, in transgenic mouse models of Alzheimer's disease, have further demonstrated that pre- and posttraumatic vitamin E supplementation reduces lipid peroxidation and amyloidosis and improves cognitive performance following repetitive concussive brain injury.[51]

Despite its considerable promise in many animal models, studies of the effectiveness of vitamin E supplementation in preventing or treating neurologic disease in human patients have yielded conflicting results. Several population-based studies have found vitamin E-associated reductions in ischemic stroke risk,[52, 191] whereas others have failed to find such an association.[23, 30, 65, 193]. Additionally, several of these studies have noted an increased risk for hemorrhagic stroke, warranting caution regarding widespread usage.[191, 193] While recent studies have reported that vitamin E supplementation in mild cognitive impairment (MCI) and Alzheimer's disease patients proved largely ineffective,[91] such claims have been controversial, and one should consider several factors when critically reviewing the results of these studies. For starters, the doses used in these trials were quite low. Additionally, these clinical trials explored the effectiveness of alpha-tocopherol, the least active form of vitamin E. Even though it is the major form of vitamin E in U.S. diets, gamma-tocopherol has received little attention compared to alpha-tocopherol, which is generally found in supplements.[219] Gamma-tocopherol is the main anti-inflammatory component and has been found to be more effective in scavenging free radicals and nitrogen oxygen species that cause inflammation. Interestingly, the use of alpha-tocopherol supplements also significantly reduces serum gamma-tocopherol; therefore, any potential health benefits of alpha-tocopherol supplements may be offset by deleterious changes in the bioavailability of other forms of potent tocopherols and tocotrienols.[219] One other point of consideration is that in neurodegenerative disease states like Alzheimer's disease and Parkinson's disease, where there are high levels of reactive oxygen species generation, vitamin E can tend to become oxidized itself. For maximal effectiveness and to maintain its antioxidant capacity, vitamin E must be given in conjunction with other antioxidants like vitamin C or flavonoids. These various factors might account for the null effects of alpha-tocopherol supplementation in patients with MCI and Alzheimer's disease.[219]

In contrast, emerging evidence has suggested that daily intravenous administration of vitamin E following TBI significantly decreases mortality and improves patient outcomes when assessed at discharge and at 2- and 6-month follow-up time points.[172] Importantly, no increase in adverse events was detected. This study also identified that high-dose vitamin C administration following injury stabilized or reduced perilesional edema and infarction in the majority of patients receiving postinjury treatment.[172] Like vitamin E, vitamin C, also known as ascorbic acid, is a potent antioxidant present in high concentrations in the CNS. Given these similarities in action, it has been speculated that combined vitamin C and E therapy may potentiate CNS antioxidation and act synergistically with regard to neuroprotection. Few studies have investigated combination therapy; however, one prospective human study has found that combined intake of vitamin C and E displays significant treatment interaction and reduces the risk of stroke.[52] Future studies are needed to confirm whether vitamin C or E monotherapy improves outcomes following TBI and whether combined therapy may further potentiate any protective benefit.

VITAMIN D

Vitamin D is structurally similar to many sterol hormones and is obtained through both dietary intake and endogenous biosynthesis from cholesterol in the skin. Following intake or biosynthesis, vitamin D undergoes enzyme-catalyzed sequential hydroxylation to yield its active form 1,25-dihydroxyvitamin D or calcitriol. Even though it has been established that vitamin D plays a vital role in calcium homeostasis peripherally, its functional role in the CNS has remained elusive. Recent research has suggested not only that the cells in the brain possess the hydroxlase responsible for vitamin D activation, but also that multiple regions in the brain abundantly express the nuclear vitamin D receptor.[69] Binding of vitamin D to its nuclear receptor, in turn, leads to its association with other transcription factors such as retinoic acid receptor. Subsequently this complex binds to vitamin D response elements in genomic DNA, thus augmenting gene transcription. Vitamin D-induced alterations in gene transcription are now believed to modulate myriad neuronal properties including proliferation, differentiation, and maintenance of calcium homeostasis.[69]

Vitamin D deficiency is endemic in the adolescent, adult, and elderly populations in the United States[38, 76, 215] and has been associated with inflammatory, autoimmune, cardiovascular, neuromuscular, and neurodegenerative diseases as well as cancer.[38] Population-based studies have suggested that vitamin D deficiency in the elderly is indeed associated with an increased prevalence of Parkinson's disease,[68] dementia, and Alzheimer's disease; an increased stroke risk; and a higher prevalence of magnetic resonance imaging findings suggestive of primary cerebrovascular lesions.[29] The association between vitamin D deficiency and elevated stroke risk or other cardiovascular disease has been confirmed in other studies.[6, 167] Furthermore, a randomized controlled trial has suggested that post-ischemic administration of vitamin D may improve endothelial cell function.[229] These studies, albeit anecdotal, suggest that vitamin D may indeed possess both neuroprotective and vasculoprotective properties.

More recent research has indicated that vitamin D supplementation and the prevention of vitamin D deficiency may have valuable roles in the treatment of TBI and may represent an important and necessary neuroprotective adjuvant for post-TBI progesterone therapy.[12, 37, 38] Progesterone is one of the few agents to demonstrate significant reductions in mortality following TBI in human patients in preliminary trials[230, 237] and phase III multicenter trials currently in progress. Similarly, in vitro and in vivo studies have suggested that vitamin D supplementation with progesterone administration may significantly enhance neuroprotection.[12] Vitamin D deficiency may increase inflammatory damage and behavioral impairment following experimental injury and attenuate the protective effects of posttraumatic progesterone treatment.[37]

SCUTELLARIA BAICALENSIS

The root Scutellaria baicalensis is one of the most widely used traditional Oriental herbal remedies. It has been used in a number of conditions including bacterial infections, inflammatory conditions, and more recently neurologic disease. At the core of its potent protective bioactivity is a trio of flavonoids, including baicalein, baicalin, and wogonin; each of these has been independently demonstrated to possess neuroprotective properties both in vitro and in vivo. Studies have demonstrated that baicalein and baicalin possess potent antioxidant abilities,[72, 84] whereas wogonin potently attenuates microglial activation and resultant neuroinflammation.[118, 165] Independent studies have further demonstrated that baicalein and baicalin may also have anti-inflammatory properties through the inhibition of the proinflammatory molecule NFκB[208, 240] and microglial activation.[123] Comparison studies have also demonstrated that baicalein may protect neurons from both excitoxic and glucose deprivation injury, while baicalin proved to be protective in excitotoxic injury and wogonin exerted no direct neuroprotective benefit in either in vitro model.[119]. Other models have suggested that wogonin does promote neurite outgrowth[128] and indeed protects neurons from oxygen–glucose deprivation,[202] in addition to excitotoxic and oxidative injury.[44] Baicalein has been shown to protect neurons from endoplasmic stress-induced apoptosis as well.[47] It remains unclear which flavonoid, if any, predominates with respect to Scutellaria-derived neuroprotection.

These potent antioxidant, anti-inflammatory, and anti-apoptotic mechanisms have been explored in a multitude of other experimental models including cerebral ischemia,[45, 88, 110, 194, 195] cerebral reperfusion injury,[240] spinal cord injury,[36, 251] Alzheimer's disease,[133] and Parkinson's disease.[133, 149] Importantly, in one model of experimental TBI, posttraumatic administration of baicalein decreased protein levels of proinflammatory cytokines, reduced cortical contusion volume, and improved neurologic outcome.[42] Whether baicalin and wogonin also possess protective effects with respect to TBI remains to be determined. Despite these positive preliminary findings in models of CNS disease, including TBI, no human studies have been conducted to evaluate whether the administration of Scutellaria provides neuroprotective benefits.

EXAMPLES OF OTHER NEUROPROTECTIVE NUTRACEUTICALS

Numerous other herbal remedies, while previously used strictly within the realm of traditional Oriental medicine, are becoming more appreciated for their multimechanistic neuroprotective benefits. One such compound, known as danshen, composed of the root Salvia miltiorrhiza, has been used for centuries as a traditional Chinese remedy for coronary artery and cerebrovascular disease. At least one study in human subjects confirmed that chronic ingestion may indeed decrease the risk of stroke as well as stroke recurrence.[1, 238] More recently, it has been shown that the bioactive compounds of Salvia miltiorrhiza extract providing much of the neuroprotective benefit are salvianic acid and lipid-soluble tanshinones.[116, 225, 226] These compounds have been shown to reduce lipid peroxidation and mitochondrial permeability,[224, 225] stabilize intracellular calcium,[85] reduce neuroinflammation,[214] and protect the blood–brain barrier.[213, 252] The neuroprotective effects have been investigated in experimental models of stroke,[116, 213] Parkinson's disease,[225] and Alzheimer's disease.[129] It is unknown whether significant benefit is associated with administration of Salvia miltiorrhiza derivatives in either experimental models of TBI or human TBI.

Another traditional remedy that has shown significant neuroprotective potential is the potent anti-inflammatory[46, 138] and antioxidant[92, 162] compound derived from the bark of the maritime pine tree - Pycnogenol. In experimental models, Pycnogenol has demonstrated the ability to slow or reduce the pathologic processes associated with Alzheimer's disease.[92, 162] Similarly, Pycnogenol administration, in a clinical study of elderly patients, led to improved cognition and reductions in markers of lipid peroxidase.[180]

Yet another example of a potential natural neuroprotective agent that has been widely studied is ginseng. Ginseng is composed of multiple neuroactive compounds, for example ginsenosides and saponins, that possess multiple mechanisms of neuroprotection including the ability to reduce brain oxidation[253] and neuroinflammation,[97, 226] protect mitochondrial function,[246] promote neurogenesis,[255] and promote expression of several neurotrophic factors.[126] In experimental models, ginsenosides or saponins have been demonstrated to exert protection in cerebral ischemia,[160] stroke,[244-246, 255] subarachnoid hemorrhage,[125] Parkinson's disease,[134] and Alzheimer's disease.[226] Ginseng is also thought to protect cognitive function during aging.[253] Preclinical studies in at least one experimental model of TBI have suggested potential benefit in improving neuropathologic and behavioral outcomes.[94] In humans, though, it remains unclear whether chronic administration of ginseng may improve cognition or slow progression of dementia.[75]

ANOTHER NATURAL APPROACH: HYPERBARIC OXYGEN THERAPY

Hyperbaric oxygen (HBO) therapy began in 1943 as a treatment for decompression sickness, also known as the bends, in U.S. naval diving personnel.[57] Since that time, HBO therapy has been demonstrated to reverse the effects of carbon monoxide poisoning, as well as to improve tissue quality and the results of surgery in previously irradiated tissue and severe diabetic foot infections involving hypoxic tissue (figure 15.1).

Recent laboratory studies suggest that HBO therapy reduces the extent of secondary brain damage following TBI and ischemic brain injury in animal models.[157, 177, 217, 247] In rodent models, posttraumatic HBO therapy significantly decreases neutrophil inflammatory infiltration and metalloproteinase (MMP)-9 levels in the injured brain.[221] Hyperbaric oxygen therapy was also shown to increase contused hippocampal vascular density and improve cognitive function following 80 low-pressure treatments in rats.[81] In other tissues of the body, HBO therapy has been found to decrease regional nitric oxide production and inhibit stimulus-induced proinflammatory cytokine production of IL-1β and tumor necrosis factor-α (TNF-α).[22]

Dosing regimens for the treatment of concussion are still under investigation. In a recent small

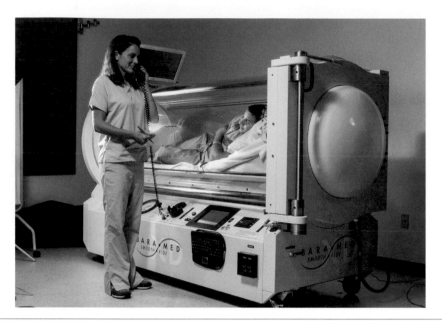

Figure 15.1   Hyperbaric oxygen therapy is an intermittent treatment of 100% oxygen at increased atmospheric pressure. Patients receive treatment while they comfortably relax in a transparent cylindrical chamber. The therapy quickly delivers high concentrations of oxygen into the bloodstream, which assists in healing.
Courtesy of the Hyperbaric Therapy of the Lowcountry.

case series of two patients with postconcussion syndrome, the researcher used HBO therapy of 100% oxygen at 1.5 atmospheric absolute (ATA) for 60 minutes once a day for 40 days.[206] Both patients found relief of their postconcussion syndrome symptoms, and normal cognitive function was restored (as measured on ImPACT neurocognitive concussion testing).

Although several studies have reported beneficial outcomes, the clinical value of HBO in treating concussion and postconcusson syndrome–prolonged postconcussion syndrome is indeterminate because the evidence is insufficient to prove effectiveness or ineffectiveness. At the time of this writing, the U.S. military was conducting a large multicenter study investigating the short-term and long-term effectiveness of HBO therapy in the treatment of TBI and post-traumatic stress disorder. The interest to understand the role HBO therapy has in postconcussion syndrome is generated from several studies that have yielded significant symptom, neuropsychological testing, and affective improvements.

There are currently no set standards for the use of HBO for postconcussion syndrome, but most clinicians treating postconcussion syndrome with HBO use 1.5 ATA and daily sessions between 1 to 2 hours. Duration of the treatment is usually associated with symptom improvement. Risks associated with HBO are mostly related to the increased pressure but are comparable to those with airplane pressurization. Ear and sinus pain can occur and, in rare cases, vision blurring due to swelling of the lens of the eye.

CONCLUDING THOUGHTS

The use of dietary supplements and herbal remedies has become more commonplace today than in the past. Several issues arise when one is considering the use of these compounds as adjuvant therapy for CNS disease. For instance, not all preparations available over the counter are standardized across the board with respect to the quantity or concentrations of compound, so quality control becomes an issue. Also, little is known about the most optimal dose or amount of consumption necessary to yield a clinical effect. Potential interactions with other nutraceuticals or prescription medications are common, and it is paramount to have a sound understanding of their biological mechanisms of action. Nonetheless, abundant preclinical studies demonstrate the neuroprotective properties of a variety of these compounds.

Multiple mechanisms lead to secondary damage after TBI, including ischemia, activation of neuronal death cascades, cerebral swelling, and inflammation. The development of neurochemical, histopathologic, and molecular techniques to study TBI has enabled researchers to gain new insights into the mechanisms underlying posttraumatic tissue damage and associated neurological dysfunction. Despite the technological advances made during the last several decades, no effective neuroprotective therapy is as yet available for mild, let alone severe, TBI. The mainstay of treatment for patients with concussions is rest; and while the majority of patients have a spontaneous resolution of their symptoms over a short period of time, a proportion of patients have persistent symptoms and develop postconcussion syndrome or prolonged postconcussion syndrome. We are also learning more about the long-term neurodegenerative processes that may result from repetitive concussive and subconcussive brain injury, including MCI, chronic traumatic encephalopathy, and dementia pugilistica. Neuroinflammation appears to be a common thread with all of these disease processes.[25] Numerous pharmacologic agents have been explored as potential therapeutic interventions aimed at ameliorating secondary damage after TBI, but without much success. It is likely that successful therapy for severe TBI may require favorable effects on multiple deleterious cascades rather than on a single pathophysiologic mechanism. One of the intriguing aspects of many of these natural approaches is that they possess multiple mechanisms of neuroprotection, particularly anti-inflammatory properties.

While an increasing number of well-designed studies are investigating the neuroprotective potential of nutraceutical preparations and natural treatment approaches, the clinical evidence is still fairly thin. There is a need for future trials exploring the potential therapeutic benefits of these compounds and hyperbaric oxygen in the treatment of TBI, particularly concussion.

ACKNOWLEDGMENT

A significant portion of this chapter is adapted from a paper published in the journal *Surgical Neurology International (SNI)*: Petraglia AL, Winkler EA, Bailes JE Stuck at the bench: Potential natural neuroprotective compounds for concussion. Surg Neurol Int 2011; 2:146.

REFERENCES

1. Danshen in ischemic stroke. Chin Med J (Engl) 1977;3(4):224-226.

2. Dietary supplementation with n-3 polyunsaturated fatty acids and vitamin E after myocardial infarction: results of the GISSI-Prevenzione trial. Gruppo Italiano per lo Studio della Sopravvivenza nell'Infarto miocardico. Lancet 1999;354(9177):447-455.

3. Aggarwal BB, Shishodia S. Suppression of the nuclear factor-kappaB activation pathway by spice-derived phytochemicals: reasoning for seasoning. Ann N Y Acad Sci 2004;1030:434-441.

4. Al Moutaery K, Al Deeb S, Ahmad Khan H, Tariq M. Caffeine impairs short-term neurological outcome after concussive head injury in rats. Neurosurgery 2003;53(3):704-711; discussion 711-702.

5. Almeida LS, Salomons GS, Hogenboom F, Jakobs C, Schoffelmeer AN. Exocytotic release of creatine in rat brain. Synapse 2006;60(2):118-123.

6. Anderson JL, May HT, Horne BD, Bair TL, Hall NL, Carlquist JF, et al. Relation of vitamin D deficiency to cardiovascular risk factors, disease status, and incident events in a general healthcare population. Am J Cardiol 2010;106(7):963-968.

7. Arendash GW, Mori T, Cao C, Mamcarz M, Runfeldt M, Dickson A, et al. Caffeine reverses cognitive impairment and decreases brain amyloid-beta levels in aged Alzheimer's disease mice. J Alzheimers Dis 2009;17(3):661-680.

8. Arendash GW, Schleif W, Rezai-Zadeh K, Jackson EK, Zacharia LC, Cracchiolo JR, et al. Caffeine protects Alzheimer's mice against cognitive impairment and reduces brain beta-amyloid production. Neuroscience 2006;142(4):941-952.

9. Ascherio A, Zhang SM, Hernan MA, Kawachi I, Colditz GA, Speizer FE, et al. Prospective study of caffeine consumption and risk of Parkinson's disease in men and women. Ann Neurol 2001;50(1):56-63.

10. Atassi N, Ratai EM, Greenblatt DJ, Pulley D, Zhao Y, Bombardier J, et al. A phase I, pharmacokinetic, dosage escalation study of creatine monohydrate in subjects with amyotrophic lateral sclerosis. Amyotroph Lateral Scler 2010;11(6):508-513.

11. Ates O, Cayli S, Altinoz E, Gurses I, Yucel N, Sener M, et al. Neuroprotection by resveratrol against traumatic brain injury in rats. Mol Cell Biochem 2007;294(1-2):137-144.

12. Atif F, Sayeed I, Ishrat T, Stein DG. Progesterone with vitamin D affords better neuroprotection against excitotoxicity in cultured cortical neurons than progesterone alone. Mol Med 2009;15(9-10):328-336.

13. Bailes JE, Mills JD. Docosahexaenoic acid reduces traumatic axonal injury in a rodent head injury model. J Neurotrauma 2010;27(9):1617-1624.

14. Baluchnejadmojarad T, Roghani M. Chronic epi-gallocatechin-3-gallate ameliorates learning and memory deficits in diabetic rats via modulation of nitric oxide and oxidative stress. Behav Brain Res 2011;224(2):305-310.

15. Baum L, Cheung SK, Mok VC, Lam LC, Leung VP, Hui E, et al. Curcumin effects on blood lipid profile in a 6-month human study. Pharmacol Res 2007;56(6):509-514.

16. Baur JA, Pearson KJ, Price NL, Jamieson HA, Lerin C, Kalra A, et al. Resveratrol improves health and survival of mice on a high-calorie diet. Nature 2006;444(7117):337-342.

17. Baur JA, Sinclair DA. Therapeutic potential of resveratrol: the in vivo evidence. Nat Rev Drug Discov 2006;5(6):493-506.

18. Beard E, Braissant O. Synthesis and transport of creatine in the CNS: importance for cerebral functions. J Neurochem 2010;115(2):297-313.

19. Bell MJ, Robertson CS, Kochanek PM, Goodman JC, Gopinath SP, Carcillo JA, et al. Interstitial brain adenosine and xanthine increase during jugular venous oxygen desaturations in humans after traumatic brain injury. Crit Care Med 2001;29(2):399-404.

20. Bender A, Auer DP, Merl T, Reilmann R, Saemann P, Yassouridis A, et al. Creatine supplementation lowers brain glutamate levels in Huntington's disease. J Neurol 2005;252(1):36-41.

21. Bender A, Koch W, Elstner M, Schombacher Y, Bender J, Moeschl M, et al. Creatine supplementation in Parkinson disease: a placebo-controlled randomized pilot trial. Neurology 2006;67(7):1262-1264.

22. Benson RM, Minter LM, Osborne BA, Granowitz EV. Hyperbaric oxygen inhibits stimulus-induced proinflammatory cytokine synthesis by human blood-derived monocyte-macrophages. Clin Exp Immunol 2003;134(1):57-62.

23. Bin Q, Hu X, Cao Y, Gao F. The role of vitamin E (tocopherol) supplementation in the prevention of stroke. A meta-analysis of 13 randomised controlled trials. Thromb Haemost 2011;105(4):579-585.

24. Blaha M, Vajnerova O, Bednar M, Vajner L, Tichy M. [Traumatic brain injuries—effects of alcohol and caffeine on intracranial pressure and cerebral blood flow]. Rozhl Chir 2009;88(11):682-686.

25. Blaylock RL, Maroon J. Immunoexcitotoxicity as a central mechanism in chronic traumatic encephalopathy—a unifying hypothesis. Surg Neurol Int 2011;2:107.

26. Bradamante S, Barenghi L, Villa A. Cardiovascular protective effects of resveratrol. Cardiovasc Drug Rev 2004;22(3):169-188.

27. Broderick JP, Viscoli CM, Brott T, Kernan WN, Brass LM, Feldmann E, et al. Major risk factors for aneurysmal subarachnoid hemorrhage in the young are modifiable. Stroke 2003;34(6):1375-1381.

28. Bromfield E, Dworetzky B, Hurwitz S, Eluri Z, Lane L, Replansky S, et al. A randomized trial of polyunsaturated fatty acids for refractory epilepsy. Epilepsy Behav 2008;12(1):187-190.

29. Buell JS, Dawson-Hughes B, Scott TM, Weiner DE, Dallal GE, Qui WQ, et al. 25-Hydroxyvitamin D, dementia, and cerebrovascular pathology in elders receiving home services. Neurology 2010;74(1):18-26.

30. Buring JE. Aspirin prevents stroke but not MI in women; vitamin E has no effect on CV disease or cancer. Cleve Clin J Med 2006;73(9):863-870.

31. Caicoya M. Fish consumption and stroke: a community case-control study in Asturias, Spain. Neuroepidemiology 2002;21(3):107-114.

32. Calderon F, Kim HY. Docosahexaenoic acid promotes neurite growth in hippocampal neurons. J Neurochem 2004;90(4):979-988.

33. Cao C, Cirrito JR, Lin X, Wang L, Verges DK, Dickson A, et al. Caffeine suppresses amyloid-beta levels in plasma and brain of Alzheimer's disease transgenic mice. J Alzheimers Dis 2009;17(3):681-697.

34. Cao D, Xue R, Xu J, Liu Z. Effects of docosahexaenoic acid on the survival and neurite outgrowth of rat cortical neurons in primary cultures. J Nutr Biochem 2005;16(9):538-546.

35. Cao DH, Xu JF, Xue RH, Zheng WF, Liu ZL. Protective effect of chronic ethyl docosahexaenoate administration on brain injury in ischemic gerbils. Pharmacol Biochem Behav 2004;79(4):651-659.

36. Cao Y, Li G, Wang YF, Fan ZK, Yu DS, Wang ZD, et al. Neuroprotective effect of baicalin on compression spinal cord injury in rats. Brain Res 2010;1357:115-123.

37. Cekic M, Cutler SM, VanLandingham JW, Stein DG. Vitamin D deficiency reduces the benefits of progesterone treatment after brain injury in aged rats. Neurobiol Aging 2011;32(5):864-874.

38. Cekic M, Stein DG. Traumatic brain injury and aging: is a combination of progesterone and vitamin D hormone a simple solution to a complex problem? Neurotherapeutics 2010;7(1):81-90.

39. Chandra V, Pandav R, Dodge HH, Johnston JM, Belle SH, DeKosky ST, et al. Incidence of Alzheimer's disease in a rural community in India: the Indo-US study. Neurology 2001;57(6):985-989.

40. Checkoway H, Powers K, Smith-Weller T, Franklin GM, Longstreth WT Jr, Swanson PD. Parkinson's disease risks associated with cigarette smoking, alcohol consumption, and caffeine intake. Am J Epidemiol 2002;155(8):732-738.

41. Chen JF, Chern Y. Impacts of methylxanthines and adenosine receptors on neurodegeneration: human and experimental studies. Handb Exp Pharmacol 2011(200):267-310.

42. Chen SF, Hsu CW, Huang WH, Wang JY. Post-injury baicalein improves histological and functional outcomes and reduces inflammatory cytokines after experimental traumatic brain injury. Br J Pharmacol 2008;155(8):1279-1296.

43. Cho HS, Kim S, Lee SY, Park JA, Kim SJ, Chun HS. Protective effect of the green tea component, L-theanine on environmental toxins-induced neuronal cell death. Neurotoxicology 2008;29(4):656-662.

44. Cho J, Lee HK. Wogonin inhibits excitotoxic and oxidative neuronal damage in primary cultured rat cortical cells. Eur J Pharmacol 2004;485(1-3):105-110.

45. Cho J, Lee HK. Wogonin inhibits ischemic brain injury in a rat model of permanent middle cerebral artery occlusion. Biol Pharm Bull 2004;27(10):1561-1564.

46. Cho KJ, Yun CH, Yoon DY, Cho YS, Rimbach G, Packer L, et al. Effect of bioflavonoids extracted from the bark of Pinus maritima on proinflammatory cytokine interleukin-1 production in lipopolysaccharide-stimulated RAW 264.7. Toxicol Appl Pharmacol 2000;168(1):64-71.

47. Choi JH, Choi AY, Yoon H, Choe W, Yoon KS, Ha J, et al. Baicalein protects HT22 murine hippocampal neuronal cells against endoplasmic reticulum stress-induced apoptosis through inhibition of reactive oxygen species production and CHOP induction. Exp Mol Med 2010;42(12):811-822.

48. Choi JY, Park CS, Kim DJ, Cho MH, Jin BK, Pie JE, et al. Prevention of nitric oxide-mediated 1-methyl-4-phenyl-1,2,3,6-tetrahydropyridine-induced Parkinson's disease in mice by tea phenolic epigallocatechin 3-gallate. Neurotoxicology 2002;23(3):367-374.

49. Choi YB, Kim YI, Lee KS, Kim BS, Kim DJ. Protective effect of epigallocatechin gallate on brain damage after transient middle cerebral artery occlusion in rats. Brain Res 2004;1019(1-2):47-54.

50. Clark RS, Carcillo JA, Kochanek PM, Obrist WD, Jackson EK, Mi Z, et al. Cerebrospinal fluid adenosine concentration and uncoupling of cerebral blood flow and oxidative metabolism after severe head injury in humans. Neurosurgery 1997;41(6):1284-1292; discussion 1292-1283.

51. Conte V, Uryu K, Fujimoto S, Yao Y, Rokach J, Longhi L, et al. Vitamin E reduces amyloidosis and improves cognitive function in Tg2576 mice following repetitive concussive brain injury. J Neurochem 2004;90(3):758-764.

52. Cook NR, Albert CM, Gaziano JM, Zaharris E, MacFadyen J, Danielson E, et al. A randomized factorial trial of vitamins C and E and beta carotene in the secondary prevention of cardiovascular events in women: results from the Women's Antioxidant Cardiovascular Study. Arch Intern Med 2007;167(15):1610-1618.

53. Costa J, Lunet N, Santos C, Santos J, Vaz-Carneiro A. Caffeine exposure and the risk of Parkinson's disease: a systematic review and meta-analysis of observational studies. J Alzheimers Dis 2010;20 Suppl 1:S221-238.

54. Cupello A, Balestrino M, Gatta E, Pellistri F, Siano S, Robello M. Activation of cerebellar granule cells GABA(A) receptors by guanidinoacetate. Neuroscience 2008;152(1):65-69.

55. Dall'Igna OP, Porciuncula LO, Souza DO, Cunha RA, Lara DR. Neuroprotection by caffeine and adenosine A2A receptor blockade of beta-amyloid neurotoxicity. Br J Pharmacol 2003;138(7):1207-1209.

56. Dash PK, Moore AN, Moody MR, Treadwell R, Felix JL, Clifton GL. Post-trauma administration of caffeine plus ethanol reduces contusion volume and improves working memory in rats. J Neurotrauma 2004;21(11):1573-1583.

57. Davis JC. Hyperbaric oxygen treatment. J Intensive Care Med 1989;4:55-57.

58. DeGiorgio CM, Miller P, Meymandi S, Gornbein JA. n-3 fatty acids (fish oil) for epilepsy, cardiac risk factors, and risk of SUDEP: clues from a pilot, double-blind, exploratory study. Epilepsy Behav 2008;13(4):681-684.

59. Della-Morte D, Dave KR, DeFazio RA, Bao YC, Raval AP, Perez-Pinzon MA. Resveratrol pretreatment protects rat brain from cerebral ischemic damage via a sirtuin 1-uncoupling protein 2 pathway. Neuroscience 2009;159(3):993-1002.

60. Dhillon N, Aggarwal BB, Newman RA, Wolff RA, Kunnumakkara AB, Abbruzzese JL, et al. Phase II trial of curcumin in patients with advanced pancreatic cancer. Clin Cancer Res 2008;14(14):4491-4499.

61. Dimpfel W, Kler A, Kriesl E, Lehnfeld R, Keplinger-Dimpfel IK. Source density analysis of the human EEG after ingestion of a drink containing decaffeinated extract of green tea enriched with L-theanine and theogallin. Nutr Neurosci 2007;10(3-4):169-180.

62. Dohare P, Garg P, Jain V, Nath C, Ray M. Dose dependence and therapeutic window for the neuroprotective effects of curcumin in thromboembolic model of rat. Behav Brain Res 2008;193(2):289-297.

63. Dyall SC, Michael-Titus AT. Neurological benefits of omega-3 fatty acids. Neuromolecular Med 2008;10(4):219-235.

64. Egashira N, Hayakawa K, Osajima M, Mishima K, Iwasaki K, Oishi R, et al. Involvement of GABA(A) receptors in the neuroprotective effect of theanine on focal cerebral ischemia in mice. J Pharmacol Sci 2007;105(2):211-214.

65. Eidelman RS, Hollar D, Hebert PR, Lamas GA, Hennekens CH. Randomized trials of vitamin E in the treatment and prevention of cardiovascular

disease. Arch Intern Med 2004;164(14):1552-1556.

66. Endres S, Ghorbani R, Kelley VE, Georgilis K, Lonnemann G, van der Meer JW, et al. The effect of dietary supplementation with n-3 polyunsaturated fatty acids on the synthesis of interleukin-1 and tumor necrosis factor by mononuclear cells. N Engl J Med 1989;320(5):265-271.

67. Eskelinen MH, Ngandu T, Tuomilehto J, Soininen H, Kivipelto M. Midlife coffee and tea drinking and the risk of late-life dementia: a population-based CAIDE study. J Alzheimers Dis 2009;16(1):85-91.

68. Evatt ML, Delong MR, Khazai N, Rosen A, Triche S, Tangpricha V. Prevalence of vitamin d insufficiency in patients with Parkinson disease and Alzheimer disease. Arch Neurol 2008;65(10):1348-1352.

69. Eyles D, Burne T, McGrath J. Vitamin D in fetal brain development. Semin Cell Dev Biol 2011;22(6):629-636.

70. Feldmann E, Broderick JP, Kernan WN, Viscoli CM, Brass LM, Brott T, et al. Major risk factors for intracerebral hemorrhage in the young are modifiable. Stroke 2005;36(9):1881-1885.

71. Gao D, Zhang X, Jiang X, Peng Y, Huang W, Cheng G, et al. Resveratrol reduces the elevated level of MMP-9 induced by cerebral ischemia-reperfusion in mice. Life Sci 2006;78(22):2564-2570.

72. Gao Z, Huang K, Yang X, Xu H. Free radical scavenging and antioxidant activities of flavonoids extracted from the radix of Scutellaria baicalensis Georgi. Biochim Biophys Acta 1999;1472(3):643-650.

73. Garbagnati F, Cairella G, De Martino A, Multari M, Scognamiglio U, Venturiero V, et al. Is antioxidant and n-3 supplementation able to improve functional status in poststroke patients? Results from the Nutristroke Trial. Cerebrovasc Dis 2009;27(4):375-383.

74. Garodia P, Ichikawa H, Malani N, Sethi G, Aggarwal BB. From ancient medicine to modern medicine: ayurvedic concepts of health and their role in inflammation and cancer. J Soc Integr Oncol 2007;5(1):25-37.

75. Geng J, Dong J, Ni H, Lee MS, Wu T, Jiang K, et al. Ginseng for cognition. Cochrane Database Syst Rev 2010(12):CD007769.

76. Gordon CM, DePeter KC, Feldman HA, Grace E, Emans SJ. Prevalence of vitamin D deficiency among healthy adolescents. Arch Pediatr Adolesc Med 2004;158(6):531-537.

77. Grobbee DE, Rimm EB, Giovannucci E, Colditz G, Stampfer M, Willett W. Coffee, caffeine, and cardiovascular disease in men. N Engl J Med 1990;323(15):1026-1032.

78. Gualano B, Artioli GG, Poortmans JR, Lancha Junior AH. Exploring the therapeutic role of creatine supplementation. Amino Acids 2010;38(1):31-44.

79. Gundimeda U, McNeill TH, Schiffman JE, Hinton DR, Gopalakrishna R. Green tea polyphenols potentiate the action of nerve growth factor to induce neuritogenesis: possible role of reactive oxygen species. J Neurosci Res 2010;88(16):3644-3655.

80. Hamaguchi T, Ono K, Yamada M. REVIEW: Curcumin and Alzheimer's disease. CNS Neurosci Ther 2010;16(5):285-297.

81. Harch PG, Kriedt C, Van Meter KW, Sutherland RJ. Hyperbaric oxygen therapy improves spatial learning and memory in a rat model of chronic traumatic brain injury. Brain Res 2007;1174:120-129.

82. Haselkorn ML, Shellington DK, Jackson EK, Vagni VA, Janesko-Feldman K, Dubey RK, et al. Adenosine A1 receptor activation as a brake on the microglial response after experimental traumatic brain injury in mice. J Neurotrauma 2010;27(5):901-910.

83. He K, Rimm EB, Merchant A, Rosner BA, Stampfer MJ, Willett WC, et al. Fish consumption and risk of stroke in men. JAMA 2002;288(24):3130-3136.

84. He XL, Wang YH, Gao M, Li XX, Zhang TT, Du GH. Baicalein protects rat brain mitochondria against chronic cerebral hypoperfusion-induced oxidative damage. Brain Res 2009;1249:212-221.

85. Hei M, Luo Y, Zhang X, Liu F. Tanshinone IIa alleviates the biochemical changes associated with hypoxic ischemic brain damage in a rat model. Phytother Res 2011;25(12):1865-1869.

86. Hersch SM, Gevorkian S, Marder K, Moskowitz C, Feigin A, Cox M, et al. Creatine in Huntington disease is safe, tolerable, bioavailable in brain and reduces serum 8OH2'dG. Neurology 2006;66(2):250-252.

87. Hogyes E, Nyakas C, Kiliaan A, Farkas T, Penke B, Luiten PG. Neuroprotective effect of developmental docosahexaenoic acid supplement against excitotoxic brain damage in infant rats. Neuroscience 2003;119(4):999-1012.

88. Hwang YK, Jinhua M, Choi BR, Cui CA, Jeon WK, Kim H, et al. Effects of Scutellaria baicalensis on chronic cerebral hypoperfusion-induced memory impairments and chronic lipopolysaccharide infusion-induced memory impairments. J Ethnopharmacol 2011;137(1):681-689.

89. Inci S, Ozcan OE, Kilinc K. Time-level relationship for lipid peroxidation and the protective effect of alpha-tocopherol in experimental mild and severe brain injury. Neurosurgery 1998;43(2):330-335; discussion 335-336.

90. Inoue H, Jiang XF, Katayama T, Osada S, Umesono K, Namura S. Brain protection by resveratrol and fenofibrate against stroke requires peroxisome

proliferator-activated receptor alpha in mice. Neurosci Lett 2003;352(3):203-206.

91. Isaac MG, Quinn R, Tabet N. Vitamin E for Alzheimer's disease and mild cognitive impairment. Cochrane Database Syst Rev 2008(3):CD002854.

92. Ishrat T, Parveen K, Hoda MN, Khan MB, Yousuf S, Ansari MA, et al. Effects of Pycnogenol and vitamin E on cognitive deficits and oxidative damage induced by intracerebroventricular streptozotocin in rats. Behav Pharmacol 2009;20(7):567-575.

93. Iso H, Rexrode KM, Stampfer MJ, Manson JE, Colditz GA, Speizer FE, et al. Intake of fish and omega-3 fatty acids and risk of stroke in women. JAMA 2001;285(3):304-312.

94. Ji YC, Kim YB, Park SW, Hwang SN, Min BK, Hong HJ, et al. Neuroprotective effect of ginseng total saponins in experimental traumatic brain injury. J Korean Med Sci 2005;20(2):291-296.

95. Jiang J, Wang W, Sun YJ, Hu M, Li F, Zhu DY. Neuroprotective effect of curcumin on focal cerebral ischemic rats by preventing blood-brain barrier damage. Eur J Pharmacol 2007;561(1-3):54-62.

96. Jones PJH, Kubow S. Lipids, sterols, and their metabolites. In: Shils ME, Olson JA, Shike M, Ross AC, eds. Modern Nutrition in Health and Disease. 2006; Baltimore, MD: Lippincott, Williams and Wilkins.

97. Jung JS, Shin JA, Park EM, Lee JE, Kang YS, Min SW, et al. Anti-inflammatory mechanism of ginsenoside Rh1 in lipopolysaccharide-stimulated microglia: critical role of the protein kinase A pathway and hemeoxygenase-1 expression. J Neurochem 2010;115(6):1668-1680.

98. Kakuda T, Yanase H, Utsunomiya K, Nozawa A, Unno T, Kataoka K. Protective effect of gamma-glutamylethylamide (theanine) on ischemic delayed neuronal death in gerbils. Neurosci Lett 2000;289(3):189-192.

99. Kalda A, Yu L, Oztas E, Chen JF. Novel neuroprotection by caffeine and adenosine A(2A) receptor antagonists in animal models of Parkinson's disease. J Neurol Sci 2006;248(1-2):9-15.

100. Kaplan S, Bisleri G, Morgan JA, Cheema FH, Oz MC. Resveratrol, a natural red wine polyphenol, reduces ischemia-reperfusion-induced spinal cord injury. Ann Thorac Surg 2005;80(6):2242-2249.

101. Karlsen A, Paur I, Bohn SK, Sakhi AK, Borge GI, Serafini M, et al. Bilberry juice modulates plasma concentration of NF-kappaB related inflammatory markers in subjects at increased risk of CVD. Eur J Nutr 2010;49(6):345-355.

102. Karuppagounder SS, Pinto JT, Xu H, Chen HL, Beal MF, Gibson GE. Dietary supplementation with resveratrol reduces plaque pathology in a transgenic model of Alzheimer's disease. Neurochem Int 2009;54(2):111-118.

103. Kelly SP, Gomez-Ramirez M, Montesi JL, Foxe JJ. L-theanine and caffeine in combination affect human cognition as evidenced by oscillatory alpha-band activity and attention task performance. J Nutr 2008;138(8):1572S-1577S.

104. Kemaloglu S, Ozkan U, Yilmaz F, Ak E, Acemoglu H, Olmez G, et al. Preventive effects of intracisternal alphatochopherol on cerebral vasospasm in experimental subarachnoid haemorrhage. Yonsei Med J 2003;44(6):955-960.

105. Kennedy DO, Wightman EL, Reay JL, Lietz G, Okello EJ, Wilde A, et al. Effects of resveratrol on cerebral blood flow variables and cognitive performance in humans: a double-blind, placebo-controlled, crossover investigation. Am J Clin Nutr 2010;91(6):1590-1597.

106. Khalatbary AR, Ahmadvand H. Anti-inflammatory effect of the epigallocatechin gallate following spinal cord trauma in rat. Iran Biomed J 2011;15(1-2):31-37.

107. Khanna S, Roy S, Slivka A, Craft TK, Chaki S, Rink C, et al. Neuroprotective properties of the natural vitamin E alpha-tocotrienol. Stroke 2005;36(10):2258-2264.

108. Kim J, Lee HJ, Lee KW. Naturally occurring phytochemicals for the prevention of Alzheimer's disease. J Neurochem 2010;112(6):1415-1430.

109. Kim TI, Lee YK, Park SG, Choi IS, Ban JO, Park HK, et al. l-Theanine, an amino acid in green tea, attenuates beta-amyloid-induced cognitive dysfunction and neurotoxicity: reduction in oxidative damage and inactivation of ERK/p38 kinase and NF-kappaB pathways. Free Radic Biol Med 2009;47(11):1601-1610.

110. Kim YO, Leem K, Park J, Lee P, Ahn DK, Lee BC, et al. Cytoprotective effect of Scutellaria baicalensis in CA1 hippocampal neurons of rats after global cerebral ischemia. J Ethnopharmacol 2001;77(2-3):183-188.

111. Kiziltepe U, Turan NN, Han U, Ulus AT, Akar F. Resveratrol, a red wine polyphenol, protects spinal cord from ischemia-reperfusion injury. J Vasc Surg 2004;40(1):138-145.

112. Kochanek PM, Vagni VA, Janesko KL, Washington CB, Crumrine PK, Garman RH, et al. Adenosine A1 receptor knockout mice develop lethal status epilepticus after experimental traumatic brain injury. J Cereb Blood Flow Metab 2006;26(4):565-575.

113. Koh SH, Lee SM, Kim HY, Lee KY, Lee YJ, Kim HT, et al. The effect of epigallocatechin gallate on suppressing disease progression of ALS model mice. Neurosci Lett 2006;395(2):103-107.

114. Kotani S, Sakaguchi E, Warashina S, Matsukawa N, Ishikura Y, Kiso Y, et al. Dietary supplementation of arachidonic and docosahexaenoic acids improves cognitive dysfunction. Neurosci Res 2006;56(2):159-164.

115. Laird MD, Sukumari-Ramesh S, Swift AE, Meiler SE, Vender JR, Dhandapani KM. Curcumin

attenuates cerebral edema following traumatic brain injury in mice: a possible role for aquaporin-4? J Neurochem 2010;113(3):637-648.

116. Lam BY, Lo AC, Sun X, Luo HW, Chung SK, Sucher NJ. Neuroprotective effects of tanshinones in transient focal cerebral ischemia in mice. Phytomedicine 2003;10(4):286-291.

117. Larsson SC, Virtamo J, Wolk A. Coffee consumption and risk of stroke in women. Stroke 2011;42(4):908-912.

118. Lee H, Kim YO, Kim H, Kim SY, Noh HS, Kang SS, et al. Flavonoid wogonin from medicinal herb is neuroprotective by inhibiting inflammatory activation of microglia. FASEB J 2003;17(13):1943-1944.

119. Lee HH, Yang LL, Wang CC, Hu SY, Chang SF, Lee YH. Differential effects of natural polyphenols on neuronal survival in primary cultured central neurons against glutamate- and glucose deprivation-induced neuronal death. Brain Res 2003;986(1-2):103-113.

120. Lee SY, Kim CY, Lee JJ, Jung JG, Lee SR. Effects of delayed administration of (-)-epigallocatechin gallate, a green tea polyphenol on the changes in polyamine levels and neuronal damage after transient forebrain ischemia in gerbils. Brain Res Bull 2003;61(4):399-406.

121. Levites Y, Weinreb O, Maor G, Youdim MB, Mandel S. Green tea polyphenol (-)-epigallocatechin-3-gallate prevents N-methyl-4-phenyl-1,2,3,6-tetrahydropyridine-induced dopaminergic neurodegeneration. J Neurochem 2001;78(5):1073-1082.

122. Li C, Yan Z, Yang J, Chen H, Li H, Jiang Y, et al. Neuroprotective effects of resveratrol on ischemic injury mediated by modulating the release of neurotransmitter and neuromodulator in rats. Neurochem Int 2010;56(3):495-500.

123. Li FQ, Wang T, Pei Z, Liu B, Hong JS. Inhibition of microglial activation by the herbal flavonoid baicalein attenuates inflammation-mediated degeneration of dopaminergic neurons. J Neural Transm 2005;112(3):331-347.

124. Li W, Dai S, An J, Li P, Chen X, Xiong R, et al. Chronic but not acute treatment with caffeine attenuates traumatic brain injury in the mouse cortical impact model. Neuroscience 2008;151(4):1198-1207.

125. Li Y, Tang J, Khatibi NH, Zhu M, Chen D, Tu L, et al. Treatment with ginsenoside rb1, a component of panax ginseng, provides neuroprotection in rats subjected to subarachnoid hemorrhage-induced brain injury. Acta Neurochir Suppl 2011;110(Pt 2):75-79.

126. Liang W, Ge S, Yang L, Yang M, Ye Z, Yan M, et al. Ginsenosides Rb1 and Rg1 promote proliferation and expression of neurotrophic factors in primary Schwann cell cultures. Brain Res 2010;1357:19-25.

127. Lim GP, Chu T, Yang F, Beech W, Frautschy SA, Cole GM. The curry spice curcumin reduces oxidative damage and amyloid pathology in an Alzheimer transgenic mouse. J Neurosci 2001;21(21):8370-8377.

128. Lim JS, Yoo M, Kwon HJ, Kim H, Kwon YK. Wogonin induces differentiation and neurite outgrowth of neural precursor cells. Biochem Biophys Res Commun 2010;402(1):42-47.

129. Liu T, Jin H, Sun QR, Xu JH, Hu HT. The neuroprotective effects of tanshinone IIA on beta-amyloid-induced toxicity in rat cortical neurons. Neuropharmacology 2010;59(7-8):595-604.

130. Liu Y, Dargusch R, Maher P, Schubert D. A broadly neuroprotective derivative of curcumin. J Neurochem 2008;105(4):1336-1345.

131. Lonergan PE, Martin DS, Horrobin DF, Lynch MA. Neuroprotective actions of eicosapentaenoic acid on lipopolysaccharide-induced dysfunction in rat hippocampus. J Neurochem 2004;91(1):20-29.

132. Lu DY, Tsao YY, Leung YM, Su KP. Docosahexaenoic acid suppresses neuroinflammatory responses and induces heme oxygenase-1 expression in BV-2 microglia: implications of antidepressant effects for omega-3 fatty acids. Neuropsychopharmacology 2010;35(11):2238-2248.

133. Lu JH, Ardah MT, Durairajan SS, Liu LF, Xie LX, Fong WF, et al. Baicalein inhibits formation of alpha-synuclein oligomers within living cells and prevents Abeta peptide fibrillation and oligomerisation. ChemBioChem 2011;12(4):615-624.

134. Luo FC, Wang SD, Qi L, Song JY, Lv T, Bai J. Protective effect of panaxatriol saponins extracted from Panax notoginseng against MPTP-induced neurotoxicity in vivo. J Ethnopharmacol 2011;133(2):448-453.

135. Maia L, de Mendonca A. Does caffeine intake protect from Alzheimer's disease? Eur J Neurol 2002;9(4):377-382.

136. Mandel S, Maor G, Youdim MB. Iron and alpha-synuclein in the substantia nigra of MPTP-treated mice: effect of neuroprotective drugs R-apomorphine and green tea polyphenol (-)-epigallocatechin-3-gallate. J Mol Neurosci 2004;24(3):401-416.

137. Mandel S, Weinreb O, Amit T, Youdim MB. Cell signaling pathways in the neuroprotective actions of the green tea polyphenol (-)-epigallocatechin-3-gallate: implications for neurodegenerative diseases. J Neurochem 2004;88(6):1555-1569.

138. Maroon JC, Bost JW, Maroon A. Natural anti-inflammatory agents for pain relief. Surg Neurol Int 2010;1:80.

139. Martinez M. Tissue levels of polyunsaturated fatty acids during early human development. J Pediatr 1992;120(4 Pt 2):S129-138.

140. Mayer K, Meyer S, Reinholz-Muhly M, Maus U, Merfels M, Lohmeyer J, et al. Short-time infusion of fish oil-based lipid emulsions, approved for parenteral nutrition, reduces monocyte pro-inflammatory cytokine generation and adhesive interaction with endothelium in humans. J Immunol 2003;171(9):4837-4843.

141. McGahon BM, Martin DS, Horrobin DF, Lynch MA. Age-related changes in synaptic function: analysis of the effect of dietary supplementation with omega-3 fatty acids. Neuroscience 1999;94(1):305-314.

142. McMorris T, Harris RC, Howard AN, Langridge G, Hall B, Corbett J, et al. Creatine supplementation, sleep deprivation, cortisol, melatonin and behavior. Physiol Behav 2007;90(1):21-28.

143. McMorris T, Mielcarz G, Harris RC, Swain JP, Howard A. Creatine supplementation and cognitive performance in elderly individuals. Neuropsychol Dev Cogn B Aging Neuropsychol Cogn 2007;14(5):517-528.

144. Menard C, Patenaude C, Gagne AM, Massicotte G. AMPA receptor-mediated cell death is reduced by docosahexaenoic acid but not by eicosapentaenoic acid in area CA1 of hippocampal slice cultures. J Neurosci Res 2009;87(4):876-886.

145. Mills JD, Bailes JE, Sedney CL, Hutchins H, Sears B. Omega-3 fatty acid supplementation and reduction of traumatic axonal injury in a rodent head injury model. J Neurosurg 2011;114(1):77-84.

146. Morley JE, Banks WA. Lipids and cognition. J Alzheimers Dis 2010;20(3):737-747.

147. Mostofsky E, Schlaug G, Mukamal KJ, Rosamond WD, Mittleman MA. Coffee and acute ischemic stroke onset: the Stroke Onset Study. Neurology 2010;75(18):1583-1588.

148. Mozaffarian D, Longstreth WT Jr, Lemaitre RN, Manolio TA, Kuller LH, Burke GL, et al. Fish consumption and stroke risk in elderly individuals: the cardiovascular health study. Arch Intern Med 2005;165(2):200-206.

149. Mu X, Hc G, Cheng Y, Li X, Xu B, Du G. Baicalein exerts neuroprotective effects in 6-hydroxydopamine-induced experimental parkinsonism in vivo and in vitro. Pharmacol Biochem Behav 2009;92(4):642-648.

150. Mukamal KJ, Ascherio A, Mittleman MA, Conigrave KM, Camargo CA Jr, Kawachi I, et al. Alcohol and risk for ischemic stroke in men: the role of drinking patterns and usual beverage. Ann Intern Med 2005;142(1):11-19.

151. Nakagawa K, Miyazawa T. Absorption and distribution of tea catechin, (-)-epigallocatechin-3-gallate, in the rat. J Nutr Sci Vitaminol (Tokyo) 1997;43(6):679-684.

152. Nasrallah F, Feki M, Kaabachi N. Creatine and creatine deficiency syndromes: biochemical and clinical aspects. Pediatr Neurol 2010;42(3):163-171.

153. Neu A, Neuhoff H, Trube G, Fehr S, Ullrich K, Roeper J, et al. Activation of GABA(A) receptors by guanidinoacetate: a novel pathophysiological mechanism. Neurobiol Dis 2002;11(2):298-307.

154. Ng TP, Chiam PC, Lee T, Chua HC, Lim L, Kua EH. Curry consumption and cognitive function in the elderly. Am J Epidemiol 2006;164(9):898-906.

155. Ng TP, Feng L, Niti M, Kua EH, Yap KB. Tea consumption and cognitive impairment and decline in older Chinese adults. Am J Clin Nutr 2008;88(1):224-231.

156. Ohtsuki S, Tachikawa M, Takanaga H, Shimizu H, Watanabe M, Hosoya K, et al. The blood-brain barrier creatine transporter is a major pathway for supplying creatine to the brain. J Cereb Blood Flow Metab 2002;22(11):1327-1335.

157. Palzur E, Vlodavsky E, Mulla H, Arieli R, Feinsod M, Soustiel JF. Hyperbaric oxygen therapy for reduction of secondary brain damage in head injury: an animal model of brain contusion. J Neurotrauma 2004;21(1):41-48.

158. Park HA, Kubicki N, Gnyawali S, Chan YC, Roy S, Khanna S, et al. Natural vitamin E {alpha}-tocotrienol protects against ischemic stroke by induction of multidrug resistance-associated protein 1. Stroke 2011;42(8):2308-2314.

159. Park JW, Hong JS, Lee KS, Kim HY, Lee JJ, Lee SR. Green tea polyphenol (-)-epigallocatechin gallate reduces matrix metalloproteinase-9 activity following transient focal cerebral ischemia. J Nutr Biochem 2010;21(11):1038-1044.

160. Park SI, Jang DK, Han YM, Sunwoo YY, Park MS, Chung YA, et al. Effect of combination therapy with sodium ozagrel and panax ginseng on transient cerebral ischemia model in rats. J Biomed Biotechnol 2010;2010:893401.

161. Park SK, Jung IC, Lee WK, Lee YS, Park HK, Go HJ, et al. A combination of green tea extract and l-theanine improves memory and attention in subjects with mild cognitive impairment: a double-blind placebo-controlled study. J Med Food 2011;14(4):334-343.

162. Peng QL, Buz'Zard AR, Lau BH. Pycnogenol protects neurons from amyloid-beta peptide-induced apoptosis. Brain Res Mol Brain Res 2002;104(1):55-65.

163. Peral MJ, Vazquez-Carretero MD, Ilundain AA. Na(+)/Cl(-)/creatine transporter activity and expression in rat brain synaptosomes. Neuroscience 2010;165(1):53-60.

164. Petraglia AL, Winkler EA, Bailes JE. Stuck at the bench: potential natural neuroprotective compounds for concussion. Surg Neurol Int 2011;2:146.

165. Piao HZ, Jin SA, Chun HS, Lee JC, Kim WK. Neuroprotective effect of wogonin: potential roles of inflammatory cytokines. Arch Pharm Res 2004;27(9):930-936.

166. Pifferi F, Jouin M, Alessandri JM, Haedke U, Roux F, Perriere N, et al. n-3 Fatty acids modulate brain glucose transport in endothelial cells of the blood-brain barrier. Prostaglandins Leukot Essent Fatty Acids 2007;77(5-6):279-286.

167. Pilz S, Dobnig H, Fischer JE, Wellnitz B, Seelhorst U, Boehm BO, et al. Low vitamin d levels predict stroke in patients referred to coronary angiography. Stroke 2008;39(9):2611-2613.

168. Poppitt SD, Howe CA, Lithander FE, Silvers KM, Lin RB, Croft J, et al. Effects of moderate-dose omega-3 fish oil on cardiovascular risk factors and mood after ischemic stroke: a randomized, controlled trial. Stroke 2009;40(11):3485-3492.

169. Puri BK, Koepp MJ, Holmes J, Hamilton G, Yuen AW. A 31-phosphorus neurospectroscopy study of omega-3 long-chain polyunsaturated fatty acid intervention with eicosapentaenoic acid and docosahexaenoic acid in patients with chronic refractory epilepsy. Prostaglandins Leukot Essent Fatty Acids 2007;77(2):105-107.

170. Quinn JF, Raman R, Thomas RG, Yurko-Mauro K, Nelson EB, Van Dyck C, et al. Docosahexaenoic acid supplementation and cognitive decline in Alzheimer disease: a randomized trial. JAMA 2010;304(17):1903-1911.

171. Raval AP, Dave KR, Perez-Pinzon MA. Resveratrol mimics ischemic preconditioning in the brain. J Cereb Blood Flow Metab 2006;26(9):1141-1147.

172. Razmkon A, Sadidi A, Sherafat-Kazemzadeh E, Mehrafshan A, Bakhtazad A. Beneficial effects of vitamin c and vitamin e administration in severe head injury: a randomized double-blind control trial. Paper presented at the Congress of Neurological Surgeons annual meeting, San Francisco, 2010.

173. Rezai-Zadeh K, Arendash GW, Hou H, Fernandez F, Jensen M, Runfeldt M, et al. Green tea epigallocatechin-3-gallate (EGCG) reduces beta-amyloid mediated cognitive impairment and modulates tau pathology in Alzheimer transgenic mice. Brain Res 2008;1214:177-187.

174. Richard T, Pawlus AD, Iglesias ML, Pedrot E, Waffo-Teguo P, Merillon JM, et al. Neuroprotective properties of resveratrol and derivatives. Ann N Y Acad Sci 2011;1215:103-108.

175. Robertson CL, Bell MJ, Kochanek PM, Adelson PD, Ruppel RA, Carcillo JA, et al. Increased adenosine in cerebrospinal fluid after severe traumatic brain injury in infants and children: association with severity of injury and excitotoxicity. Crit Care Med 2001;29(12):2287-2293.

176. Robson LG, Dyall S, Sidloff D, Michael-Titus AT. Omega-3 polyunsaturated fatty acids increase the neurite outgrowth of rat sensory neurones throughout development and in aged animals. Neurobiol Aging 2010;31(4):678-687.

177. Rockswold SB, Rockswold GL, Vargo JM, Erickson CA, Sutton RL, Bergman TA, et al. Effects of hyperbaric oxygenation therapy on cerebral metabolism and intracranial pressure in severely brain injured patients. J Neurosurg 2001;94(3):403-411.

178. Roitman S, Green T, Osher Y, Karni N, Levine J. Creatine monohydrate in resistant depression: a preliminary study. Bipolar Disord 2007;9(7):754-758.

179. Ross GW, Petrovitch H. Current evidence for neuroprotective effects of nicotine and caffeine against Parkinson's disease. Drugs Aging 2001;18(11):797-806.

180. Ryan J, Croft K, Mori T, Wesnes K, Spong J, Downey L, et al. An examination of the effects of the antioxidant Pycnogenol on cognitive performance, serum lipid profile, endocrinological and oxidative stress biomarkers in an elderly population. J Psychopharmacol 2008;22(5):553-562.

181. Saaksjarvi K, Knekt P, Rissanen H, Laaksonen MA, Reunanen A, Mannisto S. Prospective study of coffee consumption and risk of Parkinson's disease. Eur J Clin Nutr 2008;62(7):908-915.

182. Sachse KT, Jackson EK, Wisniewski SR, Gillespie DG, Puccio AM, Clark RS, et al. Increases in cerebrospinal fluid caffeine concentration are associated with favorable outcome after severe traumatic brain injury in humans. J Cereb Blood Flow Metab 2008;28(2):395-401.

183. Sakellaris G, Kotsiou M, Tamiolaki M, Kalostos G, Tsapaki E, Spanaki M, et al. Prevention of complications related to traumatic brain injury in children and adolescents with creatine administration: an open label randomized pilot study. J Trauma 2006;61(2):322-329.

184. Sakellaris G, Nasis G, Kotsiou M, Tamiolaki M, Charissis G, Evangeliou A. Prevention of traumatic headache, dizziness and fatigue with creatine administration. A pilot study. Acta Paediatr 2008;97(1):31-34.

185. Salem N Jr, Litman B, Kim HY, Gawrisch K. Mechanisms of action of docosahexaenoic acid in the nervous system. Lipids 2001;36(9):945-959.

186. Santos C, Costa J, Santos J, Vaz-Carneiro A, Lunet N. Caffeine intake and dementia: systematic review and meta-analysis. J Alzheimers Dis 2010;20 Suppl 1:S187-204.

187. Santos C, Lunet N, Azevedo A, de Mendonca A, Ritchie K, Barros H. Caffeine intake is associated with a lower risk of cognitive decline: a cohort study from Portugal. J Alzheimers Dis 2010;20 Suppl 1:S175-185.

188. Sarsilmaz M, Songur A, Ozyurt H, Kus I, Ozen OA, Ozyurt B, et al. Potential role of dietary omega-3 essential fatty acids on some oxidant/antioxidant parameters in rats' corpus striatum. Prostaglandins Leukot Essent Fatty Acids 2003;69(4):253-259.

189. Scapagnini G, Caruso C, Calabrese V. Therapeutic potential of dietary polyphenols against brain ageing and neurodegenerative disorders. Adv Exp Med Biol 2010;698:27-35.

190. Scheff SW, Dhillon HS. Creatine-enhanced diet alters levels of lactate and free fatty acids after experimental brain injury. Neurochem Res 2004;29(2):469-479.

191. Schurks M, Glynn RJ, Rist PM, Tzourio C, Kurth T. Effects of vitamin E on stroke subtypes: meta-analysis of randomised controlled trials. BMJ 2010;341:c5702.

192. Schwarzschild MA, Xu K, Oztas E, Petzer JP, Castagnoli K, Castagnoli N Jr, et al. Neuroprotection by caffeine and more specific A2A receptor antagonists in animal models of Parkinson's disease. Neurology 2003;61(11 Suppl 6):S55-61.

193. Sesso HD, Buring JE, Christen WG, Kurth T, Belanger C, MacFadyen J, et al. Vitamins E and C in the prevention of cardiovascular disease in men: the Physicians' Health Study II randomized controlled trial. JAMA 2008;300(18):2123-2133.

194. Shang Y, Cheng J, Qi J, Miao H. Scutellaria flavonoid reduced memory dysfunction and neuronal injury caused by permanent global ischemia in rats. Pharmacol Biochem Behav 2005;82(1):67-73.

195. Shang YZ, Miao H, Cheng JJ, Qi JM. Effects of amelioration of total flavonoids from stems and leaves of Scutellaria baicalensis Georgi on cognitive deficits, neuronal damage and free radicals disorder induced by cerebral ischemia in rats. Biol Pharm Bull 2006;29(4):805-810.

196. Sharma S, Ying Z, Gomez-Pinilla F. A pyrazole curcumin derivative restores membrane homeostasis disrupted after brain trauma. Exp Neurol 2010;226(1):191-199.

197. Sharma S, Zhuang Y, Ying Z, Wu A, Gomez-Pinilla F. Dietary curcumin supplementation counteracts reduction in levels of molecules involved in energy homeostasis after brain trauma. Neuroscience 2009;161(4):1037-1044.

198. Shukla PK, Khanna VK, Ali MM, Khan MY, Srimal RC. Anti-ischemic effect of curcumin in rat brain. Neurochem Res 2008;33(6):1036-1043.

199. Signoretti S, Di Pietro V, Vagnozzi R, Lazzarino G, Amorini AM, Belli A, et al. Transient alterations of creatine, creatine phosphate, N-acetylaspartate and high-energy phosphates after mild traumatic brain injury in the rat. Mol Cell Biochem 2010;333(1-2):269-277.

200. Singleton RH, Yan HQ, Fellows-Mayle W, Dixon CE. Resveratrol attenuates behavioral impairments and reduces cortical and hippocampal loss in a rat controlled cortical impact model of traumatic brain injury. J Neurotrauma 2010;27(6):1091-1099.

201. Sinha K, Chaudhary G, Gupta YK. Protective effect of resveratrol against oxidative stress in middle cerebral artery occlusion model of stroke in rats. Life Sci 2002;71(6):655-665.

202. Son D, Lee P, Lee J, Kim H, Kim SY. Neuroprotective effect of wogonin in hippocampal slice culture exposed to oxygen and glucose deprivation. Eur J Pharmacol 2004;493(1-3):99-102.

203. Songur A, Sarsilmaz M, Sogut S, Ozyurt B, Ozyurt H, Zararsiz I, et al. Hypothalamic superoxide dismutase, xanthine oxidase, nitric oxide, and malondialdehyde in rats fed with fish omega-3 fatty acids. Prog Neuropsychopharmacol Biol Psychiatry 2004;28(4):693-698.

204. Sonmez U, Sonmez A, Erbil G, Tekmen I, Baykara B. Neuroprotective effects of resveratrol against traumatic brain injury in immature rats. Neurosci Lett 2007;420(2):133-137.

205. Spector R, Johanson CE. Vitamin transport and homeostasis in mammalian brain: focus on vitamins B and E. J Neurochem 2007;103(2):425-438.

206. Stoller KP. Hyperbaric oxygen therapy (1.5 ATA) in treating sports related TBI/CTE: two case reports. Med Gas Res 2011;1(1):17.

207. Suganuma M, Okabe S, Oniyama M, Tada Y, Ito H, Fujiki H. Wide distribution of [3H](-)-epigallocatechin gallate, a cancer preventive tea polyphenol, in mouse tissue. Carcinogenesis 1998;19(10):1771-1776.

208. Suk K, Lee H, Kang SS, Cho GJ, Choi WS. Flavonoid baicalein attenuates activation-induced cell death of brain microglia. J Pharmacol Exp Ther 2003;305(2):638-645.

209. Sullivan PG, Geiger JD, Mattson MP, Scheff SW. Dietary supplement creatine protects against traumatic brain injury. Ann Neurol 2000;48(5):723-729.

210. Sung S, Yao Y, Uryu K, Yang H, Lee VM, Trojanowski JQ, et al. Early vitamin E supplementation in young but not aged mice reduces Abeta levels and amyloid deposition in a transgenic model of Alzheimer's disease. FASEB J 2004;18(2):323-325.

211. Tan EK, Tan C, Fook-Chong SM, Lum SY, Chai A, Chung H, et al. Dose-dependent protective effect of coffee, tea, and smoking in Parkinson's disease: a study in ethnic Chinese. J Neurol Sci 2003;216(1):163-167.

212. Tanaka K, Ishikawa Y, Yokoyama M, Origasa H, Matsuzaki M, Saito Y, et al. Reduction in the recurrence of stroke by eicosapentaenoic acid for hypercholesterolemic patients: subanalysis of the JELIS trial. Stroke 2008;39(7):2052-2058.

213. Tang C, Xue H, Bai C, Fu R, Wu A. The effects of Tanshinone IIA on blood-brain barrier and brain edema after transient middle cerebral artery occlusion in rats. Phytomedicine 2010;17(14):1145-1149.

214. Tang C, Xue HL, Bai CL, Fu R. Regulation of adhesion molecules expression in TNF-alpha-stimulated brain microvascular endothelial cells by tanshinone IIA: involvement of NF-kappaB and ROS generation. Phytother Res 2011;25(3):376-380.

215. Tangpricha V, Pearce EN, Chen TC, Holick MF. Vitamin D insufficiency among free-living healthy young adults. Am J Med 2002;112(8):659-662.

216. Thiyagarajan M, Sharma SS. Neuroprotective effect of curcumin in middle cerebral artery occlusion induced focal cerebral ischemia in rats. Life Sci 2004;74(8):969-985.

217. Tinianow CL, Tinianow TK, Wilcox M. Effects of hyperbaric oxygen on focal brain contusions. Biomed Sci Instrum 2000;36:275-281.

218. Travis MA, Hall ED. The effects of chronic two-fold dietary vitamin E supplementation on subarachnoid hemorrhage-induced brain hypoperfusion. Brain Res 1987;418(2):366-370.

219. Usoro OB, Mousa SA. Vitamin E forms in Alzheimer's disease: a review of controversial and clinical experiences. Crit Rev Food Sci Nutr 2010;50(5):414-419.

220. Varma MR, Dixon CE, Jackson EK, Peters GW, Melick JA, Griffith RP, et al. Administration of adenosine receptor agonists or antagonists after controlled cortical impact in mice: effects on function and histopathology. Brain Res 2002;951(2):191-201.

221. Vlodavsky E, Palzur E, Soustiel JF. Hyperbaric oxygen therapy reduces neuroinflammation and expression of matrix metalloproteinase-9 in the rat model of traumatic brain injury. Neuropathol Appl Neurobiol 2006;32(1):40-50.

222. Wakade C, King MD, Laird MD, Alleyne CH Jr, Dhandapani KM. Curcumin attenuates vascular inflammation and cerebral vasospasm after subarachnoid hemorrhage in mice. Antioxid Redox Signal 2009;11(1):35-45.

223. Wang X, Zhao X, Mao ZY, Wang XM, Liu ZL. Neuroprotective effect of docosahexaenoic acid on glutamate-induced cytotoxicity in rat hippocampal cultures. Neuroreport 2003;14(18):2457-2461.

224. Wang XJ, Wang ZB, Xu JX. Effect of salvianic acid A on lipid peroxidation and membrane permeability in mitochondria. J Ethnopharmacol 2005;97(3):441-445.

225. Wang XJ, Xu JX. Salvianic acid A protects human neuroblastoma SH-SY5Y cells against MPP+-induced cytotoxicity. Neurosci Res 2005;51(2):129-138.

226. Wang Y, Liu J, Zhang Z, Bi P, Qi Z, Zhang C. Anti-neuroinflammation effect of ginsenoside Rbl in a rat model of Alzheimer disease. Neurosci Lett 2011;487(1):70-72.

227. Washington CB, Jackson EK, Janesko KL, Vagni VA, Lefferis Z, Jenkins LW, et al. Chronic caffeine administration reduces hippocampal neuronal cell death after experimental traumatic brain injury in mice. J Neurotrauma 2005;22:366-370.

228. Wei IH, Tu HC, Huang CC, Tsai MH, Tseng CY, Shieh JY. (-)-Epigallocatechin gallate attenuates NADPH-d/nNOS expression in motor neurons of rats following peripheral nerve injury. BMC Neurosci 2011;12:52.

229. Witham MD, Dove FJ, Sugden JA, Doney AS, Struthers AD. The effect of vitamin D replacement on markers of vascular health in stroke patients - a randomised controlled trial. Nutr Metab Cardiovasc Dis 2012;22(10):864-870.

230. Wright DW, Kellermann AL, Hertzberg VS, Clark PL, Frankel M, Goldstein FC, et al. ProTECT: a randomized clinical trial of progesterone for acute traumatic brain injury. Ann Emerg Med 2007;49(4):391-402, 402 e1-2.

231. Wu A, Ying Z, Gomez-Pinilla F. Dietary curcumin counteracts the outcome of traumatic brain injury on oxidative stress, synaptic plasticity, and cognition. Exp Neurol 2006;197(2):309-317.

232. Wu A, Ying Z, Gomez-Pinilla F. Dietary omega-3 fatty acids normalize BDNF levels, reduce oxidative damage, and counteract learning disability after traumatic brain injury in rats. J Neurotrauma 2004;21(10):1457-1467.

233. Wu A, Ying Z, Gomez-Pinilla F. Omega-3 fatty acids supplementation restores mechanisms that maintain brain homeostasis in traumatic brain injury. J Neurotrauma 2007;24(10):1587-1595.

234. Wu A, Ying Z, Schubert D, Gomez-Pinilla F. Brain and spinal cord interaction: a dietary curcumin derivative counteracts locomotor and cognitive deficits after brain trauma. Neurorehabil Neural Repair 2011;25(4):332-342.

235. Wu A, Zhe Y, Gomez-Pinilla F. Vitamin E protects against oxidative damage and learning disability after mild traumatic brain injury in rats. Neurorehabil Neural Repair 2010;24(3):290-298.

236. Wyss M, Kaddurah-Daouk R. Creatine and creatinine metabolism. Physiol Rev 2000;80(3):1107-1113.

237. Xiao G, Wei J, Yan W, Wang W, Lu Z. Improved outcomes from the administration of progesterone for patients with acute severe traumatic brain injury: a randomized controlled trial. Crit Care 2008;12(2):R61.

238. Xu G, Zhao W, Zhou Z, Zhang R, Zhu W, Liu X. Danshen extracts decrease blood C reactive protein and prevent ischemic stroke recurrence: a controlled pilot study. Phytother Res 2009;23(12):1721-1725.

239. Xu K, Xu YH, Chen JF, Schwarzschild MA. Caffeine's neuroprotection against 1-methyl-4-phenyl-1,2,3,6-tetrahydropyridine toxicity shows no tolerance to chronic caffeine administration in mice. Neurosci Lett 2002;322(1):13-16.

240. Xue X, Qu XJ, Yang Y, Sheng XH, Cheng F, Jiang EN, et al. Baicalin attenuates focal cerebral ischemic reperfusion injury through inhibition of nuclear factor kappaB p65 activation. Biochem Biophys Res Commun 2010;403(3-4):398-404.

241. Yang C, Zhang X, Fan H, Liu Y. Curcumin upregulates transcription factor Nrf2, HO-1 expression and protects rat brains against focal ischemia. Brain Res 2009;1282:133-141.

242. Yang F, Lim GP, Begum AN, Ubeda OJ, Simmons MR, Ambegaokar SS, et al. Curcumin inhibits formation of amyloid beta oligomers and fibrils, binds plaques, and reduces amyloid in vivo. J Biol Chem 2005;280(7):5892-5901.

243. Yang YB, Piao YJ. Effects of resveratrol on secondary damages after acute spinal cord injury in rats. Acta Pharmacol Sin 2003;24(7):703-710.

244. Ye R, Kong X, Yang Q, Zhang Y, Han J, Li P, et al. Ginsenoside Rd in experimental stroke: superior neuroprotective efficacy with a wide therapeutic window. Neurotherapeutics 2011;8(3):515-25.

245. Ye R, Kong X, Yang Q, Zhang Y, Han J, Zhao G. Ginsenoside Rd attenuates redox imbalance and improves stroke outcome after focal cerebral ischemia in aged mice. Neuropharmacology 2011;61(4):815-824.

246. Ye R, Zhang X, Kong X, Han J, Yang Q, Zhang Y, et al. Ginsenoside Rd attenuates mitochondrial dysfunction and sequential apoptosis after transient focal ischemia. Neuroscience 2011;178:169-180.

247. Yin D, Zhou C, Kusaka I, Calvert JW, Parent AD, Nanda A, et al. Inhibition of apoptosis by hyperbaric oxygen in a rat focal cerebral ischemic model. J Cereb Blood Flow Metab 2003;23(7):855-864.

248. Yoneda H, Shirao S, Kurokawa T, Fujisawa H, Kato S, Suzuki M. Does eicosapentaenoic acid (EPA) inhibit cerebral vasospasm in patients after aneurysmal subarachnoid hemorrhage? Acta Neurol Scand 2008;118(1):54-59.

249. Yu J, Jia Y, Guo Y, Chang G, Duan W, Sun M, et al. Epigallocatechin-3-gallate protects motor neurons and regulates glutamate level. FEBS Lett 2010;584(13):2921-2925.

250. Yuen AW, Sander JW, Fluegel D, Patsalos PN, Bell GS, Johnson T, et al. Omega-3 fatty acid supplementation in patients with chronic epilepsy: a randomized trial. Epilepsy Behav 2005;7(2):253-258.

251. Yune TY, Lee JY, Cui CM, Kim HC, Oh TH. Neuroprotective effect of Scutellaria baicalensis on spinal cord injury in rats. J Neurochem 2009;110(4):1276-1287.

252. Zhang WJ, Feng J, Zhou R, Ye LY, Liu HL, Peng L, et al. Tanshinone IIA protects the human blood-brain barrier model from leukocyte-associated hypoxia-reoxygenation injury. Eur J Pharmacol 2010;648(1-3):146-152.

253. Zhao HF, Li Q, Li Y. Long-term ginsenoside administration prevents memory loss in aged female C57BL/6J mice by modulating the redox status and up-regulating the plasticity-related proteins in hippocampus. Neuroscience 2011;183:189-202.

254. Zhao J, Yu S, Zheng W, Feng G, Luo G, Wang L, et al. Curcumin improves outcomes and attenuates focal cerebral ischemic injury via anti-apoptotic mechanisms in rats. Neurochem Res 2010;35(3):374-379.

255. Zheng GQ, Cheng W, Wang Y, Wang XM, Zhao SZ, Zhou Y, et al. Ginseng total saponins enhance neurogenesis after focal cerebral ischemia. J Ethnopharmacol 2011;133(2):724-728.

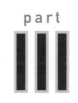

part

III

SPORT-RELATED INJURIES OF THE SPINE AND PERIPHERAL NERVOUS SYSTEM

During participation in any sport, injuries to any part of the spine are possible, as well as injuries to the soft tissue and fascia that make up the spinal unit. Though injuries that result in back pain are not the most common injury in the young athlete, they can lead to frustration, and more severe forms of injury can be a devastating source of morbidity. Most athletic injuries to the back are sprains of the ligaments or strains of the muscles. Many injuries occur after repetitive overuse of the structures of the spine. Most of the injuries affect the lumbar spine; however, cervical spine injuries are perhaps among the most feared complications of athletic activities. In this part of the book we review the important facets of an optimal response to the athlete with suspected or proven spinal injury.

Peripheral nerve injuries occur in athletes as well. These injuries can affect any peripheral nerve and can affect the athlete at any age. Certain athletes and certain nerves appear to be at higher risk for injury. Athletes may develop peripheral nerve injuries from direct trauma or chronically following repetitive trauma. Injuries can develop from compression, contusion, stretch, friction, or microtrauma. One must have a broad knowledge of peripheral nerve injuries, as at times they are serious and potentially career ending. Thus in this section we provide an overview to prepare the sports medicine practitioner to deal with these types of athletic injuries.

Cervical, Thoracic, and Lumbar Spine Injuries

Types, Causal Mechanisms, and Clinical Features

In collaboration with

Saint-Aaron L. Morris, M.D. • Wesley H. Jones, M.D.

Spinal injury is perhaps one of the most feared complications in athletic activities. Injuries can involve the soft tissues, bony structural elements, the vertebral column, the spinal cord itself, or any combination thereof. Spinal cord injuries can result in significant disability and time lost from competition and can become a source of chronic pain and functional limitation. This chapter reviews the various cervical, thoracic, and lumbar spine injuries as well as their clinical features.

BACKGROUND AND EPIDEMIOLOGY

An estimated 11% of traumatic spinal injury admissions are due to sport-related activity. Males account for three-fourths of these injuries, and individuals in their mid-20s are most frequently affected.

In a national study in Ireland, the most common causes of sport-related spinal injury were equestrian sports (41.8%), followed by rugby (16.3%), diving (15.3%), football (soccer) and hurling (9.6%), and cycling (4.2%).[5] In the United States, football, wrestling, and ice hockey account for the majority of reported athletics-related spine trauma. These injuries have the potential to be devastating, as the majority occur at the cervical level (60%).[5] Approximately one-third of all spinal injuries are associated with a neurologic deficit, and of these, at least one-third are permanent. The risks are greatest during the actual athletic contest, secondary to the use of more violent forces; the frequency trends upward in direct relationship with the level of competition.

A National Football League epidemiologic study demonstrated that spinal injuries accounted for 7% of all football-related injuries.[15] A large proportion affect the lumbar region, with soft tissue injuries accounting for the majority. An estimated 30% of athletes have sport-related low back pain, and 80% of these complaints arise during practice or training. Ligamentous sprains are common in the pediatric population, likely due to the skeletally immature spine, while discogenic disease and strains are more likely in adults. Although the majority of such injuries are not catastrophic, they generate a significant cost, with affected players missing an average of 21.4 practices and 4.4 games per injury—a significant loss to the player and team, particularly at professional levels.[10]

NORMAL ANATOMY

The spine is a complex osseous and ligamentous structure that, together with the supporting musculature, is responsible for protecting the spinal cord and nerve roots within. The exact anatomic relationships of these structures to each other are very important in clarifying the nature, extent, and potential risks of neurologic injury, as well as the urgency and extent of intervention indicated. Plain X-rays, although valuable in some instances to define stability in flexion and extension, have largely been supplanted by more revealing imaging methods. Computed tomography (CT) scans are generally best for evaluating the osseous components of the spine and to delineate any fractures or subluxation of bone, while magnetic resonance imaging (MRI) offers much better visualization of the neural elements and ligaments[8, 9, 31] (figures 16.1 and 16.2).

TYPES OF TISSUE INJURIES AND NEUROLOGIC SYNDROMES

Table 16.1 presents an outline of the various tissues that might be disrupted during a spinal injury. All would be expected to produce some degree of axial pain in the region of the spine affected. Nervous system damage, to either the spinal cord, nerve roots, or brachial plexus, represents the most severe consequence of spinal

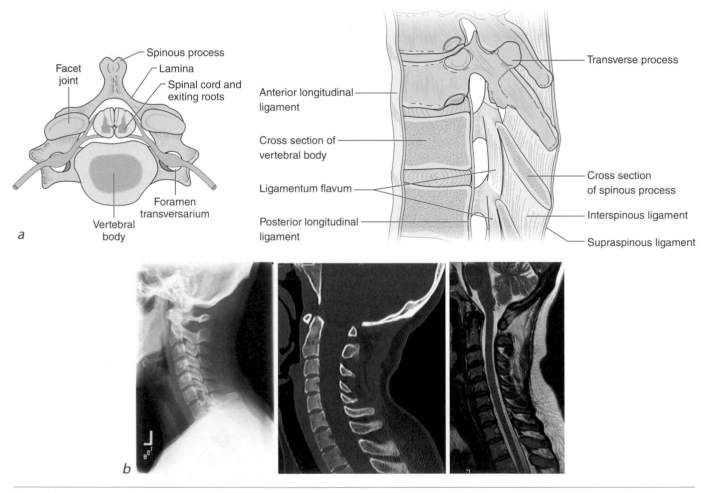

Figure 16.1 Normal spinal anatomy, cervical. (a) Schematic (axial and midsagittal views). Note the ligaments that allow flexibility while providing stability for protection of the spinal canal contents during movement (midsagittal view) and the relationship of the spinal cord and nerve roots within the spinal canal. Note also the foramen transversarium, which contains the vertebral arteries as they ascend toward the brain. (b) Neuroimaging of the cervical spine: plain X-rays, CT, and MRI. Note the integrity, alignment, and curvature of the bone anteriorly and posteriorly. The bony details are much clearer on CT scanning, while the soft tissue, discs, spinal cord, and nerve roots require MRI.

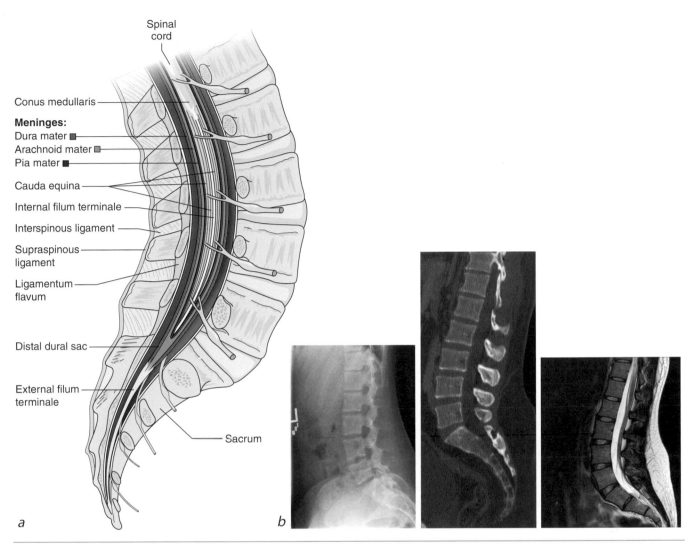

Figure 16.2   Normal spinal anatomy, lumbar (midsagittal). **(a)** Schematic (midsagittal view). Note the increased size of the vertebral bodies to provide support and a fixation point for the pelvis. **(b)** Neuroimaging of the lumbar spine: plain X-rays, CT, and MRI. Note the integrity, alignment, and curvature of the bone anteriorly and posteriorly. The bony details are much clearer on CT scanning, while the discs and other soft tissues are best seen on MRI. Note the absence of the spinal cord within the spinal fluid (CSF) in the mid and lower lumbar region as seen on MRI.

injury; having knowledge of the relationship of the various types of tissue injuries to the likelihood of nervous system compromise is imperative.

Neurologic deficits vary according to the presence or absence of spinal cord injury or the specific distribution of the nerve(s) arising and exiting the spine at that level (table 16.2, figure 16.3). Because the spinal cord generally ends at L1, lumbar injuries are not associated with spinal cord distribution deficits. The degree of any motor or cord deficits can be quantified according to the scale outlined in tables 16.3 and 16.4. Table 16.5 outlines the nomenclature and types of disc

injuries, while table 16.6 organizes the terminology and grading for fractures.

When one is faced with a potential spine injury, the initial focus is to maintain the spine in a protected unstressed position until clinical and neuroimaging studies have validated stability by regimented assessment of each portion of the affected spine region.

Whenever the spinal cord might be involved, it is imperative that the athlete not return to play until there is complete resolution of any radicular pain, sensory abnormality, weakness, and limited range of motion. Players with persistent symptoms should undergo spine immobilization

Table 16.1   Tissues Affected by Spinal Injuries

Tissue	Type of injury
Soft tissue (skin, muscle)	Sprain Strain
Ligaments	
Disc	Rupture (herniation) Spondylosis

Bone	• Congenital
	   • Stenosis
	   • Chiari malformation
	   • Bone resorption or fusion
	• Fractures
	   • Pars interarticularis (stress)
	   • Facet
	   • Spinous process
	   • Transverse process
	   • Vertebral body

Nervous system	Spinal cord Nerve root Brachial plexus

Nearby organ systems	• Vascular
	   • Carotid artery
	   • Vertebral artery
	• Renal
	   • Lung

Table 16.2   Patterns of Common Nerve Root Injuries

Level	Major muscle	Major action	Reflex	Sensation
CERVICAL				
C5	Deltoid	Abduction of arms >90 from midline		Anterior shoulder
C6	Biceps	Forearm flexion and supination	Biceps	Thumb ± index finger
C7	Triceps	Forearm extension	Triceps	Middle ± index finger
C8	Intrinsic hand muscles	Handgrip		Small finger
T1	Intrinsic hand muscles	Finger abduction		Small finger
THORACIC				
T4-10	Intercostals	Expanding chest during inhalation		Radiation paralleling rib
LUMBOSACRAL				
L1-3	Iliopsoas	Hip flexion	Cremasteric	Groin, lateral thigh
L4	Quadriceps	Knee extension	Patellar	Anterior thigh
L5	Tibialis anterior, extensor hallucis longus	Foot dorsiflexion		Dorsum of foot, great toe
S1	Gastrocnemius and soleus	Foot plantar flexion	Achilles	Lateral foot, small toe
S2-4	External anal sphincter	Rectal tone	Anal wink and bulbocavernosus	Perianal region

and CT–MR spinal imaging to assess for fractures, dislocations, or disc herniations as a source of their complaints.

Table 16.3   Muscle Strength Grading

Grade	Description
0	No movement
1	Palpable or visible contraction or both
2	Antigravity movement with assistance
3	Antigravity movement without assistance
4	Movement against some resistance
5	Movement against full resistance

Spinal Cord: Cervical Neurapraxia (Transient Quadriparesis or Quadriplegia)

Also referred to as "spinal cord concussion," this phenomenon affects as many as 1.3 per 10,000 collegiate football players. The condition is associated with temporary impairment in sensory or motor modalities (or both) of two or more extremities following spinal trauma. Burning paresthesias and weakness/paralysis of the involved extremities, often distally in the hands, generally lasts 10 to 15 minutes (74%); however, athletes may present with deficits for as long as

Table 16.4   American Spinal Injury Association (ASIA) Impairment Scale for Spinal Cord Injury

Class	Description
A	No motor or sensory function below the level of injury
B	Sensory but no motor function below the level of injury
C	>50% of the muscles innervated below the level of injury have strength grade <3
D	≥50% of the muscles innervated below the level of injury have strength grade ≥3
E	Normal motor and sensory function

Table 16.5   Types and Nomenclature for Disc Conditions

Disc term	Description
Normal	A gelatinous cartilage composed of an outer annulus fibrosus encircling a central nucleus pulposus: remnant of embryonic notochord bounded superiorly-inferiorly by adjacent vertebral bodies bounded anteriorly-posteriorly by the anterior and posterior longitudinal ligaments
Degenerative	Term describing dessication (dehydrated) and often narrowed (collapsed, irregularly thinned) disc space; associated with annulus defects, sclerotic end plates, disc "bulges," osteophytes
Bulging	In the absence of degenerative changes, a common, usually asymptomatic radiographic finding with limited amounts of disc material extending beyond the line of the posterior vertebral body toward the spinal canal in a generalized, nonfocal pattern
Herniated (ruptured)	Disc displacement beyond the confines of annulus fibrosus: Location, direction: • Dorsal, dorsolateral—central versus lateral versus "far" lateral • Intervertebral—Schmorl's node burrowing into vertebral body Degree: • Focal versus broad based • Protrusion—no "neck," fragment width greatest at herniation point • Extrusion (sequestration)—disc herniation point has narrower neck than fragment • Free fragment—herniation has potentially detached from its connection to the disc space of origin

Table 16.6 **Types and Nomenclature for Spinal Stability**

Nomenclature	Definition
Clinical	Mechanism of injury, history, and physical exam
Radiologic	Objective evidence of deviation from normal spinal anatomy that is historically consistent with biomechanically unstable spine
Biomechanical	Ability of the spine to resist ex vivo forces
Column	**Components**
Anterior	Anterior longitudinal ligament Anterior half of vertebral body Intervertebral disc including anterior annulus fibrosus
Middle	Posterior half of vertebral body Intervertebral disc including posterior annulus fibrosus Posterior longitudinal ligament Pedicles
Posterior	Posterior arch bony elements and associated ligaments including lamina and ligamentum flavum Lateral mass facet joints and joint capsule Transverse processes Spinous processes Interspinous and supraspinous ligament

1 or 2 days. Individuals with preexisting spinal stenosis (Torg ratio <0.8) have a threefold risk of developing cervical neurapraxia; however, less than half of symptomatic patients met these criteria in one study[18] (figure 16.3).

Spinal Cord: Central Cord Syndrome

The neurologic pattern of this syndrome is characterized by weakness and sensory abnormalities that are disproportionately greater in the distal upper extremities compared to the lower extremities. Sphincter dysfunction, if present, is usually transient. A mild form of this syndrome produces bilateral dysesthesias into the distal portions of the upper extremity, a syndrome known as "burning hands." This deficit distribution is caused by the somatotopic organization of the corticospinal fibers (upper extremity innervation is arranged more medially than that of the lower extremities).

Central cord syndrome is the most common incomplete spinal cord injury pattern and is typically seen after a hyperextension force has been applied to the neck. The central region of the spinal cord is susceptible to watershed ischemia that may occur from obstruction of flow within the anterior spinal artery.[3, 11, 17, 26] Hematomyelia (blood within the central portions of the spinal cord) may develop and cause progressive worsening of the symptoms over several hours. As the condition improves, lower extremity and sphincter dysfunction resolve first. The upper extremity symptoms resolve last, in a proximal to distal fashion. Approximately 90% of patients regain ambulation within 5 days of injury; however, recovery is largely dependent on the extent of injury and patient age.[2, 16]

Spinal Cord: Brown–Sequard Syndrome

Classically described as an ipsilateral loss of motor function and a contralateral loss of sensation, Brown-Sequard (hemicord) syndrome rarely presents in a pure form. Most injured athletes have a mixed presentation of both a hemicord and central cord syndrome. These individuals demonstrate ipsilateral weakness that is greater in the upper extremities; ipsilateral loss of fine touch, vibration sense, and proprioception below the level of injury; and contralateral loss of pain and temperature sensation one or two levels below the site of injury. The incidence is estimated to be 2% to 4% in spinal trauma, and this syndrome is associated with the best prognosis among the incomplete cord injuries. Approximately 90% of patients regain the ability to ambulate independently.[3, 23, 24]

Spinal Cord: Anterior Spinal Artery Syndrome

This syndrome is usually the consequence of a ventral lesion causing occlusion-disruption of flow within the anterior spinal artery. Affected patients have bilateral loss of motor function below the level of the injury, as well as bilateral loss of pain and temperature sensation one or

two levels below the insult.[3, 25] An anterior cord syndrome is likely more common than hemicord syndrome and is associated with a poorer prognosis. Only 10% to 20% of those injured recover meaningful motor function.

Nerve Root or Plexus

Cervical nerve root and brachial plexus neurapraxia are known by several colloquialisms, such as "burners" or "stingers." Stretching of the upper trunk of the brachial plexus accounts for the majority of these syndromes. Downward traction of the shoulder associated with lateral flexion of the neck to the opposite side is the proposed mechanism of injury in many cases. A

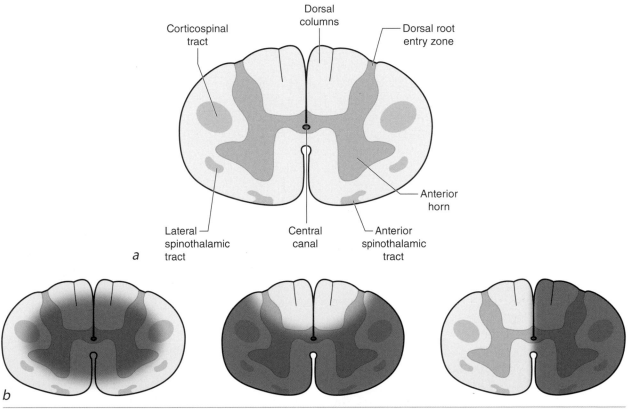

Figure 16.3 Patterns of spinal cord injury. (a) Normal spinal cord. (b) Cord syndromes. (1) Central cord syndrome: characterized by the development of weakness and sensory abnormalities that are disproportionately greater in the upper extremities compared to the lower extremities. This is secondary to the somatotopic organization of the cortico-spinal fibers (upper extremity innervation is arranged more medially than that of the lower extremities). (2) Anterior spinal cord syndrome: characterized by the development of bilateral loss of motor function below the level of the injury, as well as bilateral loss of pain and temperature sensation one or two levels below the insult. (3) Brown-Sequard syndrome: characterized by ipsilateral loss of motor function and contralateral loss of pain sensation, but rarely presents in a pure form. Individuals demonstrate ipsilateral weakness that is greater in the upper extremities; ipsilateral loss of fine touch, discriminative touch, vibration sense, and proprioception below the level of injury; and contralateral loss of pain and temperature sensation one or two levels below the site of injury.

similar pattern can be seen with a direct injury to the plexus by an external force applied to the supraclavicular area. The neurologic deficit in almost all of these cases includes the upper portion of the plexus, with weakness of the deltoid, biceps, and shoulder rotator muscles, and numbness extending down to the thumb and index finger (figure 16.4).

Any other pattern of radicular symptoms is more suggestive of an isolated nerve root injury. The C5 and C6 nerve roots are most commonly affected, due to transient neural foraminal narrowing from a compressive axial force. An underlying osteophyte or disc rupture is identified in many of these cases.

Vascular

Because the carotid and vertebral arteries traverse the neck, they are susceptible to injury whenever the spine is subjected to those forces that similarly injure the spine. The resultant neu-

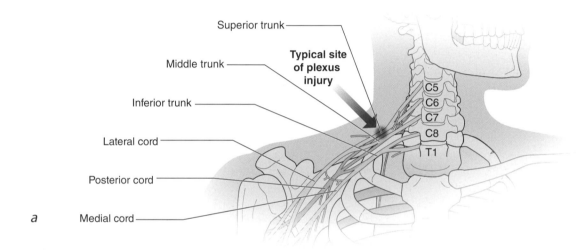

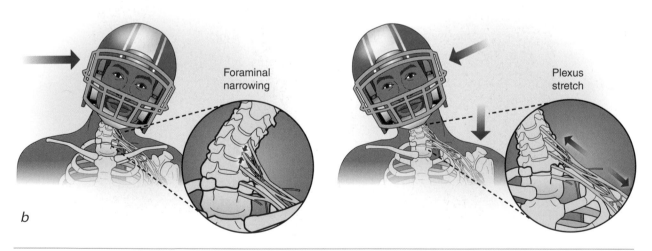

Figure 16.4 Plexus or root injuries. (a) Schematic: brachial plexus. Note its origins from the C5 through T1 nerve roots. UT = upper trunk, formed by a merger of the anterior divisions of the C5 and C6 roots. (b) Mechanisms of plexus versus root injury: The superior position of the upper trunk makes it most vulnerable to direct blows or stretching from distraction of the neck away from the shoulder. In contrast, a root may also be injured by lateral flexion of the neck toward the side of symptoms, associated with foraminal narrowing, especially in the presence of an underlying disc herniation or osteophyte.

rologic deficit pattern is quite different from those associated with the spinal cord, root, or brachial plexus; and early recognition is mandatory to prevent progressive and potentially catastrophic nervous system damage.

With carotid artery injuries, the athlete may present with ipsilateral retro-orbital headaches, pain overlying the carotid artery (carotidynia), and an incomplete Horner's syndrome (ptosis and miosis). Neurologic symptoms, often delayed, consist of cerebral hemisphere dysfunction (aphasia or contralateral hemiparesis or both, hemisensory or visual deficits) secondary to ischemia from arterial thromboembolism. Many patients return to normal, but a significant number have residual deficits or die from massive cerebral infarction and swelling.[3, 13, 37]

Injuries to the vertebral artery, which runs within the spine, can result in thromboembolic ischemia or infarction to the brain stem, cerebellum, or visual cortex, producing alterations of consciousness and cranial nerve palsies. On rare occasions, the injury may affect the vertebral artery near where it enters the CSF at the foramen magnum. The artery wall is much thinner at this site, and a subarachnoid hemorrhage may be detectable in the CSF during lumbar puncture or on early CT scans. Intracranial vertebral artery

dissections are associated with very high morbidity and rebleed rates.[12, 19, 38]

COMMON CERVICAL INJURIES AND CONDITIONS

Cervical spine injuries can present a diagnostic dilemma. The practitioner must be able to determine if a patient's symptoms are localized to the brachial plexus versus the nerve root versus a cord injury. Proper recognition is necessary to render appropriate treatment and make recommendations about future activity restrictions and return to play.

Soft Tissue

Sprains are the result of tears within the ligamentous and capsular infrastructure of the spinal column, while strains represent tears within the paraspinal musculature. Both conditions are characterized by the presence of nonradiating pain along the midline and paraspinal region of the affected segments. Focal tenderness and swelling are present in the injured area, as well as a limited range of motion with or without muscle spasm. The distinguishing feature of an

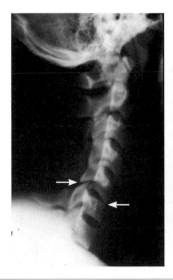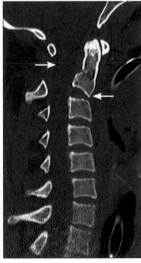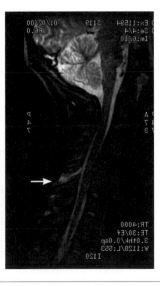

Figure 16.5 Cervical ligamentous injury. Neuroimaging with plain X-rays, CT, and MRI: Note the spine angulation at C5-6 on plain films and at C1-2 on CT scan, which makes the diagnosis of ligamentous injury evident by distortion of the normal spine alignment and curvature. Note the widened space between the spinous processes posteriorly (small arrows) and the angulation and mild subluxation of the vertebral bodies anteriorly (larger arrows). The MRI, however, can frequently demonstrate edema of the interspinous ligaments (white region with arrow) torn during the injury (arrow), making this test highly useful in athletes with severe neck strains and normal plain films.

isolated strain or sprain from spinal cord and nerve root injury is the absence of neurologic symptoms (motor–sensory deficits or radicular pain). The injured muscle groups may appear weak on examination because of pain on motion, but not in a fashion consistent with spinal cord or nerve root injury. Plain films are normal in cases of isolated sprains and strains; however, CT and MRI scans will reveal evidence of swelling and hemorrhage with more severe tears (figure 16.5).

Ligamentous injuries that threaten the stability of the anterior-to-posterior spine axis represent a serious risk to the nervous system, and can occur without any osseous injury. In the absence of neurologic complaints, the clinical presentation may be indistinguishable from a severe cervical sprain or strain. Individuals with this type of injury are at continued risk for nervous system injury until the area has been stabilized. Therefore, in either of these diagnoses, immobilization of the spinal column in neutral alignment must be maintained until neuroimaging has been performed.

Plain films and CT scans may demonstrate spinal instability (subluxation or angulation) between consecutive vertebrae. Magnetic resonance imaging of the affected spinal regions may show the edema and bleeding associated with the ligamentous disruption.[7] Some athletes have normal-appearing plain films of the spine during initial evaluation because of compensation from spasmodic spinal musculature. Once the muscle spasms have resolved, the instability becomes demonstrable on flexion–extension films. The syndrome of spinal cord injury without radiographic abnormality (SCIWORA) represents a spinal cord injury seen primarily in children less than 8 years of age, unassociated with fracture or dislocation.[4, 6, 20] "Pseudo"-subluxation or displacement of one vertebra on another, which may be up to 4 mm, is a common finding and normal variation seen on pediatric cervical imaging studies. The mechanism of neural injury in SCIWORA is presumed to be related to the inherent elasticity of the juvenile spine, which permits significant self-reducing displacement between adjacent vertebrae when subjected to flexion, extension, and distraction forces. The spinal cord is therefore vulnerable to injury even though the vertebral column is spared from disruption, and the cervical spine is the most commonly affected region.

In younger athletes, a fracture through the cartilaginous end plates (which is not seen well by X-rays) or unrecognized interspinous ligamentous injury may be among the causes of this injury. Hyperextension to the cervical spine whose vertebral canal diameter is already compromised by excessive buckling of the ligamentum flavum or osteophytes is a likely cause in older athletes. The resultant neurologic injury pattern most often resembles a central cord syndrome, with motor loss in arms greater than in the legs, and variable sensory loss. A Chiari malformation must also be considered in these patients.

Disc

Disc herniations ("ruptures") can occur in the setting of concomitant ligamentous injury or fractures, but most are independent entities. Disc herniations are associated with neck pain usually worse on the side of the disruption. Because most herniations occur posterolaterally toward the neuroforamen, clinical signs of unilateral nerve root compression are often evident, producing pain that radiates into the ipsilateral shoulder, arm, hand, or fingers, with associated weakness and sensory loss in specific patterns[1] (table 16.2). Symptoms are often worsened with neck extension. Spurling's test is a specific but insensitive maneuver whereby the examiner applies downward pressure while laterally bending the head toward the symptomatic side. A positive (Spurling's) sign is characterized by reproduction of the patient's radicular pain.[27, 29, 30] A more midline herniation can cause spinal cord compression, with resultant neurologic syndromes (figure 16.3). Magnetic resonance imaging is the most effective imaging study for the analysis of disc disease, and will confirm the level of the disc herniation and any nerve root or spinal cord compression or injury (figure 16.6).

Disc degeneration (spondylosis) represents degenerative changes of the disc that may affect spinal mobility and the size of the spinal canal (i.e., disc dessication, disc bulge, ligamentum flavum hypertrophy, facet joint hypertrophy). Spondylosis occurs with increased frequency in athletes due to the "wear and tear" that the spine experiences with training and competition. Patients may present with symptoms similar to those with disc herniation (either nerve root or spinal cord injury patterns) or with more chronic arthritic-like problems. Secondary responses to the disc degeneration include osteophyte formation above and below the affected disc space, or similar "bone spur" formation and enlargement of the facet joints. With collapse of the disc height and enlarging osteophytes both ventrally and dorsolaterally, the ligamentum flavum may clump into intervening spaces and further narrow the spinal canal or foramen.

"Spear tackler's spine" refers to an accentuated form of cervical spondylosis, with multilevel disc degeneration and ligamentous laxity as a consequence of repeated axial loading on a forwardly accelerating cervical spine. The entity is more prevalent in those who lead with their heads to make blocks and tackles during collision sports. Preexisting cervical stenosis, bony fractures, or loss of cervical lordosis may predispose to this injury. The injury results in multiple collapsed

degenerative discs and minor vertebral body compression and osteophyte formation. Any symptomatic athlete with these findings is at greater risk of catastrophic nervous system injury with return to play.[3, 35]

Bone

Cervical spine fractures are invariably associated with a significant amount of pain and soft tissue swelling. Physical examination is characterized by a limited range of motion, muscle rigidity with or without spasm, and adjacent soft tissue edema and hemorrhage. Neurologic deficits may be present secondary to neural compromise from bone or disc fragments and/or hemorrhage into adjacent ligamentous structures or the spinal cord itself (figure 16.7).

Fractures may affect the spinous process ("clay shoveler's fracture"), facets, or vertebral bodies.

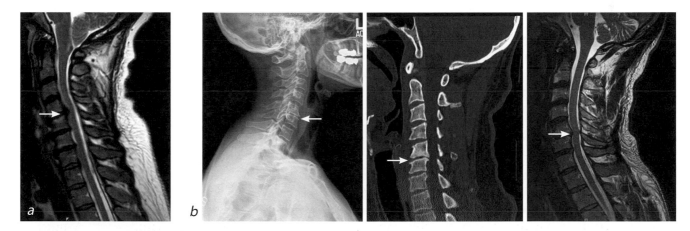

Figure 16.6 Cervical disc disease. (a) Herniation: MRI. Note central herniated disc C4-5 (arrow) producing spinal cord distortion. (b) Degeneration: neuroimaging with plain X-rays, CT, and MRI. Note collapsed disc space and secondary anterior osteophyte formation (arrows) at the site of degenerated C5-6 disc, often producing chronic neck and unilateral arm pain similar to that produced by a herniated disc.

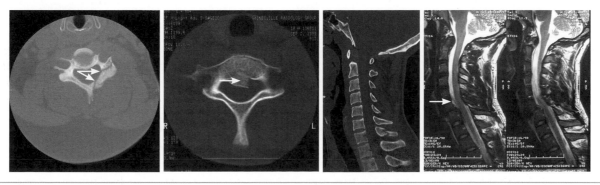

Figure 16.7 Types of cervical fractures associated with athletic injuries (arrows).

Spinal stability is dependent on the combination of the front (anterior longitudinal ligament, anterior vertebral body and disc), middle (posterior vertebral body, posterior longitudinal ligament, and facet joints), and posterior (spinous process, interspinous ligament) elements. Each injury must be carefully assayed by high-quality imaging and neurologic and physical examinations before return-to-play judgments are made. Patients with deficits or persistent spine pain must not return to play until stability is ensured and any deficit resolved. In general, any structural injury to the spinal cord, even if resolved clinically, is a serious obstacle to safe return to athletics.

Congenital narrowing of the spinal canal (figure 16.8) is a condition that exists at birth, in which a limitation of space harboring the spinal cord places the affected athlete at potentially increased risk of spinal cord injury, especially during participation in collision sports. With congenital cervical stenosis, plain radiographs demonstrate shortened pedicles and a constricted funnel-shaped spinal canal from bony compromise over many segments. Young patients with

this condition do not exhibit the degenerative changes (e.g., spondylosis, subluxation) commonly seen in older populations.

Two other types of cervical stenosis have been recognized. Bony thickening and ligamentous hypertrophy that develops diffusely over many segments and worsens with time is called developmental stenosis. Athletes involved in strength-related sports and heavy physical activity are particularly prone to this condition. Acquired cervical stenosis is caused by spondylosis, osteophytes, disc bulges and herniations, ligamentous hypertrophy, and other disease processes that contribute to focal or generalized canal narrowing.

Methods used to define cervical stenosis include sagittal canal diameter (plain X-rays), the Torg ratio (plain X-rays), and functional stenosis (MRI or myelography/CT scan). On lateral plain films, midsagittal spinal canal diameters above 15 mm are normal, and those below 13 mm are abnormal. Lateral radiographs measuring only sagittal canal diameter are subject to magnification errors, which led Torg to describe an alternative method for plain-film diagnosis, determined

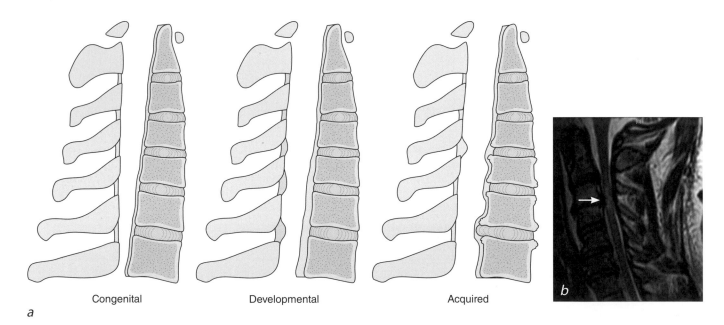

Congenital   Developmental   Acquired

a   *b*

Figure 16.8 Spinal canal stenosis. (a) Patterns: Congenital stenosis is present at birth and characterized by diffuse stenosis of the cervical spine forming a funnel-shaped canal. Developmental stenosis is due to diffuse hypertrophy of bony and ligamentous structures often found in athletes participating in collision sports. Acquired stenosis is focal (sometimes multifocal) narrowing due to ligamentous hypertrophy, spondylotic bars, or disc herniations. (b) Spinal cord injury: sagittal MRI with congenital and acquired stenosis. Note the complete loss of the CSF space around the spinal cord, representing functional stenosis with loss of functional reserve space. Also note the cord contusion (arrow) producing central cord syndrome.

by measuring the anteroposterior canal diameter and dividing this value by the vertebral body anterior–posterior diameter. Using this methodology, cervical spinal stenosis is defined as a Torg ratio less than 0.8; the reliability and significance of this ratio are variable and are of little importance since the advent of MRI.

The term "functional spinal stenosis" was coined to refer to the relationship of the cervical spinal cord to its intradural milieu (surrounding CSF), as defined by either MRI or myelography/CT scan findings. By definition, functional stenosis exists if the protective cushion of surrounding CSF around the cervical cord (the functional reserve) is obliterated.[3, 10, 35] This method is likely much more sensitive in predicting clinically significant cervical stenosis, and it represents the current standard for defining risks and management decisions regarding an athlete's ability to return to play.[7, 10, 33, 35] Cervical stenosis is present in up to 93% of cervical neurapraxia cases but has a low positive predictive value, which makes it an unsuitable means of screening at-risk players.[3, 7, 18, 33, 36]

Vascular

Carotid artery injury may result from direct compressive forces on the neck; hyperextension with extreme lateral rotation; or fractures, dislocations, or subluxations of the bony elements. The most common site of injury is several centimeters distal to the origin of the internal carotid artery as it nears the skull base. The injury causes a contusion to the vessel wall with resultant intramural hemorrhage, which may rupture into the arterial lumen. Stagnant blood within the "false" arterial lumen can embolize distally and cause a stroke or enlarge as a dissecting aneurysm[3, 13, 37] (figure 16.9).

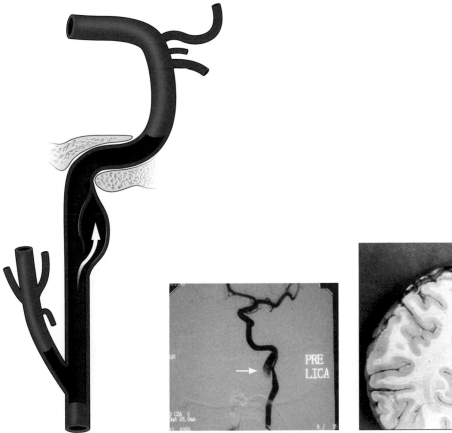
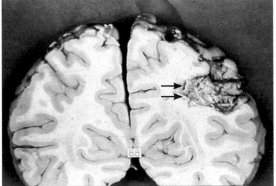

Figure 16.9 Vascular injuries associated with cervical trauma: Direct blow to the cervical carotid artery (or a cervical spine stretch or fracture) may injure the carotid or vertebral arteries, leading to a dissecting aneurysm (arrow) usually in the high cervical region. Clot within the false lumen of the vessel may embolize to the brain, causing infarction (double arrows)

The vertebral artery enters the cervical spine at C6 and runs through the foramen transversarium as it ascends to enter the skull at the foramen magnum. Its intraosseous course makes it susceptible to stretch or direct trauma associated with fractures, subluxations, and dislocations of the bony elements. As with carotid artery injuries, the most common level of injury is high in the neck, at the C1-2 vertebral level. Similarly, a dissection may embolize distally to cause brain stem, cerebellum, or visual cortex ischemia or infarction. A subarachnoid hemorrhage detectable on CT scanning may indicate an injury to the vessel after it has entered the dura, a situation associated with very high morbidity and rebleed rates.[12, 19, 38]

Brachial Plexus

This injury type is characterized by the acute onset of unilateral radicular pain that extends from the neck toward the distal upper extremity, following a direct blow to the plexus or a distraction of the cervical spine away from the shoulder. The pain, often burning, usually resolves within a few seconds or minutes, but weakness and sensory abnormalities may persist for days to weeks. The injury generally occurs at the level of the upper trunk of the brachial plexus, but cervical root compression syndromes may closely mimic its symptoms. As many as 50% of athletes participating in contact sports experience this type of injury.

Other Cervical Lesions

Chiari malformations are conditions in which, simply put, there is too much cerebellum to fit into the posterior fossa of the skull, resulting in displacement of that excess tissue through the foramen magnum at the skull base into the upper portion of the spinal canal. This "impaction" within the foramen creates a functional stenosis that may increase the likelihood of the athlete's experiencing spinal cord, medullary, and cranial nerve dysfunction after minimal trauma. About one-third of adult Chiari patients have syringo- or hydromyelia (a cyst of cerebrospinal fluid within the spinal cord), which can cause a central cord syndrome (figure 16.10).

Klippel-Feil syndrome is the congenital fusion of two or more cervical bony vertebrae. On physical exam, the patient may exhibit a low-lying posterior hairline, shortened neck, and limited neck motion. This condition poses an increased risk of spinal cord injury due to the increased cervical movement or basilar impression (or both) at either end of the defect. Some patients have an associated congenitally narrow neural foramen at the affected levels, which increases the likelihood of nerve root compression. Athletes with this condition may be more prone to developing myelopathy from spinal cord compression or radiculopathy from nerve root injury following sport-related trauma.[34]

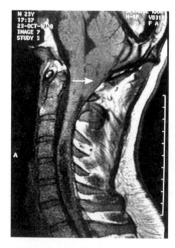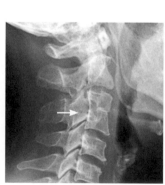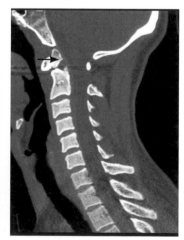

Figure 16.10 Other cervical lesions: Some conditions narrow the cervical spinal canal diameter or alter the biomechanics of normal cervical adaptation to stressful forces, which may heighten the athlete's risks of sustaining a spinal cord injury.

Os odontoideum is characterized by the presence of a nonfused but well-corticated bone ossicle at the level of the dens. This condition is usually evident in the absence of previously known trauma. Following an injury, athletes may complain of neck pain or demonstrate physical findings consistent with brain stem and spinal cord compression or injury.

COMMON THORACIC INJURIES

Athletic injuries to the thoracic spine are infrequent. Thoracic strains or sprains are more common and may occur when ligaments become torn or damaged. The seriousness of the sprain depends on how badly the ligaments are torn. Symptoms of thoracic sprain may include muscle spasms, pain that radiates to different zones of the body, stiffness, headaches, digestive issues, rib pain, and limited range of motion. Thoracic involvement of the disc and bone is of greater concern given the limited space in the spinal canal and the greater risk for neurologic deficit.

Disc

Thoracic disc herniations are very uncommon. Approximately one-fourth are traumatic, and three-fourths arise at the level of T8 or lower. [32] Few are related to athletic activities, as the chest wall provides strong support that reduces the transmission of forces on the intervertebral discs. When these herniations are present, there is often midscapular or lower spine region discomfort, associated with a band-like discomfort radiating in a dermatomal distribution paralleling the ribs toward the anterior chest wall. On occasion, the pain may be mistaken for underlying cardiac pathology. Since the thoracic spinal canal is small, there is a higher incidence of associated myelopathy compared to herniations at other levels.

Bone

Unlike the situation with the cervical spine, the thoracic spine's stability does not depend heavily on the facet joint. The ribs provide additional structural support at joints formed between the rib heads and the transverse processes and vertebral bodies. Thoracic fractures, however rare, should prompt attention to the surrounding viscera. If the ribs have been broken, local bruising, tenderness to palpation, or a flail chest may be evident signs. Rib fractures have a high association with pneumo- and hemothoraces, as well as pulmonary and cardiac contusions, which greatly complicate patient safety and management.

COMMON LUMBAR INJURIES

Lumbar spine injuries differ from those in the cervical or thoracic region in that the brain stem, spinal cord, and vascular supply to the brain are not at risk. Risks and extent of neurologic injury are generally milder. Injuries can involve soft tissues, bone, intervertebral discs, neural elements such as nerve roots, or some combination of these. Each type of injury has unique mechanisms of injury as well as signs and symptoms. Here we review the various lumbar spine injuries (table 16.7).

Table 16.7 **Lumbar Region Injuries: Predisposing Activities**

Athlete at risk	Predisposing activity	Type of spinal lesion
Contact sports	Field trauma	Transverse process, facet fracture, vertebral compression fracture
Weightlifting	Squats Poor technique	Vertebral compression fractures, disc degeneration, herniation, end plate fracture, spondylosis, spondylolysis, spondylolisthesis
Gymnastics	Repetitive axial loading	Disc degeneration
Football lineman	In hyperextension	Intraosseous disc herniation, spondylolysis, spondylolisthesis
Golf	Repetitive axial loading	Disc degeneration, herniation, spondylosis

Soft Tissue

Sprains and strains are common entities of the lumbar spine region and often reflect inadequate stretching, improper training techniques, or both. The hallmark symptom is paraspinal tenderness and pain that may radiate from the lower back to the side of the hip and thigh secondary to spasms of the lumbodorsal fascia and tensor fascia latae. The pain is unassociated with radiculopathy during positional changes such as standing, sitting, bending, or twisting.

Contusions (or bruises) are usually the result of direct trauma, such as a knee or helmet striking the lumbar area during American football, during which blood extravasates into subcutaneous structures or muscles. Focal low back pain and tenderness, confirmed later by discoloration over the painful area, confirms the diagnosis. Extensive bruising may indicate deeper injuries to a transverse process, the kidneys, ureter, or more than one of these.

No neurologic abnormalities accompany either of these injury types, as the nerve roots are well protected by the thick lumbar paraspinous musculature. Any positive neurologic finding should prompt a search for an intraspinal cause. Radiographic studies are generally normal, apart from showing straightening of the lumbar spine from spasm or the other chronic osseous abnormalities from longstanding athletic endeavors.

Disc

Lumbar disc herniations are classically associated with lower back pain and unilateral radiculopathy (sciatica) with or without neurologic deficits distally in the affected lower extremity; they are much more common with increased age. In the younger athlete, persistent back pain may be the only complaint. In the adolescent and teenage years, the disc material is more viscous and the ligamentous infrastructure is more robust, greatly reducing the incidence of free fragment herniations. In the latter age groups, the presentation is often limited to persistent back pain, muscle spasms, and hamstring tightness without "clear-cut" nerve root signs. On physical exam, the only finding may be mild scoliosis from unilateral paraspinous muscle spasm (figure 16.11).

The frequency of lumbar disc herniations is much higher in athletes who undergo repetitive axial loading, flexion, and rotation of the lumbar spine, as do competitive weightlifters and American football players. Most improve or resolve rapidly with conservative management, but for refractory cases, MRI is highly effective in delineating the anatomical relationships and integrity of the lumbar discs and nerve roots. Computed tomography or MRI studies have also shown a higher incidence of superior end plate fractures and Schmorl's nodes in this population.

Lumbar spondylosis, similar to cervical spondylosis, occurs secondary to degeneration of the lumbar spinal axis (disc dessication, osteophyte formation, ligamentum flavum clumping, and facet joint hypertrophy). Athletes are at increased risk of experiencing accelerated degenerative changes in this region because of the frequent and repetitive stresses associated with training and competition. The disc degeneration and dessication may cause low back pain, while any focal narrowing of the canal or foraminal diameter may cause radiculopathy. Symptoms usually begin with an episode of lower back pain, associated with unilateral or midline paraspinous pain and spasm that refers to one or both hips or thighs. When the condition is severe, the canal or neural foramen may narrow and become stenotic either centrally or laterally.

Plain X-rays demonstrate multiple asymmetrically collapsed discs, Schmorl's nodes, and osteophytes extending from the disc margins. An MRI scan often shows accelerated degenerative changes and loss of water content at multiple disc spaces. The discs appear to bulge but do not compromise the spinal canal and neural foramen (lumbar stenosis) until the facets have substantially hypertrophied. Computed tomography scanning can distinguish facet fractures with hemorrhage not apparent on plain films that can clinically mimic a ruptured disc. Advanced cases ultimately lead to the classic degenerative changes of lumbar stenosis, including disc desiccation and collapse, osteophyte formation along the disc spaces, multiple-level facet hypertrophy, and narrowing of the spinal canal.

Bone

Pars defects (spondylolysis with or without spondylolisthesis) reflect a disruption of bone (spondylolysis) at the level of the pars interarticularis of the lumbar spine. This condition

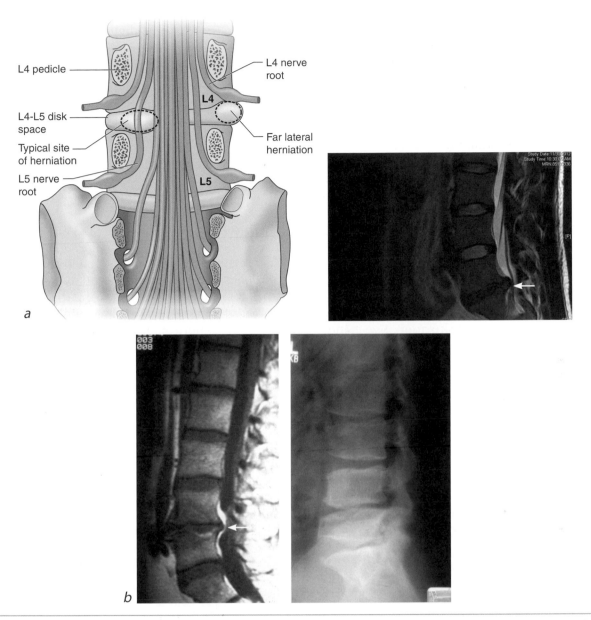

Figure 16.11 Lumbar disc disease. (a) Herniation. Schematic demonstrates lateral and far-lateral locations, which produce somewhat different clinical findings. A typical L4-5 disc rupture compresses the L5 root before its exit from the spinal canal, while a far lateral disc herniation at the same level compresses the L4 nerve root after it has exited the neural foramen. On MRI scan, note the large herniated disc at L5-S1 (arrow) in a collegiate athlete with acute onset of unrelenting low back and radicular pain associated with weightlifting (squats). (b) Degenerative: Note focal osteophyte and disc collapse (arrow, left image) in offensive lineman with low back pain and paraspinous spasm, likely in response to repetitive weightlifting and hyperextension associated with techniques required by this position. Note accelerated lumbar spondylosis (right image) in 30-year-old former gymnast. Multilevel disc collapse and vertebral body compression are evident.

occurs most commonly at L5-S1, followed by L4-5 level (figure 16.12). This disorder is associated with repetitive hyperextension forces in the lumbar region, and the highest incidence is noted in young gymnasts, ages 9 to 15 (11%), and American football players (15%), particularly linemen. Affected athletes may complain of lower back pain that worsens with extension. Lumbar muscle spasm and hamstring tightness are typical physical findings. Radiculopathy is usually absent, although there is often some discomfort in the lateral thigh due to associated tightening of the tensor fascia latae. The athlete may compensate for the pain by adopting a shortened stride in which the hips and knees are hyperflexed during ambulation (table 16.8).

Pars disruption (spondylolysis) can be preceded by a stress fracture; during this period the bone is still intact but weakened and inflamed. In suspected cases, plain films may be negative or ambiguous. Early MRI or single-photon emission computed tomography (SPECT) scanning may demonstrate a stress fracture before frank spondylolysis occurs. Both of the these studies may demonstrate a metabolically "active" pars defect with or without evidence of spondylolysis. If detected early, active lesions, especially those without sclerotic edges, have a better healing capacity with conservative therapy.

Once spondylolysis occurs, the athlete is susceptible to progressive subluxation of the affected vertebral interspace (spondylolisthesis). Depending on severity of the subluxation, five grades of spondylolisthesis have been classified as outlined in table 16.8. Since the affected lumbar area has no adjacent spinal cord nearby, continuance of play is rarely limited by neurologic risks or consequences.

Table 16.8   Spondylolisthesis Grading

Grade	Subluxation percentage
I	<25%
II	25-50%
III	50-75%
IV	75-99%
V	100%

Other Fractures

Even though the lumbar vertebrae are much stronger and are built for structural support of the spinal axis, elite athletes are at an increased risk for fractures both during training and competition. American football players and rugby players are at the greatest risk during tackling or blocking maneuvers. The mechanism of injury reflects axial loading and flexion forces applied to the lower back, producing varying degrees of compression fractures. Similarly, freestyle wres-

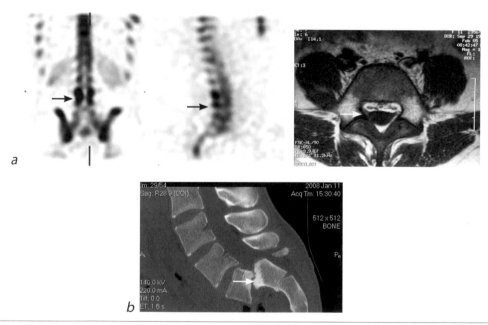

Figure 16.12   Lumbar spondylolysis and spondylolisthesis. (a) Stress fracture of pars interarticularis (spondylolysis): single-photon emission computed tomography scan (left image) in 20-year-old athlete with recent onset of lower back pain and paraspinous discomfort and tightness. Note "hot spots" at L5 vertebra in the region of the pars interarticularis (arrow). MRI (right image) shows bone edema (arrow) in response to repetitive stress. (b) Spondylolysis with spondylolisthesis: In another case, lysis of the pars interarticularis led to subluxation (arrow) of L5 on S1 (grade 3 spondylolisthesis). Athlete was asymptomatic when not training.

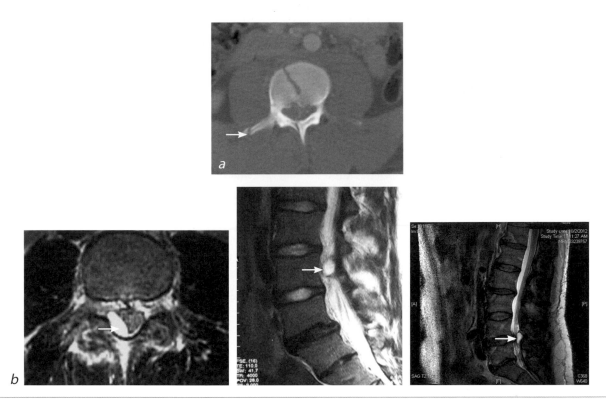

Figure 16.13 Lumbar fractures, facet injuries. (a) Transverse process fracture: upper lumbar CT scan in a 19-year-old wide receiver who complained of upper lumbar pain and tenderness after being struck in the flank by a defender's helmet. Plain X-rays demonstrated transverse process fracture. Later urinalysis revealed microscopic hematuria. (b) Repeated or forceful hyperextension related to athletics can lead to small fractures and hemorrhage from the facet joint (left, center images, arrows), best seen on MRI scan. This lesion resolved over several weeks and did not require intervention. Chronic degenerative changes in the facet joint and discs may lead to a synovial cyst (right image), which can produce unrelenting radicular symptoms.

tlers are at a heightened risk due to low-lying and hyperflexed postures assumed during competition, as well as the increased kyphotic curvature of the thoracic spine observed in this group.[10, 15, 22, 28] Winter sports such as skiing, snowboarding, and sledging are also associated with lumbar compression fractures secondary to those forces applied to the lower spine during landings.

Spinous process fractures are exceedingly rare in the lumbar spine. As with thoracic fractures, transverse process fractures are associated with a risk of adjacent visceral injury, particularly to the kidneys and ureters. Affected patients may complain of flank pain and have hematuria during initial assessment.[14, 21] Lumbar facet injuries primarily occur in athletes performing repeated forceful hyperextension motions, such as football linemen, gymnasts, wrestlers, and golfers.[2] The clinical findings of facet fractures are more often unilateral; these include ipsilateral paralumbar

tenderness and hip and buttock pain referred to the groin, hip, and posterior thigh. The pain is exacerbated by hyperextension and the neurologic examination is usually normal, although a transverse process or facet fracture may uncommonly contuse an adjacent exiting nerve root.

Mild compression fractures of the vertebral body are common, particularly in individuals who have been doing heavy weightlifting training for many years. The anterior portion of the vertebral body lacks horizontal trabeculations, and exercises such as squats or military presses can generate significant flexion–compression forces that lead to repetitive end plate fractures, collapse of the disc space, and ultimately compression fractures of the vertebral bodies. When the end plate fails, the nucleus pulposis may herniate into the fracture, producing a Schmorl's node. Most compression fractures produce acute back pain very similar to that associated with contusions or sprains. Paraspinous muscle spasm is common, is usually bilateral, may extend into the buttocks, and may be restimulated by movement or palpation of the affected region.

CONCLUDING THOUGHTS

This chapter outlines the definitions and clinical features, together with examples, of sport-related spine injuries. It is imperative that the health care team be competent in the recognition of those at risk of injury to the neuroaxis, as well as having a fundamental understanding of the pertinent anatomy and mechanisms of injury. The chapter that follows extends the reader's understanding of both on- and off-the-field management of these conditions, the rehabilitative and surgical options, and the rationale for return-to-play decision making.

REFERENCES

1. Clinical assessment after acute cervical spinal cord injury. Neurosurgery 2002;50(3 Suppl):S21-29.

2. Management of acute central cervical spinal cord injuries. Neurosurgery 2002;50(3 Suppl):S166-172.

3. Bailes JE, Petschauer M, Guskiewicz KM, Marano G. Management of cervical spine injuries in athletes. J Athl Train 2007;42(1):126-134.

4. Bondurant CP, Oro JJ. Spinal cord injury without radiographic abnormality and Chiari malformation. J Neurosurg 1993;79(6):833-838.

5. Boran S, Lenehan B, Street J, McCormack D, Poynton A. A 10-year review of sports-related spinal injuries. Ir J Med Sci 2011;180(4):859-863.

6. Callaway GH, O'Brien SJ, Tehrany AM. Chiari I malformation and spinal cord injury: cause for concern in contact athletes? Med Sci Sports Exerc 1996;28(10):1218-1220.

7. Cantu RC. Cervical spine injuries in the athlete. Semin Neurol 2000;20(2):173-178.

8. Como JJ, Diaz JJ, Dunham CM, Chiu WC, Duane TM, Capella JM, et al. Practice management guidelines for identification of cervical spine injuries following trauma: update from the Eastern Association for the Surgery of Trauma Practice Management Guidelines Committee. J Trauma 2009;67(3):651-659.

9. D'Alise MD, Benzel EC, Hart BL. Magnetic resonance imaging evaluation of the cervical spine in the comatose or obtunded trauma patient. J Neurosurg 1999;91(1 Suppl):54-59.

10. Dunn IF, Proctor MR, Day AL. Lumbar spine injuries in athletes. Neurosurg Focus 2006;21(4):E4.

11. Epstein N, Epstein JA, Benjamin V, Ransohoff J. Traumatic myelopathy in patients with cervical spinal stenosis without fracture or dislocation: methods of diagnosis, management, and prognosis. Spine 1980;5(6):489-496.

12. Halbach VV, Higashida RT, Dowd CF, Fraser KW, Smith TP, Teitelbaum GP, et al. Endovascular treatment of vertebral artery dissections and pseudoaneurysms. J Neurosurg 1993;79(2):183-191.

13. Hart RG, Easton JD. Dissections of cervical and cerebral arteries. Neurol Clin 1983;1(1):155-182.

14. Kelly M, Robinson CM. Fractures of the thoracolumbar vertebrae from sledging: a recurrent British winter problem. Injury 2003;34(12):940-941.

15. Mall NA, Buchowski J, Zebala L, Wright RW, Matava MJ. Spine and axial skeleton injuries in the National Football League. Am J Sports Med 2012;40(8):1755-1761.

16. Massaro F, Lanotte M, Faccani G. Acute traumatic central cord syndrome. Acta Neurologica 1993;15(2):97-105.

17. Merriam WF, Taylor TK, Ruff SJ, McPhail MJ. A reappraisal of acute traumatic central cord syndrome. J Bone Joint Surg Br 1986;68(5):708-713.

18. Meyer SA, Schulte KR, Callaghan JJ, Albright JP, Powell JW, Crowley ET, et al. Cervical spinal stenosis and stingers in collegiate football players. Am J Sports Med 1994;22(2):158-166.

19. Okuchi K, Watabe Y, Hiramatsu K, Tada T, Sakaki T, Kyoi K, et al. Dissecting aneurysm of the vertebral artery as a cause of Wallenberg's syndrome. No Shinkei Geka 1990;18(8):721-727.

20. Pang D, Pollack IF. Spinal cord injury without radiographic abnormality in children--the SCIWORA syndrome. J Trauma 1989;29(5):654-664.

21. Rachbauer F, Sterzinger W, Eibl G. Radiographic abnormalities in the thoracolumbar spine of young elite skiers. Am J Sports Med 2001;29(4):446-449.

22. Rajabi R, Doherty P, Goodarzi M, Hemayattalab R. Comparison of thoracic kyphosis in two groups of elite Greco-Roman and freestyle wrestlers and a group of non-athletic participants. Br J Sports Med 2008;42(3):229-232; discussion 232.

23. Roth EJ, Park T, Pang T, Yarkony GM, Lee MY. Traumatic cervical Brown-Sequard and Brown-Sequard-plus syndromes: the spectrum of presentations and outcomes. Paraplegia 1991;29(9):582-589.

24. Rumana CS, Baskin DS. Brown-Sequard syndrome produced by cervical disc herniation: case report and literature review. Surg Neurol 1996;45(4):359-361.

25. Schneider RC. The syndrome of acute anterior spinal cord injury. J Neurosurg 1955;12(2):95-122.

26. Schneider RC, Cherry G, Pantek H. The syndrome of acute central cervical spinal cord injury; with special reference to the mechanisms involved in hyperextension injuries of cervical spine. J Neurosurg 1954;11(6):546-577.

27. Scoville WB, Whitcomb BB. Lateral rupture of cervical intervertebral disks. Postgrad Med 1966;39(2):174-180.

28. Shelly MJ, Butler JS, Timlin M, Walsh MG, Poynton AR, O'Byrne JM. Spinal injuries in Irish rugby: a ten-year review. J Bone Joint Surg Br 2006;88(6):771-775.

29. Spurling RG, Scoville WB. Lateral Rupture of the Cervical Intervertebral Discs: A Common Cause if Shoulder and Arm Pain. Surg Gynecol Obstet 1944;78:350-358.

30. Spurling RG, Segerberg LH. Lateral intervertebral disk lesions in the lower cervical region. JAMA 1953;151(5):354-359.

31. Stiell IG, Clement CM, McKnight RD, Brison R, Schull MJ, Rowe BH, et al. The Canadian C-spine rule versus the NEXUS low-risk criteria in patients with trauma. New Engl J Med 2003;349(26):2510-2518.

32. Stillerman CB, Chen TC, Couldwell WT, Zhang W, Weiss MH. Experience in the surgical management of 82 symptomatic herniated thoracic discs and review of the literature. J Neurosurg 1998;88(4):623-633.

33. Torg JS, Naranja RJ Jr, Pavlov H, Galinat BJ, Warren R, Stine RA. The relationship of developmental narrowing of the cervical spinal canal to reversible and irreversible injury of the cervical spinal cord in football players. J Bone Joint Surg Am 1996;78(9):1308-1314.

34. Torg JS, Ramsey-Emrhein JA. Management guidelines for participation in collision activities with congenital, developmental, or post-injury lesions involving the cervical spine. Clin Sports Med 1997;16(3):501-530.

35. Torg JS, Sennett B, Pavlov H, Leventhal MR, Glasgow SG. Spear tackler's spine. An entity precluding participation in tackle football and collision activities that expose the cervical spine to axial energy inputs. Am J Sports Med 1993;21(5):640-649.

36. Vaccaro AR, Klein GR, Ciccoti M, Pfaff WL, Moulton MJ, Hilibrand AJ, et al. Return to play criteria for the athlete with cervical spine injuries resulting in stinger and transient quadriplegia/paresis. Spine J 2002;2(5):351-356.

37. Welling RE, Taha A, Goel T, Cranley J, Krause R, Hafner C, et al. Extracranial carotid artery aneurysms. Surgery 1983;93(2):319-323.

38. Zhao WY, Krings T, Alvarez H, Ozanne A, Holmin S, Lasjaunias P. Management of spontaneous haemorrhagic intracranial vertebrobasilar dissection: review of 21 consecutive cases. Acta Neurochir 2007;149(6):585-596; discussion 596.

Management of Spine Injuries, Including Rehabilitation, Surgical Considerations, and Return to Play

In collaboration with

Wesley H. Jones, MD • Saint Aaron-Morris, MD

The osseous spinal column, the spinal cord including the nerve roots, and the supporting soft tissue musculature and ligaments function as a unit enabling the athlete to execute complex, precise movements during athletic competition. A deficiency or imbalance of one entity can acutely hinder the athlete's abilities or cause overcompensation leading to decline in performance or risk of more serious injury. Thus, postinjury medical management and rehabilitation, including surgical treatment when necessary, must be very well understood by affected athletes and their physicians, trainers, and therapists.

Treatment and rehabilitation of the injured athlete begin as soon as the injury is recognized. An ideal treatment, whether surgical or nonsurgical, should first focus on preservation and protection of the nervous system for the remainder of the individual's life, regardless of return to competition. Once the overall safety of the athlete can be assured, treatment should focus on restoring her to an asymptomatic preinjury level of function. Finally, before an athlete is reexposed to possible recurrent injury, any preexisting underlying mechanical or structural deficiencies should be corrected.

After a spine injury, many factors must be considered before the athlete can return to play. As the level of competition increases from amateur to professional, the pressure imposed by financial and social incentives is increasingly significant. No matter how compelling other reasons might seem, the safety and neurologic health of an athlete cannot be jeopardized. The aim of this chapter is to provide guidelines for the acute management, therapy and rehabilitation goals, and surgical considerations that maximize the likelihood of a safe return to play for the affected athlete.

ON-THE-FIELD ASSESSMENT

Standard trauma protocols that address airway, breathing, and circulation should be instituted when any athlete suspected of having sustained a spine injury is first approached. The primary (initial) assessment recognizes any emergent life-threatening injuries, with immediate activation of the emergency medical system. After the primary survey is completed and actual or impending cardiopulmonary compromise is eliminated, the remaining possible scenarios facing the treating personnel depend on the presence or absence of altered mental status[5] (figure 17.1).

A player presenting with altered mental status should be evaluated with a brief neurologic exam that also includes the ability to move all extremities and any point tenderness along the neural axis. Any patient with normal mental status should undergo a neurologic spinal cord injury (SCI) assessment. An athlete with a normal neurologic exam and history but with persistent pain, point tenderness, or decreased range of motion of the spine is assumed to have occult SCI or spinal instability. All of these circumstances require removing the athlete from competition for further evaluation.

It is essential that all treating personnel recognize, react to, properly stabilize, and transport any suspected spine or SCI. The Inter-Association Task Force for Appropriate Care of the Spine–Injured Athlete and the National Athletic Trainers' Association[66] have published guides directing initial management of the head- or neck-injured

athlete[25, 55, 66] (figure 17.2). Preparation includes ensuring that all proper equipment is available and functioning, such as a spine board and cervical collar. Treating personnel should be certified and be able to execute all necessary emergency medical services. Rehearsing in order to be able to flawlessly execute an organized, efficient plan will clearly define the role of each member of the medical team. Availability of ambulance transport to a tertiary care center is also essential.

It is paramount to achieve and maintain spine stabilization as soon as possible after the injury. In contact sports such as American football, stabilization may be complicated by the presence of protective equipment; unnecessary movement during removal may potentially manipulate an unstable spine. Today, most face masks have universal removal capabilities that allow access to the airway and proper immobilization without removal of the helmet or shoulder pads. As outlined in the following list,[66] a helmet should not be removed unless it interferes with appropriate

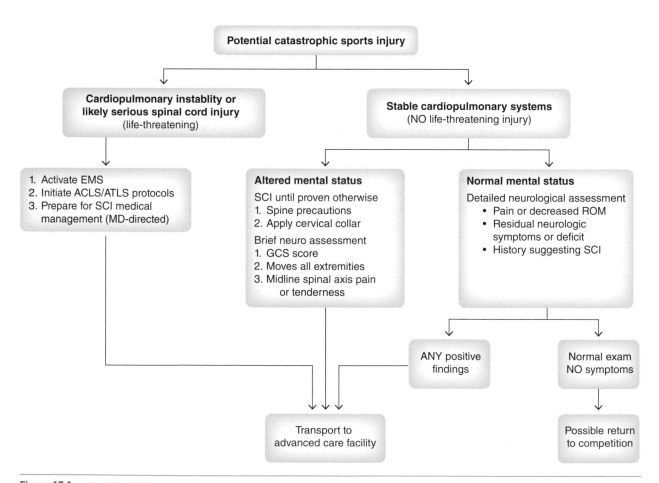

Figure 17.1 On-the-field triage.

Checklist: Preparation for and Management of Acute Cervical Spine Injuries

Component	Recommendations to be known and practiced by all appropriate personnel
1. Prevention	• Understand the sport-specific causes, underlying mechanisms, and basic acute physiological and clinical responses manifested in SCI • Be familiar with the safety rules implemented and appropriate use and maintenance of protective equipment • Educate coaches, athletes, and other medical personnel on proper technique and avoidance of dangerous maneuvers (e.g., spear tackling)
2. Planning	• Proper certification (basic life support (BLS), advanced cardiovascular life support (ACLS), pediatric advanced life support (PALS), advanced trauma life support (ATLS), and so on) • Coordination with EMS and medical doctors for availability and hospital transport • Rehearsal of required action in the event of catastrophic injury

3. Assessment	• One or more of the following heightens suspicion of SCI and initiates acute SCI protocol:
	  • Unconsciousness or altered level of consciousness
	  • Bilateral neurological findings or complaints
	  • Spinal axis pain or tenderness
	  • Obvious spinal bony deformity

4. Stabilization	• Immediate manual immobilization without cervical traction
	• Realignment to a neutral spine position unless:
	  • Resistance encountered
	  • Airway compromised
	  • Movement causes or exacerbates an acute neurological deficit, pain, or muscle spasms

5. Airway	• Immediate airway access—face mask removal guidelines • Airway management—secured by certified personnel; minimize motion (jaw thrust, not chin tilt)

6. Transfer and immobilization	• Proper position, sequence for transfer
	  • Prone athletes log roll to supine
	  • Place external rigid orthosis (cervical collar)
	  • Six-man lift and slide technique to transfer to spine board

7. Equipment removal	• Do not remove equipment before arrival to hospital (see exceptions) • Have tools for removal readily available and be knowledgeable of appropriate removal technique • Team personnel (and tools) accompany athlete to hospital to ensure proper removal

Figure 17.2 Spinal cord injury preparation checklist.

immobilization and hinders necessary access to the airway for ventilation. If removal becomes necessary, spine stabilization must be maintained throughout the process (Inter-Association Task Force for Appropriate Care of the Spine–Injured Athlete,[55] National Athletic Trainers' Association[66]). With or without equipment, neck stabilization and immobilization are achieved by a rigid cervical collar and by placement of the patient on a spine backboard with sandbags or equivalent on both sides of head, secured with an immobilizing strap. Preliminary transfer movements should maintain proper alignment by using the "log-rolling" technique. After stabilization, further evaluation and treatment must be considered during emergency medical services transport as outlined in table 17.1.

Reasons for On-the-Field Helmet Removal

- Cardiopulmonary status is unstable.
- Airway cannot be established even with the face mask removed.
- Life-threatening hemorrhage under the helmet can be controlled only by removal.
- Helmet and strap do not hold head securely, so immobilizing the helmet does not adequately immobilize the spine.
- Helmet prevents immobilization for transportation in an appropriate position.

Adapted from the NATA Guidelines

RADIOLOGICAL ASSESSMENT

Once cardiopulmonary and spinal stability is ensured, imaging is needed in all patients suspected of having a spine injury. Each type of injury has its own individual mechanisms of development, signs and symptoms, radiographic features, treatment, and return-to-play decisions. For obvious reasons, the on-the-field and early radiographic assessment phases focus on the brain and cervical spine. Thoracic spine injuries,

stabilized by the rib cage, are rarely encountered during competition. Lumbar spine injuries differ from those in the cervical or thoracic region in that the brain stem, spinal cord, and cerebral vasculature are not at risk. The larger and stronger bones in this region significantly lower the risk of instability due to a fracture. A neurologic injury is substantially milder and, when present, usually limited to a single nerve root.

A cervical collar can be cleared clinically, and radiographic studies are not indicated in an asymptomatic athlete with no mental status changes, no neck pain or posterior midline tenderness, no focal neurologic deficit, normal ROM, and no gross spinal deformities.[24] The value and details of the various imaging modalities were discussed in the previous chapter. A thin-cut, noncontrast computed tomography (CT) scan from the occiput to T1 with sagittal and coronal reconstructions is the primary modality for initial imaging in cervical spine trauma. In cases in which CT scan is unavailable, X-rays of lateral, anteroposterior (AP), and open-mouth odontoid films can be substituted; however, up to 10% to 15% of cervical spine injuries can be missed.[28] The resultant clinical algorithm, based on CT findings and the absence or presence of neurologic or radiographic abnormalities, is outlined in figure 17.3.

While CT can show bony abnormalities, it is inferior to magnetic resonance imaging (MRI)

Table 17.1 Acute Medical Management of Suspected SCI (Physician Directed)

System	Details
Airway, oxygenation, and ventilation	• Airway—maintain access with jaw thrust, not chin tilt. • Oxygenation—monitor fraction of inspired oxygen (FiO_2) • Ventilation—monitor vital capacity (may be altered in upper cervical level injuries) Intubate as necessary if any of these is compromised
Spinal shock (circulation)	Goal systolic blood pressure (SBP) >90, mean arterial pressure (MAP) >85 • Volume—IV fluids • Hypotension—pressors (dopamine) • Bradycardia—atropine
Spine	Immobilize with rigid orthosis until cleared
Temperature	Euthermia (no proven benefit of hypothermia)
ASIA exam	Document initial neurological level (see detailed ASIA exam in previous chapter)
Methylprednisolone	Current evidence suggests more harmful than beneficial

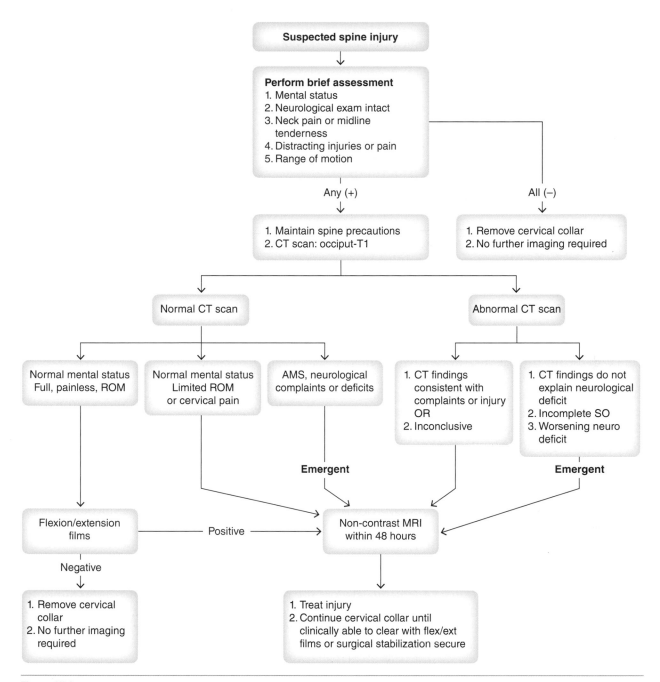

Figure 17.3 Radiographic assessment of spinal cord injury.

for evaluating nerve, soft tissue, and ligamentous injury. An emergent MRI is indicated in the setting of a neurologic deficit.[3, 4, 5] Injuries such as an acute herniated disc, intramedullary contusions or edema, ligamentous injury, epidural hemorrhage, and residual nerve or spinal cord compression are all more readily visualized on MRI (see figures in previous chapter).

TREATMENT AND REHABILITATION

Most spinal injuries occurring during athletics are benign and will resolve with conservative treatment, allowing the athlete to return to competition with no prolonged complications. With the exception of unstable spine fractures, cauda equina syndrome, and other rare emergencies that require immediate intervention, surgery is indicated only after failure of a trial of conservative measures.

As opposed to the situation with the general population, conservative management of an elite athlete with a spine injury poses a particular challenge. The athlete often has a competition or training schedule heavily influencing the timetable for which rehabilitation or recovery is expected. Coaches, organizations, and strong societal pressures may exert great influence on the decision making. Loss of time from competition can potentially have profound financial implications for the athlete or team.

Sports often require rigorous training and dedication to obtain elite physical condition to counteract the intense physical demands that place a great amount of stress on an athlete's body, predisposing him to injury.[74] The higher level of physical conditioning undoubtedly benefits athletes in their ability to rapidly progress and respond to a proper rehabilitation program. Conversely, a rather minor injury or symptoms in an elite athlete may manifest as significant dysfunction in performance compared to what is seen in the general population.

In addition to treating the primary injury, a comprehensive rehabilitation program aims to prevent further deconditioning while systematically correcting any biomechanical strength, flexibility, structural, or technique flaws or deficits. In order to advance, an athlete must demonstrate asymptomatic, biomechanically correct execution of all aspects of a particular phase before adding any degree of complexity. Both the treating clinicians and the injured athlete must embrace the principle that treatment and rehabilitation ultimately fail when primarily focused on the resolution of symptoms. Successful treatment allows the athlete to return to preinjury performance ability and corrects underlying mechanical flaws by implementing protective mechanisms that prevent recurrence or further injury.[16, 33, 44]

Initial Evaluation

The initial evaluation and assessment of an injured athlete provides an essential foundation for guiding all subsequent treatment. All evaluations should begin with a detailed subjective history from the athlete as well as any physicians, family members, trainers, and coaches who are

able to provide pertinent information about the athlete or injury. Inquiry may include such questions as these:

What was the timing of this injury?

What was the mechanism of the injury?

Has the athlete experienced these symptoms before and, if so, how were they managed and did the athlete fully recover?

Is the athlete experiencing pain, and if so how does she characterize it?

Adapted from the NATA Guidelines.

Coupled with a thorough history is a comprehensive physical examination aimed at isolating the underlying injury and objectively documenting its associated clinical signs or abnormalities. Pay particular attention to the athlete's gait, asymmetries, flexibility, and discomfort during testing. A detailed neurologic exam should also be performed, with particular attention given to accurately assessing, grading, and documenting sensation, reflexes, strength, muscle tone, and long track signs.[16, 33, 44, 49, 65]

Designing a Rehabilitation Program

No single ideal program exists for the rehabilitation of all athletes suffering a spine injury.[46, 74] The most effective treatment uses all philosophies in a multifaceted approach specifically tailored to the injury and the sport-specific functional goals of the individual athlete. A consistency among the various rehabilitation models is the division of the rehabilitative processes into different phases that the athlete will progress through while recovering from the injury[8, 33, 42, 74] (table 17.2).

The initial phase focuses on decreasing pain, controlling the inflammatory response, and promoting primary tissue healing.[8] Physical and palliative modalities such as ice, heat, and electrical stimulation are often used in combination with pharmacologic therapy to facilitate the healing process. Other possible modalities include spinal manipulation therapy, traction, ultrasound, cognitive behavioral therapy, acupuncture, and massage therapy. None have been validated with sufficient level I evidence to substantiate their use. In a review of nonpharmacologic modalities used in treating acute low back pain, the only physical treatment with good evidence of efficacy was superficial heat.[13]

Table 17.2　Common Methods of Conservative Therapy in Cervical and Lumbar Spine Injuries

Method	Description	
Physical and palliative	Rest	Bed rest for no longer than 48 h Immobilization for symptomatic muscle spasms (7-10 days) Removal from all sport-related activities
	Topical	Applied during acute injury phase No proven benefit of heat to increase circulation versus ice to decrease inflammation Avoid prolonged use (>10 min) or extreme temperatures
	Physical	Traction—no proven benefit, potentially harmful Spinal manipulations—evidence lacking, potentially harmful Massage—can be used as adjuvant therapy
Medications	Nonsteroidal anti-inflammatory drugs	Medication of choice in spine injuriesAnti-inflammatory and analgesic propertiesBenefit seen up to 7 to 10 days postinjury
	Steroids	Administered acutely to decrease inflammatory response, leading to decreased pain • Used systemically (oral or IV) to provide symptomatic relief • Local epidural injection—palliative, not therapeutic
	Narcotics	Opioids administered acutely to provide symptomatic relief Avoid long-term administration (>5 days)
	Muscle relaxants	Short-term symptomatic relief Example: benzodiazepines Placebo effect; most act as central nervous system relaxants

PHASES OF REHABILITATION

	Phase	Description
Physical therapy and rehabilitation	1. Acute	Initial healing phase to allow appropriate tissue recovery Activity modification, brief bed rest, or immobilization as necessary to facilitate recovery and prevent further tissue injury Pain control
	2. Subacute	Correct fundamental mechanical flaws Focus on flexibility and range of motion exercises Core strengthening and balance
	3. Integrative and maintenance	Sport-specific exercises using biomechanical technique from previous phases Institution of protective measures aimed at preventing injury recurrence
	4. Return to competition	Pain free No neurologic deficit Painless full range of motion Physician clearance Appropriate protective measures in place

Medications

Due to their dual anti-inflammatory effects and analgesic properties, nonsteroidal anti-inflammatory drugs (NSAIDs) are the preferred medication used to treat acute neck and back pain associated with spine injuries.[59] Opioids may be indicated in patients with severe pain but should be discontinued as soon as possible due to the possibility of tolerance and dependence. Muscle relaxants for the treatment of muscle spasms are commonly used and may provide short-term symptomatic relief.[14, 64] Corticosteroids, given either systemically or locally, can provide short-term relief in certain spine injuries. More recently, the use of localized epidural steroid injections has yielded conflicting reports regarding their long-term efficacy for treatment of low back pain. A recent small retrospective study, in NFL athletes suffering herniated lumbar discs, found that epidural steroid injections provided a safe and effective therapeutic option for lumbar disc herniation.[43] Any long-term use of analgesic or anti-inflammatory medication is potentially detrimental to the athlete. Persistent pain should warrant further investigation into the severity or cause of the athlete's injury and the potential need for surgical intervention, not serve as an indication for distributing more potent medications or prolonging their use.

Immobilization and Activity Modification

Initial immobilization of an athlete with a spine injury is essential in order to prevent severe SCI. If stability of the spine has been established, the use of a rigid orthotic collar is necessary only for providing comfort and alleviating mechanical stress placed on the injured spine and associated musculature during the acute phase. Once the acute pain (often due to muscle spasms) subsides (7-10 days), the patient can gradually begin increasing ROM and strengthening exercises. In the lumbar spine, bed rest for low back pain reduces pressure and movement on the spine and nerve roots that may have led to the symptoms. A supine position with the knees slightly flexed accomplishes this best.[52] However, in the majority of patients with low back pain, and almost never with cervical neck pain, bed rest is not indicated.

After 2 or 3 days, gradual increase in movement and activity should be encouraged. Prolonged bed rest has been shown to worsen symptoms and lengthen the time before return to normal activity.[19] Finally, activity modification with a graduated progression of exertion and ROM should be initiated at a rate dependent on the severity of the athlete's injury. The goal is to achieve a safe, tolerable level of discomfort through graduated activity in order to minimize stagnancy. Activities that stress the spine, such as heavy lifting, prolonged sitting or standing,

and excessive bending or twisting are avoided in the acute phase.

Correcting Posture

Immediate education and implementation of proper postural positioning can begin in the acute phase.[8, 27, 30, 48] Instructing an athlete about appropriate posture and ergonomics during normal activities of daily living (ADLs) will help install a posture-first (biomechanically sound) mind-set as he advances throughout the all the rehabilitative phases and incorporates sport-specific techniques.[74]

Failure of Initial Phase

The initial phase provides a strong indication that a patient may not respond to conservative therapy. Although somewhat arbitrary, 6 weeks is the most common time frame used to label an injury as "failed conservative treatment." An athlete who continues to have a significant amount of pain and dysfunction thereafter should begin considering an alternative treatment regimen or potential surgical intervention (table 17.3).

Subacute Phase

As the athlete's acute pain subsides, she can more actively participate and transition into a more dynamic phase of rehabilitation. The subacute phase of spinal rehabilitation focuses on maintaining aerobic capacity and correcting deficits with graduated stretching and strengthening exercises to improve spinal flexibility and stability, eventually incorporated into progressively performing sport-specific exercises. The subacute phase can be further divided into a restorative phase, intended to correct flexibility and strength deficits, and an integrative phase in which functional adaptations achieved are gradually incorporated into sport-specific movements.[42]

Maintenance of Physical Fitness

Athletes have often spent numerous hours conditioning and training the body in order to maximize performance. Thus, it is vital to minimize any loss of endurance and muscle strength while balancing the need to allow appropriate tissue healing and rehabilitation.[73] Cessation or reduction of a training regimen has been shown to lead to physiological and anatomical alterations in

Table 17.3   Contraindications for Return to Contact Sport—Cervical Spine (Neurologically Intact, Asymptomatic, Painless Full ROM)

None	Relative	Absolute
NONSURGICAL		
Klippel-Feil: isolated below C3, no instability Spina bifida occulta Asymptomatic congenital or acquired nonfocal stenosis Healed, nondisplaced minor fractures (e.g., clay shoveler's fracture, end plate or minimal compression)	Congenital or acquired stenosis with two or fewer episodes of spinal cord neuropraxia Minimally displaced, healed minor fractures Minor C1 or C2 fractures Minimal radiographic dynamic instability • <3.5 mm translation • <11 degrees angulation	Odontoid abnormalities • Agenesis • Hypoplasia • Os odontoidium C1-C2 anomaly or ligamentous instability Klippel-Feil (multilevel or high cervical) Radiographic dynamic instability • 3.5 mm translation • >11 degrees angulation Cord neuropraxia with: • More than two episodes • Cord injury or ligamentous instability on MRI • Duration >24-36 h Unstable spine fracture
SURGICAL		
Resolved herniated nucleus pulposis One level anterior or posterior fusion	Postop discectomy for herniated nucleus pulposus (HNP) with facet compromise Level anterior cervical discectomy and fusion (ACDF) - (low cervical)	≥3-level fusion anterior or ≥2-level posterior C1-C2 fusion

cardiopulmonary capacity, muscle performance, metabolic response, and hormonal regulation during both short-term (less than 4 weeks) and, more markedly, in long-term (>4 weeks) detraining periods.[50, 51] Peak-performance elite athletes see more marked reductions in comparison to recently trained athletes. Several exercises potentially limit the amount of "deconditioning" that can occur while simultaneously providing early rehabilitative benefits.[33] Swimming, stationary bicycles, and elliptical machines are commonly used and effective means of minimizing the deconditioning process, with minimal stress placed on the spine.[22]

Flexibility and Strengthening

Incorporating flexibility training into an athlete's rehabilitation will help correct or improve fundamental musculoskeletal biomechanics.[67, 74] Strong evidence exists to demonstrate that a multimodal approach, integrating stretching and

strengthening regimens, is highly effective for spinal rehabilitation.[38] If no contraindication to spinal motion exists, such as a fracture requiring orthosis, early mobilization and restoration of ROM can typically be initiated within the first 48 to 72 hours following acute injury. The athlete's pain tolerance, clinical signs of muscle fatigue, or inability to maintain proper mechanics should serve as indicators of how rapidly to advance.[31, 46] Initially, flexibility and strengthening are addressed in a single plane and then transitioned to multiplanar dynamic flexibility and, finally, dynamic strengthening. The athlete should maintain a neutral spine position throughout all phases, and an inability to maintain proper position during one phase prevents progression to the next.

Restoring Range of Motion and Flexibility

Three basic forms of stretching techniques are often employed, either individually or in conjunction with one another. These include static stretching, dynamic stretching, and proprioceptive neuromuscular facilitation (PNF).[32] Initially, passive ROM in a single plane with static stretching gently mobilizes the soft tissue. As patients regain full pain-free ROM, they usually transition into dynamic stretching. When the athlete transitions into higher-intensity and sport-specific rehabilitation, PNF stretching comprises more advanced, specific forms of dynamic stretching integrated with isometric contractions.[32]

Strengthening

Once general mobility has been established, strengthening of the stabilizing muscles of the spine is addressed. Isometric exercises targeting the paraspinal and core musculature are initially implemented, followed by the addition of more advanced isokinetic and dynamic exercises.[45] As the athlete advances, the activities become more dynamically complex through gradual increases in speed and repetitions and even the application of minimal resistance to promote muscle strength and endurance.[9, 33]

Core Stability and Conditioning

"Core stability" implies the ability of the trunk to maintain a fixed position or trajectory following any perturbation.[76] While the ligaments and bone provide a passive and resistive stiffness to stabilize the spine, the core musculature is essential in maintaining the dynamic and functional stability of the spine. Hence, the core is the foundation for most athletic movement by forming the center connection of the upper and lower extremities and enabling an athlete to perform precise coordinated movements.

The strength and stability of the core provide the foundation that determines the force, precision, and speed of a desired axial movement. At first, core stabilization exercises ideally should focus on reactivation of the "dormant" muscles. Functional progression emphasizes developing balance and coordination in all three cardinal planes: frontal, sagittal, and transverse. The end objective is to enhance neuromuscular control, balance, and coordination through a combination of joint stability exercises and plyometric, proprioceptive, balance, and finally sport-specific training.[1, 2, 7, 10, 30, 41, 42, 47, 53, 54, 57, 58, 60, 61]

Integrative and Maintenance Phase

Application of functional exercises for sport-specific motion marks the transition from the subacute phase into the integrative phase of rehabilitation.[26] Any deficiencies need to be corrected, and an athlete must prove that he can consistently reproduce the proper mechanics before increasing the velocity and force of the activity. The athlete and the clinician need to pay attention to signs of fatigue that may result in return to improper mechanics.[26, 42, 56]

Final Phase: Return to Competition

The treating physician ultimately must provide clearance before an athlete can return to competition. Regardless of external time pressures or the therapeutic goals met, the injury must have had appropriate time to heal, and no radiographic evidence of instability or incomplete healing should be present. An athlete must be completely free of any signs and symptoms experienced due to the original injury. Functionally, the athlete must have regained full pain-free ROM, have restored preinjury strength, and be able to demonstrate preinjury proficiency in athletic performance with no recurrence of symptoms when subjected to sport-specific maneuvers.[8, 22, 41, 42, 74]

SURGICAL CONSIDERATIONS

Before surgery is considered, all other potential pathology that may cause the athlete's symptoms must be excluded via a thorough history and a complete physical and neurologic exam, in addition to the appropriate radiological and laboratory diagnostic workup. Only when the patient's clinical history, symptoms, physical exam findings, and radiological findings are consistent should surgical intervention be discussed. For example, a radiographic abnormality at one disc level that does not correlate with the radicular dermatomal pain and myotomal weakness found during the history or physical exam should raise suspicion about other causes and warrant further investigation. It is well established that asymptomatic patients can have abnormal MRI findings, with the frequency increasing with age.[8, 71] General indications for surgery include persistent or progressive neurologic deficit, subjective symptoms or physical signs suggesting myelopathy, and pain consistent with the history, examination, and radiographic findings that persists longer than 6 to 8 weeks despite appropriate conservative treatment.[21, 61, 63, 77]

The competitive athlete has several unique attributes that need to be taken into account in relation to surgical intervention. First, athletes are often young, healthy, and highly motivated and also in elite physical condition; collectively these characteristics make them ideal surgical candidates. Second, earlier intervention can be considered in an athlete to facilitate a more rapid recovery and earlier return to competition. As opposed to the situation with members of the general population, who can often compromise their everyday activities without a dramatic change in their everyday lifestyle, minor symptoms in an athlete can dramatically affect athletic performance. Additionally, a prolonged trial of conservative treatment can come at a great cost to an athlete: Financially, loss of physical condition with restricted training and even potential career advancement opportunities are all associated with loss of active competition. Third, a surgeon must carefully consider the season- or career-altering implications of a particular procedure. The pressure to return to competition often imposes a need for earlier stability, yet the physiological stresses an athlete will place on the spine are far greater than in the general population and will ultimately test the durability of the surgical intervention to the extreme.

The philosophy of any surgery is to definitively treat the abnormal pathology while simultaneously maintaining and restoring tissue to its natural anatomical and physiological conditions. Therefore, several general tenets should be followed: (1) approach from the direction of the pathology, (2) keep in mind that less is more (3), avoid fusion when possible, and (4) preserve normal anatomy[69] (figure 17.4). Further disrupting the spine's natural anatomy and biomechanics with a decision to fuse two consecutive vertebrae, or to take a more invasive approach involving muscular dissection, may result in small changes in flexibility, muscular strength, reaction time, and postoperative pain. Such subtleties may manifest as a decline in an elite athlete's performance. The increasingly advanced application of microsurgical techniques and minimally invasive approaches has given the treating surgeon a heightened ability to minimize tissue trauma, treat the underlying pathology, and respect the spine's natural stability.

CERVICAL SPINE INJURIES AND THEIR MANAGEMENT AND TREATMENT

Athletic injuries to the cervical spine have similar biomechanics but vary somewhat according to the sport. The specific tissues disrupted and the risks of neurologic injury are outlined in the previous chapter. This section outlines the specifics of management, following diagnosis, relative to the type of injury.

Soft Tissue Injury

Sprains, strains, and contusions of the neck ligaments and musculature are all managed similarly. Only in the rare instance of an unstable ligamentous injury is any surgical intervention indicated. The athlete should be immobilized in a rigid orthosis until stability is ensured, with administration of anti-inflammatory or analgesic medication to encourage rest and healing. Prolonged immobilization may lead to atrophy and deconditioning, so flexion and extension radiographs should be performed to rule out dynamic instability as soon as the discomfort has resolved. If the dynamic studies are negative, the athlete should be weaned from the cervical collar with institution of ROM and strengthening exercises as tolerated. Flexibility training, isometric strengthening, and flexion–extension physiotherapy are commonly used to recondition and strengthen the neck to prevent further injury.[20, 34, 77]

Cervical Disc Disease or Spondylosis

In comparison to the general population, athletes in high-impact sports are likely at an increased risk for development of cervical disc disease in their lifetime.[77] As with most injuries, a trial of

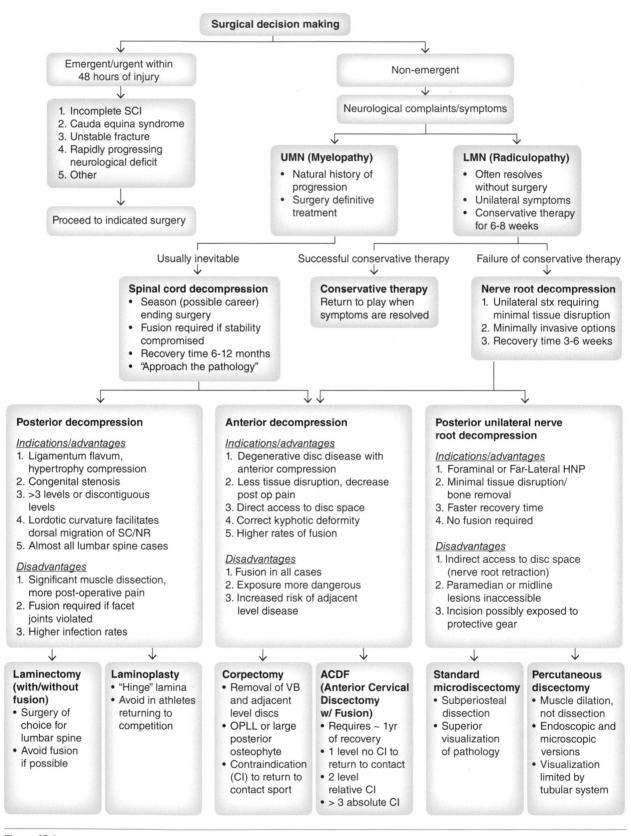

Surgical decision making

Emergent/urgent within 48 hours of injury
1. Incomplete SCI
2. Cauda equina syndrome
3. Unstable fracture
4. Rapidly progressing neurological deficit
5. Other

Proceed to indicated surgery

Non-emergent

Neurological complaints/symptoms

UMN (Myelopathy)
- Natural history of progression
- Surgery definitive treatment

LMN (Radiculopathy)
- Often resolves without surgery
- Unilateral symptoms
- Conservative therapy for 6-8 weeks

Usually inevitable

Successful conservative therapy

Failure of conservative therapy

Spinal cord decompression
- Season (possible career) ending surgery
- Fusion required if stability compromised
- Recovery time 6-12 months
- "Approach the pathology"

Conservative therapy
Return to play when symptoms are resolved

Nerve root decompression
1. Unilateral stx requiring minimal tissue disruption
2. Minimally invasive options
3. Recovery time 3-6 weeks

Posterior decompression

Indications/advantages
1. Ligamentum flavum, hypertrophy compression
2. Congenital stenosis
3. >3 levels or discontiguous levels
4. Lordotic curvature facilitates dorsal migration of SC/NR
5. Almost all lumbar spine cases

Disadvantages
1. Significant muscle dissection, more post-operative pain
2. Fusion required if facet joints violated
3. Higher infection rates

Anterior decompression

Indications/advantages
1. Degenerative disc disease with anterior compression
2. Less tissue disruption, decrease post op pain
3. Direct access to disc space
4. Correct kyphotic deformity
5. Higher rates of fusion

Disadvantages
1. Fusion in all cases
2. Exposure more dangerous
3. Increased risk of adjacent level disease

Posterior unilateral nerve root decompression

Indications/advantages
1. Foraminal or Far-Lateral HNP
2. Minimal tissue disruption/ bone removal
3. Faster recovery time
4. No fusion required

Disadvantages
1. Indirect access to disc space (nerve root retraction)
2. Paramedian or midline lesions inaccessible
3. Incision possibly exposed to protective gear

Laminectomy (with/without fusion)
- Surgery of choice for lumbar spine
- Avoid fusion if possible

Laminoplasty
- "Hinge" lamina
- Avoid in athletes returning to competition

Corpectomy
- Removal of VB and adjacent level discs
- OPLL or large posterior osteophyte
- Contraindication (CI) to return to contact sport

ACDF (Anterior Cervical Discectomy w/ Fusion)
- Requires ~ 1yr of recovery
- 1 level no CI to return to contact
- 2 level relative CI
- > 3 absolute CI

Standard microdiscectomy
- Subperiosteal dissection
- Superior visualization of pathology

Percutaneous discectomy
- Muscle dilation, not dissection
- Endoscopic and microscopic versions
- Visualization limited by tubular system

Figure 17.4   Surgical options, advantages (anterior vs. posterior).

conservative management for a minimum of 6 to 8 weeks comprises the initial management of cervical disc disease and consists of rest, activity modification, anti-inflammatory or analgesic medication, and cervical support. As the athlete's initial pain subsides, progression into the subacute phase can occur, with gentle, passive ROM exercises advanced to isometric and resistance ROM exercises. If the athlete remains asymptomatic, sport-specific training and drills begin. Return to play is allowed when a patient has pain-free full strength and ROM capabilities.

Roughly 90% of patients with cervical radiculopathy due to a herniated disc will improve without surgery.[61] Indications for surgery are persistent or recurrent radicular pain unresponsive to conservative treatment and progression or persistence of a neurologic deficit.[63, 73] For myelopathy, early surgery is usually recommended, as surgically treated patients have better outcomes compared to those under nonsurgical management.[62, 72] Surgery is rarely recommended for axial neck pain without associated radiculopathy or myelopathy.

Anterior and posterior approaches have been used to successfully treat cervical disc disease; both have advantages and disadvantages.[6, 72] In general, ventral pathologies including central disc herniation or posterior vertebral column osteophytes are approached anteriorly. Dorsally compressive pathology including posterior–lateral osteophytes or disc herniation or ligament flavum hypertrophy are approached posteriorly. For radiculopathy, the goal of surgery is to decompress the nerve root. Surgical options include (1) posterior cervical laminoforaminotomy, (2) anterior cervical discectomy with or without fusion (ACD[F]) and with or without internal fixation (plating), and (3) modified versions of these using minimally invasive microendoscopic techniques. Correspondingly, for myelopathy, where the goal of surgery is primarily spinal cord decompression, surgical options include (1) single- or multiple-level ACDF, (2) single- or multiple-level corpectomy (removal of vertebral body) with fusion, (3) posterior laminectomy with or without fusion, (4) posterior laminoplasty, and, again, (5) modified minimally invasive procedures. Less invasive, minimal reconstruction procedures are preferred

as they tend to pose the least risk, with reduced recovery time.[72]

Surgical Considerations: Cervical Spine Fractures and Spinal Cord Injury

Since most fractures are associated with some degree of ligamentous and soft tissue injury that may or may not be clinically significant, even minor fractures should elicit extended evaluation with MRI. Minimal compression fractures, spinous process fractures, and, rarely, isolated lamina fractures are usually considered stable spine fractures and can be managed conservatively. Following immobilization, typical progression through rehabilitation and return to competition should proceed as outlined earlier.[4, 5, 22, 77]

Catastrophic SCI should be managed initially according to the guidelines discussed previously.[29, 55, 66] Depending on the location, degree of injury, and neurologic compromise, unstable spine fractures usually require initial reduction with external traction and subsequent stabilization by external orthoses or surgical intervention. Emergent surgical decompression may be indicated in acute SCI. Conflicting data exist on the appropriate timing of emergent surgical intervention. A recent systematic review and a multicenter prospective randomized controlled trial indicate an advantage for early decompressive surgery (<24 hours) in the setting of spinal cord trauma.[11, 23] Any athlete sustaining a major, unstable spine fracture almost always requires surgical stabilization with return to competition absolutely contraindicated.[22]

Spinal Stenosis and Transient Spinal Cord Injury

As outlined previously, athletes experiencing a transient spinal cord injury (TSCI) should be managed as for an acute SCI until appropriate clinical and radiological evidence is obtained to clear any underlying cause of the injury. Return to play in the presence of persistent stenosis is controversial. Surgery is recommended in the setting of focal lesions with cord compression or instability demonstrated through MRI or dynamic plain films.[15] Bailes and colleagues have suggested that an athlete may be safe to return to play as long as the CSF signal around the spinal cord is preserved on MRI, in combination with rapid and complete resolution of clinical symptoms.[3, 5] Cervical stenosis complicated by evidence of ligamentous instability, multiple episodes of neuropraxia, or a single episode with evidence of SCI and symptoms that persist for greater than 36 hours represent absolute contraindications to return to play.[5, 15, 77] In patients who require operative therapy for focal causes of stenosis, such as disc herniation or segmental instability, prerequisites for returning to play include resolution of symptoms and a solid fusion with normal dynamic radiographs.[1, 13, 37]

"Stingers"

Up to 50% of athletes involved in collision and contact sports experience one or more stingers during their career. While detrimental to performance, transient isolated brachial plexus injuries are self-limiting, and an athlete is allowed to return to competition once there is pain-free resolution of neurologic symptoms. Further workup, however, is necessary if the symptoms persist for an extended length of time, if they occur repeatedly, or if SCI is a concern. Signs or symptoms that suggest SCI include bilateral symptoms, lower extremity involvement, long tract signs, or bowel or bladder dysfunction.[3, 22, 39]

Cervical Spine Injury: Return to Play

When a suspected neck injury occurs in an athlete, it is essential for medical personnel to accurately recognize and systematically classify a spine injury in order to facilitate effective management as well as return to play. Bailes and coauthors developed a system to classify cervical spine injuries in athletes. Type I injuries include those that result in permanent neurologic injury, either complete or incomplete. Type II injuries are transient neurologic injuries that resolve within 24 hours and have normal radiographic studies. With type III injuries, the athlete is neurologically intact but radiographic abnormalities are present. The relative and absolute contraindications

to return to play are outlined in table 17.3.[3, 4, 5, 20, 28, 39, 63]

THORACIC AND LUMBAR SPINE INJURIES AND THEIR MANAGEMENT

The top-level athlete with a lumbar spine problem often has specific physical, motivational, and therapy goal differences from the general population. Athletes appear to have a lower incidence of serious lower back injuries than expected, as well as a reduced severity of clinical complaints once the injury occurs. These differences may be explained by several factors, including age, natural selection, and training routines.

Since the risks of neurologic sequelae following many lumbar injuries are low, continued athletic participation, with appropriate alterations in training, can often be allowed. The goal of therapy should be to return the athlete to competition as soon as possible while maintaining the highest regard for the athlete's safety. Initially, the primary mode of therapy should be conservative, as the acute episode often resolves, allowing the athlete to gradually return to full activity and participation in sport.

Soft Tissue Injury

Low back pain is a common occurrence in athletes and is usually secondary to a muscle strain, muscle contusion, or ligamentous sprain sustained either acutely or from chronic biomechanical stress. However the injury manifests, it is important to rule out any potential structural or neuronal lesions contributing to the pain. Contusions may initially be treated with ice and cold packs to reduce pain and swelling. Later, heat, massage, anti-inflammatory drugs, and restricted activity are often useful. After the initial discomfort has improved, usually within several days, physical rehabilitation begins, with emphasis placed on correcting improper mechanics, increasing flexibility and ROM, and core strength training. With sprains or strains, the healing phase may vary depending on the severity of the injury and can sometimes be prolonged up to 6 to 8 weeks. Once the injury is resolved, the athlete may return to play without restrictions. The exercises should be maintained so as to reduce the chances of repetitive injury.

Disc Herniation

Acute lumbar disc herniations presenting with severe back and radicular pain are initially best treated with activity restriction, analgesics, muscle relaxants, and nonsteroidal anti-inflammatory medications. Once symptoms lessen, a program of lumbar and abdominal stretching and strengthening exercises can begin, followed by gradual increases in weight training and other routine practice activities that do not place the spine in extremes of axial loading, flexion, and rotation.

Surgery is a strong consideration in the management of a symptomatic ruptured lumbar disc. Urgent operative intervention should take place in athletes presenting with significant neurologic compromise (cauda equina syndrome, foot drop, or other major motor deficit). Other, nonurgent indications include severe, incapacitating back and radicular pain that does not respond to conservative therapy and chronically recurring symptoms that persist despite adequate rehabilitation.

The chances of impairing the athlete's ability to compete successfully should be weighed against the time lost in pursuing a likely unsuccessful conservative treatment regimen. The amateur athlete may be urged to discontinue the given sport indefinitely and to try to find another type of competition that is less stressful physically. In the top-level athlete, in whom years of training have been invested and potentially great financial or other rewards are in place or anticipated, cessation of competition has much greater consequences.

Once a decision for surgery has been made, the likelihood of the athlete's returning to play may be enhanced by the selection of a procedure that will relieve the patient's symptoms with minimal disruption of bony, muscular, and ligamentous structures. The standard intervention is a microdiscectomy, during which the offending fragment is directly extracted through a small incision using the surgical microscope or endoscope.[21, 22, 35-37, 70] Accompanying degenerative changes such as spondylosis or spondylolysis, if asymptomatic, should not be disturbed, as a more involved and prophylactic procedure, especially a lumbar fusion, carries a much higher likelihood of ending the athlete's career.

Spondylosis

During acute flare-ups, treatment should include rest, restricted activities, physical therapy, and anti-inflammatory drugs. If osteophytic nerve root compression is the cause of symptoms, decompression via a limited foraminotomy is often very effective. Otherwise, as there is no significant risk of neurologic injury, the athlete may return to play whenever symptoms resolve enough to allow comfortable participation. Advanced cases may ultimately lead to the classic degenerative changes of lumbar stenosis (see previous chapter). Surgery should be considered if symptoms suggestive of instability or of typical lumbar stenosis are refractory to conservative measures. Modern neurosurgery now includes minimally invasive techniques that produce less disruption of the lumbar paraspinous musculature; excellent results can be achieved with some athletes, although return to the athletic field is much more unlikely than with discectomy or foraminotomy.[28, 40, 45, 56, 69, 72]

Fractures

Thoracic and lumbar spine fractures affecting spinal stability are rarely encountered in athletics.[40] When they do occur, most are usually adequately treated with nonoperative measures. In the initial workup, particular attention must be given to the surrounding cardiac, renal, and lung parenchyma, as a complicating organ injury may also be present. After an initial period of external bracing and healing during which symptoms gradually resolve, the patient can begin a progressive rehabilitation program. Surgery is reserved for conditions causing nerve root or spinal cord compression that results in an acute or progressive neurologic deficit or severe or intractable radicular pain. Emergent or urgent surgery is indicated only in an acute spinal column fracture resulting in spinal instability.[40, 68] Facet fractures are not uncommon, particularly in sports requiring forceful hyperextension activities or training regimens. Bleeding from the disrupted bone edges may resemble a synovial cyst as seen with advanced spondylosis (see previous chapter). Most facet fractures resolve without a need for surgical intervention.

Pars Interarticularis Disease: Spondylolysis and Spondylolisthesis

For stress fractures involving the pars interarticularis, treatment is conservative and should include rest and avoidance of the inciting activity, if this has been clarified, combined with antiinflammatory drugs and bracing. Treatment should continue until symptoms resolve, and ideally until the single-photon emission computed tomography (SPECT) scan has returned to normal. A similar treatment regimen is also indicated for athletes with symptomatic spondylolysis without spondylolisthesis, although the pars defect will not likely heal once the fracture becomes established.[72, 75]

Treatment of spondylolisthesis is based on the degree of slippage and the clinical symptoms. In asymptomatic patients with low-grade subluxation (less than 25%), the risk of increased displacement from intensive training is minimal, and continued activity is not contraindicated.[20] Management is aimed at alleviating an athlete's pain while preventing progression and instability. In most cases, a conservative treatment approach is warranted, consisting of rest until pain subsides with gradual increase in activity. Incorporating an aggressive core-strengthening, lower limb flexibility rehabilitation program usually allows athletes with low-grade slips to return to competition. External orthosis may aid the initial healing process by providing support and stability.

Surgical intervention is indicated only for athletes with persistent pain for more than 6 months, progressing spondylolisthesis, traumatic spondylolisthesis, or neurological deficit or for symptomatic patients with a high-grade slip.[21, 40] Surgical treatment involving a multilevel spinal fusion or a direct repair of the pars defect, each with various techniques and optional interventions depending on the injury and surgeon's preference, may be performed. Due to the extent of tissue injury, increased stress on adjacent structures, and motion limitation associated with multilevel fusions, the athlete's likelihood of returning to heavy contact sports or peak training capability is diminished.[21]

Thoracic and Lumbar Spine Injury: Return to Play

Many lumbar spinal injuries are related to training errors, while others are caused by the demands of a specific type of athletic activity. The athlete will invariably be returning to the exact type of activity that precipitated the injury. Initially, the primary mode of therapy should be conservative, as the acute episode will often resolve. As with cervical spine injuries, protection and preservation of the nervous system for the remainder of the individual's life are the primary treatment objective. Since the risks of neurologic sequelae following many lumbar injuries are low, however, continued athletic participation, with appropriate alterations in training, can often be allowed.

To be considered for return to competition, the athlete must be pain free through a full ROM, be free of any neurologic deficit, and have completed a successful rehabilitation program. Because the risks of neurologic compromise are low, many athletes continue to participate while still having some symptoms. While published recommendations are intended to serve as a guide, clinicians should rely on their good judgment as well as case-specific individual attributes of the athlete when making any recommendation. The exact timing of return after a surgical procedure should be based on a number of factors but can be as early as 4 to 6 weeks and during the same season. Future training would include maintenance of strong paraspinous muscular support and flexibility so as to minimize the chance of recurrence.[21, 28, 40, 42, 66]

CONCLUDING THOUGHTS

Spinal injuries can be devastating for both the patient and the patient's family. When a spinal injury occurs, it is the role of the team physician and trainers to rapidly assess the situation, immobilize the spine, and prepare the athlete for transfer to a facility where definitive diagnosis and management can occur. Lumbar spinal injuries are far more common, although they can be equally disabling. Undoubtedly, prevention of spinal injury is of primary concern. Education can help achieve this; however, sometimes the demands of a specific type of athletic activity precipitate such injuries. Treatment options will vary depending on the type of injury sustained. The goals for management of any spinal injury are protecting and preserving neurological function, which can be achieved through an immediate and proper response on the part of the practitioner.

REFERENCES

1. Adams MA, Dolan P, Hutton WC. Diurnal variations in the stresses on the lumbar spine. Spine 1987;12(2):130-137.

2. Akuthota V, Ferreiro A, Moore T, Fredericson M. Core stability exercise principles. Curr Sports Med Rep 2008;7(1):39-44.

3. Bailes JE. Experience with cervical stenosis and temporary paralysis in athletes. J Neurosurg Spine 2005;2(1):11-16.

4. Bailes JE, Warren WL. Cervical spine injuries in athletes. In: Neurological Sports Medicine. Rolling Mcadows, IL: Thieme/AANS; 2001.

5. Bailes JE, Petschauer M, Guskiewicz KM, et al. Management of cervical spine injuries in athletes. J Athl Train 2007;42(1):126-134.

6. Baron EM, Young WF. Cervical spondylotic myelopathy. Neurosurgery 2007;60(1 Suppl 1):S35-S41.

7. Barr KP, Griggs M, Cadby T. Lumbar stabilization. Am J Phys Med Rehabil 2007;86(1):72-80.

8. Beazell JR, Magrum EM. Rehabilitation of head and neck injuries in the athlete. Clin Sports Med 2003;22(3):523-557.

9. Behm DG, Drinkwater EJ, Willardson JM, et al. The role of instability rehabilitative resistance training for the core musculature. Strength Cond J 2011;33(3):72.

10. Belavý DL, Armbrecht G, Richardson CA, et al. Muscle atrophy and changes in spinal morphology. Spine 2011;36(2):137-145.

11. Carreon LY, Dimar JR. Early versus late stabilization of spine injuries. Spine 2011;36(11):E727-E733.

12. Castinel BH, Adam P, Milburn PD, et al. Epidemiology of cervical spine abnormalities in asymptomatic adult professional rugby union players using static and dynamic MRI protocols: 2002 to 2006. Br J Sports Med 2010;44(3):194-199.

13. Chou R, Huffman LH; American Pain Society; American College of Physicians. Nonpharmacologic therapies for acute and chronic low back pain: a review of the evidence for an American Pain Society/American College of Physicians clinical practice guideline. Ann Intern Med 2007;147(7):492-504.

14. Chou R, Huffman LH; American Pain Society; American College of Physicians. Medications for acute and chronic low back pain: a review of the evidence for an American Pain Society/American College of Physicians clinical practice guideline. Ann Intern Med 2007;147(7):505-514.

15. Clark AJ, Auguste KI, Sun PP. Cervical spinal stenosis and sports-related cervical cord neurapraxia. Neurosurg Focus 2011;31(5):E7.

16. Crockett B. Rehabilitation of the athlete. Mo Med 2011;108(3):173-175.

17. Danneels LA, Vanderstraeten GG, Cambier DC, et al. Effects of three different training modalities on the cross sectional area of the lumbar multifidus muscle in patients with chronic low back pain. Br J Sports Med 2001;35(3):186-191.

18. Demoulin C, Crielaard JM, Vanderthommen M. Spinal muscle evaluation in healthy individuals and low-back-pain patients: a literature review. Joint Bone Spine 2007;74(1):9-13.

19. Deyo RA, Diehl AK, Rosenthal M. How many days of bed rest for acute low back pain? New Engl J Med 1986;315(17):1064-1070.

20. Dorshimer GW, Kelly M. Cervical pain in the athlete: common conditions and treatment. Prim Care 2005;32(1):231-243.

21. Dunn IF, Proctor MR, Day AL. Lumbar spine injuries in athletes. Neurosurg Focus 2006;21(4):E4.

22. Eddy D, Congeni J, Loud K. A review of spine injuries and return to play. Clin J Sport Med 2005;15(6):453-458.

23. Fehlings MG, Vaccaro A, Wilson JR, et al. Early versus delayed decompression for traumatic cervical spinal cord injury: results of the Surgical Timing in Acute Spinal Cord Injury Study (STASCIS). PLoS ONE 2012;7(2):e32037.

24. Ghanta MK, Smith LM Polin RS, et al. An analysis of Eastern Association for the Surgery of Trauma practice guidelines for cervical spine evaluation in a series of patients with multiple imaging techniques. Am Surg 2002;68(6):563-567; discussion 567-568.

25. Ghiselli G, Schaadt G, McAllister DR. On-the-field evaluation of an athlete with a head or neck injury. Clin Sports Med 2003;22(3):445-465.

26. Gluck GS, Bendo JA, Spivak JM. The lumbar spine and low back pain in golf: a literature review of swing biomechanics and injury prevention. Spine J 2008;8(5):778-788.

27. Grant R. Physical Therapy of the Cervical and Thoracic Spine. St. Louis, MO: Churchill Livingstone; 2002.

28. Greenberg MS. Handbook of Neurosurgery. New York, NY: Thieme; 2010.

29. Hadley MN, Walters BC, Grabb PA, et al. Guidelines for the management of acute cervical spine and spinal cord injuries. Clin Neurosurg 2002;49:407-498.

30. Hodges PW, Richardson CA. Inefficient muscular stabilization of the lumbar spine associated with low back pain. A motor control evaluation of transversus abdominis. Spine 1996;21(22):2640-2650.

31. Holt LE, Pelham TW, Holt J. Stretching the major muscle groups of the trunk and neck. In: Flexibility: A Concise Guide. Totowa, NJ: Humana Press; 2008.

32. Holt LE, Pelham TW, Holt J. Flexibility: A Concise Guide. Totowa, NJ: Humana Press; 2008.

33. Hopkins TJ, White AA. Rehabilitation of athletes following spine injury. Clin Sports Med 1993;12(3):603-619.

34. Hovis WD, Limbird TJ. An evaluation of cervical orthoses in limiting hyperextension and lateral flexion in football. Med Sci Sports Exerc 1994;26(7):872-876.

35. Hsu WK. Performance-based outcomes following lumbar discectomy in professional athletes in the National Football League. Spine 2010;35(12):1247-1251.

36. Hsu WK. Outcomes following nonoperative and operative treatment for cervical disc herniations in National Football League athletes. Spine 2011;36(10):800-805.

37. Hsu WK, McCarthy KJ, Savage JW, et al. The Professional Athlete Spine Initiative: outcomes after lumbar disc herniation in 342 elite professional athletes. Spine J 2011;11(3):180-186.

38. Kay TM, Gross A, Goldsmith C, et al. Exercises for mechanical neck disorders. Cochrane Database Syst Rev 2005;3.

39. Kepler CK, Vaccaro AR. Injuries and abnormalities of the cervical spine and return to play criteria. Clin Sports Med 2012;31(3):499-508.

40. Khan N, Husain S, Haak M. Thoracolumbar injuries in the athlete. Sports Med Arthrosc 2008;16(1):16-25.

41. Krabak BJ, Kanarek SL. Cervical spine pain in the competitive athlete. Phys Med Rehabil Clin North Am 2011;22(3):459-471.

42. Krabak B, Kennedy DJ. Functional rehabilitation of lumbar spine injuries in the athlete. Sports Med Arthrosc 2008;16(1):47-54.

43. Krych AJ, Richman D, Drakos M, et al. Epidural steroid injection for lumbar disc herniation in NFL athletes. Med Sci Sports Exerc 2012;44(2):193-198.

44. Labruyère R, Agarwala A, Curt A. Rehabilitation in spine and spinal cord trauma. Spine 2010;35(Suppl):S259-S262.

45. Lawrence JP, Greene HS, Grauer JN. Back pain in athletes. J Am Acad Orthop Surg 2006;14(13):726-735.

46. Machado LAC, de Souza MVS, Ferreira PH, et al. The McKenzie method for low back pain. Spine 2006;31(9):E254-E262.

47. Mannion AF. Fibre type characteristics and function of the human paraspinal muscles: normal values and changes in association with low back pain. J Electromyogr Kinesiol 1999;9(6):363-377.

48. Mayoux-Benhamou MA, Revel M, Vallée C, et al. Longus colli has a postural function on cervical curvature. SRA 1994;16(4):367-371.

49. Montgomery S, Haak M. Management of lumbar injuries in athletes. Sports Med 1999;27(2):135-141.

50. Mujika I, Padilla S. Detraining: loss of training-induced physiological and performance adaptations. Part I: Short term insufficient training stimulus. Sports Med 2000;30(2):79-87.

51. Mujika I, Padilla S. Detraining: loss of training-induced physiological and performance adaptations. Part II: Long term insufficient training stimulus. Sports Med 2000;30(3):145-154.

52. Nachemson AL. Newest knowledge of low back pain. A critical look. Clin Orthop Relat Res 1992;(279):8-20.

53. Niemeläinen R, Briand M-M, Battié MC. Substantial asymmetry in paraspinal muscle cross-sectional area in healthy adults questions its value as a marker of low back pain and pathology. Spine 2011;36(25):2152-2157.

54. Peter Reeves N, Narendra KS, Cholewicki J. Spine stability: the six blind men and the elephant. Clin Biomech 2007;22(3):266-274.

55. Prehospital care of the spine-injured athlete. A document from the Inter-Association Task Force for Appropriate Care of the Spine-Injured Athlete. 1998.

56. Reed JJ, Wadsworth LT. Lower back pain in golf: a review. Curr Sports Med Rep 2010;9(1):57-59.

57. Renkawitz T, Boluki D, Grifka J. The association of low back pain, neuromuscular imbalance, and trunk extension strength in athletes. Spine J 2006;6(6):673-683.

58. Richardson CA, Snijders CJ, Hides JA, et al. The relation between the transversus abdominis muscles, sacroiliac joint mechanics, and low back pain. Spine 2002;27(4):399-405.

59. Roelofs PD, Deyo RA, Koes BW, et al. Non-steroidal anti-inflammatory drugs for low back pain. Cochrane Database of Systematic Reviews 2008, Issue 1. Art. No.: CD000396.

60. Saal JA, Saal JS. Nonoperative treatment of herniated lumbar intervertebral disc with radiculopathy. An outcome study. Spine 1989;14(4):431-437.

61. Saal JS, Saal JA, Yurth EF. Nonoperative management of herniated cervical intervertebral disc with radiculopathy. Spine 1995;21(16):1877-1883.

62. Sampath P, Bendebba M, Davis JD, et al. Outcome of patients treated for cervical myelopathy. A prospective, multicenter study with independent clinical review. Spine 2000;25(6):670-676.

63. Scherping SC. Cervical disc disease in the athlete. Clin Sports Med 2002;21(1):37-47- vi.

64. See S, Ginzburg R. Choosing a skeletal muscle relaxant. Am Fam Physician 2008;78(3):365-370.

65. Standaert CJ, Herring SA, Pratt TW. Rehabilitation of the athlete with low back pain. Curr Sports Med Rep 2004;3(1):35-40.

66. Swartz EE, Boden BP, Courson RW, et al. National Athletic Trainers' Association position statement: acute management of the cervical spine–injured athlete. J Athl Train 2009;44(3):306-331.

67. Tallarico RA, Madom IA, Palumbo MA. Spondylolysis and spondylolisthesis in the athlete. Sports Med Arthrosc 2008;16(1):32-38.

68. Vaccaro AR, Lehman RA, Hurlbert RJ, et al. A new classification of thoracolumbar injuries: the importance of injury morphology, the integrity of the posterior ligamentous complex, and neurologic status. Spine 2005;30(20):2325-2333.

69. Van der Veer CA. Minimally invasive treatment options for athletes with spine injuries. In: Neurological Sports Medicine. Rolling Meadows, IL: Thieme/AANS; 2001.

70. Weinstein JN, Lurie JD, Tosteson TD, et al. Surgical vs nonoperative treatment for lumbar disk herniation: the Spine Patient Outcomes Research Trial (SPORT) observational cohort. JAMA 2006;296(20):2451-2459. 71.   Weis EB. Abnormal magnetic-resonance scans of the cervical spine in asymptomatic subjects. J Bone Joint Surg Am 1991;73(7):1113.

71. Winn HR. Youmans Neurological Surgery. Philadelphia: Saunders; 2011.

72. Witwer BP, Trost GR. Cervical spondylosis. Neurosurgery 2007;60(1 Suppl 1):S130-S136.

73. Young JL, Press JM, Herring SA. The disc at risk in athletes: perspectives on operative and non-operative care. Med Sci Sports Exerc 1997;29(7 Suppl):S222-232.

74. Young W, d'Hemecourt P. Back pain in adolescent athletes. Phys Sportsmed 2011;39(4):80-89. Zazulak B, Cholewicki J, Reeves, NP. Neuromuscular control of trunk stability: clinical implications for sports injury prevention. J Am Acad Orthop Surg 2008;6(9):497-505.

75. Zmurko MG, Tannoury TY, Tannouty CA, et al. Cervical sprains, disc herniations, minor fractures, and other cervical injuries in the athlete. Clin Sports Med 2003;22(3):513-521.

Peripheral Nerve Injuries in Athletes

In collaboration with

Fabio V. C. Sparapani, MD, PhD • Robert J. Spinner, MD

Peripheral nerve injuries can occur in all athletes and in all sports. Their prevalence is likely to increase given the current widespread popularity of amateur and professional sports as well as weightlifting or resistance training, personal fitness, and other forms of healthy recreational activity.[14] Some sports have their own characteristic injuries.[25] However, all sports share a potential for a broad spectrum of injuries. A multidisciplinary approach to athletes and their injuries may involve neurologists, physiatrists, sports medicine physicians, psychologists, orthopedic and plastic surgeons, and neurosurgeons.

EPIDEMIOLOGY

In 2010, the National Electronic Surveillance System (NEISS) reported an estimated 1,987,774 injuries in the United States related to six sports (football, baseball, cycling, basketball, wrestling, and snow activities), based on 57,767 cases reported in a predetermined sample of hospitals.[1] In Australia, the activities that most commonly caused sport-related injury for all ages were cycling, Australian football, basketball, soccer, cricket, netball, and rugby. The nerve injuries occurred during competitions or practice sessions, and the common types of nerve injury were associated with fractures, strains, and sprains.[12,

13] In another study, ice hockey was a principal cause of injuries in those under 16 years of age.[23]

A retrospective study based on electrophysiological parameters, involving 180 athletes with 216 nerve root, plexus, or peripheral nerve injuries, found that 86% of these injuries affected the upper extremity and principally the median nerve, followed by axillary, ulnar, and suprascapular mononeuropathies. In the lower extremity, the peroneal nerve was the most affected.[18] More than 33% of injuries were sustained during football.

PATHOGENESIS

Factors associated with the sport activity include vibration and mechanical pressure. These and other physical factors can augment the development of pathophysiological changes and, if persistently affecting the surrounding tissue, can lead to vasoconstriction, development of inflammatory processes, and microlesions. These in turn can affect the function or structure of nerves.[11] Injuries in athletes may occur as a result of extrinsic forces such as repetitive microtrauma, friction, compression, contusion, and traction. Traction may produce different degrees of stretch injury, often in continuity, but can lead to rupture or avulsion.[2] As several groups have reported, training-induced changes in peripheral nerves can occur even in noninjured athletes.[6, 20, 21] Table 18.1 presents a list of peripheral nerve injuries that have been related to particular sports.

Different temporal patterns of presentation can be described and are often correlated with the forces involved in the injuries.

Acute Injuries

These injuries are immediate and typically are easily identified. Open injuries may affect peripheral nerves in superficial locations, such as the peroneal nerve near the fibular neck or the median and ulnar nerves at the wrist. These open injuries may result in lacerations of nerves and associated vascular structures and may require urgent treatment.

A closed injury can occur with or without bony injury via the transfer of kinetic energy following direct impact. For example, the peroneal nerve may be directly injured at the fibular neck, such as after a tackle in American football, soccer, or rugby. In some cases this is associated with

a fibular neck fracture. Knee dislocations may result in a wide array of neurovascular injuries accompanying the orthopedic issues. These closed stretch injuries in severe cases can rupture the peroneal nerve and popliteal artery. Peroneal nerve palsy due to indirect trauma has also been reported. Even in mild ankle sprains, forces may be transmitted from the ankle up the leg to the peroneal nerve at the fibular neck.

After violent accidents during contact sports or motorized sports (snowmobiles), acute traction injuries may occur to the brachial plexus. They can vary, in the most benign form, from "stingers" to "prolonged burners" through to avulsion with permanent sequelae. Stingers, despite being underreported, are quite common (figure 18.1). They are well known in football players but also occur in wrestlers, weightlifters, boxers, and gymnasts. An injured player complains of transient pain, numbness, and weakness of the affected shoulder (C5) and arm (C6) that can last a few seconds to minutes and then resolve completely. Weakness affects the deltoids, spinati,

Table 18.1 Peripheral Nerve Injuries Associated With Particular Sports

Nerve	Type of injury	Site	Sports
Spinal accessory	Direct trauma Traction		Lacrosse, hockey, football
Suprascapular	Direct trauma Traction		DT—boxing, backpacking, fencing, parasailing T—volleyball, handball, wrestling
Long thoracic	Direct trauma Traction Inflammation		DT—football, wrestling, boxing T—golf (after missing the ball), gymnastics, rappelling
Axillary	Direct trauma Traction Entrapment	T—anterior shoulder dislocation E—quadrilateral space syndrome, hypertrophic teres minor	DT—football, wresting, hockey T—anterior shoulder dislocation E—baseball, volleyball, overhead throwing
Musculocutaneous	Traction Entrapment	T—shoulder dislocation E—coracobrachialis and biceps	E—ice hockey, bodybuilding
Radial	Direct trauma Traction Entrapment	DT—humerus fracture	T—arm wrestling FB—tennis, weightlifting, discus throw
Posterior interosseous	Entrapment Inflammation	FB—arcade of Frohse (leading supinator edge)	FB—tennis, racquetball, Frisbee

Nerve	Type of injury	Site	Sports
Median and branches	Direct trauma Entrapment	DT—carpal tunnel E—elbow region: pronator teres, flexor digitorum superficialis, lacertus fibrosus, Struther's ligament Wrist Carpal tunnel	E—weightlifting, baseball, golf
Digital	Direct trauma	DT—thumb	DT—mountain climbing, bowling (bowler's thumb), archery, tennis
Anterior interosseous	Traction Inflammation	E—proximal forearm fibrous bands	
Ulnar	Direct trauma Traction	DT—wrist (Guyon's canal) and elbow (cubital tunnel)	DT—wrist Wheelchair athletes, cyclists Elbow Weightlifting, wheelchair athletes, rowers, gymnasts, T-tennis
Pudendal	Direct trauma		Cyclists
Lateral femoral cutaneous	Direct trauma Traction	Inguinal ligament	DT—weightlifting belts, SCUBA T—gymnastics, rope skipping
Femoral	Direct trauma Traction	DT—retroperitoneal hematoma Femur fracture	DT and T—gymnastics, dancing, figure skating, long jump, football
Sciatic	Direct trauma Traction	DT—hip dislocation Femur fracture	DT—rugby, football T—yoga, cycling
Common peroneal and branches	Direct trauma Traction	T—knee dislocation DT—proximal fibula Anterior tarsal tunnel syndrome	T—knee dislocation DT—fibula: ice hockey, football, soccer, martial arts, surfing Anterior tarsal tunnel syndrome: tight footwear, ballet, skiing, skating
Tibial and branches	Direct trauma Traction	T—knee dislocation DT—foot Tarsal tunnel syndrome Foot Medial plantar nerve	T—knee dislocation DT—foot Running, hiking, hockey, jogger's foot (medial plantar nerve)
Digital	Direct trauma Traction	Toes Morton's neuroma, Joplin's neuroma	Toes Morton's neuroma, Joplin's neuroma Running, dance, stair stepping, martial arts

SCUBA, self-contained underwater breathing apparatus; T, traction; DT, direct trauma; E, entrapment, FB, fibrous band.

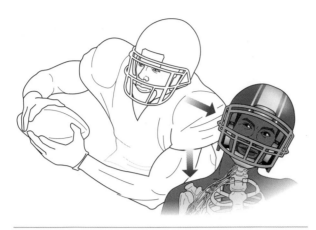

Figure 18.1 A "stinger" or "burner."

and biceps. It probably reflects a neuropraxia to C5 and C6 roots or nerves or the upper trunk. The exact mechanism and localization are not known. Approximately 10% of stingers may be prolonged. A small percentage of injuries may result in severe brachial plexus injuries in that distribution or even the entire distribution (C5-T1). Repeated stingers are common, affecting 50% of athletes with a previous stinger. These individuals may be at an increased risk for permanent injury and disability.

Subacute Injuries

Any delayed neurological symptom described many days or weeks after a sport-related injury should be evaluated thoroughly to rule out an important differential diagnosis that could be related or unrelated to the sport activity.

Vascular Lesions

Expanding masses, for example from hematomas from injured arteries or veins or pseudoaneurysms, should be remembered as potential causes of delayed nerve injury.

Swelling

Edema, hematoma, or muscle contusion can occur in a subacute manner too, but may require urgent treatment if it is within a closed anatomic location, such as at a "tunnel" or within a compartment.

Inflammatory Conditions

Inflammatory conditions are quite rare but may occur during this subacute time period. The

most common is Parsonage-Turner syndrome or idiopathic brachial plexitis or plexopathy. It is thought to be an inflammatory or immune-mediated disorder that must be considered as a differential diagnosis of upper limb injuries. Injuries (such as those occurring in sport) or surgery may trigger it. It typically begins with an intense periscapular pain that characteristically awakens the patient during the night and lasts about 2 weeks. When the pain disappears, the patient experiences weakness, often affecting certain nerves: dorsal scapular, suprascapular, axillary, long thoracic, anterior interosseous, and posterior interosseous. Weakness may take upward of 18 months to improve. On occasion, weakness and pain may persist.

Tumors

A long-distance runner with a schwannoma of the peroneal nerve was misdiagnosed as having exertional compartment syndrome of the leg. [20] Maceroli and colleagues reported an athletic adult with a history of recurrent knee pain with an expanding mass in the vicinity of the involved nerve who was treated for multifocal schwannomatosis.[19] Our group has described the association of peroneal intraneural ganglion cysts derived from the superior tibiofibular joint in individuals who suffered ankle sprains.

Chronic Injuries

Chronic injuries have one or more mechanisms, may be static or dynamic, and can manifest after months or years.[8] The increasing popularity of weight training and fitness among the population can explain these lesions in nonathletic patients as well.[4]

Overuse (Direct Microtrauma)

Overuse can be a major cause of neuropathy. Morton's metatarsalgia and Joplin's neuroma, both plantar digital nerve injuries, occur in runners and may result from cumulative trauma. With the recent great popularity of the martial arts, more traumatic neuralgia at the pressure points of strike has also been reported.[17]

Misuse

Some sports involve unusual movements reaching the extremes of the range of movement in a joint. These movements can occur against or without great resistance. Volleyball players and baseball pitchers, with their characteristic overhead hand movements and repetitive scapular rotation, may injure the suprascapular nerve at the suprascapular ligament.

Underlying Anatomical or Pathological Factors

Anatomical (congenital) variations and acquired pathologies may also result in nerve entrapment at common or uncommon sites. An anomalous fibrous band can constrict the nerve or impede its normal gliding. Any mass lesion could compromise the normal space, particularly within a tunnel—whether due to bone (such as a congenitally narrowed bony tunnel, an extra bone or bony fragment[24]), soft tissues (e.g., hypertrophied muscles or tenosynovitis), or mass lesions (ganglion cysts).

Scar tissue from previous trauma over a period of time can constrict and narrow the normal nerve gliding space, leading to compression. Examples of delayed neuropathy can occur after rupture of the semimembranosus muscle due to tethering of the sciatic nerve by a muscular branch,[3] or tearing of the external oblique muscle resulting in compression of the ilioinguinal nerve (so-called hockey groin syndrome).[15]

CLINICAL EVALUATION

The diagnosis of a sport-related peripheral nerve injury is mainly clinical. Knowledge of peripheral nerve anatomy and experience with these types of nerve injuries are essential. The clinician should be aware of the common sites and modalities of nerve injury, and the specialist should also be aware of anatomical variations and specifics unique to each sport.

A detailed history should address the type, mechanism, and timing of the injury. Historical information can be obtained from all sources, including videotapes, which if available can provide further insight into the mechanism of injury. The sequence of events that resulted in an injury, the site and the grade of injury, and its management must be clearly established, confirmed by supplementary tests, and discussed with the patient or responsible . For example, if

a patient has a foot drop following a hip dislocation, the clinician should be able to determine whether this deficit occurred immediately after the injury, or after the closed reduction or during open surgery or postoperatively, and whether the foot drop is a complete or partial injury to the peroneal and tibial divisions. A detailed history should be taken to specifically assess changes in motor and sensory function and the presence of pain.

The physical examination in the emergent setting should address the "ABCs." It is imperative to rule out life-threatening injuries including trauma to the head, spine, and major vessels after an accident. The neurological examination should focus on the evaluation of motor, sensory, and even autonomic function, as well as pain. Such a comprehensive assessment should allow establishment of the diagnosis and the correct localization of a lesion. The patient should be examined for atrophy (figure 18.2). Muscle power must be accurately assessed based not only on myotomes but also on detailed nerve distributions. A consistent grading scale should be used to record serial examinations and to minimize interobserver inconsistencies. Sensation must be checked in dermatomes and autonomous zones as well.

The presence of hypersensitivity (allodynia) should be noted following a peripheral nerve injury. Percussion tenderness, elicited by tapping along the anatomical course of the nerve, provides information relative to the level of injury. A Tinel's sign should be assessed by percussion of the nerve from distal to proximal along its course, checking for the extent of recovery. Note, however, that the presence of a Tinel's sign by itself, while it is a good sign, does not necessarily predict useful, functional recovery. Other provocative maneuvers may help localize the site of a nerve injury (e.g., Phalen's sign for carpal tunnel syndrome, elbow flexion test for cubital tunnel syndrome, Adson test for thoracic outlet syndrome). Autonomic changes may be noted, such as the absence of sweat in a peripheral nerve distribution, or even a Horner's syndrome following a brachial plexus injury (particularly to lower trunk elements). Areflexia is one of the hallmarks of a peripheral nerve injury. The presence of a brisk tendon reflex or an abnormal reflex (e.g., Babinski sign, clonus) must alert the surgeon to an upper motor neuron lesion; a peripheral

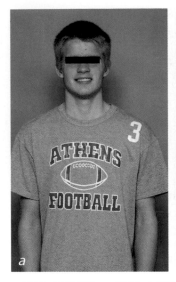
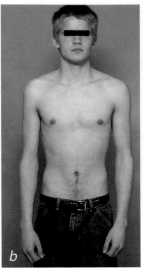
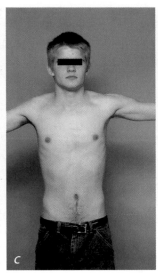
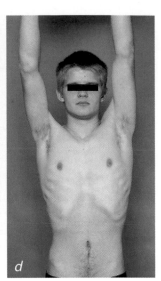

Figure 18.2 This young man (a) sustained a football-related injury. He presented with fatigability and decreased strength subjectively in his right shoulder. Because of his full range of motion, the diagnosis was delayed. He was found to have deltoid atrophy (b) and weakness (c) on testing of resisted shoulder abduction. A complete axillary nerve paralysis was confirmed clinically and electrophysiologically. Like many young athletes, he had full active range of motion (d). He compensated for the absent deltoid by using his supraspinatus muscle.

nerve injury can coexist with an associated spinal cord injury. Associated musculoskeletal injuries, such as tendon injury, can confuse and mimic a peripheral nerve injury, and these may occur in tandem.

ADDITIONAL TESTING

While the diagnosis of a peripheral nerve injury is essentially clinical, adjuvant studies often are invaluable in the complete assessment. They supplement, but do not replace, a good clinical examination. Electrophysiology can help localize the lesion or determine the severity and may be useful to compare to a prior examination. Imaging may allow "visualization" of pathology. These additional tests may be important for evaluating patients for recovery and for planning treatment.

Electrophysiological Testing

The timing of electromyography (EMG) and nerve conduction studies (NCS) is crucial to making a reliable diagnosis. There is little value in doing EMG until the process of Wallerian degeneration is complete (2-4 weeks). As denervated

muscles at this point, EMG will demonstrate fibrillations and positive sharp waves at rest. A thorough sampling of muscles is necessary. The neurophysiologist should work closely with the treating physician to ensure that the questions are answered. For example, paraspinal muscle should be carefully assessed if nerve root avulsion or proximal brachial plexus injury is a concern. As an evaluation of the recovery, the first sign of reinnervation shows up in the form of small nascent units. As with the Tinel's sign just discussed, the presence of motor units does not guarantee useful recovery of function.

Nerve conduction tests evaluate sensory and motor nerve conduction velocities and latency. Decreased or absent values signify peripheral nerve lesions. They are helpful in differentiating between nerve rupture and root avulsion, as the sensory nerve action potentials are absent in the rupture and present in the avulsion. Return of action potentials presages recovery after peripheral nerve injuries.

Radiology

While the clinical exam is the mainstay of diagnosis, a variety of neuroimaging options can be used as adjuncts in the assessment of athletes with suspected peripheral nerve injuries.

• Plain radiographs. Patients with acute nerve injuries must have X-rays of all bones suspected of being fractured or joints that may be dislocated. Radiographs might also be of value in patients with chronic traumatic neuralgia, revealing a small displaced fracture segment or an un- or malunited fracture or callus in the region of a nerve. A chest film might reveal a cervical rib or an elongated transverse process in patients diagnosed with thoracic outlet syndrome.

• Computed tomography (CT). Computed tomography is performed in some cases of associated bony injuries; CT myelography (or high-resolution magnetic resonance imaging) is widely used to determine nerve root avulsion(s) in a brachial plexus injury.

• Magnetic resonance imaging (MRI). This is an excellent imaging modality to visualize nerve and the related soft tissues following trauma. Its interpretation may be affected by the size of the nerve trunk imaged and the timing of the study,[10] not to mention the experience of the radiologist. High-resolution MRI (neurography) has expanded the role of imaging peripheral nerve.

• Ultrasound. Ultrasound is being used increasingly to image nerves related to entrapments, injuries, and mass lesions. It is a relatively simple technique that is readily available, reasonably priced, and well tolerated by the patient. It is noninvasive and radiation free. It can be done easily in the emergency room, the clinic, or the operating room. Ultrasonography may show nerve architecture and shape. Acutely, ultrasound can be used to distinguish a nerve in continuity from a transection or rupture or to show the presence of hematoma. In the chronic lesion, it could show a stump neuroma, a neuroma in continuity, and perilesional scar tissue.[7]

• Angiography. Magnetic resonance angiography can be used to document or rule out an associated vascular injury. It can clarify if there is a vascular component in patients with unclear clinical findings, such as those with suspected thoracic outlet or quadrilateral space syndromes. In select cases imaging may be performed with the limb in different positions. In some cases, invasive angiography may be necessary.

MANAGEMENT RATIONALE

The same principles and techniques used in the management of other types of peripheral nerve injuries should be applied to sport-related injuries. Early surgery (within days) is performed in rare circumstances. It is indicated in treating sharp and clean lacerations affecting nerve that can be primarily repaired. Most commonly, these nerve injuries can be repaired in an end-to-end fashion, without intervening nerve grafts (figure 18.3). Early surgery should also be considered for nerve lesions that evolve under observation, such as an expanding hematoma. Trauma associated with nerve injuries that need open reduction and internal fixation or vascular surgery may also benefit from exploration of the nerve to document the extent of injury or its continuity. At early surgery, nerves that are injured but in continuity should be decompressed. These patients should be observed closely, as described later, using serial clinical and electrophysiologic examinations.

Contaminated wounds can be debrided first. In this case, if nerve stumps are identified, they may be tacked down on some tension to fascial edges (diminishing the retraction of the stumps). Use of a long nonabsorbable suture or a radiopaque material may facilitate the safe identification of the nerve ends days later, after satisfactory treatment of the wound. Nerves with jagged ends from a blunt contusive injury may be similarly treated in a secondary fashion several weeks later when the full extent of the zone of injury is better demarcated.

Other injuries are managed nonoperatively, at least initially. These may include complete or incomplete lesions. During this period of time, management is based on rest, cessation of the offending activity, and the judicious use of pain medication or nonsteroidal anti-inflammatory agents or both. Pain should be addressed aggressively, sometimes requiring a multidisciplinary approach. Splints can be used to minimize contractures. Patients should receive a course of physical therapy for muscle strengthening and

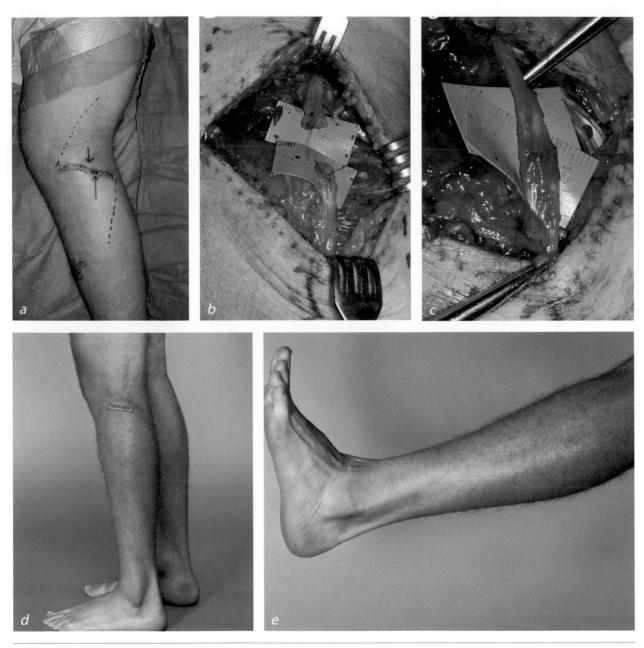

Figure 18.3 This hockey goalie sustained a skate injury to his popliteal crease. He had a foot drop and was found at routine exploration of the wound to have a lacerated common peroneal nerve near the popliteal crease (a). Sutures had been placed to identify the nerve ends (b). The common peroneal nerve was repaired directly (c) 1 week later at the time of his transfer to the authors' facility. He had an excellent recovery (d) with strong foot dorsiflexion, toe extension (e), and eversion. He returned to competitive sport.

maintenance or improvement in the range of motion. Appropriate changes should be made in the athlete's training regimen. Faulty equipment and unsound biomechanics should also be corrected. Equal importance should be given to maintaining the athlete's morale and psyche, as a nerve injury in a young adult can mean the end of a promising and possibly lucrative career and comfortable lifestyle.

Patients are closely monitored every 6 weeks clinically and, if required, electrophysiologically. Progressive improvement in motor and sensory function is the treatment goal. Spontaneous recovery has the highest rate of success. Absence of improvement (3-6 months after injury), severe or persistent pain, and delayed neurological deterioration are all indications for surgery in peripheral nerve lesions. In select cases, patients with persistent pain may benefit from nerve blocks. Depending on the agent, these can be used for diagnostic and occasionally therapeutic purposes. Positive responses to blocks may be helpful in their overall management.

SURGICAL OPTIONS: PRIMARY NERVE SURGERY

For the majority of injuries, a period of nonoperative care is suggested. Patients should have serial clinical and electrical studies during the 3 to 6 months following an injury to evaluate for any signs of reinnervation. For patients without timely evidence of reinnervation or with persistent symptoms or worsening exam, surgery is indicated.

• Decompression or neurolysis. Decompression generally refers to an unroofing procedure, such as the carpal tunnel or cubital tunnel. This can be performed acutely or chronically. External neurolysis involves a 360-degree mobilization of the nerve. As such, the nerve is freed up from any regional anatomic or pathologic structure. When surgery is performed several months after injury, nerve action potentials (NAPs) are widely used to assess neurologic function across a neural lesion. This intraoperative electrophysiologic technique may reveal recovery earlier than conventional preoperative EMG-NCS by measuring potentials across a lesion rather than in a distal target organ. Nerve action potentials have implications for treatment and outcomes.[2] An NAP across a lesion has been shown to result in good recovery after neurolysis in 90% of cases (figure 18.4). An absent NAP would not be expected to result in good recovery with neurolysis alone and therefore is better treated with a reconstructive procedure.

• Nerve reconstruction. With a variety of specialized surgeries, attempts can be made to restore a significant degree of function to patients who have suffered peripheral nerve injuries during athletic participation. Nerve reconstruction involves either direct surgical repair of nerves,

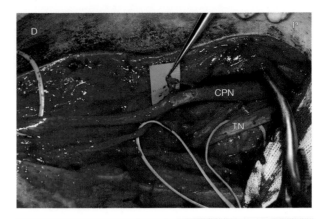

Figure 18.4 This young man sustained a football injury with a knee dislocation and multiple knee ligamentous disruptions. He had a complete foot drop that did not improve clinically or electrophysiologically. We were expecting the typical longitudinal stretch injury. At operation 6 months after the injury, we found a focal neuroma with some scarring (as seen on microbackground). External neurolysis was performed of the common peroneal nerve (CPN) and tibial nerve (TN) in the popliteal fossa. The CPN was decompressed at the fibular neck. To our surprise, nerve action potentials (NAPs) were obtained across the lesion. The patient demonstrated good return of function over the next 2 years. P, proximal; D, distal.

the use of nerve grafts, or performance of nerve transfers or ablations to help the patient regain function. The following is a list of the general types of nerve reconstruction.

• Direct repair. This is performed for a short nerve gap (transection, or after resection of a focal neuroma). This technique is preferred, whenever possible, as there is only one suture line across which axons need to grow. To minimize the nerve gap, the nerve stumps are mobilized. Where possible, to gain length, the ulnar nerve at the elbow or the radial nerve may be transposed. The stumps are recut until good fascicular structure is seen. The ends are then aligned using external and internal features. The microsurgical repair can be done with fine suture without tension (figure 18.3b and c).

• Nerve grafts. These are used to span a larger gap between nerve ends (either from a retracted transection-rupture or following the resection of a neuroma in continuity as assessed with NAPs). One or more (cable) grafts may be interposed to maximize cross-sectional area at the nerve ends. A variety of donor nerves can be used. Most commonly, the sural nerve is selected. Up to 40 cm of sural nerve can be safely harvested from an adult leg (figure 18.5).

- Nerve transfers. Transfers are used either in cases of preganglionic injuries in which no other options exist for nerve reconstruction (i.e., nerve grafting is not feasible) or for postganglionic injuries (i.e., to try to speed up recovery). An expendable functioning nerve, branch, or fascicle may be transferred to a more important but nonfunctioning recipient. First introduced for brachial plexus injuries, the use of nerve transfers has been extended to peripheral nerve injuries, due to improved outcomes with distal nerve transfers (i.e., closer to the target muscle) introduced in the past decade.

- Nerve ablation surgery. Resection of a painful nerve or a neuroma (such as from a cutaneous nerve, e.g., lateral femoral cutaneous nerve at the inguinal ligament) may occasionally be considered. The goal would be to position the newly sectioned nerve end in a more optimal location with the hope that the neuroma that forms will be painless. The management of neuropathic pain is controversial.

SURGICAL OPTIONS: SECONDARY SURGERY (SOFT TISSUE OR BONY RECONSTRUCTION)

In patients referred late (approximately >1 year from injury) or in those in whom primary nerve surgery has failed, other reconstructive techniques may be useful to augment or provide some degree of function. These include tendon–muscle or free-functioning muscle transfers, as well as joint fusions or osteotomies that can be performed by orthopedic or plastic surgeons.

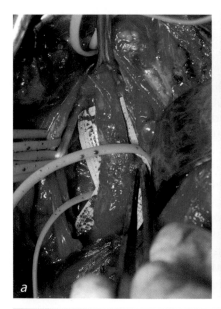 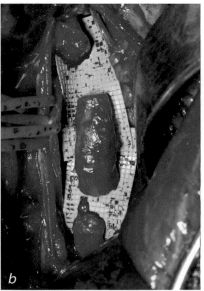 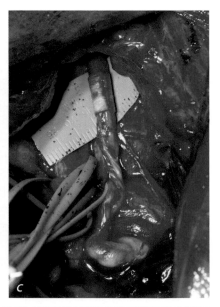

Figure 18.5 This college-level football player sustained a "prolonged" stinger after a blow from behind to his neck–shoulder region. He regained function within days but had persistent loss of shoulder strength. He continued to play despite subsequent stingers that resolved within minutes. He presented to the authors after not recovering deltoid function at 4 months. At exploration, a 6 cm lesion of the axillary nerve was noted (a). Stimulating and recording across it did not produce a nerve action potential. The neuroma was resected (b). Interpositional grafting was done using the sural nerve. Three cables were placed (c).

POSTOPERATIVE MANAGEMENT AND RETURN TO PLAY

After nerve reconstruction, patients are typically immobilized for several weeks. Following this period of time, they should resume physical therapy as previously described.

Nerve regeneration is a slow and laborious process. Athletes are not usually resigned to this. Their motivation and keen inclination to return to activity must be tempered by the necessity to heal. The patient should understand the time needed for recovery and should have realistic expectations of achievable goals, including the likelihood of returning not only to sport but also to the preinjury status. The treating physician must keep in mind that is what is acceptable or even a good result to the physician or a more sedentary patient may be a deep disappointment to the athlete, team members, and fans.

Athletes need to be treated on an individual basis, as there are only recommendations for these injuries and no specific evidence-based guidelines. Because the range of injuries and the demands based on level of participation are so diverse, return to sport is a very complicated issue.[5, 9, 16, 22] The simple notion of return to sport does not address return to all sports, all positions, or all levels of participation, let alone the temporal aspect—return during or after that game, that season, or a career? A single nerve injury cannot be compared to brachial plexus injury. For example, an athlete with an isolated axillary nerve lesion may have full active motion, compensating with a (hypertrophied) supraspinatus muscle. On the other extreme, a severe brachial plexus injury may result in significant global impairment of the limb. An amateur is not the same as a professional athlete. A recreational bicyclist is not exposed to the same demands as a football lineman. Predisposed risks are impossible to quantify. There are no easy answers.

In general, athletes in whom symptoms have resolved and examination and range of motion have normalized may return to sport. Normalization of EMG is not a requirement, as there may be persistent changes even when full strength is present. When it has been determined that players are able to return to play, they should be reexamined after the game and in the next few weeks. In general, athletes with neurologic deficits, persistent

pain, or restricted range of motion should not play and should be rehabilitated before return. Athletes should be instructed in proper techniques (e.g., for blocking or tackling), and their equipment can be modified. They should undergo strengthening and range of motion exercises. Persistent symptoms should signal further workup, serial exams, and adjuvant studies. All this aside, there are high-level athletes with neurologic deficits (e.g., even axillary nerve palsies) who compete.

In athletes who have experienced stingers, there are no contraindications for those with fewer than three episodes lasting <24 hours, full cervical range of motion, and no neurological deficit. A relative contraindication would be for those with three or more prior stingers or a prolonged stinger (lasting >24 hours). There are no absolute contraindications, and common sense must rule. The athlete's confidence should be reinforced with learning how to prevent further recurrence. Psychosocial support should be provided to encourage self-determination. The rehabilitation program should be closely supervised, hopefully facilitating a smooth and gradual progression to return to competitive activity.

LEGAL IMPLICATIONS

Suffice it to say that there are legal implications for the athlete and those treating the athlete with peripheral nerve injuries. A nerve injury in a young adult can curtail a promising and possibly lucrative career and glamorous lifestyle. Coaches, trainers, and physicians are potentially involved in important decisions related to returning to sport or ending careers that have serious ramifications. Neurologic injuries can also predispose to other neurologic or musculoskeletal injuries that must be considered. Frank discussions must be held. Good documentation is critical, and second opinions may be beneficial and supportive.

CONCLUDING THOUGHTS

Sport-related peripheral nerve injuries are common, occurring in a large number of sports and with a broad spectrum of presentations. They can occur as a result of micro- or macrotrauma, acutely or chronically. Acute nerve injuries are usually secondary to direct impact with great kinetic power involved. The diagnosis is primarily clinical but is often supplemented by additional electrophysiological or radiological tests. Initial management depends of the type of injury and the presence of associated lesions. Athletes with peripheral nerve injuries may benefit from mind and body rehabilitation, pain relief, and education to prevent reinjury. Surgery may be indicated for those with symptoms or findings that fail to improve or who have untreatable pain. Return to play depends on the results achieved with rehabilitation and the requirements of each sport.

REFERENCES

1. National Electronic Injury Surveillance System (NEISS) [https://www.cpsc.gov/cgibin/NEISS-Query/home.aspx]. 2010. Accessed October 25, 2012.

2. Neurological Sports Medicine: A Guide for Physicians and Athletic Trainers. Rolling Meadows, IL: American Association of Neurological Surgeons; 2001.

3. Bosnjak R, Mofardin S, Derham C. Delayed sciatic neuropathy after distal semimembranosus muscle rupture associated with tethering of the sciatic nerve by a rare distal muscular branch. Injury 2009;40(2):226-229.

4. Busche K. Neurologic disorders associated with weight lifting and bodybuilding. Neurol Clin 2008;26(1):309-324, xii.

5. Cantu RC. Stingers, transient quadriplegia, and cervical spinal stenosis: return to play criteria. Med Sci Sports Exerc 1997;29(7 Suppl):S233-235.

6. Capitani D, Beer S. Handlebar palsy—a compression syndrome of the deep terminal (motor) branch of the ulnar nerve in biking. J Neurol 2002;249(10):1441-1445.

7. Cokluk C, Aydin K. Ultrasound examination in the surgical treatment for upper extremity peripheral nerve injuries: part I. Turk Neurosurg 2007;17(4):277-282.

8. Colak T, Bamac B, Alemdar M, Macit Selekler H, Ozbek A, Colak S, et al. Nerve conduction studies of the axillary, musculocutaneous and radial nerves in elite ice hockey players. J Sports Med Phys Fitness 2009;49(2):224-231.

9. Cummins CA, Schneider DS. Peripheral nerve injuries in baseball players. Phys Med Rehabil Clin North Am 2009;20(1):175-193, x.

10. Du R, Auguste KI, Chin CT, Engstrom JW, Weinstein PR. Magnetic resonance neurography for the evaluation of peripheral nerve, brachial plexus, and nerve root disorders. J Neurosurg 2010;112(2):362-371.

11. Farkkila M, Pyykko I. Blood flow in the contralateral hand during vibration and hand grip contractions of lumberjacks. Scand J Work Environ Health 1979;5(4):368-374.

12. Finch C, Cassell E. The public health impact of injury during sport and active recreation. J Sci Med Sport 2006;9(6):490-497.

13. Finch C, Valuri G, Ozanne-Smith J. Sport and active recreation injuries in Australia: evidence from emergency department presentations. Br J Sports Med 1998;32(3):220-225.

14. Hirasawa Y, Sakakida K. Sports and peripheral nerve injury. Am J Sports Med 1983;11(6):420-426.

15. Irshad K, Feldman LS, Lavoie C, Lacroix VJ, Mulder DS, Brown RA. Operative management of "hockey groin syndrome": 12 years of experience in National Hockey League players. Surgery 2001;130(4):759-764; discussion 764-756.

16. Jeyamohan S, Harrop JS, Vaccaro A, Sharan AD. Athletes returning to play after cervical spine or neurobrachial injury. Curr Rev Musculoskelet Med 2008;1(3-4):175-179.

17. Kelly MD. Traumatic neuralgia from pressure-point strikes in the martial arts: results from a retrospective online survey. J Am Osteopath Assoc 2008;108(6):284-287.

18. Krivickas LS, Wilbourn AJ. Peripheral nerve injuries in athletes: a case series of over 200 injuries. Semin Neurol 2000;20(2):225-232.

19. Maceroli M, Uglialoro AD, Beebe KS, Benevenia J. Recurrent knee pain in an athletic adult: multiple schwannomas secondary to schwannomatosis: a case report. Am J Orthop (Belle Mead NJ) 2010;39(11):E119-122.

20. Paladini D, Dellantonio R, Cinti A, Angeleri F. Axillary neuropathy in volleyball players: report of two cases and literature review. J Neurol Neurosurg Psychiatry 1996;60(3):345-347.

21. Pawlak M, Kaczmarek D. Field hockey players have different values of ulnar and tibial motor nerve conduction velocity than soccer and tennis players. Arch Ital Biol 2010;148(4):365-376.

22. Podlog L, Eklund RC. Returning to competition after a serious injury: the role of self-determination. J Sports Sci 2010;28(8):819-831.

23. Spinks AB, McClure RJ. Quantifying the risk of sports injury: a systematic review of activity-specific rates for children under 16 years of age. Br J Sports Med 2007;41(9):548-557; discussion 557.

24. Spinner RJ, Atkinson JL, Wenger DE, Stuart MJ. Tardy sciatic nerve palsy following apophyseal avulsion fracture of the ischial tuberosity. Case report. J Neurosurg 1998;89(5):819-821.

25. Toth C, McNeil S, Feasby T. Peripheral nervous system injuries in sport and recreation: a systematic review. Sports Med 2005;35(8):717-738.

part V

OTHER SPORTS-RELATED NEUROLOGICAL ISSUES

Headaches are common in the general population. The athlete, though, may present with one of three types of headache: (1) headaches unrelated to athletic activity; (2) headaches that are exertion or activity related; and (3) those that are posttraumatic. An understanding of the various types of headaches allows for accurate diagnosis and subsequently effective treatment. The workup of an athlete presenting with headaches is reviewed in this part of the book.

Another neurologic issue that affects athletes is heat illness, including heat-stroke. Heatstroke is the most serious form of heat injury and is a medical emergency. Heatstroke often occurs as a progression from milder heat-related illnesses such as heat cramps, heat syncope (fainting), and heat exhaustion. It results from prolonged exposure to high temperatures, usually in combination with dehydration, which leads to failure of the body's temperature control system. In this section we also review the evaluation and management of the athlete with heat illness or heatstroke.

Headaches in Athletics

Headaches are extremely common, affecting millions of people each year. They vary in pain intensity, pattern, and location from individual to individual. In men, the lifetime prevalence is 93% for headache of any kind, 8% for migraine, and 69% for tension-type headache.[46] For women, the lifetime prevalence is 99% for headache of any kind, 25% for migraine, and 88% for tension-type headache.[46] In children, headache prevalence increases from 39% at the age of 6 to 70% at the age of 15 years.[46] Clearly widespread, headache is a costly public health problem. Despite the substantial impact, the needs of many people with headache are unmet.[14, 20] Although irritating, the majority of headaches do not require medical intervention. Athletes arc a particular subset of patients who can experience headaches specific to their sports.[35] Despite the high prevalence of headache in community populations, the epidemiology of sport-related headache is unclear. One study surveyed 178 medical students and 190 physical education students and demonstrated that 35% of both groups suffered from sport- and exercise-related headaches.[51, 52] In any case, headache can have an impact on sport at both the amateur and elite levels, and an understanding of the relationship between sport and headache, as well as options for management, is important for health care practitioners at all levels.

CLINICAL APPROACH AND ASSESSMENT

Headache is a nonspecific symptom, which means that it may have many possible causes. The brain does not have pain receptors on its surface, so headaches are usually due to disturbance of pain-sensitive structures around the brain, which can include the dural pain fibers, periosteum of the skull, muscles, nerves, arteries and veins, subcutaneous tissue, mucous membranes, and sinuses.

The key to correct diagnosis and effective treatment of an athlete with headaches lies in a detailed history.[35] A thorough assessment will aid the practitioner in trying to narrow down what type of headache is being experienced. The evaluation should include eliciting a detailed history of symptoms—namely, the location, severity, and frequency of the headache as well as the characteristic nature of the pain (e.g., throbbing, pressure-like, sharp, stabbing). Questioning about medication history and alleviating or aggravating factors also provides useful information. Preceding or other associated symptoms should also be considered, such as nausea, vomiting, diarrhea, vertigo, nasal congestion, lacrimation, weakness, sensory symptoms, dysarthria, confusion, or visual disturbances. Other factors that must be considered include history of non–sport-related headaches, family history of headaches, prior and current illnesses, excessive caffeine intake, psychosocial factors, and substance abuse.[35] In addition to a thorough neurological evaluation, a percentage of athletes with headaches will need to have a magnetic resonance imaging (MRI) scan of the brain.[35] One study found that in 103 patients with exertional headaches, 10 had an organic lesion that was identified on imaging as accounting for the headaches.[44]

There are numerous classification systems for headaches that have strict diagnostic criteria; however, these are undoubtedly more relaxed in practical clinical practice. While these classification systems have been instrumental in helping to establish uniform terminology and consistent diagnostic criteria for a range of headache disorders, they are sometimes inadequate to distinguish between different subtypes of sport headaches. The most well-recognized system is that of the International Headache Society (IHS).[1] The IHS classification has been endorsed by the World Health Organization (WHO) and incorporated into the International Classification of Diseases (ICD). Still, others think about sport headache in terms of a framework similar to that proposed by Williams and Nukada.[52] Kernick and Goadsby agreed that from a practical perspective, the classification can be somewhat cumbersome in specific settings such as sport; in their paper they defined four categories of sport-related headache, providing a pragmatic organization for practitioners.[23] The following overview of the most common types of headache and those associated with sporting activities is an attempt to bridge these different classification schemes.

International Headache Society (IHS) Classification of Headaches

Primary Headaches

- Migraine
- Tension-type headache
- Cluster headache and other trigeminal autonomic cephalgias
- Other primary headaches

Secondary Headaches

- Headache attributed to head or neck trauma or both
- Headache attributed to cranial or cervical vascular disorder
- Headache attributed to nonvascular intracranial disorder
- Headache attributed to a substance or its withdrawal
- Headache attributed to infection
- Headache attributed to disorder of homeostasis
- Headache or facial pain attributed to disorder of cranium, neck, eyes, ears, nose, sinuses, teeth, mouth, or other facial or cranial structures
- Headache attributed to psychiatric disorder

Cranial Neuralgias, Central and Primary Facial Pain, and Other Headaches

- Cranial neuralgias and central causes of facial pain
- Other headache, cranial neuralgia, central or primary facial pain

Note: Each of these categories has subcategories within that are beyond the scope of this discussion. Further detailed information and classification can be found at http://ihs-classification.org/en/.

Headache Framework Proposed by Williams and Nukada

- Effort–exertional headache
- Effort migraine
- Trauma-triggered migraine
- Posttraumatic headache

Adapted from Williams and Nukada 1994.

Sport-Related Headache Classification as Proposed by Kernick and Goadsby

- A recognized headache syndrome (migraine, tension-type headache, cluster headache) coincidental to sporting activity
- A recognized headache syndrome (migraine, tension-type headache) induced by sporting activity
- Headache arising from mechanisms that occur during exertion (these can be primary where the exact mechanism is not understood, or secondary where a direct causal factor can be demonstrated):
  - Headache related to changes in cardiovascular parameters (increase in cardiac output and raised venous pressure)

- Headache related to trauma
- Headache arising from structures in the neck
- Headache arising from mechanisms that are specific to an individual sport

Reprinted, by permission, from D.P. Kernick and P.J. Goadsby, 2011, "Guidance for the management of headache in sport on behalf of The Royal College of General Practitioners and The British Association for the Study of Headache," Cephalalgia 31(1): 106-111.

COMMONLY RECOGNIZED HEADACHE SYNDROMES COINCIDENTAL TO SPORTING ACTIVITY

The most common types of headache are the "primary headache disorders"; these include headaches such as migraine, tension-type headache, and cluster headaches. They all have typical features and are relatively common. These headaches may occur coincidental to athletic participation, and it is important to recognize their characteristic features to help guide management.

Migraine

Migraine is a common primary headache disorder that affects 15% of women and 6% of men.[29] The lifetime prevalence of migraine is 16%; however, the prevalence can vary with age and is at its highest between the ages of 25 to 55 years for both males and females.[42, 43] After the age of 55, prevalence falls for both sexes. Before the age of 12, migraine is more common in boys; but postpuberty, migraine is substantially more common in females.[42, 43] At 20 years of age, the ratio approaches 2 to 1 (females to males).[29] This ratio peaks at ages 40 to 44, approximating a ratio of 3 to 1 (females to males), and then drops to 2.5 to 1 (females to males) by the age of 70.[29] Although regular exercise can help reduce the frequency, intensity, and duration of migraine attacks,[12, 13] migraine is likely to be the most common coincidental primary headache during sport.[23]

Migraine headaches are characterized by an intense, throbbing, or pounding pain that is felt periodically in the forehead, temple, ear, or jaw or around the eye. It is often unilateral. Migraines are also frequently called vascular headaches because of the vascular system abnormalities thought to possibly give the headache its throbbing or pulsatile characteristic. A migraine headache can last anywhere from 3 hours to 3 days (and in some cases even longer). Often there is a prodrome or early headache. Sometimes, before the pain, patients experience an aura that may consist of seeing flashing lights, stars, or other white objects. If it occurs, an aura can last about 15 to 20 minutes. This type is often referred to as a classic migraine.

The symptoms that occur before the migraine can vary, though. They may involve the autonomic nervous system (symptoms such as flushing), the neurological system (i.e., numbness, tingling, problems with speech and even temporary paralysis on one side of the body), or the muscular system (spasm and muscle pain typically in the neck). Nausea and vomiting may also occur during or after the migraine attack. Factors that commonly predispose people to migraine headaches can include changes in altitude, metabolic changes, changes in medications, changes in blood pressure, hormonal changes, changes in sleeping patterns, and even variations in diet.

For the acute attack, triptans, serotonin 5-HT1B/1D receptor agonists, are the mainstay of treatment.[23] The experience of administration during sport is limited. McCrory and colleagues studied the use of intranasal sumatriptan for 38 migraine attacks in Australian rules football players.[37] There was a good response with no major side effects, but minor side effects were reported in over 70% of cases. Apart from the potential impact of triptans on cognitive performance, there are theoretical concerns regarding the potential for coronary vasoconstriction.[23] For the amateur player, a nonsteroidal anti-inflammatory, with or without an antiemetic, would be a simple and generally safe first choice.[23] If triptans were to be needed during sport in amateurs or in elite players, underlying cardiac pathology such as ischemic heart disease, conduction abnormalities, and cardiomyopathy should be excluded with an exercise electrocardiogram (ECG) and echocardiogram. If cleared for use, any of the first-line triptans, such as sumatriptan, almotriptan, eletriptan, rizatriptan, or zolmitriptan, represent reasonable first choices.[23] Nasal sprays have the theoretical advantage of faster action and to some extent are able to bypass gastrointestinal absorption limitations. A poor response or lack thereof to a triptan may not represent a class effect, and an alternative from the class should be tried. Abortive treatment of a migraine also can begin with nonsteroidal anti-inflammatory drugs (NSAIDs), although these are often ineffective. Combination drugs that contain butalbital and caffeine (Fiorinal, Fiori-cet, Esgic) or ergotamine and caffeine (Wigraine tablets, Cafergot) can alternatively be used. [35] The amount of these medications should be limited, as excessive NSAID use and caffeine intake, including dietary caffeine and caffeine in over-the-counter drugs, can cause refractory rebound headaches.

In routine practice, the first-line medications to use for the preventive treatment of migraine are beta-blockers. Propranolol is commonly used, but atenolol is convenient and cheap and probably works just as well. The use of beta-blockers in many sports, though, has obvious implications, including limitation of performance (by limiting the heart rate increase necessary for strenuous activities) and the fact that that they are banned in many professional sports. For that reason, calcium channel blockers such as verapamil are sometimes preferred for migraine headache prophylaxis. Although the evidence is limited across the board, topiramate, sodium valproate, and gabapentin are reasonable alternative choices so long as appropriate monitoring for potential side effects is undertaken.

Tension–Type Headaches

Tension-type headaches are the most common type of primary headache disorder. As with migraine, this is a disorder of middle life, with a peak prevalence between the ages of 20 and 50 years, followed by a decline. These headaches tend to occur more frequently in women, with a ratio of 1.4:1 (females to males).[46] Studies have shown that episodic tension-type headaches account for approximately 90% of all head-aches.[1, 39, 46] These headaches can be classified as either episodic or chronic. Individuals with episodic tension-type headaches may also be at an increased risk of developing chronic tension-type headaches. This condition, although less common, affects 2.6% of females and 1.6% of males.[46]

Tension-type headaches are typically dull, occipital, and bilateral. The pain is often described as a constant pressure, as if the head were being squeezed in a vice, and it can radiate from the lower back of the head, the neck, the eyes, or other muscle groups in the body. Tension-type headache pain is typically mild to moderate but may be severe. The headaches can interfere with daily living, and many patients report having to discontinue or significantly limit their normal activity. Episodic tension-type headaches are defined as tension-type headaches occurring fewer than 15 days a month, whereas chronic tension headaches occur 15 days or more a month for at least 6 months.[1] The headaches can last from minutes to days, months, or even years, though a typical tension headache lasts 4 to 6 hours.

The exact cause or causes of tension headache are unknown. Prior popular belief maintained that the pain of tension headache stemmed from muscle contraction in the face, neck and scalp, perhaps as a result of heightened emotions, tension, or stress; however, current research suggests that there doesn't appear to be a significant increase in muscle tension in people diagnosed with tension headache. Other common theories support interference or "mixed signals" involving nerve pathways to the brain, which is demonstrated by a heightened sensitivity to pain in people who have tension headaches. Thus increased muscle tenderness, a common symptom of tension headache, may actually be the result of overactive pain receptors. Potential triggers can include stress, depression and anxiety, poor posture, working in awkward positions or holding one position for a long time, jaw clenching, eyestrain, or sleep deprivation.

Episodic tension-type headaches generally respond well to over-the-counter analgesia and are even usually improved by exercise.[23] Amitriptyline is usually a first-line pharmacologic treatment option for the management of chronic tension-type headaches. Tricyclic antidepressants are effective, although they can produce somnolence and dry mouth, which can interfere with athletic performance.[35] Newer selective serotonin reuptake inhibitor (SSRI)-type antidepressants can be effective with fewer side effects, although controlled studies in headache patients have not been done.[35] In 2009, a Cochrane

Database review concluded that acupuncture could serve as a valuable nonpharmacologic option in patients with frequent episodic or chronic tension-type headaches.[28] In general, these types of headaches are unlikely to be a problem in athletics.[23]

Cluster Headaches

Cluster headache is a rare condition that involves, as its most prominent feature, an immense degree of pain that is almost always on only one side of the head. The primary headache disorder is uncommon, affecting approximately 0.1% to 0.4% of the general population. The headache occurs predominantly in males, with a 9:1 ratio (males to females).[46, 49] Some have described the pain resulting from cluster headaches as the most intense pain a human can endure—worse than burns, broken bones, or childbirth. Many cluster headache sufferers have committed suicide, leading to the nickname "suicide headache" for this type of headache.

Cluster headaches are excruciating unilateral headaches of extreme intensity.[4, 9] The pain is usually periorbital and occurs in short bursts over a "cluster period." The duration of the common cluster headache ranges from as little as 15 minutes to 3 hours or more. The onset of an attack is rapid and most often without the preliminary signs that are characteristic of a migraine. The majority of attacks occur daily for 6 to 8 weeks, typically once or twice a year, with spontaneous resolution. Cluster headaches often occur periodically with spontaneous remissions interrupting active periods of pain, although there are 20% of sufferers whose cluster headaches never remit. The cause of the condition is currently unknown.

These headaches are frequently accompanied by associated autonomic symptoms. Usually at least one of the following autonomic symptoms occurs: ptosis (drooping eyelid), miosis (pupil constriction), conjunctival injection (redness of the conjunctiva), lacrimation (tearing), rhinorrhea (runny nose), and, less commonly, facial blushing, swelling, or sweating, all appearing on the same side of the head as the pain.[4, 9] The attack can also be associated with restlessness and, less frequently, photo- or phonophobia. Nausea rarely accompanies a cluster headache, though it has been reported.

Sporting activity is unlikely during the cluster period.[23] Although frequently used as a symptomatic agent in the general population, short-term oral steroids are contraindicated for the elite athlete. During the onset of a cluster headache, many people respond to inhalation of 100% oxygen, and in studies this has been found to be quite an effective treatment.[11] Triptans, either intranasal sumatriptan or zolmitriptan or subcutaneous sumatriptan, are effective at improving symptoms during an attack or even in aborting attacks.[17, 26] Cardiovascular concerns are the same as those outlined for the treatment of migraine. For prolonged bouts of episodic or for chronic cluster headache, verapamil is the preventive agent of choice but may cause cardiac conduction delays, and monthly ECGs should be undertaken.[23] It is best avoided in elite athletes, though, where lithium or topirimate can be used. Greater occipital nerve injection may be a useful intervention in episodic cluster headache, but again, steroids are contraindicated for the elite athlete.[2, 23]

PROLONGED SPORTING ACTIVITY AS A TRIGGER FOR COMMONLY RECOGNIZED HEADACHE SYNDROMES

It is not uncommon for people to experience these primary headache disorders as a result of athletic participation. There is no evidence that cluster headache is induced by sporting activity, and most tension-type headaches are self-limiting and do not restrict athletic participation. Athletes with predisposition to migraine, however, may have prolonged exertion as one trigger for a typical migraine. It has been noted that over 20% of people with a migraine headache disorder experience migraines precipitated by physical activity.[22] In one report, exercise- or effort-induced migraine was seen in 9% of 128 patients studied.[51] The authors reported that in the study participants, such headaches often began in childhood or adolescence, with average age at onset of 15. Aura was noticed by all and nausea by the majority, and vomiting and neck stiffness were frequent. The headache was typical of migraine headaches, with a characteristic moderate to severe throbbing, and lasted for hours. The authors suggested that low oxygen tension could possibly trigger effort-induced migraine in these patients by an as yet unknown mechanism.[51]

The exercise- or effort-induced migraine headache does not typically resolve when the activity is discontinued. The headache may occur minutes or hours into the activity or after cessation of activity. For a headache to occur with prolonged exertion, additional triggers may be required, such as heat, altitude, bright light, dehydration, low blood sugar, or some combination of these. [25] The evaluation of the athlete with exertion as one trigger for migraine is the same as that for any patient presenting with headache.[25] Special emphasis on triggers related to the sporting activity should be reviewed; these may include the use of equipment, environmental factors (e.g., sunlight or altitude), or diet.[25]

Although the evidence is fairly thin, it has been reported that exercise-induced migraine can be prevented by aerobic warm-up before activity. [24] Another reasonable approach would be to treat with indomethacin 1 hour before onset of exertion. If this is not successful, titrating the dose up and treating over the 24-hour period before exertion may be considered. Alternatively, one could consider a triptan dosed appropriately before exertion.[23] Similarly, if the elite athlete has consistent problems, a triptan administered 30 to 60 minutes before activity, with the aforementioned caveats, could be tried; however, the experience with triptans used in this way is not positive. Therefore, if an athlete has consistent problems with sport-induced migraine, it may be best to start preventive pharmacotherapy as outlined earlier.

PRIMARY EXERTIONAL HEADACHE

The IHS criteria classify a primary exertional headache as a pulsating headache lasting from 5 minutes to 48 hours and brought on by and occurring only during or after physical exertion, for which no underlying cause can be identified. [1] Exertional- and effort-induced headaches are grouped together in the IHS classification. While they have many features in common, there are some clear differences between the two.

Exertional headache appears to be a response to lifting, pushing, pulling, or a similar activity. Included, as precipitating causes, are also sexual activity, coughing, sneezing, or straining at stool. The Valsalva maneuver is a common denominator among all of these activities. Exertional headaches are seen in a variety of sports. They are not necessarily in response to maximal physical effort; very often a headache occurs at submaximal activity and even at the beginning of exercise.[35] Effort-induced headache is a type of headache described by several authors as a response to aerobic activities such as running or swimming.[32, 35] The majority of these patients have a headache of a migraine type. The cardiovascular physiological processes that occur during sport can induce primary exertional headaches and can be separated most simply into those that occur with increased cardiac output and increased venous pressure.

Headache Associated With Increased Cardiac Output

Headache associated with exercise when cardiac output is raised is the most common type of sporting headache.[23] The true underlying mechanism is unknown. The headache is often described as migraine-like in character, exacerbated in hot weather and at altitude and typically occurring during the period of maximum effort, although it can be experienced during warm-up or after exertion.[23] A possible mechanism of these headaches is hyperventilation leading to vasoconstriction that triggers a reactive vasodilation with a resultant migraine-type headache.[35]

To investigate possible structural abnormalities and hence a secondary headache disorder, all effort-induced headaches should be investigated with an MRI of the brain; blood pressure and ECG; and screening labs for renal and liver function, thyroid disease, and diabetes. Sending urine to be evaluated for catecholamines may also be warranted. Arnold-Chiari malformations, a structural abnormality that involves cerebellar ectopia through the foramen magnum and neoplasms, are the most common secondary pathologies.

When a secondary cause has been excluded, evidence for the treatment of primary exercise-induced headache is anecdotal.[23] As mentioned earlier, gradual warm-up exercise routines have been advocated.[24] As also noted previously, indomethacin is the treatment of choice, but if the headaches occur more frequently, a beta-blocker can be used as a preventive pharmacotherapy providing there is no contraindication for the athlete. The evidence supporting pharmacotherapy specifically for sport-induced migraine headaches is limited; however, most medications used for the nonathlete are also alternative options.

Headache Associated With Increased Venous Pressure

This headache is more common in sports such as weightlifting and presumably caused by distension of the cerebral venous system.[23] The prevalence is unknown in sport, as most combine this type of headache with exercise- or effort-induced headache. Prior IHS criteria have typically classified this type of headache as a subform of primary exertional headache; but because of its sudden onset and presumed mechanism, it may have more similarities to primary cough headache. An important secondary cause is an Arnold-Chiari malformation, which must be excluded with a MRI of the head. The diagnostic criteria for this type of headache comprise sudden onset lasting from 1 second to 30 minutes, brought on and occurring only in association with coughing, straining, or Valsalva maneuver.[1] As with exercise-induced headaches, indomethacin is claimed to be effective in some instances.[23]

HEADACHES ATTRIBUTED TO HEAD OR NECK TRAUMA

The IHS views headaches related to trauma as secondary headache disorders. Acute posttraumatic headaches can be due to mild, moderate, or severe head injury. Headaches related to mild traumatic brain injury carry considerable overlap with those headaches seen in postconcussion syndrome. According to the IHS criteria, acute posttraumatic headache attributed to moderate or severe head injury involves moderate or severe head trauma with at least one of the following: loss of consciousness for >30 minutes, Glasgow Coma Scale (GCS) <13, posttraumatic amnesia

for >48 hours, or imaging demonstration of a traumatic brain lesion (contusion, intracerebral or subarachnoid hemorrhage or both, skull fracture).[1] The headache typically develops within 7 days after head trauma or after the regaining of consciousness following head trauma, and resolves within 3 months after head trauma. Chronic posttraumatic headache is a headache that persists for 3 months after head trauma and may be due to maladaptive central sensitization.

The mechanisms that generate pain in these posttraumatic headaches are poorly understood.[48] The headaches may be due to direct stress acting on dural structures or secondary mechanisms due to bleeding or axonal damage. A variety of pain patterns may develop, most of which resemble those of primary headache disorders such as tension-type headache, migraine headache (footballer's migraine), or rarely a cluster-like syndrome.[16, 18, 30, 33, 34, 45, 50] Alternatively, a preexisting primary headache can be made worse in close temporal relationship to trauma. The degree of injury does not always correlate with headache symptoms. Management of prolonged posttraumatic headaches is similar to that in nontraumatic cases.

Headache can arise from trauma to structures in the neck as well. Trauma to the neck can induce or exacerbate a cervical lesion with subsequent referred pain to the head via the upper cervical nerves. Cervicogenic headache is a syndrome characterized by chronic hemicranial pain that is referred to the head from either bony structures or soft tissues of the neck. The condition's pathophysiology and source of pain have been debated, but the pain is likely referred from one or more muscular, neurogenic, osseous, articular, or vascular structures in the neck.[5-8, 15, 27, 41] The trigeminocervical nucleus is a region of the upper cervical spinal cord where sensory nerve fibers in the descending tract of the trigeminal nerve (trigeminal nucleus caudalis) are believed to interact with sensory fibers from the upper cervical roots. This functional convergence of upper cervical and trigeminal sensory pathways allows the bidirectional referral of painful sensations between the neck and trigeminal sensory receptive fields of the face and head.[7, 8] A functional convergence of sensorimotor fibers in the spinal accessory nerve (CN XI) and upper cervical nerve roots ultimately converge with the descending tract of the trigeminal nerve and might also be responsible for the referral of cervical pain to the head.[7, 8]

Diagnostic criteria have been established for cervicogenic headache, but its presenting characteristics occasionally may be difficult to distinguish from primary headache disorders such as migraine or tension-type headache. A comprehensive history, review of systems, and physical examination including a complete neurological assessment is necessary. Patients with cervicogenic headache often have altered neck posture or restricted cervical range of motion.[19] The head pain can be triggered or reproduced by active neck movement, passive neck positioning especially in extension or extension with rotation toward the side of pain, or application of digital pressure to the involved facet regions or over the ipsilateral greater occipital nerve.[5] Additionally, muscular trigger points are usually found in the suboccipital, cervical, and shoulder musculature. These trigger points can also refer pain to the head when manually or physically stimulated. There are no neurological findings of cervical radiculopathy, though the patient might report scalp paresthesia or dysesthesia.[5] Imaging and laboratory studies may also aid in the diagnosis of cervicogenic headache. Zygapophyseal joint, cervical nerve, or medial branch blockade is used to confirm the diagnosis of cervicogenic headache and predict the treatment modalities that will most likely provide the greatest efficacy.[5]

The successful treatment of cervicogenic headache usually requires a multifaceted approach using pharmacologic, nonpharmacologic, manipulative, anesthetic, and occasionally surgical interventions.[31] Medications alone are often ineffective or provide only modest benefit for this condition.[5]

HEADACHES ATTRIBUTED TO SPORT–SPECIFIC MECHANISMS

A number of headaches unique to a sport have been described that have specific mechanistic etiologies. For example, any type of constrictive headwear can cause an external compression headache. This includes headwear that places pressure on the head—including tight hats, helmets, headbands, and goggles. It is not known why some people are more sensitive than others

to this type of pressure. The headaches seem to be more common among people who have migraines. This supraorbital neuralgia is also referred to as "swimmer's headache" or "swim-goggle headache," as it has been described frequently in swimmers due to pressure from their goggles[38, 40] (figure 19.1). It has also been described in hockey players due to the pressure of their helmets.[35] This type of headache is usually dull and located in the temporal and occipital areas, but it can have features of a migraine headache with all the typical manifestations, including an aura.[35] Loosening or avoiding the constrictive equipment (i.e., goggles or helmet) can prevent or stop a headache. Another example of sport-specific headache is in spinning figure skaters. The headache is thought to be due to a centrifugal effect that causes microscopic intracranial ischemia.[47] "Diver's headache" is another sport-specific headache that occurs as a result of carbon dioxide intoxication during diving.[10, 36] Headaches in divers can also be induced by a cold stimulus or can be a symptom associated with decompression illness.

Another common form of headache in sport is the muscle contraction type. It is described as an achy or tight sensation, pressure, or constriction, especially in the back of the neck, that often causes headaches in the back of the head and the temple region. Muscle contraction headache has been described that is triggered by the gripping of a mouthpiece, causing strain of facial and cervical muscles.[35] The neck and head pain is increased with tension and stress and often occurs daily. A high association of temporomandibular joint syndrome has been noted with this type of headache. Massage therapy or physical therapy is often helpful for this condition.

High-altitude headache is recognized as an accompaniment of acute mountain sickness and is thought to be due to a vascular phenomenon.[3] A study by Jokl and colleagues described a migraine-like headache in runners at the 1968 Olympics in Mexico City (7,000 feet [2,134 m] above sea level).[21] The authors went on to note an absence of headaches in these well-trained athletes at sea level. Altitude-triggered headache typically begins at approximately 3,000 meters above sea level.[35] Above 5,000 meters, patients can develop acute cerebral edema and may need prompt medical intervention with immediate, rapid descent, oxygen, and steroids.[35] The mildest mountain sickness syndrome also includes nausea, vomiting, and fatigue. The headache is throbbing in character, increases with any physical activity, and occurs after 6 to 96 hours of exposure. These headaches can resolve with acclimatization but may require treatment.

CONCLUDING THOUGHTS

The burden of illness associated with headache disorders is substantial and includes an individual as well as a societal burden. The individual burden is determined by the symptoms during the attack, by anticipation of symptoms between attacks, and by decreased quality of life in individuals who suffer from headache. The societal burden includes both direct (i.e., cost of medical care) and indirect (i.e., impact on work, school) economic costs. In the case of headaches and sport, clearly these painful disorders can affect recreational activities.

The pathogenesis of the majority of these headaches is poorly understood, and different types of activity may lead to different pathophysiological mechanisms. Further research is needed to define more accurately the scope of the problem. A better understanding of the pathophysiological mechanisms involved in sport-related headaches will lead to improved options for management. An awareness of the role of headaches in athletics on the part of the general practitioner, the sports physician, and those involved in sport at all levels will allow for more efficient and effective care.

REFERENCES

1. The International Classification of Headache Disorders: 2nd edition. Cephalalgia 2004;24 Suppl 1:9-160.
2. Ambrosini A, Vandenheede M, Rossi P, Aloj F, Sauli E, Pierelli F, et al. Suboccipital injection with a mixture of rapid- and long-acting steroids in cluster headache: a double-blind placebo-controlled study. Pain 2005;118(1-2):92-96.
3. Appenzeller O. Altitude headache. Headache 1972;12(3):126-129.
4. Beck E, Sieber WJ, Trejo R. Management of cluster headache. Am Fam Physician 2005;71(4):717-724.
5. Biondi DM. Cervicogenic headache: a review of diagnostic and treatment strategies. J Am Osteopath Assoc 2005;105(4 Suppl 2):16S-22S.
6. Biondi DM. Cervicogenic headache: diagnostic evaluation and treatment strategies. Curr Pain Headache Rep 2001;5(4):361-368.
7. Biondi DM. Cervicogenic headache: mechanisms, evaluation, and treatment strategies. J Am Osteopath Assoc 2000;100(9 Suppl):S7-14.
8. Bogduk N. The anatomical basis for cervicogenic headache. J Manipulative Physiol Ther 1992;15(1):67-70.
9. Capobianco DJ, Dodick DW. Diagnosis and treatment of cluster headache. Semin Neurol 2006;26(2):242-259.
10. Cheshire WP Jr, Ott MC. Headache in divers. Headache 2001;41(3):235-247.
11. Cohen AS, Burns B, Goadsby PJ. High-flow oxygen for treatment of cluster headache: a randomized trial. JAMA 2009;302(22):2451-2457.
12. Darling M. Exercise and migraine. A critical review. J Sports Med Phys Fitness 1991;31(2):294-302.
13. Darling M. The use of exercise as a method of aborting migraine. Headache 1991;31(9):616-618.
14. Dowson A, Jagger S. The UK migraine patient survey: quality of life and treatment. Curr Med Res Opin 1999;15(4):241-253.
15. Edmeads J. The cervical spine and headache. Neurology 1988;38(12):1874-1878.
16. Espir ML, Hodge IL, Matthews PH. Footballer's migraine. BMJ 1972;3(5822):352.
17. Goadsby PJ, Cittadini E, Burns B, Cohen AS. Trigeminal autonomic cephalalgias: diagnostic and therapeutic developments. Curr Opin Neurol 2008;21(3):323-330.
18. Haas DC, Lourie H. Trauma-triggered migraine: an explanation for common neurological attacks after mild head injury. Review of the literature. J Neurosurg 1988;68(2):181-188.
19. Hall T, Robinson K. The flexion-rotation test and active cervical mobility—a comparative measurement study in cervicogenic headache. Man Ther 2004;9(4):197-202.
20. Harpole LH, Samsa GP, Matchar DB, Silberstein SD, Blumenfeld A, Jurgelski AE. Burden of illness and satisfaction with care among patients with headache seen in a primary care setting. Headache 2005;45(8):1048-1055.
21. Jokl E, Jokl P, Seaton DC. Effect of altitude upon 1968 Olympic Games running performances. Int J Biometeorol 1969;13(3):309-311.
22. Kelman L. The triggers or precipitants of the acute migraine attack. Cephalalgia 2007;27(5):394-402.
23. Kernick DP, Goadsby PJ. Guidance for the management of headache in sport on behalf of the

Royal College of General Practitioners and the British Association for the Study of Headache. Cephalalgia 2011;31(1):106-111.

24. Lambert RW Jr, Burnet DL. Prevention of exercise induced migraine by quantitative warm-up. Headache 1985;25(6):317-319.

25. Lane JC. Migraine in the athlete. Semin Neurol 2000;20(2):195-200.

26. Law S, Derry S, Moore RA. Triptans for acute cluster headache. Cochrane Database Syst Rev 2010(4):CD008042.

27. Leone M, D'Amico D, Grazzi L, Attanasio A, Bussone G. Cervicogenic headache: a critical review of the current diagnostic criteria. Pain 1998;78(1):1-5.

28. Linde K, Allais G, Brinkhaus B, Manheimer E, Vickers A, White AR. Acupuncture for tension-type headache. Cochrane Database Syst Rev 2009(1):CD007587.

29. Lipton RB, Stewart WF. Migraine in the United States: a review of epidemiology and health care use. Neurology 1993;43(6 Suppl 3):S6-10.

30. Lucas RN. Footballer's migraine. BMJ 1972;2(5812):526.

31. Martelletti P, van Suijlekom H. Cervicogenic headache: practical approaches to therapy. CNS Drugs 2004;18(12):793-805.

32. Massey EW. Effort headache in runners. Headache 1982;22(3):99-100.

33. Matthews WB. Footballer's migraine. BMJ 1972;2(5809):326-327.

34. Matthews WB. Footballer's migraine. Am Heart J 1973;85(2):279-280.

35. Mauskop A, Leybel B. Headache in sports. In: Jordan B, ed. Sports Neurology. Philadelphia: Lippincott; 1998.

36. McCrory P. Recognizing exercise-related headache. Phys Sportsmed 1997;25(2):33-43.

37. McCrory P, Heywood J, Ugoni A. Open label study of intranasal sumatriptan (Imigran) for footballer's headache. Br J Sports Med 2005;39(8):552-554.

38. O'Brien JC Jr. Swimmer's headache, or supra-orbital neuralgia. Proc (Bayl Univ Med Cent) 2004;17(4):418-419.

39. Olesen J, Tfelt-Hansen P, Ramadan N, Goadsby PJ, Welch KMA. The Headaches. Philadelphia: Lippincott, Williams & Wilkins; 2005.

40. Pestronk A, Pestronk S. Goggle migraine. New Engl J Med 1983;308(4):226-227.

41. Pollmann W, Keidel M, Pfaffenrath V. Headache and the cervical spine: a critical review. Cephalalgia 1997;17(8):801-816.

42. Rasmussen BK. Epidemiology of headache. Cephalalgia 1995;15(1):45-68.

43. Rasmussen BK. Epidemiology of migraine. Biomed Pharmacother 1995;49(10):452-455.

44. Rooke ED. Benign exertional headache. Med Clin North Am 1968;52(4):801-808.

45. Sandyk R. Footballer's migraine—a report of 2 cases. S Afr Med J 1983;63(12):434.

46. Saper JR, Silberstein SD, Gordon CD, Hamel RL, Swidan S. Handbook of Headache Management. 2nd ed. Philadelphia: Lippincott Williams & Wilkins; 1999.

47. Schmidt C. Cerebral blood flow and migraine incidence in spinning figure skaters. Headache Q-Curr Trea 1998;9(3):249-254.

48. Seifert TD, Evans RW. Posttraumatic headache: a review. Curr Pain Headache Rep 2010;14(4):292-298.

49. Sjaastad O, Bakketeig LS. Cluster headache prevalence. Vaga study of headache epidemiology. Cephalalgia 2003;23(7):528-533.

50. Turkewitz LJ, Wirth O, Dawson GA, Casaly JS. Cluster headache following head injury: a case report and review of the literature. Headache 1992;32(10):504-506.

51. Williams SJ, Nukada H. Sport and exercise headache: part 1. Prevalence among university students. Br J Sports Med 1994;28(2):90-95.

52. Williams SJ, Nukada H. Sport and exercise headache: part 2. Diagnosis and classification. Br J Sports Med 1994;28(2):96-100.

Heat Illness
in Sport

Heat injury is a common occurrence in athletes participating in warm weather activities. There are many types of injury, ranging from mild heat cramps and heat illness to life-threatening heatstroke. Heat illness can advance quickly in athletes, and early diagnosis and proper therapy can save lives. Proper precautions must be taken for athletes at risk for hyperthermia illness; and if one is prepared, conditions such as exertional heatstroke (EHS) should be preventable. All athletes, coaches, athletic trainers, parents and guardians, and practitioners should be aware of the risk factors and causes for heat illness, follow recommended strategies, and be prepared to respond quickly to symptoms of illness.[54]

BACKGROUND

Heat illness encompasses a spectrum of illness that includes muscle and heat cramps, heat syncope, heat exhaustion, EHS, and exertional hyponatremia.[8, 54] The spectrum of illness and clinical manifestations depend on many factors, including degree of heat and especially the extent of heat exposure; the humidity level; and the athlete's level of conditioning and underlying health status, caloric expenditure, and amount of total body water loss (among other things).[5] While the causes of heat illness and ultimately EHS are multifactorial, the basic underlying mechanism is an increase in cellular metabolism that exceeds the ability of the cardiovascular system to provide sufficient circulation to the major organs and keep internal body temperature at a normal level—an overwhelming of the thermoregulatory system.[2, 5, 8, 20]

Depending on the amount of environmental heat gain and endogenous heat production, there is a progressive increase in internal body temperature, with an estimated 13% increase in cellular metabolism for every 1° C increase in body temperature.[5] It has been reported that at a core body temperature of 40.5° C (105 °F), cellular metabolism is at 50% above normal level.[5] As normal heat dissipation mechanisms begin to fail, heat-related conditions can arise.

CONTRIBUTORY FACTORS IN HEAT ILLNESS

During exercise, our body's main mechanism of cooling off is sweating; during exercise up to 90% of the energy produced is released by heat. Many factors can hinder heat release and perspiration. Environmental factors play a large role in how we are able to release heat during exercise. Air temperature, combined with humidity, wind speed, and sun, affects how well our bodies cool themselves. Direct exposure to the sun with no available shade can increase an athlete's core body temperature. As air temperature increases, thermal strain increases; but if relative humidity increases as well, the body loses its ability to use evaporation as a cooling method.[17, 20, 23, 41, 42] Humidity influences how easily sweat can evaporate, with higher levels of humidity (greater than 60%) making evaporation more difficult. Kulka and Kenney reported that heatstroke is possible at any combination of ambient temperature above 26.7 °C (80 °F) and relative humidity above 40%.[34]

Clothing can also play a role in athletes' developing heat illness. For starters, any dark clothing can increase heat absorption, which can significantly increase the chance of heat stress. Additionally, full body clothing, heavy or extensive protective equipment, and helmets can increase the potential risk, not only because of the extra weight but also as a barrier to evaporation and cooling.

An individual's level of fitness is an important consideration when one weighs potential causes of heat illness. Before exercising in the heat, athletes must be in good physical condition. Athletes with a higher percentage of body fat have greater difficulty cooling off. Extra body fat increases exertional heat production. Particularly at the elite level, it is not uncommon for athletes to weigh 300 pounds (136 kg) or more. Even athletes who weigh less but carry more muscle bulk may be at risk, as they can still generate more heat production and have an increased load to work with but may not have the increased body surface area to shed the extra heat. Also, any concomitant fevers or illness (current or recent) may increase an athlete's risk. Age should also be taken into consideration; younger athletes, in general, adjust to heat more slowly than adults. Their bodies are less effective overall at regulating body heat and need longer periods of time to adjust to warmer temperatures.

Athletes of all ages should be allowed to acclimatize to heat before a graded increase in exercise intensity. Acclimatization is a physiologic response to repeated heat exposure during exercise over the course of 10 to 14 days.[3, 15, 19-21, 55] When allowed to acclimatize, the body is able to cope better with thermal stressors, including increases in stroke volume, sweat output,

sweat rate, and evaporation of sweat, as well as decreases in heart rate, core body temperature, skin temperature, and sweat salt losses.[3, 21, 55]

Hydration status plays a large contributory role in heat illness. As athletes perspire, they lose necessary body fluids that, if not replaced, can lead to dehydration. Dehydration makes it difficult to sweat and subsequently cool down, which can result in a heat illness. Even mild levels of dehydration can impair athletic performance and mechanisms of temperature regulation. It has been reported that dehydration of as little as 2% of body weight has a negative effect on performance and thermoregulation.[41] Athletes who start activities in an already dehydrated state are at greater risk for heat injury; thus preactivity hydration status is important. Factors that can affect preactivity hydration status include inadequate rehydration after a previous exercise session; alcohol consumption; and fever, vomiting, or diarrhea.

The use of diuretics, stimulants, anabolic steroids, and performance-enhancing substances has become a temptation and a practiced behavior among many amateur, school, and professional athletes and may also increase the risk of heat illness.[1, 5] Football, wrestling, and hockey are the sports most often associated with the use of dietary supplements.[39] Ephedrine alkaloids are amphetamine-like compounds with potentially significant stimulatory properties that act on the heart and central nervous system.[5] These alkaloids are derived from various species of herbs of the genus **Ephedra**, also referred to as Ma-huang (**Ephedra equisetina**), and are often found in products advertised to promote weight loss and increased energy. These products may also contain amphetamine-like compounds such as phenylpropanolamine, pseudoephedrine, and phentermine.

The most severe adverse side effects related to amphetamine and amphetamine-like compounds (including cocaine) center on adverse cardiovascular events including lethal arrhythmias, acute myocardial infarction, and severe hypertension.[5, 31] Rhabdomyolysis and acute neurological events such as seizures and hemorrhagic–ischemic stroke have also been reported with the use of these compounds.[11, 12, 31, 33, 52] These side effects can be aggravated by the use of caffeine. Ephedra and related alkaloid compounds have been linked to thermoregulatory dysfunction. These compounds can result in increased metabolism, heat production, and core body temperature elevation.[29, 49] Such substances can cause cutaneous vasoconstriction, diminishing one's ability to conduct heat outside of the body. The compounds can also mask fatigue, which could result in athletes' pushing themselves beyond a recognizable danger point.[5]

Another common performance-enhancing supplement used by athletes is creatine monohydrate. Most athletes use creatine to promote muscle mass development and enhance energy use. While the overall safety profile of creatine is favorable, several reports have implicated its use in the development of heat illness. Creatine may cause shifts of water into skeletal muscle that could deplete intravascular volume.[27] There have been numerous reports of diarrhea, muscular cramps, heat intolerance, and dehydration associated with creatine use in athletes.[6, 30, 37, 38, 45, 46, 51]

PREVENTION

There are many ways to reduce the risk for heat injury. Dr. Douglas J. Casa has done excellent and extensive work in the realm of heat illness in athletes, and the National Athletic Trainers' Association (NATA) position statement on preventing sudden death in sports nicely outlines recommendations for preventing EHS (see the following list). Exercise intensity can increase core body temperature faster and to a higher extent than any other factor.[43] Thus, it is essential to be flexible with regard to exercise intensity and to be conscious of rest periods when environmental or other factors may present a potential hazard. Extreme or new environmental conditions should be approached with caution, and practices should be altered and events canceled as appropriate.[21] Athletes should be given time to gradually adapt to a new activity or climate. The intensity and duration of exercise can be increased in a graded fashion. It may be beneficial for athletes to avoid wearing heavy protective equipment until they have acclimatized. Consideration should be given to scheduling outdoor exercise at the coolest time of day, either early morning or after sunset.

National Athletic Trainers' Association Recommendations on Preventing Exertional Heatstroke

- In conjunction with preseason screening, athletes should be questioned about risk factors for heat illness or a history of heat illness. Evidence Category: C
- Special considerations and modifications are needed for those wearing protective equipment during periods of high environmental stress. Evidence Category: B
- Athletes should be acclimatized to the heat gradually over a period of 7 to 14 days. Evidence Category: B
- Athletes should maintain a consistent level of euhydration and replace fluids lost through sweat during games and practices. Athletes should have free access to readily available fluids at all times, not only during designated breaks. Evidence Category: B
- The sports medicine staff must educate relevant personnel (eg, coaches, administrators, security guards, EMS staff, athletes) about preventing exertional heatstroke (EHS) and the policies and procedures that are to be followed in the event of an incident. Signs and symptoms of a medical emergency should also be reviewed. Evidence Category: C

Reprinted, by permission, from D.J. Casa et al., 2012, "National athletic trainers' association position statement: Preventing sudden death in sports," Journal of Athletic Training 47(1): 96-118.

In general, one can consult the athletic trainer and physician before starting any new exercise activity to discuss any preexisting medical conditions (especially cardiac or pulmonary), recent illnesses, or medications that can contribute to dehydration or heat illness. Athletes can wear light-colored clothing and use plenty of sunscreen or sunblock to protect against sun exposure. Fluid replacement is essential to preventing heat injury. Hydration can help reduce heart rate, fatigue, and core body temperature while improving performance and cognitive functioning.[17, 19, 23, 42, 50] Athletes should make sure they remain well hydrated before, during, and after exercise. Fluids that are lost during exercise or practice should be replaced whether the athlete feels thirsty or not. Monitoring the color of one's urine is an easy and quick way to assess hydration status; darker urine is a sign of less hydration.

THE SPECTRUM OF HEAT ILLNESS AND MANAGEMENT

When normal thermoregulatory mechanisms start to fail, several minor and moderate heat-related conditions can arise as an individual progresses to more severe heat injury.

Heat Cramps

One mild heat-related condition commonly seen in athletes is heat cramps. Heat cramps are painful involuntary spasms of the major muscle groups used in exercise (i.e., stomach, arm, and leg muscles) that are thought to occur when sodium and water are not replaced during intense, prolonged exercise in the heat. This depletion results in an alkalosis and increased osmolality and lactate levels, which are thought to cause the spasms. Treatment generally involves cessation of the exercise activity and administration of oral or intravenous fluid replacement. In addition to rest, gentle stretching of the affected muscles can sometimes also provide symptomatic relief. When recognized and treated promptly, the symptoms of heat cramps are ordinarily adequately controlled and not serious.[3, 5]

Heat Syncope and Heat Exhaustion

More moderate forms of heat illness include heat syncope and heat exhaustion. Heat syncope is typically characterized by symptoms of weakness, fatigue, and fainting. These symptoms are typically brought on by significant exercise in the heat. Heat syncope often occurs during the first 5 days of adjusting to a new activity, especially when sodium and water losses are not replaced. Those taking diuretics and young athletes returning to play after time off for injury are at greater risk for heat syncope. Another condition that may be considered in the differential diagnosis is exercise-associated collapse (EAC); however, the underlying cause may be more distinct. Exercise-associated collapse occurs in a conscious athlete after completion of an exertional event or after stopping exercise; the athlete is unable to stand or walk unaided as light-headedness, faintness

and dizziness, or syncope causes the collapse.[47] The mechanism of EAC is multifactorial and has previously been attributed to hyperthermia or dehydration.[13, 48, 53] Currently, however, EAC is believed to be principally the result of transient postural hypotension caused by lower extremity pooling of blood once the athlete stops exercising or running and the resultant impairment of cardiac baroreflexes.[4, 28, 32]

Heat exhaustion is an intermediate step in heat illness wherein heat overload produces symptoms such as nausea, vomiting, significant fatigue, hyperventilation, excessive weakness, headache, excessive thirst, heavy sweating, and a fast, weak pulse. While temperature elevation does occur, signs of dehydration may not appear prominent, and central nervous system (CNS) function remains normal.[5] The condition is a reversible one. The mainstay of treatment for heat exhaustion includes recognizing the symptoms, stopping the activity, moving the individual to a cooler environment, administration of fluids, and observation. If nausea or vomiting prevents the affected individual from drinking enough fluids, intravenous administration may be required.

Heatstroke

Exertional heatstroke is the most severe form of heat injury and is a medical emergency that is often irreversible. Exertional heatstroke is classically characterized as a core body temperature greater than 40.0 °C (104 °F) with associated CNS dysfunction.[2, 5, 16, 21, 41, 43] The CNS dysfunction may present as headache, disorientation, confusion, dizziness, vomiting, diarrhea, loss of balance, staggering, irritability, irrational or unusual behavior, apathy, aggressiveness, hysteria, delirium, incoherent speech, seizure, collapse, loss of consciousness, decerebrate posturing, and coma. In addition to elevated temperature and CNS dysfunction, athletes can show other signs and symptoms that may raise the suspicion of EHS, including hypotension, a widened pulse pressure, tachycardia, hyperventilation, and hot, dry skin. It has been reported, though, that most athletes with EHS have hot, sweaty skin as opposed to the dry skin classically described as accompanying EHS.[2, 7, 43] Although body temperature is classically elevated above 40.0 °C (104 °F), heatstroke is not necessarily related to the extent of fever.

[5] An acute-phase response results in cells liberating heat shock proteins and other inflammatory mediators; but as the condition progresses, there is usually rapid multisystem organ failure (hepatic, renal, coagulation cascade) and final cardiovascular collapse.[5]

Heatstroke may occur as a progression from heat syncope and heat exhaustion; however, it can also occur without prodromal or warning signs or symptoms of more minor and moderate heat injury. Hence recognition and assessment of EHS are of paramount importance. The two main criteria for diagnosis of EHS are (1) a core body temperature greater than 40.0 °C to 40.5 °C (104 °F to 105 °F), taken via a rectal thermometer soon after collapse, and (2) CNS dysfunction.[5, 10, 15, 19, 21, 40] In some cases of EHS, patients have a lucid interval during which they are cognitively normal, followed by rapidly deteriorating symptoms.[16, 21] Rectal temperature and gastrointestinal temperature (via ingestible thermistors) are the only methods proven valid for accurate temperature measurement in a patient with EHS. [18, 21] Other temperature assessment devices, such as oral, axillary, aural canal, and temporal artery thermometers, are inferior and inaccurate in an exercising person and should not be relied on in the absence of a valid device.[16, 21] In some settings, obtaining a rectal temperature may not be feasible; however, because of the importance of immediate action, the practitioner should rely on other key diagnostic indicators. Ultimately, if EHS is suspected, treatment should be started at once.

The mainstay of treatment for this condition is removal of the patient from the heat source and rapid cooling and hydration. The goal for any EHS victim is to lower the body temperature to 38.9 °C (102 °F) or less within 30 minutes of collapse.[21] The length of time body temperature is above the critical core temperature of 40.0 °C to 40.5 °C (104 °F to 105 °F) dictates the morbidity and risk of death from EHS.[21, 26] Cold-water

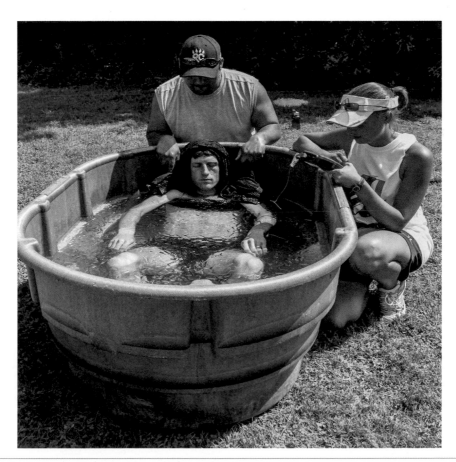

Figure 20.1 A cold-water immersion tub should be the primary piece of equipment used for the treatment of EHS, to cool the athlete rapidly to a temperature of 38.9 °C (102 °F) or less within 30 minutes of collapse.

immersion is the most effective cooling modality for EHS[14, 22] (figure 20.1). The water should be approximately 1.7 °C to 15.0 °C (35 °F to 59 °F) and continuously stirred to maximize cooling; and the athlete should be removed when core body temperature reaches 38.9 °C (102 °F) to prevent overcooling.[21] If cold-water immersion is not available, cold-water dousing or wet ice towel rotation placed over the entire body may be used to assist with cooling, although these methods have not been shown to be as effective as cold-water immersion. Policies and procedures for cooling athletes before transport to the hospital must be explicitly clear and must be shared with potential emergency medical services responders so that treatment by all the involved medical professionals is coordinated.[21] In general, though, athletes should be cooled first and then transported to a hospital unless cooling and proper medical care are unavailable on-site.

RETURN TO PLAY

When treated with oral or intravenous fluid replacement and rest, most minor and moderate heat illnesses are not serious, and most athletes can return to play once medically stable. Structured guidelines for return to play after EHS are lacking. The main considerations are treating any associated sequelae and, if possible, identifying the cause of the EHS so that future episodes can be prevented.[21] Many patients with EHS are cooled effectively and, once sent home, may be able to resume modified activity within 1 to 3 weeks.[21] When treatment is delayed, patients may experience residual complications for months or years after the event. Most guidelines suggest that after a period of no activity, the athlete should be asymptomatic with normal blood enzyme levels before a gradual return to activity is initiated, although no tools are available to truly assess whether the thermoregulatory system is fully recovered.[44] The most recent NATA guidelines state that in all cases of EHS, after the athlete has completed a 7-day rest period and obtained normal blood work and physician clearance, an athlete may begin a progression of physical activity, supervised by the athletic trainer, from low intensity to high intensity and increasing duration in a temperate environment, followed by the same progression in a warm to hot environment.[21] In some cases, full recovery may not be possible; and if the athlete experiences any side effects or negative symptoms with training, the progression should be slowed or delayed indefinitely.

CONCLUDING THOUGHTS

The exact science and pathophysiology of dehydration and heatstroke in athletes are incompletely understood; however, our understanding of the thermoregulatory mechanisms involved with intense exercise in warm climates has improved vastly. However, great advances have been made in the past few decades in the management of hydration, electrolytes, and practice session strategies, and this has contributed to progressively diminishing fatality rates due to heatstroke in athletes.[5] Ultimately, increased education at all levels, early recognition, and proper treatment can prevent the serious consequences of heat-related illness from occurring.

In the near future, further work should emerge on a new generation of cooling devices and techniques for patients with neurological injury, particularly postcardiac arrest. These innovative cooling techniques and devices, which comprise cooling catheters, helmets, and sophisticated cooling blankets, should prove to be of some benefit to patients with heatstroke. Moving forward, their efficacy will have to be rigorously tested in hyperthermic patients. In addition to improving the cooling techniques, it will be necessary to develop therapies based on modulation of the inflammatory and coagulation responses as well.[9] Immunomodulators such as interleukin-1 receptor antagonists, glucocorticoids, and recombinant activated protein C improve survival in animal models of heatstroke but have yet to be studied in humans.[9, 24, 25, 35, 36]

REFERENCES

1. Applegate EA, Grivetti LE. Search for the competitive edge: a history of dietary fads and supplements. J Nutr 1997;127(5 Suppl):869S-873S.

2. Armstrong LE, Casa DJ, Millard-Stafford M, Moran DS, Pyne SW, Roberts WO. American College of Sports Medicine position stand. Exertional heat illness during training and competition. Med Sci Sports Exerc 2007;39(3):556-572.

3. Armstrong LE, Maresh CM. The induction and decay of heat acclimatisation in trained athletes. Sports Med 1991;12(5):302-312.

4. Asplund CA, O'Connor FG, Noakes TD. Exercise-associated collapse: an evidence-based review and primer for clinicians. Br J Sports Med 2011;45(14):1157-1162.

5. Bailes JE, Cantu RC, Day AL. The neurosurgeon in sport: awareness of the risks of heatstroke and dietary supplements. Neurosurgery 2002;51(2):283-286; discussion 286-288.

6. Barrette EP. Creatine supplementation for enhancement of athletic performance. Alternative Med Alert 1998;1:73-84.

7. Bergeron MF, McKeag DB, Casa DJ, Clarkson PM, Dick RW, Eichner ER, et al. Youth football: heat stress and injury risk. Med Sci Sports Exerc 2005;37(8):1421-1430.

8. Binkley HM, Beckett J, Casa DJ, Kleiner DM, Plummer PE. National Athletic Trainers' Association position statement: exertional heat illnesses. J Athl Train 2002;37(3):329-343.

9. Bouchama A, Dehbi M, Chaves-Carballo E. Cooling and hemodynamic management in heatstroke: practical recommendations. Crit Care 2007;11(3):R54.

10. Bouchama A, Knochel JP. Heat stroke. New Engl J Med 2002;346(25):1978-1988.

11. Brody SL, Wrenn KD, Wilber MM, Slovis CM. Predicting the severity of cocaine-associated rhabdomyolysis. Ann Emerg Med 1990;19(10):1137-1143.

12. Bruno A, Nolte KB, Chapin J. Stroke associated with ephedrine use. Neurology 1993;43(7):1313-1316.

13. Cade JR, Free HJ, De Quesada AM, Shires DL, Roby L. Changes in body fluid composition and volume during vigorous exercise by athletes. J Sports Med Phys Fitness 1971;11(3):172-178.

14. Casa DJ, Anderson JM, Armstrong LE, Maresh CM. Survival strategy: acute treatment of exertional heat stroke. J Strength Cond Res 2006;20(3):462.

15. Casa DJ, Anderson SA, Baker L, Bennett S, Bergeron MF, Connolly D, et al. The inter-association task force for preventing sudden death in collegiate conditioning sessions: best practices recommendations. J Athl Train 2012;47(4):477-480.

16. Casa DJ, Armstrong LE, Ganio MS, Yeargin SW. Exertional heat stroke in competitive athletes. Curr Sports Med Rep 2005;4(6):309-317.

17. Casa DJ, Armstrong LE, Hillman SK, Montain SJ, Reiff RV, Rich BS, et al. National athletic trainers' association position statement: fluid replacement for athletes. J Athl Train 2000;35(2):212-224.

18. Casa DJ, Becker SM, Ganio MS, Brown CM, Yeargin SW, Roti MW, et al. Validity of devices that assess body temperature during outdoor exercise in the heat. J Athl Train 2007;42(3):333-342.

19. Casa DJ, Clarkson PM, Roberts WO. American College of Sports Medicine roundtable on hydration and physical activity: consensus statements. Curr Sports Med Rep 2005;4(3):115-127.

20. Casa DJ, Csillan D, Armstrong LE, Baker LB, Bergeron MF, Buchanan VM, et al. Preseason heat-acclimatization guidelines for secondary school athletics. J Athl Train 2009;44(3):332-333.

21. Casa DJ, Guskiewicz KM, Anderson SA, Courson RW, Heck JF, Jimenez CC, et al. National athletic trainers' association position statement: preventing sudden death in sports. J Athl Train 2012;47(1):96-118.

22. Casa DJ, McDermott BP, Lee EC, Yeargin SW, Armstrong LE, Maresh CM. Cold water immersion: the gold standard for exertional heatstroke treatment. Exerc Sport Sci Rev 2007;35(3):141-149.

23. Casa DJ, Stearns RL, Lopez RM, Ganio MS, McDermott BP, Walker Yeargin S, et al. Influence of hydration on physiological function and performance during trail running in the heat. J Athl Train 2010;45(2):147-156.

24. Chen CM, Hou CC, Cheng KC, Tian RL, Chang CP, Lin MT. Activated protein C therapy in a rat heat stroke model. Crit Care Med 2006;34(7):1960-1966.

25. Chiu WT, Kao TY, Lin MT. Interleukin-1 receptor antagonist increases survival in rat heatstroke by reducing hypothalamic serotonin release. Neurosci Lett 1995;202(1-2):33-36.

26. Costrini A. Emergency treatment of exertional heatstroke and comparison of whole body cooling techniques. Med Sci Sports Exerc 1990;22(1):15-18.

27. Demant TW, Rhodes EC. Effects of creatine supplementation on exercise performance. Sports Med 1999;28(1):49-60.

28. Eichna LW, Horvath SM, Bean WB. Post-exertional orthostatic hypotension. Am J Med Sci 1947;213(6):641-654.

29. Gill ND, Shield A, Blazevich AJ, Zhou S, Weatherby RP. Muscular and cardiorespiratory effects of pseudoephedrine in human athletes. Br J Clin Pharmacol 2000;50(3):205-213.

30. Greenwood M, Farris J, Kreider R, Greenwood L, Byars A. Creatine supplementation patterns and perceived effects in select division I collegiate athletes. Clin J Sports Med 2000;10(3):191-194.

31. Haller CA, Benowitz NL. Adverse cardiovascular and central nervous system events associated with dietary supplements containing ephedra alkaloids. New Engl J Med 2000;343(25):1833-1838.

32. Holtzhausen LM, Noakes TD. Collapsed ultraendurance athlete: proposed mechanisms and an approach to management. Clin J Sports Med 1997;7(4):292-301.

33. Kernan WN, Viscoli CM, Brass LM, Broderick JP, Brott T, Feldmann E, et al. Phenylpropanolamine and the risk of hemorrhagic stroke. New Engl J Med 2000;343(25):1826-1832.

34. Kulka TJ, Kenney WL. Heat balance limits in football uniforms how different uniform ensembles alter the equation. Phys Sportsmed 2002;30(7):29-39.

35. Lin MT, Liu HH, Yang YL. Involvement of interleukin-1 receptor mechanisms in development of arterial hypotension in rat heatstroke. Am J Physiol 1997;273(4 Pt 2):H2072-2077.

36. Liu CC, Chien CH, Lin MT. Glucocorticoids reduce interleukin-1 concentration and result in neuroprotective effects in rat heatstroke. J Physiol 2000;527 Pt 2:333-343.

37. Lopez RM, Casa DJ. The influence of nutritional ergogenic aids on exercise heat tolerance and hydration status. Curr Sports Med Rep 2009;8(4):192-199.

38. Lopez RM, Casa DJ, McDermott BP, Ganio MS, Armstrong LE, Maresh CM. Does creatine supplementation hinder exercise heat tolerance or hydration status? A systematic review with meta-analyses. J Athl Train 2009;44(2):215-223.

39. Massad SJ, Shier NW, Koceja DM, Ellis NT. High school athletes and nutritional supplements: a study of knowledge and use. Int J Sport Nutr 1995;5(3):232-245.

40. McDermott BP, Casa DJ, Yeargin SW, Ganio MS, Armstrong LE, Maresh CM. Recovery and return to activity following exertional heat stroke: considerations for the sports medicine staff. J Sport Rehabil 2007;16(3):163-181.

41. Montain SJ, Coyle EF. Influence of graded dehydration on hyperthermia and cardiovascular drift during exercise. J Appl Physiol 1992;73(4):1340-1350.

42. Montain SJ, Sawka MN, Latzka WA, Valeri CR. Thermal and cardiovascular strain from hypohydration: influence of exercise intensity. Int J Sports Med 1998;19(2):87-91.

43. Mora-Rodriguez R, Del Coso J, Estevez E. Thermoregulatory responses to constant versus variable-intensity exercise in the heat. Med Sci Sports Exerc 2008;40(11):1945-1952.

44. O'Connor FG, Casa DJ, Bergeron MF, Carter R III, Deuster P, Heled Y, et al. American College of Sports Medicine Roundtable on exertional heat stroke—return to duty/return to play: conference proceedings. Curr Sports Med Rep 2010;9(5):314-321.

45. Pecci MA, Lombardo JA. Performance-enhancing supplements. Phys Med Rehabil Clin North Am 2000;11(4):949-960.

46. Poortmans JR, Francaux M. Adverse effects of creatine supplementation: fact or fiction? Sports Med 2000;30(3):155-170.

47. Roberts WO. Exercise-associated collapse care matrix in the marathon. Sports Med 2007;37(4-5):431-433.

48. Rowell LB, Marx HJ, Bruce RA, Conn RD, Kusumi F. Reductions in cardiac output, central blood volume, and stroke volume with thermal stress in normal men during exercise. J Clin Invest 1966;45(11):1801-1816.

49. Savdie E, Prevedoros H, Irish A, Vickers C, Concannon A, Darveniza P, et al. Heat stroke following Rugby League football. Med J Aust 1991;155(9):636-639.

50. Sawka MN, Latzka WA, Matott RP, Montain SJ. Hydration effects on temperature regulation. Int J Sports Med 1998;19 Suppl 2:S108-110.

51. Silver MD. Use of ergogenic aids by athletes. J Am Acad Orthop Surg 2001;9(1):61-70.

52. Welch RD, Todd K, Krause GS. Incidence of cocaine-associated rhabdomyolysis. Ann Emerg Med 1991;20(2):154-157.

53. Wyndham CH, Strydom NB. The danger of an inadequate water intake during marathon running. S Afr Med J 1969;43(29):893-896.

54. Yard EE, Gilchrist J, Haileyesus T, Murphy M, Collins C, McIlvain N, et al. Heat illness among high school athletes—United States, 2005-2009. J Safety Res 2010;41(6):471-474.

55. Yeargin SW, Casa DJ, Judelson DA, McDermott BP, Ganio MS, Lee EC, et al. Thermoregulatory responses and hydration practices in heat-acclimatized adolescents during preseason high school football. J Athl Train 2010;45(2):136-146.

American Spinal Injury Association (ASIA) Standard Neurological Classification of Spinal Cord Injury

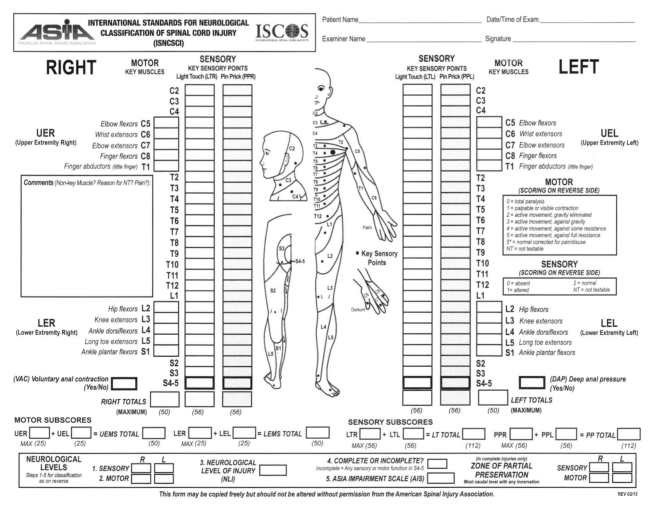

American Spinal Injury Association: International Standards for Neurological Classification of Spinal Cord Injury, revised 2013; Atlanta, GA. Reprinted 2013.

Muscle Function Grading

0 = total paralysis

1 = palpable or visible contraction

2 = active movement, full range of motion (ROM) with gravity eliminated

3 = active movement, full ROM against gravity

4 = active movement, full ROM against gravity and moderate resistance in a muscle specific position.

5 = (normal) active movement, full ROM against gravity and full resistance in a functional muscle position expected from an otherwise unimpaired person.

5* = (normal) active movement, full ROM against gravity and sufficient resistance to be considered normal if identified inhibiting factors (i.e. pain, disuse) were not present.

NT = not testable (i.e. due to immobilization, severe pain such that the patient cannot be graded, amputation of limb, or contracture of > 50% of the normal range of motion).

Sensory Grading

0 = Absent

1 = Altered, either decreased/impaired sensation or hypersensitivity

2 = Normal

NT = Not testable

Non Key Muscle Functions (optional)

May be used to assign a motor level to differentiate AIS B vs. C

Movement	Root level
Shoulder: Flexion, extension, abduction, adduction, internal and external rotation **Elbow:** Supination	C5
Elbow: Pronation **Wrist:** Flexion	C6
Finger: Flexion at proximal joint, extension. **Thumb:** Flexion, extension and abduction in plane of thumb	C7
Finger: Flexion at MCP joint **Thumb:** Opposition, adduction and abduction perpendicular to palm	C8
Finger: Abduction of the index finger	T1
Hip: Adduction	L2
Hip: External rotation	L3
Hip: Extension, abduction, internal rotation **Knee:** Flexion **Ankle:** Inversion and eversion **Toe:** MP and IP extension	L4
Hallux and Toe: DIP and PIP flexion and abduction	L5
Hallux: Adduction	S1

ASIA Impairment Scale (AIS)

A = Complete. No sensory or motor function is preserved in the sacral segments S4-5.

B = Sensory Incomplete. Sensory but not motor function is preserved below the neurological level and includes the sacral segments S4-5 (light touch or pin prick at S4-5 or deep anal pressure) AND no motor function is preserved more than three levels below the motor level on either side of the body.

C = Motor Incomplete. Motor function is preserved below the neurological level**, and more than half of key muscle functions below the neurological level of injury (NLI) have a muscle grade less than 3 (Grades 0-2).

D = Motor Incomplete. Motor function is preserved below the neurological level**, and at least half (half or more) of key muscle functions below the NLI have a muscle grade ≥ 3.

E = Normal. If sensation and motor function as tested with the ISNCSCI are graded as normal in all segments, and the patient had prior deficits, then the AIS grade is E. Someone without an initial SCI does not receive an AIS grade.

** For an individual to receive a grade of C or D, i.e. motor incomplete status, they must have either (1) voluntary anal sphincter contraction or (2) sacral sensory sparing with sparing of motor funtion more than three levels below the motor level for that side of the body. The International Standards at this time allows even non-key muscle function more than 3 levels below the motor level to be used in determining motor incomplete status (AIS B versus C).

NOTE: When assessing the extent of motor sparing below the level for distinguishing between AIS B and C, the *motor level* on each side is used; whereas to differentiate between AIS C and D (based on proportion of key muscle functions with strength grade 3 or greater) the *neurological level of injury* is used.

Steps in Classification

The following order is recommended for determining the classification of individuals with SCI.

1. Determine sensory levels for right and left sides.
The sensory level is the most caudal, intact dermatome for both pin prick and light touch sensation.

2. Determine motor levels for right and left sides.
Defined by the lowest key muscle function that has a grade of at least 3 (on supine testing), providing the key muscle functions represented by segments above that level are judged to be intact (graded as a 5).
Note: in regions where there is no myotome to test, the motor level is presumed to be the same as the sensory level, if testable motor function above that level is also normal.

3. Determine the neurological level of injury (NLI)
This refers to the most caudal segment of the cord with intact sensation and antigravity (3 or more) muscle function strength, provided that there is normal (intact) sensory and motor function rostrally respectively.
The NLI is the most cephalad of the sensory and motor levels determined in steps 1 and 2.

4. Determine whether the injury is Complete or Incomplete.
(i.e. absence or presence of sacral sparing)
*If voluntary anal contraction = **No** AND all S4-5 sensory scores = **0** AND deep anal pressure = **No**, then injury is Complete.*
*Otherwise, injury is **Incomplete**.*

5. Determine ASIA Impairment Scale (AIS) Grade:

Is injury Complete? **If YES, AIS=A** and can record ZPP (lowest dermatome or myotome on each side with some preservation)

NO ↓

Is injury Motor Complete? If YES, AIS=B

NO ↓ (No=voluntary anal contraction OR motor function more than three levels below the motor level on a given side, if the patient has sensory incomplete classification)

Are at least half (half or more) of the key muscles below the neurological level of injury graded 3 or better?

NO ↓ YES ↓

AIS=C AIS=D

If sensation and motor function is normal in all segments, AIS=E
Note: AIS E is used in follow-up testing when an individual with a documented SCI has recovered normal function. If at initial testing no deficits are found, the individual is neurologically intact; the ASIA Impairment Scale does not apply.

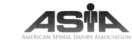

INTERNATIONAL STANDARDS FOR NEUROLOGICAL CLASSIFICATION OF SPINAL CORD INJURY

American Spinal Injury Association: International Standards for Neurological Classification of Spinal Cord Injury, revised 2013; Atlanta, GA. Reprinted 2013.

Sample Concussion
Symptom Checklist

Graded Symptom Checklist (GSC)

Symptom	Time of injury	2 to 3 h postinjury	24 h postinjury	48 h postinjury	72 h postinjury
Blurred vision					
Dizziness					
Drowsiness					
Excess sleep					
Easily distracted					
Fatigue					
Feel "in a fog"					
Feel "slowed down"					
Headache					
Inappropriate emotions					
Irritability					
Loss of consciousness					
Loss of orientation					
Memory problems					
Nausea					
Nervousness					
Personality change					
Poor balance-coordination					
Poor concentration					
Ringing in ears					
Sadness					
Seeing stars					
Sensitivity to light					
Sensitivity to noise					
Sleep disturbance					
Vacant stare—glassy eyed					
Vomiting					

Note: The GSC should be used not only for the initial evaluation but also for each subsequent follow-up assessment until all signs and symptoms have cleared at rest and during physical exertion. In lieu of simply checking each symptom present, the certified athletic trainer can ask the athlete to grade or score the severity of the symptoms on a scale of 0 to 6, where 0 = not present, 1 = mild, 3 = moderate, and 6 = most severe.

Reprinted, by permission, from K.M. Guskiewicz et al., 2004, "National Athletic Trainers' Association position statement: Management of sport-related concussion," *Journal of Athletic Training* 29(3): 280-297.

Sport Concussion Assessment Tool (SCAT3)

SCAT3™

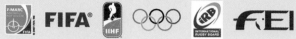

Sport Concussion Assessment Tool – 3rd Edition

For use by medical professionals only

Name _____ Date/Time of Injury: _____ Examiner: _____

Date of Assessment: _____

What is the SCAT3?[1]

The SCAT3 is a standardized tool for evaluating injured athletes for concussion and can be used in athletes aged from 13 years and older. It supersedes the original SCAT and the SCAT2 published in 2005 and 2009, respectively[2]. For younger persons, ages 12 and under, please use the Child SCAT3. The SCAT3 is designed for use by medical professionals. If you are not qualified, please use the Sport Concussion Recognition Tool[1]. Preseason baseline testing with the SCAT3 can be helpful for interpreting post-injury test scores.

Specific instructions for use of the SCAT3 are provided on page 3. If you are not familiar with the SCAT3, please read through these instructions carefully. This tool may be freely copied in its current form for distribution to individuals, teams, groups and organizations. Any revision or any reproduction in a digital form requires approval by the Concussion in Sport Group.

NOTE: The diagnosis of a concussion is a clinical judgment, ideally made by a medical professional. The SCAT3 should not be used solely to make, or exclude, the diagnosis of concussion in the absence of clinical judgement. An athlete may have a concussion even if their SCAT3 is "normal".

What is a concussion?

A concussion is a disturbance in brain function caused by a direct or indirect force to the head. It results in a variety of non-specific signs and/or symptoms (some examples listed below) and most often does not involve loss of consciousness. Concussion should be suspected in the presence of **any one or more** of the following:

- Symptoms (e.g., headache), or
- Physical signs (e.g., unsteadiness), or
- Impaired brain function (e.g. confusion) or
- Abnormal behaviour (e.g., change in personality).

SIDELINE ASSESSMENT

Indications for Emergency Management

NOTE: A hit to the head can sometimes be associated with a more serious brain injury. Any of the following warrants consideration of activating emergency procedures and urgent transportation to the nearest hospital:

- Glasgow Coma score less than 15
- Deteriorating mental status
- Potential spinal injury
- Progressive, worsening symptoms or new neurologic signs

Potential signs of concussion?

If any of the following signs are observed after a direct or indirect blow to the head, the athlete should stop participation, be evaluated by a medical professional and **should not be permitted to return to sport the same day** if a concussion is suspected.

Any loss of consciousness?	Y	N
"If so, how long?" _____		
Balance or motor incoordination (stumbles, slow/laboured movements, etc.)?	Y	N
Disorientation or confusion (inability to respond appropriately to questions)?	Y	N
Loss of memory:	Y	N
"If so, how long?" _____		
"Before or after the injury?" _____		
Blank or vacant look:	Y	N
Visible facial injury in combination with any of the above:	Y	N

1 Glasgow coma scale (GCS)

Best eye response (E)	
No eye opening	1
Eye opening in response to pain	2
Eye opening to speech	3
Eyes opening spontaneously	4
Best verbal response (V)	
No verbal response	1
Incomprehensible sounds	2
Inappropriate words	3
Confused	4
Oriented	5
Best motor response (M)	
No motor response	1
Extension to pain	2
Abnormal flexion to pain	3
Flexion/Withdrawal to pain	4
Localizes to pain	5
Obeys commands	6
Glasgow Coma score (E + V + M)	of 15

GCS should be recorded for all athletes in case of subsequent deterioration.

2 Maddocks Score[3]

"I am going to ask you a few questions, please listen carefully and give your best effort."

Modified Maddocks questions (1 point for each correct answer)

What venue are we at today?	0	1
Which half is it now?	0	1
Who scored last in this match?	0	1
What team did you play last week/game?	0	1
Did your team win the last game?	0	1
Maddocks score		of 5

Maddocks score is validated for sideline diagnosis of concussion only and is not used for serial testing.

Notes: Mechanism of Injury ("tell me what happened"?):

_____

_____

_____

_____

Any athlete with a suspected concussion should be REMOVED FROM PLAY, medically assessed, monitored for deterioration (i.e., should not be left alone) and should not drive a motor vehicle until cleared to do so by a medical professional. No athlete diagnosed with concussion should be returned to sports participation on the day of Injury.

BACKGROUND

Name: _____ Date: _____
Examiner: _____
Sport/team/school: _____ Date/time of injury: _____
Age: _____ Gender: [ ] M [ ] F
Years of education completed: _____
Dominant hand: [ ] right [ ] left [ ] neither
How many concussions do you think you have had in the past? ____
When was the most recent concussion? _____
How long was your recovery from the most recent concussion? ____
Have you ever been hospitalized or had medical imaging done for a head injury? [ ] Y [ ] N
Have you ever been diagnosed with headaches or migraines? [ ] Y [ ] N
Do you have a learning disability, dyslexia, ADD/ADHD? [ ] Y [ ] N
Have you ever been diagnosed with depression, anxiety or other psychiatric disorder? [ ] Y [ ] N
Has anyone in your family ever been diagnosed with any of these problems? [ ] Y [ ] N
Are you on any medications? If yes, please list: [ ] Y [ ] N

SCAT3 to be done in resting state. Best done 10 or more minutes post excercise.

SYMPTOM EVALUATION

3 How do you feel?

"You should score yourself on the following symptoms, based on how you feel now".

	none	mild		moderate		severe	
Headache	0	1	2	3	4	5	6
"Pressure in head"	0	1	2	3	4	5	6
Neck Pain	0	1	2	3	4	5	6
Nausea or vomiting	0	1	2	3	4	5	6
Dizziness	0	1	2	3	4	5	6
Blurred vision	0	1	2	3	4	5	6
Balance problems	0	1	2	3	4	5	6
Sensitivity to light	0	1	2	3	4	5	6
Sensitivity to noise	0	1	2	3	4	5	6
Feeling slowed down	0	1	2	3	4	5	6
Feeling like "in a fog"	0	1	2	3	4	5	6
"Don't feel right"	0	1	2	3	4	5	6
Difficulty concentrating	0	1	2	3	4	5	6
Difficulty remembering	0	1	2	3	4	5	6
Fatigue or low energy	0	1	2	3	4	5	6
Confusion	0	1	2	3	4	5	6
Drowsiness	0	1	2	3	4	5	6
Trouble falling asleep	0	1	2	3	4	5	6
More emotional	0	1	2	3	4	5	6
Irritability	0	1	2	3	4	5	6
Sadness	0	1	2	3	4	5	6
Nervous or Anxious	0	1	2	3	4	5	6

Total number of symptoms (Maximum possible 22) ____
Symptom severity score (Maximum possible 132) ____

Do the symptoms get worse with physical activity? [ ] Y [ ] N
Do the symptoms get worse with mental activity? [ ] Y [ ] N

[ ] self rated   [ ] self rated and clinician monitored
[ ] clinician interview   [ ] self rated with parent input

Overall rating: If you know the athlete well prior to the injury, how different is the athlete acting compared to his/her usual self?
Please circle one response:
no different   very different   unsure   N/A

Scoring on the SCAT3 should not be used as a stand-alone method to diagnose concussion, measure recovery or make decisions about an athlete's readiness to return to competition after concussion. Since signs and symptoms may evolve over time, it is important to consider repeat evaluation in the acute assessment of concussion.

COGNITIVE & PHYSICAL EVALUATION

4 Cognitive assessment
Standardized Assessment of Concussion (SAC)[4]

Orientation (1 point for each correct answer)
What month is it?	0	1
What is the date today?	0	1
What is the day of the week?	0	1
What year is it?	0	1
What time is it right now? (within 1 hour)	0	1

Orientation score ____ of 5

Immediate memory
List	Trial 1	Trial 2	Trial 3	Alternative word list		
elbow	0 1	0 1	0 1	candle	baby	finger
apple	0 1	0 1	0 1	paper	monkey	penny
carpet	0 1	0 1	0 1	sugar	perfume	blanket
saddle	0 1	0 1	0 1	sandwich	sunset	lemon
bubble	0 1	0 1	0 1	wagon	iron	insect
Total						

Immediate memory score total ____ of 15

Concentration: Digits Backward
List	Trial 1	Alternative digit list		
4-9-3	0 1	6-2-9	5-2-6	4-1-5
3-8-1-4	0 1	3-2-7-9	1-7-9-5	4-9-6-8
6-2-9-7-1	0 1	1-5-2-8-6	3-8-5-2-7	6-1-8-4-3
7-1-8-4-6-2	0 1	5-3-9-1-4-8	8-3-1-9-6-4	7-2-4-8-5-6
Total of 4				

Concentration: Month in Reverse Order (1 pt. for entire sequence correct)
Dec-Nov-Oct-Sept-Aug-Jul-Jun-May-Apr-Mar-Feb-Jan   0   1

Concentration score ____ of 5

5 Neck Examination:
Range of motion   Tenderness   Upper and lower limb sensation & strength
Findings: _____

6 Balance examination
Do one or both of the following tests.
Footwear (shoes, barefoot, braces, tape, etc.) _____

Modified Balance Error Scoring System (BESS) testing[5]
Which foot was tested (i.e. which is the non-dominant foot) [ ] Left [ ] Right
Testing surface (hard floor, field, etc.) _____
Condition
Double leg stance: ____ Errors
Single leg stance (non-dominant foot): ____ Errors
Tandem stance (non-dominant foot at back): ____ Errors

And/Or
Tandem gait[6,7]
Time (best of 4 trials): ____ seconds

7 Coordination examination
Upper limb coordination
Which arm was tested: [ ] Left [ ] Right
Coordination score ____ of 1

8 SAC Delayed Recall[4]
Delayed recall score ____ of 5

INSTRUCTIONS

Words in *Italics* throughout the SCAT3 are the instructions given to the athlete by the tester.

Symptom Scale

"You should score yourself on the following symptoms, based on how you feel now".

To be completed by the athlete. In situations where the symptom scale is being completed after exercise, it should still be done in a resting state, at least 10 minutes post exercise.
For total number of symptoms, maximum possible is 22.
For Symptom severity score, add all scores in table, maximum possible is $22 \times 6 = 132$.

SAC[4]

Immediate Memory

"I am going to test your memory. I will read you a list of words and when I am done, repeat back as many words as you can remember, in any order."

Trials 2 & 3:

"I am going to repeat the same list again. Repeat back as many words as you can remember in any order, even if you said the word before."

Complete all 3 trials regardless of score on trial 1 & 2. Read the words at a rate of one per second. **Score 1 pt. for each correct response.** Total score equals sum across all 3 trials. Do not inform the athlete that delayed recall will be tested.

Concentration
Digits backward

"I am going to read you a string of numbers and when I am done, you repeat them back to me backwards, in reverse order of how I read them to you. For example, if I say 7-1-9, you would say 9-1-7."

If correct, go to next string length. If incorrect, read trial 2. **One point possible for each string length.** Stop after incorrect on both trials. The digits should be read at the rate of one per second.

Months in reverse order

"Now tell me the months of the year in reverse order. Start with the last month and go backward. So you'll say December, November … Go ahead"

1 pt. for entire sequence correct

Delayed Recall

The delayed recall should be performed after completion of the Balance and Coordination Examination.

"Do you remember that list of words I read a few times earlier? Tell me as many words from the list as you can remember in any order."

Score 1 pt. for each correct response

Balance Examination

Modified Balance Error Scoring System (BESS) testing[5]

This balance testing is based on a modified version of the Balance Error Scoring System (BESS)[5]. A stopwatch or watch with a second hand is required for this testing.

"I am now going to test your balance. Please take your shoes off, roll up your pant legs above ankle (if applicable), and remove any ankle taping (if applicable). This test will consist of three twenty second tests with different stances."

(a) Double leg stance:

"The first stance is standing with your feet together with your hands on your hips and with your eyes closed. You should try to maintain stability in that position for 20 seconds. I will be counting the number of times you move out of this position. I will start timing when you are set and have closed your eyes."

(b) Single leg stance:

"If you were to kick a ball, which foot would you use? [This will be the dominant foot] Now stand on your non-dominant foot. The dominant leg should be held in approximately 30 degrees of hip flexion and 45 degrees of knee flexion. Again, you should try to maintain stability for 20 seconds with your hands on your hips and your eyes closed. I will be counting the number of times you move out of this position. If you stumble out of this position, open your eyes and return to the start position and continue balancing. I will start timing when you are set and have closed your eyes."

(c) Tandem stance:

"Now stand heel-to-toe with your non-dominant foot in back. Your weight should be evenly distributed across both feet. Again, you should try to maintain stability for 20 seconds with your hands on your hips and your eyes closed. I will be counting the number of times you move out of this position. If you stumble out of this position, open your eyes and return to the start position and continue balancing. I will start timing when you are set and have closed your eyes."

Balance testing – types of errors

1. Hands lifted off iliac crest
2. Opening eyes
3. Step, stumble, or fall
4. Moving hip into > 30 degrees abduction
5. Lifting forefoot or heel
6. Remaining out of test position > 5 sec

Each of the 20-second trials is scored by counting the errors, or deviations from the proper stance, accumulated by the athlete. The examiner will begin counting errors only after the individual has assumed the proper start position. **The modified BESS is calculated by adding one error point for each error during the three 20-second tests. The maximum total number of errors for any single condition is 10.** If an athlete commits multiple errors simultaneously, only one error is recorded but the athlete should quickly return to the testing position, and counting should resume once subject is set. Subjects that are unable to maintain the testing procedure for a minimum of **five seconds** at the start are assigned the highest possible score, ten, for that testing condition.

OPTION: For further assessment, the same 3 stances can be performed on a surface of medium density foam (e.g., approximately 50 cm x 40 cm x 6 cm).

Tandem Gait[6,7]

Participants are instructed to stand with their feet together behind a starting line (the test is best done with footwear removed). Then, they walk in a forward direction as quickly and as accurately as possible along a 38mm wide (sports tape), 3 meter line with an alternate foot heel-to-toe gait ensuring that they approximate their heel and toe on each step. Once they cross the end of the 3m line, they turn 180 degrees and return to the starting point using the same gait. A total of 4 trials are done and the best time is retained. Athletes should complete the test in 14 seconds. Athletes fail the test if they step off the line, have a separation between their heel and toe, or if they touch or grab the examiner or an object. In this case, the time is not recorded and the trial repeated, if appropriate.

Coordination Examination

Upper limb coordination
Finger-to-nose (FTN) task:

"I am going to test your coordination now. Please sit comfortably on the chair with your eyes open and your arm (either right or left) outstretched (shoulder flexed to 90 degrees and elbow and fingers extended), pointing in front of you. When I give a start signal, I would like you to perform five successive finger to nose repetitions using your index finger to touch the tip of the nose, and then return to the starting position, as quickly and as accurately as possible."

Scoring: 5 correct repetitions in < 4 seconds = 1
Note for testers: Athletes fail the test if they do not touch their nose, do not fully extend their elbow or do not perform five repetitions. Failure should be scored as 0.

References & Footnotes

1. This tool has been developed by a group of international experts at the 4th International Consensus meeting on Concussion in Sport held in Zurich, Switzerland in November 2012. The full details of the conference outcomes and the authors of the tool are published in The BJSM Injury Prevention and Health Protection, 2013, Volume 47, Issue 5. The outcome paper will also be simultaneously co-published in other leading biomedical journals with the copyright held by the Concussion in Sport Group, to allow unrestricted distribution, providing no alterations are made.

2. McCrory P et al., Consensus Statement on Concussion in Sport – the 3rd International Conference on Concussion in Sport held in Zurich, November 2008. British Journal of Sports Medicine 2009; 43: i76-89.

3. Maddocks, DL; Dicker, GD; Saling, MM. The assessment of orientation following concussion in athletes. Clinical Journal of Sport Medicine. 1995; 5(1): 32–3.

4. McCrea M. Standardized mental status testing of acute concussion. Clinical Journal of Sport Medicine. 2001; 11: 176–181.

5. Guskiewicz KM. Assessment of postural stability following sport-related concussion. Current Sports Medicine Reports. 2003; 2: 24–30.

6. Schneiders, A.G., Sullivan, S.J., Gray, A., Hammond-Tooke, G. & McCrory, P. Normative values for 16-37 year old subjects for three clinical measures of motor performance used in the assessment of sports concussions. Journal of Science and Medicine in Sport. 2010; 13(2): 196–201.

7. Schneiders, A.G., Sullivan, S.J., Kvarnstrom. J.K., Olsson, M., Yden. T. & Marshall, S.W. The effect of footwear and sports-surface on dynamic neurological screening in sport-related concussion. Journal of Science and Medicine in Sport. 2010; 13(4): 382–386

ATHLETE INFORMATION

Any athlete suspected of having a concussion should be removed from play, and then seek medical evaluation.

Signs to watch for

Problems could arise over the first 24–48 hours. The athlete should not be left alone and must go to a hospital at once if they:

- Have a headache that gets worse
- Are very drowsy or can't be awakened
- Can't recognize people or places
- Have repeated vomiting
- Behave unusually or seem confused; are very irritable
- Have seizures (arms and legs jerk uncontrollably)
- Have weak or numb arms or legs
- Are unsteady on their feet; have slurred speech

Remember, it is better to be safe.
Consult your doctor after a suspected concussion.

Return to play

Athletes should not be returned to play the same day of injury.
When returning athletes to play, they should be **medically cleared and then follow a stepwise supervised program**, with stages of progression.

For example:

Rehabilitation stage	Functional exercise at each stage of rehabilitation	Objective of each stage
No activity	Physical and cognitive rest	Recovery
Light aerobic exercise	Walking, swimming or stationary cycling keeping intensity, 70 % maximum predicted heart rate. No resistance training	Increase heart rate
Sport-specific exercise	Skating drills in ice hockey, running drills in soccer. No head impact activities	Add movement
Non-contact training drills	Progression to more complex training drills, eg passing drills in football and ice hockey. May start progressive resistance training	Exercise, coordination, and cognitive load
Full contact practice	Following medical clearance participate in normal training activities	Restore confidence and assess functional skills by coaching staff
Return to play	Normal game play	

There should be at least 24 hours (or longer) for each stage and if symptoms recur the athlete should rest until they resolve once again and then resume the program at the previous asymptomatic stage. Resistance training should only be added in the later stages.

If the athlete is symptomatic for more than 10 days, then consultation by a medical practitioner who is expert in the management of concussion, is recommended.

Medical clearance should be given before return to play.

Scoring Summary:

Test Domain	Score		
	Date:	Date:	Date:
Number of Symptoms of 22			
Symptom Severity Score of 132			
Orientation of 5			
Immediate Memory of 15			
Concentration of 5			
Delayed Recall of 5			
SAC Total			
BESS (total errors)			
Tandem Gait (seconds)			
Coordination of 1			

Notes:

_____
_____
_____
_____
_____
_____
_____
_____
_____
_____
_____
_____
_____
_____
_____
_____

✂- -

CONCUSSION INJURY ADVICE

(To be given to the **person monitoring** the concussed athlete)

This patient has received an injury to the head. A careful medical examination has been carried out and no sign of any serious complications has been found. Recovery time is variable across individuals and the patient will need monitoring for a further period by a responsible adult. Your treating physician will provide guidance as to this timeframe.

If you notice any change in behaviour, vomiting, dizziness, worsening head-ache, double vision or excessive drowsiness, please contact your doctor or the nearest hospital emergency department immediately.

Other important points:

- Rest (physically and mentally), including training or playing sports until symptoms resolve and you are medically cleared
- No alcohol
- No prescription or non-prescription drugs without medical supervision.
  Specifically:
    · No sleeping tablets
    · Do not use aspirin, anti-inflammatory medication or sedating pain killers
- Do not drive until medically cleared
- Do not train or play sport until medically cleared

Clinic phone number

Patient's name _____

Date/time of injury _____

Date/time of medical review _____

Treating physician _____

Contact details or stamp

McCrory P, Meeuwisse W, Aubry M, Cantu R.C., Dvorak J, Echemendia R, Engebretsen L, Johnston K, Ktcher J, Raftery M, Sills A, Benson B, Davis G, Ellenbogen R, Guskeiwicz K, Herring SA, Iverson G, Jordan B, Kissick J, McCrea M, McIntosh A, Maddocks D, Makdissi M, Purcell L, Putukian M, Schneider K, Tator C, Turner M. Consensus statement on concussion in sport: The 4th International Conference on Concussion in Sport held in Zurich, November 2012. Br J Sports Med 2013; 47: 250-258

Sport Concussion Assessment Tool for Children

Child-SCAT3™

Sport Concussion Assessment Tool for children ages 5 to12 years

For use by medical professionals only

What is childSCAT3?[1]

The ChildSCAT3 is a standardized tool for evaluating injured children for concussion and can be used in children aged from 5 to 12 years. It supersedes the original SCAT and the SCAT2 published in 2005 and 2009, respectively[2]. For older persons, ages 13 years and over, please use the SCAT3. The ChildSCAT3 is designed for use by medical professionals. If you are not qualified, please use the Sport Concussion Recognition Tool[1].Preseason baseline testing with the ChildSCAT3 can be helpful for interpreting post-injury test scores.

Specific instructions for use of the ChildSCAT are provided on page 3. If you are not familiar with the ChildSCAT3, please read through these instructions carefully. This tool may be freely copied in its current form for distribution to individuals, teams, groups and organizations. Any revision and any reproduction in a digital form require approval by the Concussion in Sport Group.
NOTE: The diagnosis of a concussion is a clinical judgment, ideally made by a medical professional. The ChildSCAT3 should not be used solely to make, or exclude, the diagnosis of concussion in the absence of clinical judgement. An athlete may have a concussion even if their ChildSCAT3 is "normal".

What is a concussion?

A concussion is a disturbance in brain function caused by a direct or indirect force to the head. It results in a variety of non-specific signs and/or symptoms (like those listed below) and most often does not involve loss of consciousness. Concussion should be suspected in the presence of any one or more of the following:

- Symptoms (e.g., headache), or
- Physical signs (e.g., unsteadiness), or
- Impaired brain function (e.g. confusion) or
- Abnormal behaviour (e.g., change in personality).

SIDELINE ASSESSMENT

Indications for Emergency Management

NOTE: A hit to the head can sometimes be associated with a more severe brain injury. If the concussed child displays any of the following, then do not proceed with the ChildSCAT3; instead activate emergency procedures and urgent transportation to the nearest hospital:

- Glasgow Coma score less than 15
- Deteriorating mental status
- Potential spinal injury
- Progressive, worsening symptoms or new neurologic signs
- Persistent vomiting
- Evidence of skull fracture
- Post traumatic seizures
- Coagulopathy
- History of Neurosurgery (eg Shunt)
- Multiple injuries

1 Glasgow coma scale (GCS)

Best eye response (E)	
No eye opening	1
Eye opening in response to pain	2
Eye opening to speech	3
Eyes opening spontaneously	4
Best verbal response (V)	
No verbal response	1
Incomprehensible sounds	2
Inappropriate words	3
Confused	4
Oriented	5
Best motor response (M)	
No motor response	1
Extension to pain	2
Abnormal flexion to pain	3
Flexion/Withdrawal to pain	4
Localizes to pain	5
Obeys commands	6
Glasgow Coma score (E + V + M)	of 15

GCS should be recorded for all athletes in case of subsequent deterioration.

Potential signs of concussion?

If any of the following signs are observed after a direct or indirect blow to the head, the child should stop participation, be evaluated by a medical professional and **should not be permitted to return to sport the same day** if a concussion is suspected.

Any loss of consciousness?	Y	N
"If so, how long?"		
Balance or motor incoordination (stumbles, slow/laboured movements, etc.)?	Y	N
Disorientation or confusion (inability to respond appropriately to questions)?	Y	N
Loss of memory:	Y	N
"If so, how long?"		
"Before or after the injury?"		
Blank or vacant look:	Y	N
Visible facial injury in combination with any of the above:	Y	N

2 Sideline Assessment – child-Maddocks Score[3]

"I am going to ask you a few questions, please listen carefully and give your best effort."

Modified Maddocks questions (1 point for each correct answer)

Where are we at now?	0	1
Is it before or after lunch?	0	1
What did you have last lesson/class?	0	1
What is your teacher's name?	0	1
child-Maddocks score		of 4

Child-Maddocks score is for sideline diagnosis of concussion only and is not used for serial testing.

Any child with a suspected concussion should be REMOVED FROM PLAY, medically assessed and monitored for deterioration (i.e., should not be left alone). No child diagnosed with concussion should be returned to sports participation on the day of Injury.

BACKGROUND

Name:	Date/Time of Injury:
Examiner:	Date of Assessment:
Sport/team/school:	
Age:	Gender: M F
Current school year/grade:	
Dominant hand:	right left neither
Mechanism of Injury ("tell me what happened"?):	

For Parent/carer to complete:

How many concussions has the child had in the past?

When was the most recent concussion?

How long was the recovery from the most recent concussion?

Has the child ever been hospitalized or had medical imaging done (CT or MRI) for a head injury?	Y	N
Has the child ever been diagnosed with headaches or migraines?	Y	N
Does the child have a learning disability, dyslexia, ADD/ADHD, seizure disorder?	Y	N
Has the child ever been diagnosed with depression, anxiety or other psychiatric disorder?	Y	N
Has anyone in the family ever been diagnosed with any of these problems?	Y	N
Is the child on any medications? If yes, please list:	Y	N

SYMPTOM EVALUATION

3 Child report

Name: _____

	never	rarely	sometimes	often
I have trouble paying attention	0	1	2	3
I get distracted easily	0	1	2	3
I have a hard time concentrating	0	1	2	3
I have problems remembering what people tell me	0	1	2	3
I have problems following directions	0	1	2	3
I daydream too much	0	1	2	3
I get confused	0	1	2	3
I forget things	0	1	2	3
I have problems finishing things	0	1	2	3
I have trouble figuring things out	0	1	2	3
It's hard for me to learn new things	0	1	2	3
I have headaches	0	1	2	3
I feel dizzy	0	1	2	3
I feel like the room is spinning	0	1	2	3
I feel like I'm going to faint	0	1	2	3
Things are blurry when I look at them	0	1	2	3
I see double	0	1	2	3
I feel sick to my stomach	0	1	2	3
I get tired a lot	0	1	2	3
I get tired easily	0	1	2	3

Total number of symptoms (Maximum possible 20)
Symptom severity score (Maximum possible 20 x 3 = 60)

☐ self rated   ☐ clinician interview   ☐ self rated and clinician monitored

4 Parent report

The child	never	rarely	sometimes	often
has trouble sustaining attention	0	1	2	3
Is easily distracted	0	1	2	3
has difficulty concentrating	0	1	2	3
has problems remembering what he/she is told	0	1	2	3
has difficulty following directions	0	1	2	3
tends to daydream	0	1	2	3
gets confused	0	1	2	3
is forgetful	0	1	2	3
has difficulty completing tasks	0	1	2	3
has poor problem solving skills	0	1	2	3
has problems learning	0	1	2	3
has headaches	0	1	2	3
feels dizzy	0	1	2	3
has a feeling that the room is spinning	0	1	2	3
feels faint	0	1	2	3
has blurred vision	0	1	2	3
has double vision	0	1	2	3
experiences nausea	0	1	2	3
gets tired a lot	0	1	2	3
gets tired easily	0	1	2	3

Total number of symptoms (Maximum possible 20)
Symptom severity score (Maximum possible 20 x 3 = 60)

Do the symptoms get worse with physical activity?   ☐ Y ☐ N
Do the symptoms get worse with mental activity?   ☐ Y ☐ N

☐ parent self rated   ☐ clinician interview   ☐ parent self rated and clinician monitored

Overall rating for parent/teacher/coach/carer to answer.
How different is the child acting compared to his/her usual self?
Please circle one response:

no different	very different	unsure	N/A

Name of person completing Parent-report: _____
Relationship to child of person completing Parent-report: _____

Scoring on the ChildSCAT3 should not be used as a stand-alone method to diagnose concussion, measure recovery or make decisions about an athlete's readiness to return to competition after concussion.

COGNITIVE & PHYSICAL EVALUATION

5 Cognitive assessment
Standardized Assessment of Concussion – Child Version (SAC-C)[4]

Orientation (1 point for each correct answer)

What month is it?	0	1
What is the date today?	0	1
What is the day of the week?	0	1
What year is it?	0	1
Orientation score		of 4

Immediate memory

List	Trial 1	Trial 2	Trial 3	Alternative word list		
elbow	0 1	0 1	0 1	candle	baby	finger
apple	0 1	0 1	0 1	paper	monkey	penny
carpet	0 1	0 1	0 1	sugar	perfume	blanket
saddle	0 1	0 1	0 1	sandwich	sunset	lemon
bubble	0 1	0 1	0 1	wagon	iron	insect
Total						

Immediate memory score total   of 15

Concentration: Digits Backward

List	Trial 1	Alternative digit list		
6-2	0 1	5-2	4-1	4-9
4-9-3	0 1	6-2-9	5-2-6	4-1-5
3-8-1-4	0 1	3-2-7-9	1-7-9-5	4-9-6-8
6-2-9-7-1	0 1	1-5-2-8-6	3-8-5-2-7	6-1-8-4-3
7-1-8-4-6-2	0 1	5-3-9-1-4-8	8-3-1-9-6-4	7-2-4-8-5-6
Total of 5				

Concentration: Days in Reverse Order (1 pt. for entire sequence correct)

Sunday-Saturday-Friday Thursday-Wednesday-Tuesday-Monday   0   1

Concentration score   of 6

6 Neck Examination:

Range of motion   Tenderness   Upper and lower limb sensation & strength
Findings: _____

7 Balance examination

Do one or both of the following tests.
Footwear (shoes, barefoot, braces, tape, etc.) _____
Modified Balance Error Scoring System (BESS) testing[5]
Which foot was tested (i.e. which is the non-dominant foot)   ☐ Left ☐ Right
Testing surface (hard floor, field, etc.) _____
Condition
Double leg stance: Errors
Tandem stance (non-dominant foot at back):   Errors

Tandem gait[6,7]
Time taken to complete (best of 4 trials): _____ seconds
If child attempted, but unable to complete tandem gait, mark here   ☐

8 Coordination examination
Upper limb coordination
Which arm was tested: ☐ Left ☐ Right
Coordination score   of 1

9 SAC Delayed Recall[4]
Delayed recall score   of 5

Since signs and symptoms may evolve over time, it is important to consider repeat evaluation in the acute assessment of concussion.

INSTRUCTIONS

Words in *Italics* throughout the ChildSCAT3 are the instructions given to the child by the tester.

Sideline Assessment – child-Maddocks Score

To be completed on the sideline/in the playground, immediately following concussion. There is no requirement to repeat these questions at follow-up.

Symptom Scale[8]

In situations where the symptom scale is being completed after exercise, it should still be done in a resting state, at least 10 minutes post exercise.

On the day of injury
- the child is to complete the Child Report, according to how he/she feels now.

On all subsequent days
- the child is to complete the Child Report, according to how he/she feels today, **and**
- the parent/carer is to complete the Parent Report according to how the child has been over the previous 24 hours.

Standardized Assessment of Concussion – Child Version (SAC-C)[4]

Orientation
Ask each question on the score sheet. A correct answer for **each question scores 1 point.** If the child does not understand the question, gives an incorrect answer, or no answer, then the score for that question is 0 points.

Immediate memory
"I am going to test your memory. I will read you a list of words and when I am done, repeat back as many words as you can remember, in any order."

Trials 2 & 3:
"I am going to repeat the same list again. Repeat back as many words as you can remember in any order, even if you said the word before."

Complete all 3 trials regardless of score on trial 1 & 2. Read the words at a rate of one per second. **Score 1 pt. for each correct response.** Total score equals sum across all 3 trials. Do not inform the child that delayed recall will be tested.

Concentration
Digits Backward:
"I am going to read you a string of numbers and when I am done, you repeat them back to me backwards, in reverse order of how I read them to you. For example, if I say 7-1, you would say 1-7."

If correct, go to next string length. If incorrect, read trial 2. **One point possible for each string length.** Stop after incorrect on both trials. The digits should be read at the rate of one per second.

Days in Reverse Order:
"Now tell me the days of the week in reverse order. Start with Sunday and go backward. So you'll say Sunday, Saturday … Go ahead"

1 pt. for entire sequence correct

Delayed recall

The delayed recall should be performed after completion of the Balance and Coordination Examination.
"Do you remember that list of words I read a few times earlier? Tell me as many words from the list as you can remember in any order."

Circle each word correctly recalled. **Total score equals number of words recalled.**

Balance examination

These instructions are to be read by the person administering the childSCAT3, and each balance task **should be demonstrated to the child.** The child should then be asked to copy what the examiner demonstrated.

Modified Balance Error Scoring System (BESS) testing[5]

This balance testing is based on a modified version of the Balance Error Scoring System (BESS)[5]. A stopwatch or watch with a second hand is required for this testing.

"I am now going to test your balance. Please take your shoes off, roll up your pant legs above ankle (if applicable), and remove any ankle taping (if applicable). This test will consist of two different parts."

(a) Double leg stance:
The first stance is standing with the feet together with hands on hips and with eyes closed. The child should try to maintain stability in that position for 20 seconds. You should inform the child that you will be counting the number of times the child moves out of this position. You should start timing when the child is set and the eyes are closed.

(b) Tandem stance:
Instruct the child to stand heel-to-toe with the non-dominant foot in the back. Weight should be evenly distributed across both feet. Again, the child should try to maintain stability for 20 seconds with hands on hips and eyes closed. You should inform the child that you will be counting the number of times the child moves out of this position. If the child stumbles out of this position, instruct him/her to open the eyes and return to the start position and continue balancing. You should start timing when the child is set and the eyes are closed.

Balance testing – types of errors - Parts (a) and (b)

1. Hands lifted off iliac crest
2. Opening eyes
3. Step, stumble, or fall
4. Moving hip into > 30 degrees abduction
5. Lifting forefoot or heel
6. Remaining out of test position > 5 sec

Each of the 20-second trials is scored by counting the errors, or deviations from the proper stance, accumulated by the child. The examiner will begin counting errors only after the child has assumed the proper start position. **The modified BESS is calculated by adding one error point for each error during the two 20-second tests. The maximum total number of errors for any single condition is 10.** If a child commits multiple errors simultaneously, only one error is recorded but the child should quickly return to the testing position, and counting should resume once subject is set. Children who are unable to maintain the testing procedure for a minimum of **five seconds** at the start are assigned the highest possible score, ten, for that testing condition.

OPTION: For further assessment, the same 2 stances can be performed on a surface of medium density foam (e.g., approximately 50cm x 40cm x 6cm).

Tandem Gait[6,7]

Use a clock (with a second hand) or stopwatch to measure the time taken to complete this task. Instruction for the examiner – **Demonstrate the following to the child:**

The child is instructed to stand with their feet together behind a starting line (the test is best done with footwear removed). Then, they walk in a forward direction as quickly and as accurately as possible along a 38mm wide (sports tape), 3 meter line with an alternate foot heel-to-toe gait ensuring that they approximate their heel and toe on each step. Once they cross the end of the 3m line, they turn 180 degrees and return to the starting point using the same gait. A total of 4 trials are done and the best time is retained. Children fail the test if they step off the line, have a separation between their heel and toe, or if they touch or grab the examiner or an object. In this case, the time is not recorded and the trial repeated, if appropriate.

Explain to the child that you will time how long it takes them to walk to the end of the line and back.

Coordination examination

Upper limb coordination
Finger-to-nose (FTN) task:

The tester should **demonstrate it to the child.**

"I am going to test your coordination now. Please sit comfortably on the chair with your eyes open and your arm (either right or left) outstretched (shoulder flexed to 90 degrees and elbow and fingers extended). When I give a start signal, I would like you to perform five successive finger to nose repetitions using your index finger to touch the tip of the nose as quickly and as accurately as possible."

Scoring: 5 correct repetitions in < 4 seconds = 1
Note for testers: Children fail the test if they do not touch their nose, do not fully extend their elbow or do not perform five repetitions. **Failure should be scored as 0.**

References & Footnotes

1. This tool has been developed by a group of international experts at the 4th International Consensus meeting on Concussion in Sport held in Zurich, Switzerland in November 2012. The full details of the conference outcomes and the authors of the tool are published in The BJSM Injury Prevention and Health Protection, 2013, Volume 47, Issue 5. The outcome paper will also be simultaneously co-published in other leading biomedical journals with the copyright held by the Concussion in Sport Group, to allow unrestricted distribution, providing no alterations are made.

2. McCrory P et al., Consensus Statement on Concussion in Sport – the 3rd International Conference on Concussion in Sport held in Zurich, November 2008. British Journal of Sports Medicine 2009; 43: i76-89.

3. Maddocks, DL; Dicker, GD; Saling, MM. The assessment of orientation following concussion in athletes. Clinical Journal of Sport Medicine. 1995; 5(1): 32–3.

4. McCrea M. Standardized mental status testing of acute concussion. Clinical Journal of Sport Medicine. 2001; 11: 176–181.

5. Guskiewicz KM. Assessment of postural stability following sport-related concussion. Current Sports Medicine Reports. 2003; 2: 24–30.

6. Schneiders, A.G., Sullivan, S.J., Gray, A., Hammond-Tooke, G. & McCrory, P. Normative values for 16-37 year old subjects for three clinical measures of motor performance used in the assessment of sports concussions. Journal of Science and Medicine in Sport. 2010; 13(2): 196–201.

7. Schneiders, A.G., Sullivan, S.J., Kvarnstrom. J.K., Olsson, M., Yden. T. & Marshall, S.W. The effect of footwear and sports-surface on dynamic neurological screening in sport-related concussion. Journal of Science and Medicine in Sport. 2010; 13(4): 382–386

8. Ayr, L.K., Yeates, K.O., Taylor, H.G., & Brown, M. Dimensions of post-concussive symptoms in children with mild traumatic brain injuries. Journal of the International Neuropsychological Society. 2009; 15:19–30.

Concussion in Sports
Palm Card

Concussion in Sports

This palm card provides information and tools to help medical staff with the on-field recognition and management of concussion.

Concussion Signs and Symptoms[1]

Signs Observed by Medical Staff	Symptoms Reported by Athlete
Appears dazed or stunned	Headache or "pressure" in head
Is confused about assignment	Nausea
Forgets sports plays	Balance problems or dizziness
Is unsure of game, score, opponent	Double or fuzzy vision
Moves clumsily	Sensitivity to light
Answers questions slowly	Sensitivity to noise
Loses consciousness (even briefly)	Feeling sluggish or slowed down
Shows behavior or personality changes	Feeling foggy or groggy
Can't recall events prior to hit or fall (retrograde amnesia)	Does not "feel right"
Can't recall events after hit or fall (anterograde amnesia)	

[1]This palm card is part of the "Heads Up: Brain Injury in Your Practice" tool kit developed by the Centers for Disease Control and Prevention (CDC). For more information, visit: www.cdc.gov/injury.

Signs of Deteriorating Neurological Function

An athlete should be taken to the emergency department if any of the following signs and/or symptoms are present:

- Headaches that worsen
- Seizures
- Focal neurologic signs
- Looks very drowsy or can't be awakened
- Repeated vomiting
- Slurred speech
- Can't recognize people or places
- Increasing confusion or irritability
- Weakness or numbness in arms or legs
- Neck pain
- Unusual behavior change
- Significant irritability
- Any loss of consciousness greater than 30 seconds or longer. (Brief loss of consciousness (under 30 seconds) should be taken seriously and the patient should be carefully monitored.)

No Return to Play

Any athlete who exhibits signs and symptoms of concussion should be removed from play and should not participate in games or practices until they have been evaluated and given permission by an appropriate health care provider. Research indicates that high school athletes with less than 15 minutes of on-field symptoms exhibited deficits on formal neuropsychological testing and re-emergence of active symptoms, lasting up to one week post-injury.[2]

Exertion

Symptoms will typically worsen or re-emerge with exertion, indicating incomplete recovery. If the athlete is symptom-free, provoking with exertion is recommended (e.g. 5 push-ups, 5 sit ups, 5 knee bends, 40 yard sprint).

Return to play should occur gradually. Individuals should be monitored by an appropriate health care provider for symptoms and cognitive function carefully during each stage of increased exertion.

Repeated Evaluation

On-field, follow-up evaluation (e.g. every 5 minutes) is important, as signs and symptoms of concussion may evolve over time.

Off-Field Management

The physician should provide information to parents/caregivers regarding the athlete's condition. For example, the athlete:

- Should not operate a motor vehicle or participate in activities such as sports, PE class, riding a bicycle, riding carnival rides, etc.
- May experience cognitive/behavioral difficulties at home, making it necessary to reduce physical and cognitive exertion (e.g., running, lifting weights, intensive studying) until fully recovered.
- Should receive follow-up medical and neuropsychological evaluation, both for managing injury and determining return to sports.

[1]Adapted from: Lovell MR, Collins MW, Iverson GL, Johnston KM, Bradley JP. Grade 1 or "ding" concussions in high school athletes. The American Journal of Sports Medicine 2004;32(1):47-54.

[2]Lovell MR, Collins MW, Bradley J. Return to play following sports-related concussion. Clinics in Sports Medicine 2004;23(3):421-41.

On-Field Mental Status Evaluation

(This mental status assessment is recommended for high school-age athletes and older. Any inability of the athlete to respond correctly to the questions below should be considered abnormal.)

Orientation

What period/quarter/half are we in?
What stadium/field is this?
What city is this?
Who is the opposing team?
Who scored last?
What team did we play last?

Anterograde Amnesia

Ask the athlete to repeat the following words: Girl, Dog, Green

Retrograde Amnesia

Ask the athlete the following:
Do you remember the hit?
What happened in the play prior to the hit?
What happened in the quarter/period prior to the hit?
What was the score of the game prior to the hit?

Concentration

Ask the athlete to do the following:
Repeat the days of the week backwards (starting with today)
Repeat the months of the year backward (starting with December)
Repeat these numbers backward 63 (36), 419 (914), 6294 (4926)

Word List Memory

Ask the athlete to repeat the three words from earlier: Girl, Dog, Green

From CDC, Heads up: Brain injury in your practice toolkit.

Index

Page numbers followed by an *f* or a *t* indicate a figure or table, respectively.

NJCAA (National Junior College Athletic Association) 5
N-methyl-D-aspartate (NMDA) 89, 90-91
NOC (New Orleans Criteria) 122
nocebo effect 184
NOCSAE (National Operating Committee for Standards in Athletic Equipment) 4, 81
nonsteroidal anti-inflammatory drugs (NSAIDs) 327, 358

O

Olympic Games 3
Omalu, Bennet 43, 189
Omalu-Bailes histomorphology subtypes of CTE 195*t*
Os odontoideum 313

P

Pahulu v. University of Kansas 51-52
palm card 378-381
paper-pencil testing in concussion assessment 144-145
Parkinson's disease (PD)
  in boxers 199
  CTE versus 194, 198
  natural neuroprotective approaches to treatment 278, 279-280, 282
  prior brain injury as a cause 236
paroxetine 260
pars interarticularis 9, 11, 302*f*, 314, 316*f*, 316, 336. *See also* spondylolysis
Parsonage-Turner syndrome 344
pathophysiology of concussions
  axonal injury 91*f*, 91
  blood-brain barrier breakdown 92-93
  cerebral blood flow dynamics 92
  immunoexcitotoxicity 93-94, 94*f*
  neurometabolic cascade 89-91, 90*f*
PCS. *See* postconcussion syndrome
PD. *See* Parkinson's disease
perineural fibrosis 11
peripheral nerve injury
  acute injuries 342-344
  archery 6
  association with particular sports 342-343*t*
  bony reconstruction 350
  chronic injuries 344-345
  clinical evaluation 345*f*, 345-346, 346*f*
  concluding thoughts 351-352
  dance 9
  electrophysiology testing 345-346
  epidemiology 341
  hockey 22, 341, 345
  legal implications 351
  martial arts and mixed martial arts 24
  mountain climbing and hiking 25
  pathogenesis 341-342
  postoperative management and return to play 351

primary nerve surgery 349*f*, 349-351, 350*f*
  radiological assessment 346
  rowing 27
  shooting sports 27
  snowmobiling and ATVs 28
  soft tissue surgery 350
  subacute injuries 344
  surgery decision 347-349, 348*f*
  volleyball 30
peroneal neuropathy 6
PET (positron emission tomography) 133
Phalen's sign 345
pharmacologic therapy
  cognitive symptoms 260, 261*t*, 262
  concluding thoughts 264
  decision to treat 251-252
  emotional symptoms 258, 259*t*, 260
  natural alternatives to. *See* natural neuroprotective approaches to concussion
  role of education in patient management 251
  sleep disturbance symptoms 257-258, 258*t*
  for somatic symptoms 253*t*, 253-257, 256*t*, 259*t*
physical education 3
pinched nerve syndrome 5-6
Pinson v. State of Tennessee 51
PNF (proprioceptive neuromuscular facilitation) 330
Polamalu, Troy 54
Pop Warner Football (PWF) 238
positron emission tomography (PET) 133
postconcussion neurosis-traumatic encephalitis 190*t*, 190
postconcussion syndrome (PCS)
  biopsychosocial conceptualization of 183-184
  clinical care 237
  concluding thoughts 184
  decision to treat pharmacologically 251-252
  definitions of 179-180
  neuroanatomical substrate for symptoms 181-182
  psychogenesis of 182
  scope of the problem 181
posterior interosseous nerve entrapment 26
posttraumatic encephalopathy (PTE) 192, 193*f*
posttraumatic myelopathy (PTM) 192
posttraumatic stress disorder (PTSD) 152, 198
postural equilibrium 163-164
pramiracetam 262
prazosin 257
"Preventing Sudden Death in Sports" 48
process fractures 317
progesterone 282

prolonged postconcussion syndrome (PPCS)
  biopsychosocial conceptualization of 183-184
  decision to treat pharmacologically 251-252
  defined 237
  psychogenesis of 182-183
propranolol 255, 358
proprioceptive neuromuscular facilitation (PNF) 330
proximate cause 48
PTM (posttraumatic myelopathy) 192
PTSD (posttraumatic stress disorder) 152, 198
pudendal nerve injury 17
PWF (Pop Warner Football) 238
Pycnogenol 283

Q

quadriplegia 303-304

R

racket sports 25-26
radial nerve palsy 26
radiculopathy (sciatica) 314, 333
radiological assessment
  peripheral nerve injury 346-347
  spine injuries management 324-325, 325*f*
  subconcussions 213-214
RBANS (Repeatable Battery for the Assessment of Neuropsychological Status) 213
RCI (reliable change indices) 148
reaction time assessments 172
reasonable person standard 45
recovery from injury. *See* injury recovery process
Regan v. State of New York 51
rehabilitation in concussion management 262-264. *See also* injury recovery process
reliable change indices (RCI) 148
Repeatable Battery for the Assessment of Neuropsychological Status (RBANS) 213
resveratrol 275-276, 276*t*
return to sport participation
  after heat illness 370
  with brain abnormalities 240-244, 241*f*, 242*f*, 243*f*
  cervical spine injury management and 334
  checklist use 239
  clinical presentation and 239-240
  concluding thoughts 249
  concussion and TBI history 245-247
  contraindications after spine injury 329*t*
  cumulative dose considerations 240
  development of return-to-play assessments 141-142
  history of return to play 235-237
  neuroimaging use 239

About the Authors

Anthony L. Petraglia, MD, graduated from the University of Chicago in 2002 with a BA in neuroscience and earned his medical degree from the University of Rochester School of Medicine and Dentistry in 2007. He completed his residency in neurological surgery at the University of Rochester Medical Center in 2014. Petraglia was the first neurosurgery resident to complete a neurological sports medicine fellowship, and is currently an attending neurosurgeon at Unity Health System in Rochester, New York, where he is also the director of the concussion program.

Petraglia has presented nationally and internationally on neurological sports medicine, has published numerous manuscripts and book chapters on various aspects of neurological surgery, and performs editorial duties for several medical journals. His membership in professional organizations includes the Congress of Neurological Surgeons (CNS) and the American Association of Neurological Surgeons (AANS), and he has served as an assistant to the Sports Medicine Section of the AANS/CNS. He has worked as a physician with several collegiate and high school football teams, as a neurosurgical consultant for the Webster Youth Sports Council, and as a medical director for cyclocross racing.

Julian E. Bailes, Jr., MD, earned a BS from Louisiana State University in 1978, and his MD from Louisiana State University School of Medicine in New Orleans in 1982. He completed a general surgery internship at Northwestern Memorial Hospital in 1983 and a neurological surgery residency at Northwestern University in Chicago in 1987, as well as a fellowship in cerebrovascular surgery at the Barrow Neurological Institute in Phoenix.

Bailes was director of cerebrovascular surgery at Allegheny General Hospital in Pittsburgh from 1988 until 1997 and later at Celebration Health Hospital in Orlando, where he also was the director of emergency medical services at

both the city and county levels. In 2000, Bailes assumed the position of professor and chair in the department of neurosurgery at West Virginia University School of Medicine in Morgantown. He most recently assumed the position of chair of the department of neurosurgery at NorthShore University Health System in Chicago and is co-director of thc Ncurological Institute.

Bailes is a past chair of the Sports Medicine Section for the American Association of Neurological Surgeons. He has more than 100 publications concerning various aspects of neurological surgery, including three books on neurological sports medicine, and performs editorial duties for numerous medical journals. He is an internationally recognized expert on neurological athletic injuries and has been a team physician at either the National Football League (NFL) or collegiate level for more than 20 years. Since 1992, he has been the neurological consultant to the NFL Players' Association (NFLPA), which has sponsored his research on the effects of head injuries on professional athletes. He is the director of the NFLPA's Second Opinion Network. He is the medical director of the Center for Study of Retired Athletes, which is affiliated with the NFLPA and the University of North Carolina, and is the medical director of Pop Warner Football, the nation's largest youth football association.

Arthur L. Day, MD, graduated from Louisiana State University Medical School in 1972. He completed his surgical internship in Birmingham, Alabama, and subsequently completed his residency in neurological surgery and fellowship in brain tumor immunology at the University of Florida College of Medicine in Gainesville, Florida.

Day practiced at the University of Florida for 25 years, ultimately rising to the positions of professor, co-chair, and program director of the department of neurological surgery at the University of Florida. In 2002, he moved to Boston to assume a position as a professor of surgery at Harvard Medical School with a clinical practice at Brigham and Women's Hospital. While there, he served as the associate chair and residency program director of the department of neurological surgery at Brigham and Women's and Children's Hospital in Boston. Subsequently, he was the chair of the department and also the director of the Cerebrovascular Center and the Neurologic Sports Injury Center at Brigham and Women's Hospital. He co-founded and directed an annual meeting at Fenway Park addressing the latest knowledge and treatments of athletic-related neurological injuries. He currently is professor, vice chair, residency program director, and director of clinical education in the department of neurosurgery at the University of Texas Medical School at Houston.

Day has held leadership positions in many medical professional societies and has received numerous awards and honors. He has published almost 170 journal articles and book chapters and has co-edited a book about neurological sports injuries. He is an internationally recognized expert in neurological sports medicine. For the past 30 years, he has served as a consulting physician for multiple NCAA and National Football League (NFL) teams.

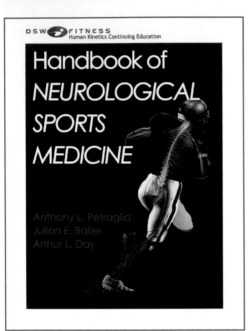
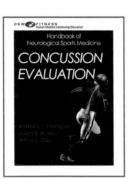
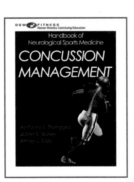
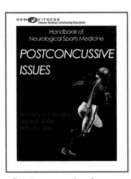
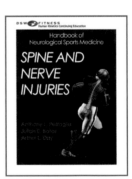